ATLAS OF ORTHOSES AND ASSISTIVE DEVICES

Third Edition

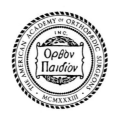

ATLAS OF ORTHOSES
AND ASSISTIVE DEVICES

THIRD EDITION

EDITORS:

Bertram Goldberg, M.D.

John D. Hsu, M.D.
Chairman
Department of Surgery
Chief of Orthopaedics
Rancho Los Amigos Medical Center
Clinical Professor, Orthopaedics
University of Southern California
School of Medicine
Downey, California

with 968 illustrations

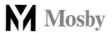 Mosby

St. Louis Baltimore Boston
Carlsbad Chicago Naples New York Philadelphia Portland
London Madrid Mexico City Singapore Sydney Tokyo Toronto Wiesbaden

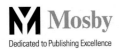

Dedicated to Publishing Excellence

A Times Mirror
Company

Publisher: Anne Patterson
Editor: Robert Hurley
Developmental Editor: Lauranne Billus
Project Manager: Linda Clarke
Senior Production Editor: Allan S. Kleinberg
Manufacturing Supervisor: Bill Winneberger
Designer: Carolyn O'Brien

THIRD EDITION
Copyright © 1997 by Mosby–Year Book, Inc.
A Mosby imprint of Mosby–Year Book, Inc.

Previous editions copyrighted 1985, 1975

Printed in the United States of America
Composition by Graphic World, Inc.
Printing/binding by Maple–Vail York

Mosby–Year Book, Inc.
11830 Westline Industrial Drive
St. Louis, Missouri 63146

Library of Congress Cataloging in Publication Data
Atlas of orthoses and assistive devices / American Academy of
  Orthopaedic Surgeons ; editors, Bertram Goldberg, John D. Hsu.—
  3rd ed.
      p.   cm.
   Rev. ed. of: Atlas of orthotics. 2nd ed. 1985.
   Includes bibliographical references and index.
   ISBN 0-8151-0052-3.
   1. Orthopedic apparatus.   I. Goldberg, Bertram, 1938-1995.
 II. Hsu, John D.   III. American Academy of Orthopaedic Surgeons.
 IV. Atlas of orthotics.
      [DNLM: 1. Orthotic Devices.   2. Biomechanics.   3. Orthopedic
 Fixation Devices.   4. Self-Help Devices.   WE 26A881 1996]
 RD755.A85   1996
 617.3'07—dc20
 DNLM/DLC
 for Library of Congress   96-29147
                                                                     CIP

97 98 99 00 01 / 9 8 7 6 5 4 3 2 1

SECTION EDITORS

William W. Eversmann, Jr., M.D.
Hand Surgeon
Iowa Medical Clinic
Cedar Rapids, Iowa

John R. Fisk, M.D.
Associate Professor of Surgery
Southern Illinois University School of Medicine
Springfield, Illinois

†Bertram Goldberg, M.D.

John D. Hsu, M.D.
Chairman
Department of Surgery
Chief of Orthopaedics
Rancho Los Amigos Medical Center
Clinical Professor, Orthopaedics
University of Southern California
School of Medicine
Downey, California

John E. Lonstein, M.D.
Clinical Associate Professor
Department of Orthopaedics
University of Minnesota
Fairview Riverside Medical Center
Minneapolis, Minnesota;
Gillette Children's Hospital
St. Paul, Minnesota

John W. Michael, M.Ed., C.P.O., F.I.S.P.O.
Director of Professional and Technical Service
Otto Bock, USA
Minneapolis, Minnesota

Thomas J. Moore, M.D.
Associate Professor of Orthopaedic Surgery
Emory University School of Medicine
Atlanta, Georgia

CONTRIBUTORS

Kai-Nan An, Ph.D.
Professor of Bioengineering
Director, Biomechanics Laboratory
Chair, Division of Orthopaedic Research
Mayo Clinic
Mayo Foundation
Rochester, Minnesota

Sam Andrews, B.S., C.T.R.S.
Director, Therapeutic Recreation
Craig Hospital

David F. Apple, Jr., M.D.
Associate Clinical Professor of Orthopaedic Surgery
and Rehabilitation Medicine
Emory University
Shepherd Center, Medical Director
Atlanta, Georgia
Englewood, California

Judy Askins, C.T.R.S.
Shepherd Spinal Center
Atlanta, Georgia

Rita Ayyangar, M.B.B.S.
Assistant Professor of Physical Medicine and
 Rehabilitation and Clinical Pediatrics
University of Cincinnati
Attending Physician, Department of Pediatric
 Rehabilitation
Children's Hospital Medical Center
Cincinnati, Ohio

Jane M. Baumgarten, B.S., O.T.R.
Occupational Therapy Clinical Instructor
Rancho Los Amigos Medical Center
Downey, California

Courtney W. Brown, M.D.
Associate Clinical Professor
University of Colorado
Lakewood Orthopaedic Clinic, PC
Lakewood, Colorado

†Deceased.

Wilton H. Bunch, M.D., Ph.D.
Church Divinity School of the Pacific
Berkeley, California

Scott J. Calhoun, M.D.
Orthopaedic Resident
University of Illinois at Chicago
Chicago, Illinois

James H. Campbell, Ph.D.
Prosthetist and Orthotist
Manager of Clinical Services
Remploy Healthcare
Leeds, England

Richard B. Chambers, M.D.
Associate Clinical Professor of Orthopaedic Surgery
University of Southern California
Rancho Los Amigos Medical Center
Downey, California

Joseph B. Chandler, M.D.
Staff Physician
Peachtree Orthopaedic Clinic, P.A.
Team Orthopaedist
Atlanta Braves
Atlanta, Georgia

Gregory H. Chow, M.D.
Assistant Clinical Professor of Orthopedic Surgery
Department of Surgery
University of Hawaii
Orthopedic Associates of Hawaii
Queen's Medical Center
Honolulu, Hawaii

Darrell R. Clark, B.S., C.O.
Assistant Professor
California State University
Dominguez Hills, California;
Director of Orthotics
Rancho Los Amigos Medical Center
Downey, California

Mary Williams Clark, M.D.
Associate Professor of Orthopaedic Surgery
and Rehabilitation
Associate Professor of Pediatrics
The Milton S. Hershey Medical Center
Penn State University
Hershey, Pennsylvania

Ann Cody, C.T.R.S.
Atlanta Paralympic Organizing Committee
Atlanta, Georgia

Alvin H. Crawford, M.D.
Professor and Director, Pediatric Orthopaedics
University of Cincinnati
The Children's Hospital Medical Center
Cincinnati, Ohio

John Dorris, M.D.
Orthopaedic Resident
Emory University School of Medicine
Atlanta, Georgia

James C. Drennan, M.D.
Professor of Orthopaedics and Pediatrics
University of New Mexico School of Medicine
Medical Director/CEO
Carrie Tingley Hospital
Albuquerque, New Mexico

Gregory L. Durrett, C.O.
Crestview Hills, Kentucky

Joan E. Edelstein, M.A., P.T., F.I.S.P.O.
Associate Professor of Clinical Physical Therapy
    and Director
Program in Physical Therapy
Columbia University College of Physicians
    and Surgeons
New York, New York

Robert E. Eilert, M.D.
Professor of Orthopaedic Surgery
University of Colorado Health Sciences Center
Chairman, Department of Orthopaedic Surgery
The Children's Hospital
Denver, Colorado

Nancy Elftman, B.A., B.S.C.O., C.Ped.
Orthotic Department
Rancho Los Amigos Medical Center
Downey, California

Douglas Elson, B.S.
Certified Orthotist
Rancho Los Amigos Medical Center
Downey, California

William W. Eversmann, Jr., M.D.
Hand Surgeon
Iowa Medical Clinic
Cedar Rapids, Iowa

Colin W. Fennell, M.D., F.R.C.S.C.
Clinical Assistant Professor
University of Calgary
Orthopaedic Staff
Foothills Hospital
Calgary, Alberta

Laura Fenwick, C.O.
Instructor
Northwestern University Medical School
Consulting Orthotist
Rehabilitation Institute of Chicago
Chicago, Illinois

John R. Fisk, M.D.
Associate Professor of Surgery
Southern Illinois University School of Medicine
Springfield, Illinois

Richard A. Foulds, Ph.D.
Director, Applied Science and Engineering
    Laboratories
Research Professor—CIS and ME
University of Delaware
Alfred I. duPont Institute, Director
Wilmington, Delaware

Carol Frey, M.D.
Associate Clinical Professor of Orthopaedic Surgery
University of Southern California
Director, Orthopaedic Foot and Ankle Center
Orthopaedic Hospital
Los Angeles, California

Jan Furumasu, B.S., P.T.
Physical Therapist
Clinical Specialist
Rancho Los Amigos Medical Center
Downey, California

Donna Q. Gavin, C.O.
Director of Orthotics
BioConcepts, Inc.
Orthotic-Prosthetic Center
Burr Ridge, Illinois

Thomas M. Gavin, C.O.
BioConcepts, Inc.
Orthotic-Prosthetic Center
Burr Ridge, Illinois;
Orthopaedic Biomechanics Laboratory
Rehabilitation Research and Development Center
Veterans Administration Hospital
Hines, Illinois;
Prosthetic-Orthotic Center
Northwestern University Medical School
Chicago, Illinois

Gail Gilinsky, O.T.R.
Director, Occupational Therapy
Craig Hospital
Englewood, Colorado

Bertram Goldberg, M.D.†

Letha Y. Griffin, M.D., Ph.D.
Staff Physician
Peachtree Orthopaedic Clinic, P.A.
Team Physician
Georgia State University
Agnes Scott College
Piedmont Hospital
Atlanta, Georgia

John A. I. Grossman, M.D., F.A.C.S.
Assistant Professor of Surgery
New York University Medical Center
Attending Physician
Bellevue Hospital
Director of Hand Therapy
Rusk Institute of Rehabilitation Medicine
Manhattan Eye, Ear, and Throat Hospital
New York, New York

William S. Harwin, M.A., M.S.C., Ph.D.
Department of Cybernetics
University of Reading
Reading, England

Howard S. Hirsch, M.D.
Attending Orthopaedic Surgeon
Miriam Hospital
Providence, Rhode Island

†Deceased.

John D. Hsu, M.D.
Chairman
Department of Surgery
Chief of Orthopaedics
Rancho Los Amigos Medical Center
Clinical Professor, Orthopaedics
University of Southern California
School of Medicine
Downey, California

James C. Johns, Jr., M.D.
Iowa Medical Clinic, P.C.
Cedar Rapids, Iowa

Marjorie E. Johnson, M.S., P.T.
Instructor in Bioengineering
Mayo Medical School
Supervisor, Orthopaedic Biomechanics Laboratory
Mayo Clinic, Mayo Foundation
Rochester, Minnesota

Deena Garrison Jones, O.T.R.
Adjunct Faculty Member
Virginia Commonwealth University
Occupational Therapy Educational Supervisor
Woodrow Wilson Rehabilitation Center
Fishersville, Virginia

Mary Ann Keenan, M.D.
Professor of Orthopaedic Surgery
Professor of Physical Medicine and Rehabilitation
Temple University School of Medicine
Chairman, Department of Orthopaedic Surgery
Albert Einstein Medical Center
Philadelphia, Pennsylvania

Betti J. Krapfl, R.P.T., B.S., P.T.
RESNA
University of North Carolina
Chapel Hill, North Carolina;
Assistant Director, Physical Therapy Department
Craig Hospital
Englewood, Colorado

Melvin D. Law, Jr., M.D.
Clinical Instructor, Chattanooga Unit
University of Tennessee College of Medicine
Baptist Hospital Medical Center
Nashville, Tennessee

Maurice LeBlanc, M.S.M.E., C.P.
Lecturer
Stanford University School of Engineering
REC Director of Research
Packard Children's Hospital
Palo Alto, California

Robert D. Leffert, M.D.
Professor of Orthopaedic Surgery
Harvard Medical School
Visiting Orthopaedic Surgeon and Chief of the
    Surgical Upper Extremity of Rehabilitation Unit
Massachusetts General Hospital
Boston, Massachusetts

Judy Leonard, O.T.R., O.H.T.
Director
Regional Hand Rehabilitation Services, Inc.
Grand Rapids, Michigan

Phyllis D. Levine, P.T.
Chicagoland Orthopaedic Rehabilitation Services
Palos Heights, Illinois

Robert S. Lin, C.O.
Newington Orthotic and Prosthetic Systems
Children's Hospital Center
Newington, Connecticut

John E. Lonstein, M.D.
Clinical Associate Professor
Department of Orthopaedics
University of Minnesota
Fairview Riverside Medical Center
Minneapolis, Minnesota;
Gillette Children's Hospital
St. Paul, Minnesota

Timothy S. Loth, M.D.
Department of Orthopaedics
Iowa Medical Clinic, PC
Cedar Rapids, Iowa

Paul A. Lotke, M.D.
Professor of Orthopaedic Surgery
Chief of the Implant Service
Hospital of the University of Pennsylvania
Philadelphia, Pennsylvania

Colleen Lowe, M.P.H., O.T.R./L., C.H.T.
Coordinator, Hand Therapy Service
Massachusetts General Hospital
Boston, Massachusetts

Thomas R. Lunsford, M.S.E., C.O.
Assistant Professor
Baylor College of Medicine
Certified Orthotist
Lone Star Orthotics
The Institute for Rehabilitation and Research
Houston, Texas

Jeffrey A. Mann, M.D.
Foot and Ankle Fellow
Oakland Foot and Ankle Fellowship Program
Oakland, California

Roger A. Mann, M.D.
Associate Clinical Professor Orthopaedic Surgery
University of California at San Francisco
Director, Reconstructive Foot and Ankle Fellowship
San Francisco, California

John W. Michael, M.Ed., C.P.O., F.I.S.P.O.
Director of Professional and Technical Service
Otto Bock, USA
Minneapolis, Minnesota

Thomas J. Moore, M.D.
Associate Professor of Orthopaedic Surgery
Emory University School of Medicine
Atlanta, Georgia

Manohar M. Panjabi
Director of Biomechanics Research
Professor of Orthopaedics and Research and
    Mechanical Engineering
Yale University School of Medicine
New Haven, Connecticut

Avinash G. Patwardhan, Ph.D.
Professor, Department of Orthopaedic Surgery
Loyola University Medical School
Maywood, Illinois;
Orthopaedic Biomechanics Laboratory
Rehabilitation Research and Development Center
Veterans Administration Hospital
Hines, Illinois;
Prosthetic-Orthotic Center
Northwestern University Medical School
Chicago, Illinois

Grant Peacock
Atlanta Paralympic Organizing Committee
Atlanta, Georgia

Jacquelin Perry, M.D.
Professor of Orthopaedics
University of Southern California
Los Angeles, California;
Chief, Pathokinesiology/Polio Service
Rancho Los Amigos Medical Center
Downey, California

Troy D. Pierce, M.D.
Private Practice
The Bone & Joint Center
Bismarck, North Dakota

Tariq Rahman, Ph.D.
Research Assistant Professor
University of Delaware
Research Engineer
A.I. duPont Institute
Wilmington, Delaware

Lorna E. Ramos, M.A., O.T.R./L.
Clinical Supervisor, Hand Therapy Unit
Rusk Institute of Rehabilitation Medicine
New York University Medical Center
New York, New York

John A. Reister, M.D.
Associate Clinical Professor of Orthopaedics
Texas A&M University School of Medicine
Uniformed Services University for the Health
    Sciences
Scott and White Hospital
Staff Orthopaedic Surgeon
Brooke Army Medical Center
Scott and White Hospital
Darnell Army Community Hospital
Ft. Hood, Texas

John F. Ritterbusch, M.D.
Associate Professor of Orthopaedics and Pediatrics
University of New Mexico School of Medicine
Associate Medical Director
Carrie Tingley Hospital
Albuquerque, New Mexico

Enricho B. Robotti, M.D.
Division of Plastic Surgery
Hospedali Riuniti do Bergamo
Bergamo, Italy

Theodore F. Schlegel, M.D.
Orthopaedic Surgeon
Steadman Hawkins Denver Clinic
Denver, Colorado;
Vail Valley Medical Center
Vail, Colorado;
Swedish Hospital
Englewood, Colorado

John M. Snowden, C.P.O.
Director of Orthotics/Prosthetics Department
Massachusetts General Hospital
Harvard Medical School
Boston, Massachusetts

J. Richard Steadman, M.D.
Clinical Professor
University of Texas Southwestern
Dallas, Texas;
Chairman, Medical Group
United States Ski Team
Orthopaedic Surgeon
Steadman Hawkins Clinic
Vail Valley Medical Center
Vail, Colorado

Terry J. Supan, C.P.O.
Associate Professor
Department of Surgery
Division of Orthopaedics and Rehabilitation
Southern Illinois University School of Medicine
Director of Orthotics and Prosthetics
Southern Illinois University School of Medicine
Springfield, Illinois

Alfred B. Swanson, M.D.
Professor of Surgery
Michigan State University
East Lansing, Michigan;
Director of Orthopaedic Surgery Residency Training
    Program of the Grand Rapids Hospitals
Director of Hand Surgery Fellowship and
    Orthopaedic Research
Blodgett Memorial Medical Center
Grand Rapids, Michigan

Geneviève de Groot Swanson, M.D.
Assistant Clinical Professor of Surgery
Michigan State University
East Lansing, Michigan;
Coordinator
Orthopaedic Research Department
Blodgett Memorial Medical Center
Grand Rapids, Michigan

Barbara Trader
Atlanta Paralympic Organizing Committee
Atlanta, Georgia

Cathleen S. Van Buskirk, M.D.
Resident Physician in Orthopaedic Surgery
University of New Mexico School of Medicine
Albuquerque, New Mexico

John M. Wallace, C.O.
Vice President
Lone Star Orthotics Inc.
Houston, Texas

Robert L. Waters, M.D.
Clinical Professor of Orthopaedic Surgery
University of Southern California
Chief Medical Officer
Rancho Los Amigos Medical Center
Downey, California

Augustus A. White III, M.D., Dr. Med. Sci.
Professor of Orthopaedic Surgery
Harvard Medical School
Director, Spine Fellowship Program
Beth Israel Hospital
Boston, Massachusetts

Kent K. Wu, M.D.
Henry Ford Hospital
Detroit, Michigan

Arlene N. Yang, M.S.P.T.
Adjunct Instructor
University of Southern California
Department of Biokinesiology and Physical Therapy
Physical Therapist II/Neurologic Resource Clinician
Rancho Los Amigos Medical Center
Downey, California

Y. Lynn Yasuda, M.S.Ed., O.T.R., F.A.O.T.A.
Honorary Clinical Faculty
OT Department, University of Southern California
OT Coordinator of Clinical Education
Rancho Los Amigos Medical Center
Downey, California

Bertram Goldberg passed away of complications resulting from myeloma on June 2, 1995, in Denver, Colorado. A short period before his death, he was an actively practicing orthopedic surgeon in Englewood, Colorado, and secretary of the Orthopaedic Rehabilitation Association. He was an extremely courageous man who lived with his illness for over ten years. Sadly, it became active and began interfering with his practice, orthopedic teaching activities, and travel during his last year.

Bertram Goldberg was born June 30, 1938, and raised in Philadelphia. He graduated from the U.S. Military Academy at West Point in 1962 and served his country as an Air Defense Officer before entering medical school. He graduated from Duke University School of Medicine in 1969, completed his residency through Walter Reed Army Medical Center, and became an orthopaedic surgeon, certified by the American Board of Orthopaedic Surgery, in 1974.

He continued to serve in the U.S. Army Medical Corps and became Chief of Spine Service at Fitzsimmons Army Medical Center. He retired from military service with the rank of Colonel, M.C.

In 1982, Dr. Goldberg began his private practice in Denver, Colorado, where he was affiliated with such institutions as Swedish Medical Center, Porter Memorial Hospital, Littleton, Hospital, Children's Hospital, Craig Rehabilitation Hospital, and Spaulding Rehabilitation Hospital. He had a special interest in the care of amputees and diabetic patients with foot problems and was co-director of the amputee clinic at Denver General Hospital, director of the amputee clinic at Fitzsimmons Army Medical Center, and a consultant to the Institute for Limb Preservation at Presbyterian Hospital. He was also an active member of the American Academy of Orthopaedic Surgeons Committee on Rehabilitation, Prosthetics and Orthotics.

To his colleagues, Bert was a very friendly person. He was very energetic and displayed a zest for life. His enthusiasm carried over to, and stimulated, those who worked with him. He could be counted on. When he accepted a task or project, all those who had had the opportunity to work with him knew it was going to be well organized, well supervised, precise, accurate, well done, and "on time." Bert was also extremely loyal to his friends. Along with those many friends, he leaves his wife, Susan, of 33 years, and three children, Eric, Julia, and David.

He is greatly missed.

J.D.H.

IN MEMORIAM

Bertram Goldberg

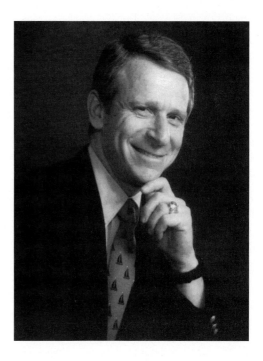

To Mrs. Francine Hsu for her love, encouragement and support;

To the late Bertram Goldberg, M.D., who started this project, and to his wife, Susan; and

To John Michael, M.Ed., C.P.O., whose friendship, professional advice, and help with this volume is greatly appreciated.

PREFACE

The word *orthosis* is derived from the Greek meaning "to make straight." Many decades ago, orthoses were used solely to either straighten limbs or straighten the spine. The science of orthotics has now evolved. Orthoses are now used to prevent deformities (AFO to prevent contractures following traumatic brain injury), to enhance gait (a reciprocating gait orthosis for ambulation in paraplegics), to facilitate activities of daily living (a wrist/hand orthosis for quadriplegia), to alleviate pain (spinal orthoses for degenerative arthritis of the spine), to protect desensate limbs (orthoses for neuropathic feet), to promote osteogenesis (functional brace for extremity fractures), and of course to strengthen limbs and spines. The goal of Doctors Hsu and Goldberg in editing the *AAOS Atlas of Orthoses and Assistive Devices* was to assemble a cross section of experts from multiple fields—orthopedists, orthotists, occupational therapists, and physical therapists—to gain a broad perspective in the usage of orthoses for various diseases. The orthotic management reported in this volume reflects present clinical practices. Available controlled studies have been cited whenever possible to provide scientifically valid justification for the opinions expressed. Alternative methods of treatment to orthoses, especially if more effective, have been emphasized (e.g., intramedullary nailing for femoral fractures in contrast to functional bracing).

The year 1995 marked the fiftieth anniversary of the death of President Franklin D. Roosevelt. During his Presidency, Roosevelt, a survivor of polio, was adamant about not allowing photographs of himself in either long leg braces or a wheelchair. The political climate at that time precluded a "disabled" President. In contrast, over 3,500 disabled athletes from 100 nations participated before millions of spectators at the 1996 Atlanta Paralympic Games.

The purpose of this book is to provide the scientific basis for usage of orthoses. The emphasis is on the restoration and preservation of function.

Thomas J. Moore

CONTENTS

BASICS

INTRODUCTION
John D. Hsu

The orthotic prescription needs to be a document that can be clearly understood by both the prescriber and the Certified Orthotist. The prescriber must understand the problem, the specific disability, the overall condition of the patient, the abnormal biomechanical or physiologic condition, and the area where the orthosis is to function and assist. For optimal results, the prescription needs to be individualized and comprehensive. This is the *blueprint* for what needs to be done. An obscure plan brings about a variable result. This is not good enough for the patient.

A systematic review of the biomechanics by region is included in the first section. Hip and knee motion is essential for gait. Its clinical impact is highlighted by the chapter on normal and pathologic gait (Chapter 3), but for more details on knee joint biomechanics the reader is referred to Chapter 28.

Specific foot and ankle motions and relationships are complex. They are appropriately described in the chapter on biomechanics of the foot (Chapter 7). When joints do not function normally and are impaired by pathologic changes and arthrodesis, additional stresses are applied, which results in additional pressures, deformities, or breakdown requiring orthotic support.

The chapter on biomechanics of the spine (Chapter 4) relates to spinal motion from the anatomic standpoint, namely, the ligamentous and muscle support. It complements Chapter 8 in Section Two on how the orthosis influences the damaged spine and the biomechanics of the orthosis.

Similarly, motion in the upper extremity, described as a linkage system for hand placement, is complex to analyze. Dynamic shoulder joint stability is important and affected by ligamentous constraints and muscle action. The illustrations for the chapter on biomechanics of the hand (Chapter 6) are appropriate representations of the author's concept for better reader understanding.

As we recognize and better understand the underlying physiologic changes in disorders of the musculoskeletal system, the need to comprehend and apply biomechanical principles has increased. Biomechanical knowledge needs to be integrated into patient care and in the design of orthoses. We are fortunate that this leadership has been taken by engineers involved in the rehabilitation field, frequently referred to by Vernon L. Nickel, a leader in the development of this orthopedic subspecialty, as *engineering orthopedics.*[1-3]

REFERENCES

1. Kozole KP: Rehabilitation engineering and assistive technology. In Nickel VL, Botte MJ (eds): Orthopaedic rehabilitation, 2nd ed, New York, 1992, Churchill Livingstone, pp 145–159.
2. Nickel VL: Orthopedic rehabilitation—challenges and opportunities, Clin Orthop Rel Res 63:153–161, 1969.
3. Reswick JB, Simoes N: Application of engineering principles in management of spinal cord injured patients, Clin Orthop Rel Res 112:124–129, 1975.

The Orthotic Prescription

Thomas R. Lunsford
John M. Wallace

The clinical setting of the mid-1990s has entered a period of rapid change as health care providers respond to the increasingly complex demands of various participants. The current practice environment is a fiercely competitive one in which the pressures to reduce costs require that services be provided in a fast-paced and time-budgeted atmosphere. An explosion of technologic advances has spurred a race to apply new materials, components, and designs to meet treatment objectives. The clinician must also follow the requirements and procedures of a complex array of third-party payers and case managers. Additionally, an increasingly litigious society demands thorough documentation of each interaction between the clinician and the patient. Finally, as consumers become more educated, they are demanding a greater role in determining their treatment course. As a result, clinicians must maximize productivity while increasing the accuracy, efficiency and quality of the services they provide. A clear, concise, and complete orthotic prescription can be the mechanism for achieving these objectives.

This chapter focuses on collaboration as the key to composing the optimum orthotic prescription, defines the orthotic prescription, and describes the process by which it is produced. The orthotic team's role and conventions in terminology are reviewed. Particular attention is given to transforming and synthesizing patient evaluation information into an orthotic prescription. A sample format for the orthotic prescription is presented, including a discussion of essential elements. Finally, examples of prescriptions are presented to illustrate the entire process, including effective justification to third-party payers.

DEFINITION OF ORTHOTIC PRESCRIPTION

The *orthotic prescription* is a written directive from a physician for the preparation and use of an orthosis as a remedy or treatment for a specific patient's pathologic condition. The prescription must identify the patient for whom the prescription is written and should contain patient's age, gender, diagnosis, funding resources, and origin of the referral. It must include a description of the orthosis, treatment objectives to be met by the orthosis, and a lucid justification. Finally, it must identify the prescribing physician and contain his or her signature and identification number(s).

ORTHOTIC TEAM

The orthotic team and its multidisciplinary approach to solving the complex problems of patients with biomechanical deficits was first described by Cary and associates in 1975.[1] They described the orthotic team as a physician, therapist, and Certified Orthotist working together to devise orthotic solutions. Today, the patient is added to the team. For the team to operate effectively and efficiently, the professional members must be familiar with the language of the other's discipline and acknowledge the other's strengths and expertise.

Physician

The physician is generally the team leader and is responsible for generating the prescription. The physician should provide the diagnosis, precautions, and medical objectives. Knowledge of orthotic management is useful, but with rapid advances in materials, components, and orthotic design it is prudent for the physician to develop a relationship with a qualified Certified Orthotist who can propose orthotic options with comparative advantages and disadvantages.

Therapist

When the treatment objective is one of functional improvement, such as gait mechanics or hand use, the physical or occupational therapist may contribute to the orthotic plan by identifying specific biomechanical deficits. The therapist might also recommend specific therapeutic objectives for orthotic treatment. The therapist can ensure long-term success of the orthotic treatment by providing training to the patient in all aspects of using the orthosis and by providing follow-up.

Patient

The input of the patient is often overlooked in the generation of the orthotic prescription. Early patient involvement and input about function, aesthetics, material, or weight concerns are critical to later acceptance and compliance.

Orthotist

The role of the orthotist is to integrate the information from the physician, therapist, and patient and to make decisions about design and materials. Once a particular approach has been agreed on by the orthotic team, the orthotist finalizes the design, fabricates, fits, and critiques the orthosis.

TERMINOLOGY

The use of standard terminology by the orthotic team is key to clear and effective communication. In addition, it enables the involved fee-paying agency to identify what is being prescribed.

A standard for orthotic terminology was developed in the early 1970s.[2] Before this time, orthoses were identified by proper names, or eponyms, derived from the place of origin, the developer, or sometimes a name unrelated to either. There are scores of such names, such as the Milwaukee brace, the Klenzak, and the Scottish Rite orthosis. A frequent problem with eponyms is that they do not identify the scope of the orthosis or its purpose and may only be known regionally to clinicians.

Learning about eponymous orthoses was a process of rote memory, which could not be done logically or systematically. Fee-paying agencies had difficulties in developing a fee schedule that reflected the service provided by the orthotist and the function of the orthosis.

Harris was author of a report in 1973 prepared by the Task Force on Standardization of Prosthetic-Orthotic Terminology.[2] Its primary objective was to develop terms based on logical systems to communicate the functions desired. A secondary objective was to provide a logical system for teaching physicians, therapists, and orthotists and for use in fee schedules. The task force agreed that proper names and eponyms should be eliminated and that orthoses should be described first by the principal joints that they encompass. Harris

listed many practical recommendations, which have proven over time to be logical and sound. *Orthoses* is the proper term for the group of devices variously called orthopedic appliances, braces, splints, calipers, and supports. Orthosis is defined as "any medical device applied to, or around, a bodily segment in the case of physical impairment or disability." For the sake of classification, the body is divided into three major anatomic areas: (1) upper limbs, (2) lower limbs, and (3) spine. The development of specialized craniofacial orthoses, for burn scar management and plagiocephaly, was not anticipated in this classification.

Acronyms

The task force recommended that the major joints encompassed be used to describe the orthosis. The initial letters of the joints are combined to create acronyms. Examples include the long-leg brace, which became the knee-ankle-foot orthosis (KAFO), and the short-leg brace, which became the ankle-foot orthosis (AFO). Examples of upper limb orthoses include the short and long opponens, which became the static hand orthosis (HdO) and the static wrist-hand orthosis (WHO), respectively. Other upper limb orthoses were named elbow orthosis (EO) and shoulder-elbow-wrist-hand orthosis (SEWHO). This terminology has been endorsed by ISO and is now accepted worldwide.

In practice, the use of eponyms has not disappeared. There are frequently several orthotic options to manage a given clinical situation. Use of eponyms in conjunction with standard terminology can help clarify the preferred design. For example, an adolescent idiopathic scoliosis may be managed with one of several orthotic designs. Depending on the specifics of the case and the preference of the physician, a Boston-type TLSO might be provided. This use of the eponym as an adjective distinguishes the Boston-type TLSO from a Charleston-type or other low-profile TLSO also suitable for scoliosis treatment.

For simplicity, the terminology groups certain joint complexes, such as the hand, wrist, and foot, as units for descriptive purposes. Only if an orthosis is prescribed to provide specific controls to the intrinsic joints of these complexes is it necessary to specify in more detail. An orthosis designed to control subtalar motion would be specified as a foot orthosis (FO) for subtalar control.

The hand is subdivided into metacarpal phalangeal (MCP), proximal interphalangeal (PIP), and distal interphalangeal (DID) joints, and thumb carpo metacarpal (CM), MCP, and IP joints. A wrist hand orthosis with metacarpal phalangeal extension assists of fingers 2-5 would be termed a "WHO with MCP 2–5 extension assist."

The spine is subdivided into cervical, thoracic, lumbar, and sacral regions. A neck brace is a cervical orthosis

(CO), an orthopedic corset is a lumbosacral orthosis (LSO) and a Milwaukee brace is a cervicothoracic-lumbosacral orthosis (CTLSO). Acronyms longer than five letters are uncommon. Although a body jacket connected to bilateral full-leg braces is theoretically known as a TLSHKAFO, it is often referred to as a "TLSO plus bilateral HKAFOs." One variant, which provides a reciprocal gait, is colloquially abbreviated as RGO (reciprocating gait orthosis).

Control

Specific terminology is used to describe the type of joint control desired: free motion (no control), assisted motion, resisted motion, stopped motion, and re-strained motion.

An orthosis may permit *free* or unencumbered motion in a given plane. For example, an AFO with a free motion mechanical ankle joint might be used for me-diolateral (inversion/eversion) control. In the sagittal plane, however, it allows free motion throughout the range of dorsiflexion and plantar flexion.

An orthosis may *assist* motion by the application of an external force to increase the range, velocity, or force of a desired motion, using a spring, elastic band, motor, or weighted counterbalance to compensate for the effects of gravity. Common examples include the dorsiflexion assist AFO and wrist extension assist WHO. When elastic devices, such as springs or rubber bands, are used to *assist* motion, it is important to note that the comple-mentary motion is *resisted*. For example, the use of a rubber band to provide wrist extension assist for a patient with a radial nerve injury automatically in-creases the effort required to produce wrist flexion.

An orthosis may also deliberately *resist* motion to decrease the velocity or force of an undesirable motion. To illustrate, the AFO with plantar flexion resist is used to prevent foot slap during loading in the presence of weak anterior compartment musculature or sensory loss. As the heel strikes the floor, the normal eccentric action of the anterior compartment musculature is replaced with a plantar flexion resist spring.

An orthosis may *stop* motion or limit the range of motion. The prescription should indicate the specific motion to be stopped and when the stop is to be engaged. A knee orthosis (KO) with 90-degree flexion stop and −20-degrees extension stop may be used postoperatively to limit knee motion. The prescription should specify whenever adjustable stops are required: KO with adjustable range of motion stops—set range initially from 90-degree flexion to −20 degrees exten-sion.

An orthosis may also *hold* by eliminating all motion of the joint at a specific position. For the patient with weak anterior compartment musculature and a weak calf, a solid plastic AFO that completely restrains ankle mo-

tion may be indicated. This could be described as a rigid plastic AFO to hold the ankle in 5 degrees dorsiflexion.

Additional descriptors

There are three additional descriptors. The term *variable* may be used with the term *stop*, *resist*, or *assist* to indicate the need for an adjustable system, with the desired range of motion specified. A *lock* is an optional mechanism that, when engaged, holds the joint in a fixed position. One example of locked motion is the ring or drop lock system used for knee control on some KAFOs. Mechanical hip and elbow joints may also be locked.

On rare occasions, an orthosis may be prescribed to partially *deweight* the lower limb. In practice, secondary discomfort at the deweighting force sites is the main limitation to deweighting. When this is an objective for a prescribed orthosis, however, the amount of loading to be carried by the orthosis can be expressed as a percent-age of the normal load: "Bivalved AFO to reduce axial loading at calcaneus 15 percent."

EVALUATION AND PRESCRIPTION

The medical community is indebted to Newton C. McCollough III for his creative and significant contri-bution in developing and presenting *biomechanical anal-ysis systems*, a systematic and logical approach to patient evaluation and orthotic prescription.[3] These systems emphasize the importance of an accurate, objective biomechanical analysis of the body segments as the foundation for determining orthotic needs. This bio-mechanical system is useful for precisely documenting biomechanical deficits, particularly for controlled re-search.

A systematic functional evaluation of the impaired limb or body segment is the basis for a rational prescrip-tion. Even though the technical analysis forms are often considered too detailed and time consuming to be routinely used in a clinical setting, familiarity with the concepts is essential for creating sound orthotic pre-scriptions. Because of their thoroughness and overall importance, the reader is referred to the two previous editions of this *Atlas* for complete descriptions and instructions for using the technical analysis forms for the lower limb, upper limb, and spine.[3,4]

Elements of orthotic prescription

Patient-specific information appears at the top of most prescriptions. This may include, but not be lim-ited to, name, institution identification number, ad-dress, telephone number, age, gender, diagnosis, and date of prescription. This information is essential for medical chart creation or entry, subsequent appointments, financial screening, and developing an overall sense of the patient's pathomechanical condition (e.g., T-12 complete paraplegia, hemiplegia, adult-onset rheumatoid arthritis). Having an accurate diagnosis and history allows the practitioner to plan for likely changes in the patient's clinical picture based on the natural history of the pathology. Knowing that a patient has had poliomyelitis, spinal cord injury, stroke, brain injury, or diabetes orients the clinician to a constellation of sensory deficits, muscle weakness potential, hypertonicity, and potential for deformities.

Sufficient reimbursement information must be obtained if financial clearance is to be obtained in a timely fashion. This should include carrier, plan identification, deductions, percent payable, and any other information that expedites financial screening. Clinicians consider themselves fortunate when they are spared this issue. The trend, however, is to increase the clinician's involvement. Some institutions perform this function during the admissions process, and only the patient's identification number and carrier may need to be identified.

The text of the prescription is, of course, the main element. The convenient "leg brace" phrase, for example, written diagonally across a prescription is rarely sufficient. On the other hand, a lengthy prescription detailing every component dimension, shape, and placement is neither necessary nor desirable.

A brief acronym (e.g., AFO, KAFO, WHO) with the key therapeutic or functional objectives developed as a team documents the rationale clearly and simultaneously permits the Certified Orthotist to use his or her skills and knowledge to design the most cost-effective orthosis. For example, the prescription may read "KAFO with knee hyperextension stop at −10°, restrain dorsiflexion to 15° at terminal stance, and allow adjustability for growth." This acknowledgment of the orthotist's expertise fosters creativity and maximizes the benefit to the patient.

Justification

The justification is written to provide funding agencies or other interested parties a clear explanation of why orthotic treatment is necessary. Treatment objectives fall under one or more general categories: prevention or correction of deformity, protection of a weak or painful musculoskeletal segment, improvement of function, etc.

The original treatment objectives that emerged from the evaluation of the patient's pathomechanical condition can also be used as the basis for the justification. For example, a patient who exhibits excessive dorsiflexion in terminal stance because of a weak calf requires an AFO to restrain excessive dorsiflexion. The justification in this case is that without the AFO, the patient is at risk of knee buckle and possibly falling or at risk of overstretching the pathologic calf musculature making full recovery unlikely.

A justification can be compelling when it shows that orthotic treatment will either reduce the cost of rehabilitation or increase independence and self-care. Moreover, justification is particularly convincing when it can be stated that withholding orthotic treatment can be deleterious to a patient's health.

Examples

Even though patient evaluation has been enhanced with modern instruments for performing objective measurements, it remains, for the most part, an art form. This art form requires structured didactic training and clinical mentoring to master.

Three examples are presented here to illustrate how to convert evaluative data and interview information into a prescription. The premise of these examples is that the diagnosis is known (physician), a relatively short list of treatment objectives has been identified (therapist), and an interview with the patient has revealed specific preferences.

- *Example 1*—J.W. is a 65-year-old female who had a spinal tumor. The tumor was surgically excised and her condition post-operatively was T-8 incomplete paraplegia. One month postoperatively she presented with the clinical findings listed below.

- **Strength**

		Right	*Left*
Stance	Hip ext./abd.	P−	F+
	Knee extension	P	G
	Plantar flexion	P	P
Swing	Hip flexion	F	F+
	Knee flexion	P	F
	Dorsiflexion	P	G

- **Proprioception**

Hip	impaired	normal
Knee	impaired	normal
Ankle	absent	normal
Toes	absent	impaired

- **Tone**
  Right: mild plantar flexion clonus
  Left: normal
- **Range of motion**—Hip, knee, and ankle within normal limits.
- **Gait analysis**

Right	Weight acceptance	Excessive knee flexion
	Single limb support	Excessive knee extension thrust and excessive plantar flexion
	Swing limb advancement	Increased hip flexion, with excessive plantar flexion
Left	Weight acceptance	Limited knee flexion
	Single limb support	Excessive knee flexion and excessive dorsiflexion, no heel off
	Swing limb advancement	Normal

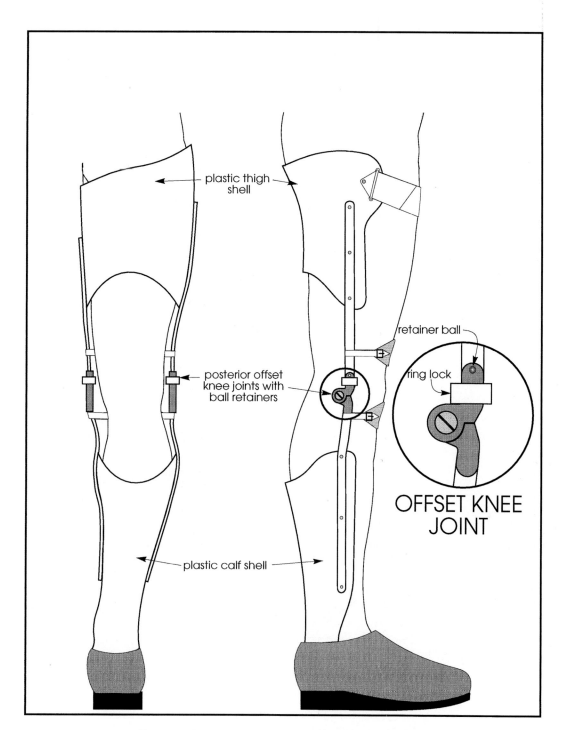

Fig. 1.1. Plastic KAFO (with posterior offset knee joints).

• **Synthesis**—The right lower limb lacks both muscle control and sensory awareness. There are three reasons to lock the ankle: weak musculature, spasticity, and absent proprioception. There are three reasons to lock the knee: weak hip and knee extensors, impaired proprioception, and the resulting extension thrust during single-limb support. Therefore, a KAFO should be prescribed for the right lower limb. Because this patient is an incomplete paraplegic and may continue to improve, the orthotist has recommended a posterior offset knee joint with a ring lock and retainers so that if the patient makes significant gains in quadriceps strength and/or

proprioception, she may unlock the mechanical knee joints for unencumbered knee flexion during swing phase (Fig. 1.1). However, the KAFO will still be required to check knee extension thrust until enough return allows the KAFO to be reduced to an AFO.

The left lower limb suffers from a weak calf. The limited knee flexion at weight acceptance is an indication that the quadriceps alone cannot withstand the flexion challenge without support from the calf. The excessive dorsiflexion in single limb support with no heel off in terminal stance confirms that the weak calf is

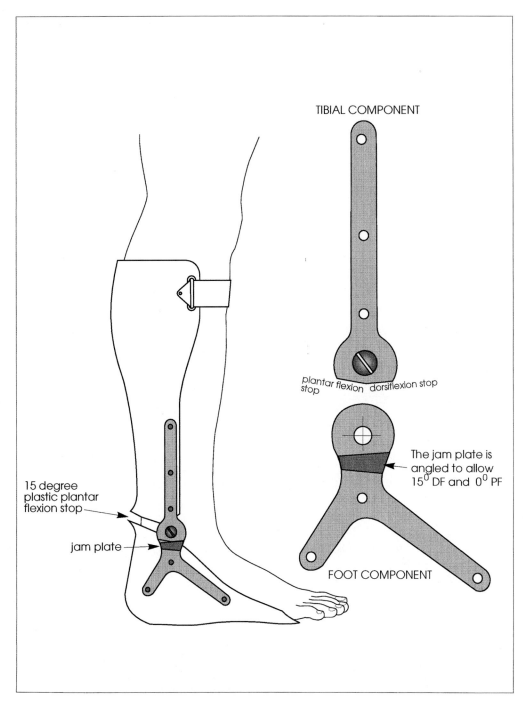

TIBIAL COMPONENT

plantar flexion dorsiflexion stop
stop

The jam plate is
angled to allow
15⁰ DF and 0⁰ PF

15 degree
plastic plantar
flexion stop

jam plate

FOOT COMPONENT

Fig. 1.2.   Plastic AFO (with mechanical ankle joint).

the main problem. Because there is adequate strength and pro-prioception at the knee and hip on the left, only an AFO is prescribed to restrain excessive dorsiflexion in stance. It is not desirable, however, to lock the ankle and restrain plantar flexion because the left anterior compartment musculature and ankle proprioception are sufficiently intact to withstand the demands of plantar flexion during loading. The orthotist suggested a custom plastic AFO with a special adjustable mechanical ankle joint, which restrains excessive dorsiflexion and allows free plantar flexion (Fig. 1.2).

- **Prescription**—The prescription for J.W. is shown in Figure 1.3. The information is divided into four sections. The first contains the patient's name, address, telephone number, ID number, diagnosis, and prescription date. The second contains the orthoses required and the specific treatment objectives. In this case, a KAFO and AFO are being prescribed, and the associated treatment objectives are noted. The third section contains the justification for the KAFO and AFO in terms of the rehabilitation goals of the physician and therapist. The fourth section contains the prescribing physician's signature and printed name, the date needed, and reason.

Patient Name ___*J. W.*___   Date __11_/_28_/_94__

Patient No. _51372_   Diagnosis ___*T - 8 (incomlete)*___

☐ Inpatient (Nursing Unit _____)   Current Address:
                                                   123 *Main St.*
☒ Outpatient (Telephone No. _(123_456-7890_____) *Anywhere, USA*   98765

Orthotic Service Needed:

Ⓡ *KAFO to prevent knee extension thrust and excessive dorsiflexion in stance.*

Ⓛ *AFO to prevent excessive dorsiflexion in stance and allow free plantar flexion during loading.*

Precautions: DC date: _NA_/ _ / _

Justification: Ⓡ *KAFO is required to protect weak musculature of the knee and ankle. KAFO will also provide stability during gait. Total contact plastic is required at foot and ankle for positioning, control of spasticity, and proprioceptive input.*

Ⓛ *AFO is required to protect weak calf musculature during stance and to provide optimum stride characteristics. The adjustable ankle joint will allow clinical adjustments to be made as the patient's strength improves. Plastic is required to match the KAFO side.*

Date Needed: __12_/_15_/_94__   Reason: *Patient leaving area*

Recommended By __*Tom Lunsford, CO*__

Physician's Signature __*John Smith, MD*__   Print: John Smith, MD   Ext. _1234_

Fig. 1.3. Orthotic prescription sheet for previous orthoses.

- *Example 2*—R.T. is a 35-year-old female who is diagnosed with C-4 incomplete spinal cord injury secondary to a motor vehicle accident. Currently she is ambulatory in a halo vest apparatus with a painful subluxation of her left shoulder. The subluxation of her shoulder occurred after the initial injury secondary to gravitational forces acting on weak shoulder musculature. Two weeks postinjury she presented with the clinical findings listed below.

- **Strength**

		Right	Left
Stance	Hip ext./abd.	G/P	G/F+
	Knee extension	N	G
	Plantar flexion	N	G
Swing	Hip flexion	G	G
	Knee flexion	N	G
	Dorsiflexion	N	G
Upper limb	Shoulder (general)	G	P−
	Elbow (general)	F+	G
	Wrist (flexion/extension)	F+/G	F+/F+

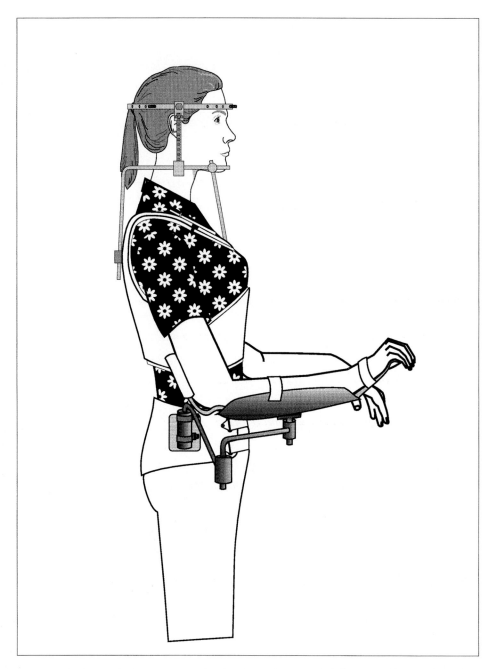

Fig. 1.4.   Shoulder-elbow-wrist orthosis (gunslinger type with mobile arm support attachment).

	Right	*Left*
Hand		
Thumb	G	F+
Fingers	F+	F−

- **Proprioception**—Upper limbs within normal limits.
- **Tone**—None.
- **Range of motion**—Halo-vest limited shoulder motion, otherwise within normal limits throughout.
- **Gait analysis**—Walked with rolling walker to support painful shoulder. Endurance generally low, but improving. No significant gait deviations.
- **Synthesis**—The orthotic treatment objectives relate to R.T.'s painful shoulder. Residual effects of her spinal cord injury include a weakened and subluxed left glenohumeral joint that is painful

and at risk of further damage if left unsupported. To walk, she must support her weak shoulder with her contralateral hand or with a rolling walker with a forearm trough limiting the use of her upper limb. Her present condition offers little opportunity for functional tasks and her rehabilitation is slowed. Therefore, the orthotic treatment objectives for her shoulder include alleviating pain, preventing subluxation, promoting healing of the traumatized tissues, facilitating hand function on the left, and freeing the right hand for independent activities. The orthotist suggested a shoulder-elbow-wrist orthosis (SEWO) of the gunslinger[5] type (Fig. 1.4). This orthosis consists of forearm and wrist trough linked to a plastic iliac cap. The linkage is similar to a mobile arm support and allows maximum shoulder and elbow motion while minimizing gravitational tension on the soft tissues of the glenohumeral joint.

Patient Name _R. T._	Date _11_/_23_/_94_
Patient No. _27315_	Diagnosis _C - 4 Brown Sequard_
[X] Inpatient (Nursing Unit _503 - 2_)	Current Address: _321 First St._
[ ] Outpatient (Telephone No. (___) ___)	_Anytown, USA 87654_

Orthotic Service Needed:

SEWHO ("gunslinger" type)   *Shoulder-elbow-wrist orthosis to alleviate shoulder pain, take tension off the glenohumeral joint, and mobilize and protect UE for positioning of "intrinsic +" hand.*

Precautions: *UE orthosis must be compatible with halo-vest*   DC date: _12_/_10_/_94_

Justification:

R.T. needs shoulder support to alleviate pain secondary to gh subluxation. It is necessary to protect the traumatized soft tissues so her rehabilitation can proceed. The SEWHO will allow her to ambulate without a walker and to position her hand for table top tasks and independent living activities. Also, this will free her contralateral UE for additional self-care.

Date Needed: _12_/_10_/_94_	Reason: *Patient to be discharged*
Recommended By _Tom Lunsford, CO_	Ext. _4321_
Physician's Signature _Robert Brown, MD_	Print: Robert Brown, MD

Fig. 1.5. Orthotic prescription sheet.

- **Prescription**—The prescription for R.T. is shown in Figure 1.5. Unique to this prescription is the use of both a generic name and an eponym adjective as well as the treatment objectives. The justification is compelling in this case, because the therapeutic needs are closely tied to the functional objectives.

- *Example 3*—D.D. is a 9-year-old male with Duchenne's muscular dystrophy. This young patient has come to the outpatient clinic with complaints of difficult breathing and exhibits poor sitting posture. D.D. is nonambulatory and uses a wheelchair for mobility. The patient exhibits a flaccid spinal posture with lateral bending and kyphosis.

- **Strength**
    Lower limbs: poor or weaker
    Upper limbs: fair with poor endurance
    Trunk
        Extensors: fair
        Flexors: poor
        Lateral flexors: fair
        Rotation: absent

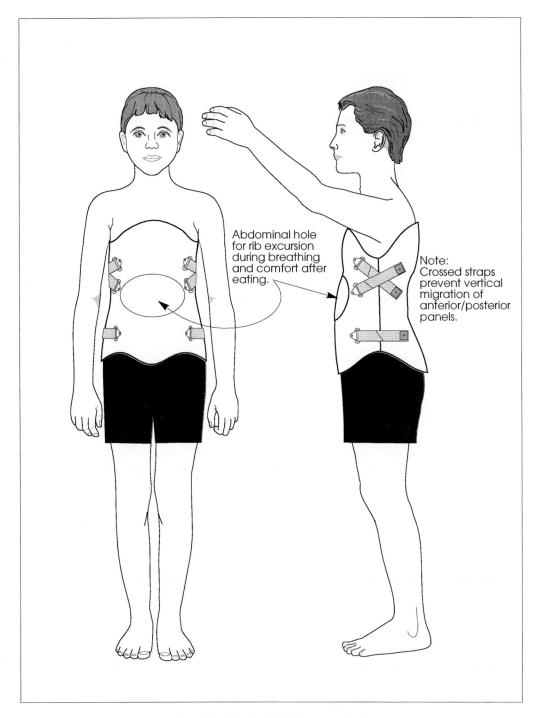

Abdominal hole
for rib excursion
during breathing
and comfort after
eating.

Note:
Crossed straps
prevent vertical
migration of
anterior/posterior
panels.

Fig. 1.6. Plastic TLSO (body jacket).

- **Pulmonary function**
     Vital capacity: 1.3 L
     Tidal volume: 250 cc
     Inspiration pressure: 18 mm Hg
- **Range of motion**
     Bilateral hip flexion contractures (20°)
     Bilateral plantar flexion contractures (40°)
- **Gait analysis**—Nonambulatory.
- **Synthesis**—The orthotic treatment objective is to maximize
 pulmonary function and improve sitting posture. This will be done

by aligning the spine so that the trunk and abdominal accessory
musculature can assist breathing without the restriction associated
with the spinal flaccidity. A plastic, total contact type of thoraco-
lumbo-sacral orthosis (TLSO) is one approach (Fig. 1.6). The
TLSO must be designed so that the normal rib excursion during
breathing is not restricted. Also, an anterior modification is required to avoid discomfort after eating. Lastly, the design should
permit changes in the girth of the patient with growth.

- **Prescription**—The prescription for D.D. is shown in Figure 1.7.
 The orthosis required in this case is a TLSO of the plastic body

Patient Name *D. D..* Date *11 / 17 / 94*

Patient No. *23456* Diagnosis *DMD*

☐ Inpatient (Nursing Unit ______________)

☒ Outpatient (Telephone No. *(999) 876-5432*)

Current Address:
890 Center St.
Someplace, USA 77771

Orthotic Service Needed:

TLSO (body jacket) *Total contact type of body jacket to support paralytic spine, facilitate breathing, and allow for lower abdominal expansion after meal time (discomfort).*

Precautions: *Limited pulmonary function* DC date: *NA / /*

Justification:

This patient requires trunk support to facilitate breathing. Without a trunk support the patient's spine collapses and he has difficulty breathing..

Date Needed: *12/ 20 / 94* Reason: *Patient to be discharged*

Recommended By *Tom Lunsford, CO* Ext. *4321*

Physician's Signature *S. Page, MD* Print: Suzanne Page, MD

Fig. 1.7. Orthotic prescription sheet.

jacket type. This TLSO has horizontal rib relief along the anterolateral margin of the lower ribs to accommodate rib excursion during breathing. Also, the anterior panel of the TLSO has a large hole in the structural plastic bridged by the liner to prevent discomfort after eating.

SUMMARY

The orthotic prescription is defined as a written directive from the physician. However, an effective prescription must also meet the needs of funding agencies, incorporate clinical input from therapist and patient, and indicate specific treatment objectives so that the Certified Orthotist can design the optimum orthotic system to fully meet all needs. This requires close collaboration and ongoing communication between the prescribing physician, therapist, patient, and orthotist.

The entire process is enhanced by the use of standardized terminology and nomenclature so that there is effective communication between the professional members of the orthotic team as well as with funding agencies.

A prescription format is presented with specific examples illustrating the essential elements. The raw clinical data are synthesized to illustrate the transition from treatment objectives to a specific orthotic design.

REFERENCES

1. Cary JM, Lusskin R, Thompson RG: Prescription principles. In Atlas of orthotics: biomechanical principles and application, St. Louis, 1975, CV Mosby.
2. Harris EE: A new orthotic terminology: a guide to its use for prescription and fee schedules, Orthot Prosthet 27:6–9, 1973.
3. McCollough NC: Biomechanical analysis systems for orthotic prescription. In Atlas of orthotics: biomechanical principles and application, 2nd ed, St. Louis, 1985, CV Mosby.
4. McCollough NC: Biomechanical analysis systems for orthotic prescription. In Atlas of orthotics: biomechanical principles and application, St. Louis, 1975, CV Mosby.
5. Perry J: Prescription principles. In Atlas of orthotics: biomechanical principles and application, St. Louis, 1975, CV Mosby.

Strength and Materials

Thomas R. Lunsford

Metals and plastics are the principal materials used in orthotics and prosthetics. To understand recommended design and fabrication procedures, it is important to have basic knowledge of the properties of the various available materials. One must be familiar with these materials to cope with both standard and difficult design and fabrication problems.

Selection of the correct material for a given design depends partially on understanding the elementary principles of mechanics and materials, concepts of forces, deformation and failure of structures under load, improvement in mechanical properties by heat treatment or other means, and design of structures. For example, the choices for a knee-ankle-foot orthosis (KAFO) may include several types of steels, numerous alloys of aluminum, and titanium and its alloys. Important but minor uses of other metals include copper or brass rivets and successive platings of copper, nickel, and chromium. Plastics, fabrics, rubbers, and leathers have wide indications, and composite structures (plastic matrix with reinforcing fibers) are beginning to be used.

Despite publicity for exotic materials, no single material is a panacea. One explanation for this is that frequently a single design might require divergent mechanical properties (e.g., stiffness and flexibility required in an ankle-foot orthosis (AFO) for dorsiflexion restraint and free plantar flexion).

In general, understanding of mechanics and strength of materials, even if intuitive, is important to the practitioner during the design stage. A general understanding of stresses arising from loading of structures, particularly from the bending of beams, is needed. Then the practitioner can appreciate the importance of simple methods to allow controlled deformation during fitting, to provide stiffness or resiliency as prescribed, and to reduce breakage whether from impact or from repeated loading. A general discussion of materials and

specific theory related to design, fabrication, and riveting guidelines follows.

STRENGTH AND STRESS

The strength of the material selected for the fabrication of the orthoses or prostheses is one of the practitioner's main considerations. *Strength* is defined as the ability of a material to resist forces. When comparative studies are made of the strength of materials, the concept of stress must be introduced.

Stress relates to both the magnitude of the applied forces and the amount of material resisting the forces. It is defined as force per unit cross-sectional area of material and is usually expressed in pounds per square inch (psi). The amount of stress, σ, is computed using the equation

$$\sigma = \frac{F}{A} \qquad (1)$$

where
F = applied force, lbs, and
A = cross-sectional area, in.^{2}

The same amount of force applied over different areas causes radically different stresses. For example, a one pound weight is placed on a cylindrical test bar having a cross-sectional area of 1 square inch. According to Eq 1, the compressive stress, σ_c, in the cylindrical test bar is 1 pound per square inch (Fig. 2.1). When the same 1-lb weight is placed on a needle having a cross-sectional area of 0.001 square inch, however, the compressive stress, σ_c, in the needle is 1000 psi (Fig. 2.2).

A force exerted on a small area always causes more stress than the same force acting on a larger area. When a woman is wearing high heels, her weight is supported

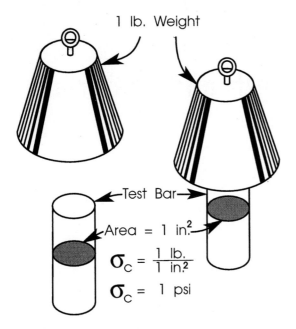

Fig. 2.1.   Compressive stress on a cylinder.

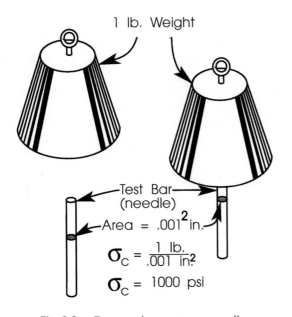

Fig. 2.2.   Compressive stress on a needle.

by the narrow heels having an area of only a fraction of a square inch. With flat shoes, the same weight or force is spread over a heel having a larger cross-sectional area. The stress in the heel of the shoe is much greater when high heels are worn because there is less material resisting the applied forces.

Similar problems are encountered in orthoses and prostheses. A child weighing 100 lb and wearing a weight-bearing orthosis with a 90-degree posterior stop (Fig. 2.3) can exert forces at initial contact that create stresses of thousands of pounds per square inch. If the

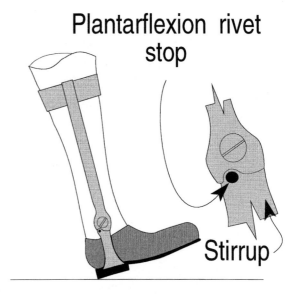

Fig. 2.3.   AFO with 90-degree plantar flexion stop.

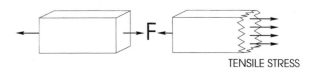

Fig. 2.4.   Tension.

child jumps, the force would increase with the height of the jump. The stress at the stop or on the rivet could be great enough to cause failure.

Tensile, compressive, shear, and flexural stresses

Materials are subject to several types of stress depending upon the way that the forces are applied. These are tensile, compressive, shear, and flexural stresses.

Tensile stresses.   Tensile stresses act to pull apart an object or cause it to be in tension. Tensile stresses occur parallel to the line of force but perpendicular to the area in question (Fig. 2.4). If an object is pulled at both ends, it is in tension and sufficient force will pull it apart. Two children fighting over a fish scale, and exerting opposing forces, put it in tension as shown by the indicator on the scale (Fig. 2.5).

Compressive stresses.   Compressive stresses act to squeeze or compress objects. They also occur parallel to the line of force and perpendicular to the cross-sectional area (Fig. 2.6).

A blacksmith shapes metal by hitting the material with a hammer to squeeze or compress the metal into the desired shape. In the same manner, clay yields to low compressive stress; clay is distorted and squeezed out of shape by comparatively small forces.

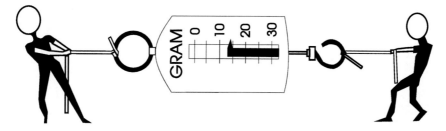

Fig. 2.5. A spring scale can be used to demonstrate tension.

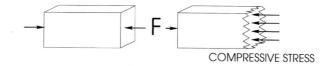

Fig. 2.6. Compression.

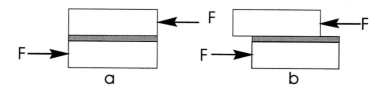

Fig. 2.7. Shear.

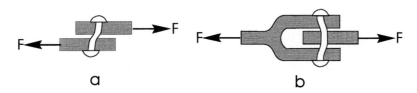

Fig. 2.8. Joint shear.

Shear stresses. Shear stresses act to scissor or shear the object causing the planes of the material to slide over each other. Shear stresses occur parallel to the applied forces. Consider two blocks (Fig. 2.7, *a*) with their surfaces bonded together. If forces acting in opposite directions are applied to these blocks, they tend to slide over each other. If these forces are great enough, the bond between the blocks will break (Fig. 2.7, *b*). If the area of the bonded surfaces were increased, however, the effect of the forces would be distributed over a greater area. The average stress would be decreased, and there would be increased resistance to shear stress.

A common lap joint and clevis joint are examples of where a shear pin is used as the axis of the joint (Fig. 2.8). The lap joint has one shear area of the rivet resisting the forces applied to the lap joint (Fig. 2.8, *a*), and the rivet in the box joint (clevis) has an area resisting the applied forces that is twice as great as the area in the lap joint (assuming that the rivets in both joints are the same size; Fig. 2.8, *b*). Consequently the

clevis joint will withstand twice as much shear force as the lap joint. The lap joint also has less resistance to fatigue (fluctuating stress of relatively low magnitude, which results in failure) because it is more susceptible to flexing stresses.

Flexural stress. Flexural stress (bending) is a combination of tension and compression stresses. Beams are subject to flexural stresses. When a beam is loaded transversely, it will sag. The top fibers of a beam are in maximum compression while the bottom side is in maximum tension (Fig. 2.9). The term *fiber*, as used here, means the geometric lines that compose the prismatic beam. The exact nature of these compressive and tensile stresses are discussed later.

Ultimate stress

Ultimate stress is the stress at which a material ruptures. The strength of the material before it ruptures also depends on the type of stress to which it is subjected. For example, ultimate shear stresses are usually lower than ultimate tensile stresses (i.e., less

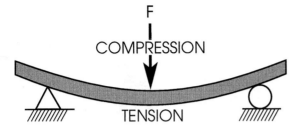

Fig. 2.9. Flexure.

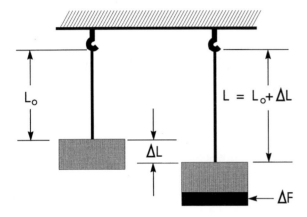

Fig. 2.10. Strain.

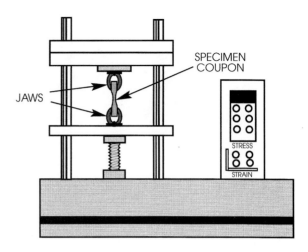

Fig. 2.11. Tension test.

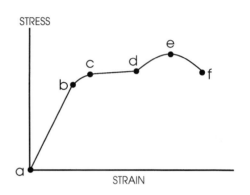

Fig. 2.12. Stress-strain.

shear stress has to be applied before the material ruptures than in the case of tensile or compressive stress).

Strain

Materials subjected to sufficient stress will deform or change their shape. If a material lengthens or shortens in response to stress, it is said to experience *strain*. Strain is denoted by ϵ and may be found by dividing the total elongation (or contraction) ΔL by the original length L_0 of the structure being loaded:

$$\epsilon = -\frac{\Delta L}{L_0} \qquad (2)$$

Consider a change in length ΔL of a wire or rod caused by a change in stretching force F (Fig. 2.10). The amount of stretch is proportional to the original length of wire. A wire 5 inches long stretches twice as much as a wire 2.5 inches long, other things being equal.

Stress-strain curve

The most widely used means of seeking knowledge of the mechanical properties of materials is the tension test. Much can be learned from observing the data collected from such a test. In the tension test, the dimensions of the specimen coupon are fixed by standardization, so that the results may be universally understood, no matter where, or by whom, the test is

conducted. The specimen coupon is mounted between the jaws of a tensile testing machine, which is simply a device for stretching the specimen at a controlled rate. Usually the cross-sectional area of the coupon is smaller in the center to avoid failures where the coupon is gripped. The resistance that the specimen offers to being stretched and the linear deformations are measured by sensitive instrumentation (Fig. 2.11).

The force of resistance divided by the cross-sectional area of the specimen is the *stress* in the specimen (Eq 1). The *strain* is the total deformation divided by the original length (Eq 2). If the stresses in the specimen are plotted as ordinates of a graph, with the accompanying strains as abscissae, a number of the mechanical properties are graphically revealed. Figure 2.12 shows such a stress-strain diagram for a mild steel specimen.

The shape and magnitude of the stress-strain curve of a metal depend on its composition; heat treatment; prior history of plastic deformation; and the strain rate, temperature, and state of stress imposed during testing. The parameters that are used to describe the stress-strain curve of a metal are tensile strength, yield strength or yield point, percent elongation, and reduc-

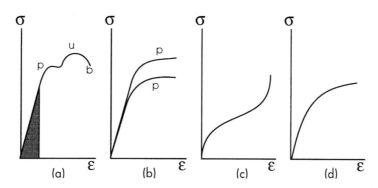

Fig. 2.13. Stress-strain diagrams for different materials.

Table 2.1. Modulus of elasticity

MATERIAL	E ($\times 10^6$ psi)	MATERIAL	E ($\times 10^6$ psi)
Steel	30	Magnesium	6.5
Carbon composite	18.5	Bone	2.85
Copper	16	Polyester–Dacron	2
Brass	15	Polyester (4110)	0.65
Bronze	12	Surlyn	0.34
Aluminum	10.3	Polypropylene	0.23
Kevlar	9	HD polypropylene	0.113
Glass	8.4	LD polypropylene	0.018

tion in area. The first two are strength parameters; the last two indicate ductility.

The general shape of the stress-strain curve (see Fig. 2.12) requires further explanation. In the region from *a* to *b*, the stress is linearly proportional to strain and the strain is elastic (i.e., the stressed part returns to its original shape when the load is removed). When the applied stress exceeds the yield strength, *b*, the specimen undergoes plastic deformation. If the load is subsequently reduced to zero, the part remains permanently deformed. The stress required to produce continued plastic deformation increases with increasing plastic strain (points *c*, *d*, and *e* on Fig. 2.12), that is, the metal strain hardens. The volume of the part remains constant during plastic deformation, and as the part elongates, its cross-sectional area decreases uniformly along its length until point *e* is reached. The ordinate of point *e* is the tensile strength of the material. After point *e*, further elongation requires less applied stress until the part ruptures at point *f* (breaking or fracture strength).

Stress-strain diagrams assume widely differing forms for various materials. Figure 2.13, *a*, is the stress-strain diagram for a medium-carbon structural steel. The ordinates of points *p*, *u*, and *b* are the yield point, tensile strength, and breaking strength. The lower curve of Figure 2.13, *b*, is for an alloy steel, the higher curve for hard steels. For nonferrous alloys and cast iron the diagram has the form indicated in Figure 2.13, *c*,

while the plot of Figure 2.13, *d*, is typical for rubber.

For any material having a stress-strain curve of the form shown in Figure 2.13, *a* to *d*, it is evident that the relation between stress and strain is linear for comparatively small values of the strain. This linear relationship between elongation and the axial force causing it was first reported by Sir Robert Hooke in 1678 and is called *Hooke's law*. Expressed as an equation, Hooke's law becomes

$$\sigma = \epsilon E \qquad (3)$$

where

σ = stress, psi,

ϵ = strain, inch/inch, and

E = constant of proportionality between stress and strain. This constant is also called *Young's modulus* or the *modulus of elasticity*.

The slope of the stress-strain curve from the origin to point *p* (see Fig. 2.13, *a* and *b*) is the modulus of elasticity of that particular material, *E*. This region where the slope is a straight line is called the *elastic region*. The ordinate of a point coincident with *p* is known as the *elastic limit* (i.e., the maximum stress that may be developed during a simple tension test such that there is no permanent or residual deformation when the load is entirely removed). Values for *E* are shown in Table 2.1.

In a routine tension test (Fig. 2.14), which illustrates

Hooke's law, a bar of area A is placed between two jaws of a vise and a force F is applied to compress the bar. Combining Eqs 1, 2, and 3 and solving for the shortening, ΔL, gives

$$\Delta L = \frac{FL_0}{AE} \qquad (4)$$

Because the original length L_0, cross-sectional area A, and modulus of elasticity E are constants, the shortening ΔL depends solely on F. As F doubles, so does ΔL.

The operation of a steel spring scale is another practical illustration of Hooke's law (Fig. 2.15). The amount of deflection of the spring for every pound of force of the load remains constant. In Figure 2.15, a, the scale indicates 3 units (pounds, ounces, grams). With

one weight added (Fig. 2.15, b), the scale indicates 5, or 2 additional units. A second weight added (Fig. 2.15, c) causes the scale to indicate 7, or a total of 4 additional units, and a third weight stretches the spring 2 more units (Fig. 2.15, d). Therefore, it is possible to make uniform gradations for every unit of force to the point beyond the range of elasticity where the spring would distort or break. Scales are manufactured with springs strong enough to bear certain predetermined maximum loads. A compression spring scale designed to remain within the elastic range, recording weights to about 250 lb and then returning back to 0, is the common type used for weighing people.

Plastic range. Plastic range is beyond the elastic range (b to past e on the stress-strain diagram of Fig. 2.12), and the material behaves plastically. That is, the material has a set or permanent deformation when externally applied loads are removed—it has "flowed" or become plastic. In the case of the steel spring scale, if the weight did not actually break the spring, it would stretch it permanently so that the readings on the scale would be no longer accurate. Some steels in the plastic range behave just like taffy being stretched.

For most materials, the stress-strain curve has an initial linear elastic region in which deformation is reversible. Note the load σ_2 in Figure 2.16. This load will cause strain ϵ_E; when the load is removed the strain disappears (i.e., point X (σ_2, ϵ_E) moves linearly down the proportional portion of the curve to the origin). Similarly, when load σ_1 is applied, strain ϵ_T results. When load σ_1 is removed, however, point Y does not move back along the original curve to the origin but moves to the strain axis along a line parallel to the original linear region intersecting the strain axis at ϵ_P. Therefore, with no load, the material has a residual or permanent strain of ϵ_P. This quantity, ϵ_P,

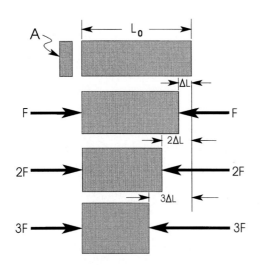

Fig. 2.14. Linearity.

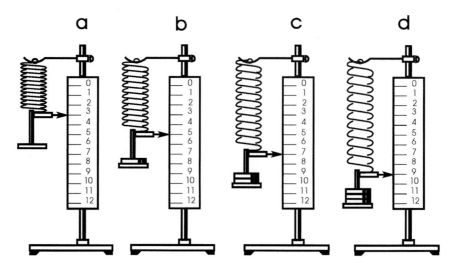

Fig. 2.15. Linear relationship between stretch and weight.

is the plastic strain and $(\epsilon_T - \epsilon_P)$ is the elastic strain, ϵ_E, or:

$$\epsilon_T - \epsilon_P = \epsilon_E \qquad (5)$$

where

ϵ_T = total strain under load,

ϵ_P = plastic (or permanent) strain, and

ϵ_E = elastic strain.

Yield point. Yield point (point *b* on the stress-strain diagram of Fig. 2.12) refers to that point at which a marked increase in strain occurs without a corresponding increase in stress. The horizontal portion of the stress-strain curve (*b-c-d*, Fig. 2.12) indicates the yield stress corresponding to this yield point. The yield point is the "knee" in the stress-strain curve for a material and separates the elastic from the plastic portions of the curve.

Tensile strength. The tensile strength of a material is obtained by dividing the maximum tensile force reached during the test (*e* on the stress-strain diagram of Fig. 2.12) by the original cross-sectional area of the test specimen.

Toughness and ductility. The area under the curve to the point of maximum stress (*a-b-c-d-e* on diagram of Fig. 2.12) indicates the *toughness* of the material, or its ability to withstand shock loads before rupturing. The supporting arms of a car bumper are an example of when toughness is of great value as a

mechanical property. *Ductility* is the ability of a material to sustain large permanent deformations in tension, as drawing a rod into a wire. The distinction between ductility and toughness is that ductility deals only with the ability to deform, whereas toughness considers both the ability to deform and the stress developed during the deformation.

Thermal stress

When a material is subjected to a change in temperature, its dimensions increase or decrease as the temperature rises or falls. If the material is constrained by neighboring structures, stress is produced.

The influence of temperature change is noted through the medium of the coefficient of thermal expansion (α), which is defined as the unit strain produced by a temperature change of one degree. This physical constant is a mechanical property of each material, and values of α for several materials are given in Table 2.2.

If the temperature of a bar of length L_0 inches is increased ΔT degrees Fahrenheit, the elongation in inches, ΔL, of the unrestrained bar is given by

$$\Delta L = \alpha L_0 \Delta T \qquad (6)$$

If the heated rod is compressed back to its original length, then it will be experiencing compression given by Eq 4:

$$\Delta L = \frac{F L_0}{AE} \qquad (7)$$

Combining Eqs 6 and 7 and solving for stress, $\sigma = F/A$, gives

$$\sigma = \alpha \Delta T E \qquad (8)$$

Equation 8 allows the calculation of stress in a rod as a function of the increase in temperature ΔT, the modulus of elasticity E (Table 2.1), and the coefficient of thermal expansion α (Table 2.2). The concept of change in dimension as the result of temperature rise is illustrated in Example 1 in Appendix A.

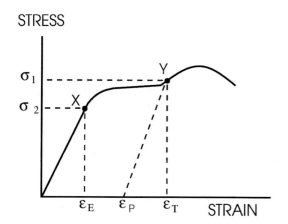

Fig. 2.16. Plastic strain.

MATERIAL	COEFFICIENT, α ($\times 10^{-6}$ in./in.-°F)	MATERIAL	COEFFICIENT, α ($\times 10^{-6}$ in./in.-°F)
Steel	6.5	Brass	10.4
Cast iron	6.0	Bronze	10.0
Wrought iron	6.7	Aluminum	12.5
Copper	9.3	Magnesium	14.5

Table 2.2. Coefficient of thermal expansion

Centroids and center of gravity

The centroid and center of gravity of objects play an important role in their mechanical properties. The center of gravity and centroid of two identically shaped objects are the same if the density is uniform in each object. The centroid is a geometrical factor and center of gravity depends on mass.

For an object of uniform density, the term *center of gravity* is replaced by the *centroid of the area*. The centroid of an area is defined as the point of application of the resultant of a uniformly distributed force acting on the area. An irregularly shaped plate of material of uniform thickness *(t)* is shown in Figure 2.17. Two elemental areas (*a* and *b*) are shown with centroids $(\bar{x}_1, \bar{y}_1)$ and $(\bar{x}_2, \bar{y}_2)$, respectively. If the large, irregularly shaped plate is divided into small elemental areas, each having its own centroid, then the centroid for the irregularly shaped plate is $(\bar{x}, \bar{y})$, where

$$\bar{x} = \Sigma_i \frac{\bar{x}_i a_i}{A}$$

$$\bar{y} = \Sigma_i \frac{\bar{y}_i a_i}{A}$$

and

$$\bar{x} = \frac{\bar{x}_1 a_1 + \bar{x}_2 a_2 + \cdots}{A}$$

$$\bar{y} = \frac{\bar{y}_1 a_1 + \bar{y}_2 a_2 + \cdots}{A}$$

The *y*-centroids for several common geometrical shapes are given in Table 2.3. The general equations for the *x*- and *y*-components of the centroid are shown in Example 2 in Appendix A.

Moment of inertia

The moment of inertia of a finite area about an axis in the plane of the area is given by the summation of the moments of inertia about the same axis of all elements of the area contained in the finite area. In general, the moment of inertia is defined as the product of the area and the square of the distance between the area and the given axis. The moments of inertia about the centroidal axes, I_{cc}, of a few simple but important geometrical shapes are determined by integral calculus and are given in Table 2.3.

Parallel axis theorem. When the moment of inertia has been determined with respect to a given axis, such as the centroidal axis above, the moment of

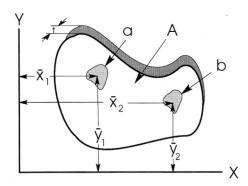

Fig. 2.17. Centroids.

Table 2.3.	Geometric factors for common shapes			
	RECTANGLE	**TRIANGLE**	**CIRCLE**	**SEMICIRCLE**
$\bar{y}_c$	$h/2$	$h/3$	r	$0.425r$
I_{cc}	$bh^3/12$	$bh^3/36$	$0.785r^4$	$0.11r^4$
I_{xx}	$bh^3/3$	$bh^3/12$	$3.93r^4$	$0.393r^4$
Z	$bh^2/6$	$bh^3/24$	$0.785r^3$	$0.19r^3$
c	$h/2$	$2h/3$ (top)	r	$0.575r$ (top)
		$h/3$ (bottom)		$0.425r$ (bottom)

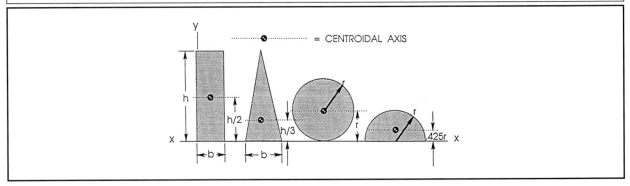

inertia with respect to a parallel axis can be obtained by means of the *parallel axis theorem*, provided that one of the axes passes through the centroid of the area. The parallel axis theorem states that *the moment of inertia with respect to any axis is equal to the moment of inertia with respect to a parallel axis through the centroid added to the product of the area and the square of the distance between the two axes* (Fig. 2.18):

$$I_{xx} = I_{cc} + Ad^2 \qquad \text{or} \qquad I_{cc} = I_{xx} - Ad^2 \qquad (9)$$

where

I_{xx} = moment of inertia about x-axis,
I_{cc} = moment of inertia about centroid,
A = area, and
d = distance between axes.

An illustration of the moment of inertia concept using the parallel axis theorem is given in Example 3 in Appendix A.

Stresses in beams

If forces are applied to a beam as shown in Figure 2.19, downward bending of the beam occurs. It is convenient to imagine a beam to be composed of an infinite number of thin longitudinal rods or fibers. Each longitudinal fiber is assumed to act independently of every other fiber (i.e., there are no lateral stresses [shear] between fibers). The beam of Figure 2.19 will deflect downward and the fibers in the lower part of the beam undergo extension, whereas those in the upper part are shortened. These changes in the lengths of the fibers set up stresses in the fibers. Those that are extended have tensile stresses acting on the fibers in the direction of the longitudinal axis of the beam, whereas those that are shortened are subject to compression stresses.

There always exists one surface in the beams that contains fibers that do not undergo any extension or compression, and thus are not subject to any tensile or compressive stress. This surface is called the *neutral surface* of the beam. The intersection of the neutral surface with any cross section of the beam perpendicular to its longitudinal axis is called the *neutral axis*. All fibers on one side of the neutral axis are in a state of tension, whereas those on the opposite side are in compression.

For any beam having a longitudinal plane of symmetry and subject to a bending torque T at a certain cross section, the normal stress σ, acting on a longitudinal fiber at a distance y from the neutral axis of the beam (see Fig. 2.20), is given by

$$\sigma = \frac{Ty}{I} \qquad (10)$$

where I = moment of inertia of the cross-sectional area about the neutral or centroidal axis in inches[4].

These stresses vary from zero at the neutral axis of the beam ($y = 0$) to a maximum at the outer fibers (Fig. 2.20). These stresses are called *bending*, *flexure*, or *fiber stresses*.

Section modulus. The value of y at the outer fibers of the beam is frequently denoted by c. At these fibers, the bending stress is a maximum and is given by

$$\sigma = \frac{Tc}{I} = \frac{T}{I/c} \qquad (11)$$

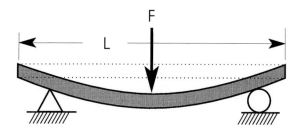

Fig. 2.19. Beam stress.

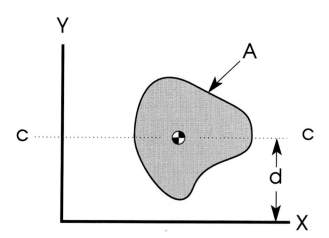

Fig. 2.18. Parallel axis theorem.

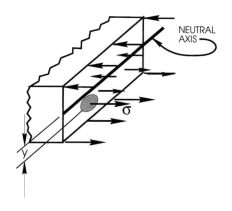

Fig. 2.20. Neutral axis (zero stress).

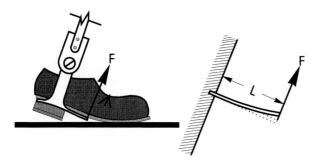

Fig. 2.21.   Free body diagram of cantilevered beam.

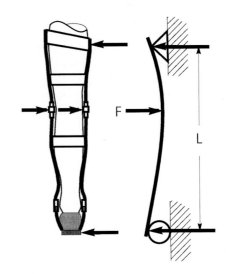

Fig. 2.22.   Free body diagram of freely supported beam.

The ratio I/c is called the *section modulus* and is usually denoted by the symbol Z. The section modulus for the shapes shown in Table 2.3 are obtained by dividing the moment of inertia about the centroidal axis by the length of the centroid. For example, the moment of inertia for a rectangle about its centroidal axis is $bh^3/12$ and the length of the centroid is $h/2$; therefore, the section modulus is $bh^2/6$. Section moduli are shown in Table 2.3.

Beam torque. Most structural elements in orthoses can be represented by either a cantilever beam loaded transversely with a perpendicular force at the end (such as a stirrup in terminal stance; Fig. 2.21) or by a beam freely supported at the ends and centrally loaded (such as a KAFO prescribed to control valgum; Fig. 2.22).

The maximum *torque* in cantilevered (see Fig. 2.21) and freely supported (see Fig. 2.22) *beams* is given by

$$T_{\max} = FL \tag{12}$$

$$T_{\max} = \frac{FL}{4} \tag{13}$$

Figure 2.23 gives the maximum torque for a few simple beams. If more than one external force acts on a beam, the bending torque is the sum of the torques caused by all the external forces acting on either side of the beam.

Beam stress.   The *stress* in a cantilevered or freely supported *beam* can now be determined by substituting Eqs 12 or 13 into Eq 11, which gives

$$\sigma = \frac{FLc}{I} \quad \text{(cantilevered beam)} \tag{14}$$

and

$$\sigma = \frac{FLc}{4I} \quad \text{(freely supported beam)} \tag{15}$$

If the aforementioned beams have rectangular cross sections with height h and base b (i.e., $c = h/2$ and

$I = bh^3/12$), then the expressions for stress can be rewritten as

$$\sigma = \frac{6FL}{bh^2} \quad \text{(cantilevered beam)} \tag{16}$$

and

$$\sigma = \frac{3FL}{2bh^2} \quad \text{(freely supported beam)} \tag{17}$$

As the cross-sectional area of the beam changes shape, so does the expression for the moment of inertia *(I)* and the outer fiber-to-neutral axis distance *(c)*.

Beam deflection. The maximum *deflection* of *beams* (sidebars, stirrups) is important to practitioners because the biomechanical objective of prescribed devices frequently depends on either the ability of a device to not deflect or to deflect a given amount. Excessive deflection (bending) of a device may either disturb alignment or prevent successful operation.

Deflection theory provides a technique of analysis for evaluating the nature and magnitude of deformations in beams. The cantilevered beam (Fig. 2.24) carries a concentrated downward load F at the free end. A cantilevered beam is, by definition, rigidly supported at the other end. The general expression for the downward deflection *(y)*, anywhere along the length (*x*-axis) of the beam is given by

$$y(x) = -\frac{Fx^3}{6EI} + \frac{FxL^2}{2EI} - \frac{FL^3}{3EI} \tag{18}$$

The maximum deflection of the cantilevered beam $(y_{\max})$ occurs at the free end when $x = 0$:

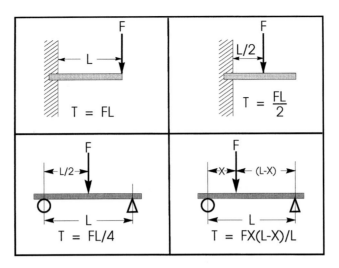

Fig. 2.23. Maximum bending torques of common beams.

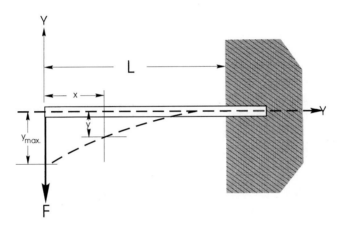

Fig. 2.24. Cantilevered beam.

$$y_{max} = -\frac{FL^3}{3EI} \qquad (19)$$

The general expression for the deflection of the freely supported beam with the midspan load (Fig. 2.25) is given by

$$y(x) = \frac{Fx^3}{12EI} - \frac{FxL^2}{16EI} \qquad (20)$$

The maximum deflection of the freely supported beam (y_{max}) occurs at the midspan when $x = L/2$:

$$y_{max} = -\frac{FL^3}{48EI} \qquad (21)$$

The negative sign in Eqs 19 and 21 indicates that this maximum deflection is downward from the unloaded position. Example 4 in Appendix A provides an illustration of calculating KAFO stress and deflection using the concepts of moment of inertia and centroid.

METALS

A *metal* is defined as a chemical element that is lustrous, hard, malleable, heavy, ductile, and tenacious and is usually a good conductor of heat and electricity. Of the 93 elements, 73 are classified as metals. The elements oxygen; chlorine; iodine; bromine; hydrogen; and the inert gases (helium, neon, argon, krypton, xenon, and radon) are considered nonmetallic. There is, however, a group of elements, such as carbon, sulfur, silicon, and phosphorus, that is intermediate between the metals and nonmetals. These elements portray under certain circumstances the characteristics of metals and, under other circumstances, the characteristics of nonmetals. They are referred to as *metalloids*.

The most widely used metallic elements include iron, copper, lead, zinc, aluminum, tin, nickel, and magnesium. Some of these are used extensively in the pure state, but by far the largest amount is used in the form of alloys. An *alloy* is a combination of elements that exhibits the properties of a metal. The properties of alloys differ appreciably from those of the constituent elements, and improvement of strength, ductility, hardness, wear resistance, and corrosion resistance may be obtained in an alloy by combinations of various elements.

Crystallinity

One of the important characteristics of all metals is their crystallinity. A *crystalline substance* is one in which the atoms are arranged in definite and repeating order in a three-dimensional pattern. This regular arrangement of atoms is called a *space-lattice*. Space-lattices are characteristic of all crystalline materials. Most metals crystallize in one of three types of space-lattices:

- *Cubic system*—three contiguous edges of equal length and at right angles—simple lattice, body-centered lattice, and face-centered lattice (Fig. 2.26).

- *Tetragonal system*—three contiguous edges, two of equal length, all at right angles—simple lattice and body-centered lattice (Fig. 2.27).
- *Hexagonal system*—three parallel sets of equal length horizontal axes at 120E and a vertical axis—close-packed hexagonal (Fig. 2.28).

This orderly state is also described as balanced, unstrained, or annealed. Some metals can exist in several lattice forms, depending on the temperature. Examples of metals that normally exist in only one form are:

- *Face-centered cubic:* Ca, Ni, Cu, Ag, Au, Pb, Al
- *Body-centered cubic:* Li, Na, K, V, W
- *Face-centered tetragonal:* In
- *Close-packed hexagonal:* Be, Mg, Zn, Cd

Common iron is an example of one of many metals that may exist in more than one lattice form:

- *Body-centered cubic:* Below 1663EF

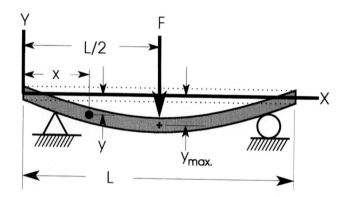

Fig. 2.25.   Freely supported beam.

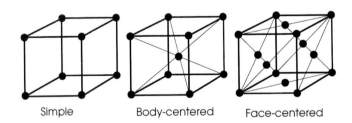

Simple   Body-centered   Face-centered

Fig. 2.26.   Space lattices for cubes.

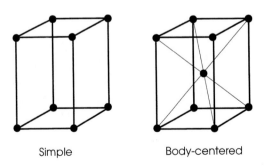

Simple   Body-centered

Fig. 2.27.   Space lattices for tetragonals.

- *Face-centered cubic:* 1663EF to 2557EF
- *Body-centered cubic:* 2557EF to 2795EF

A metal in the liquid state is noncrystalline, and the atoms move freely among one another without regard to interspatial distances. The internal energy that these atoms possess prevents them from approaching one another closely enough to come under the control of their attractive electrostatic fields. As the liquid cools, however, and loses energy, the atoms move more sluggishly. At a certain temperature, for a particular pure metal, certain atoms are arranged in the proper position

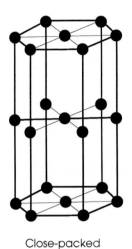

Close-packed

Fig. 2.28. Space lattice for a hexagon.

to form a single lattice typical of metal. The temperature at which atoms begin to arrange themselves in a regular geometrical pattern (lattice) is called the *freezing point.* As heat is removed from metal, crystallization continues, and the lattices grow about each center. This growth continues at the expense of the liquid, with the lattice structure expanding in all directions until development is stopped by interference with other space-lattices or with the walls of the container. If a space-lattice is permitted to grow freely without interference, a single crystal is produced that has an external shape typical of the system in which it crystallizes.

Crystallization centers form at random throughout the liquid mass by the aggregation of a proper number of atoms to form a space-lattice. Each of these centers of crystallization enlarges as more atoms are added, until interference is encountered. A diagrammatic representation of the process of solidification is shown in Figure 2.29. In this diagram, the squares represent space-lattices. In *a*, crystallization has begun at four centers.

As crystallization continues, more centers appear and develop with space-lattices of random orientation. Successive stages in the crystallization are shown by *b, c, d, e,* and *f.* Small crystals join large ones, provided that they have about the same orientation (i.e., their axes are nearly aligned). During the last stages of formation, crystals meet, and there are places at the surface of intersections where it is impossible for another space-lattice to develop. Such interference accounts for the

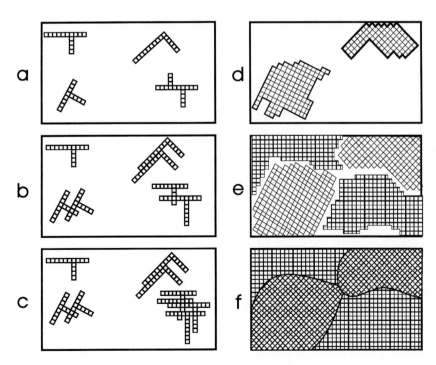

Fig. 2.29.   Stages in the process of solidification of metals.

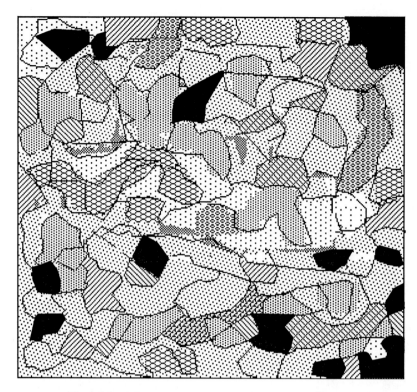

Fig. 2.30.   Microscopic schematic of iron grain structure.

irregular appearance of crystals in a piece of metal when polished and etched (Fig. 2.30).

Grain structure

If, during the growth process, the development of external features, such as regular faces, is prevented by interference from the growth of other centers, each unit is called a *grain* rather than a crystal. The term *crystal* is usually applied to a group of space-lattices of the same orientation that show symmetry by the development of regular faces. Each grain is essentially a single crystal. The size of the grain depends on the temperature from which the metal is cast, the cooling rate, and the nature of the metal. In general, however, slow cooling leads to coarse grain and rapid cooling to fine grain metals.

Slip planes

When a force is applied to a crystal, the space-lattice is distorted as evidenced by a change in dimension of the crystal. This distortion causes some of the atoms in the lattice to be closer together and others to be farther apart. The magnitude of the applied force necessary to cause the distortion depends on the forces that act between the atoms in the lattice and tends to restore it to its normal configuration. If the applied force is removed, the atomic forces return the atoms to their normal positions in the lattice. Cubic patterns (lattices) characterize the more ductile or workable materials. Hexagonal and more complex patterns tend to be more brittle or more rigid. The force required to bring about the first permanent displacement corresponds to the elastic limit. This permanent displacement, or slip, occurs in the lattice on certain specified planes called *slip planes*. The ability of a crystal to slip in this manner without separation is the criterion of plasticity. Practically all metals are plastic to a certain degree. During plastic deformations, the lattice undergoes distortion, thus becoming highly stressed and hardened.

There are certain planes with a space-lattice along which this slip, or plastic deformation, can take place more easily than along others. Those planes that have the greatest population of atoms and, likewise, have the greatest separation of atoms on each side of the planes under consideration are usually the ones of easiest slip. Therefore, slip takes place along these planes first when the elastic limit is exceeded. Sliding movements tend to take place at 45° angles to the direction of the applied load because much higher stresses are required to pull atoms directly apart or to push them straight together.

A particular characteristic of crystalline materials is that slip is not necessarily confined to one set of planes during the process of deformation. Some of the com-

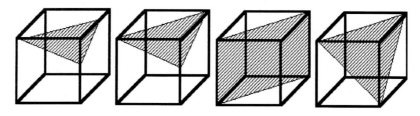

Fig. 2.31. Typical planes of slip in a cubic lattice.

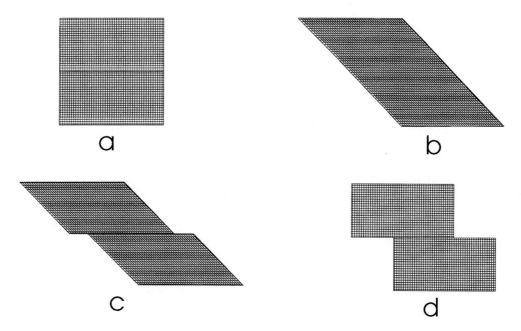

Fig. 2.32. Deformation of a cubic crystal lattice. *a*, unstrained condition. *b*, elastic deformation. *c*, plastic deformation. *d*, permanent set as a result of slip.

mon planes of slip in the simple cubic system are shown in Figure 2.31.

Mechanical properties

The mechanical properties of metals depend on their lattice structures. In general, metals that exist with the face-centered cubic structure are ductile throughout a wide range of temperatures. Those metals that are of the close-packed hexagonal type of lattice (see Fig. 2.28) are appreciably hardened by cold working, and plastic deformation takes place most easily on planes parallel to the base of the lattice.

Of the many qualities of metals, the most significant are the related properties of elasticity and plasticity. Plasticity depends on the ability to shape and contour aluminum and stainless steel to match body contours; elasticity governs their safe and economical use as load-bearing members.

As discussed in the section on Strength and Stress, a body is said to be *elastic* if, after change in shape when externally loaded, it returns to its original shape with removal of the load. The *elastic limit* is the maximum

stress at which the body behaves elastically. The *proportional limit* is the stress at which strain ceases to be proportional to applied stress; it is practically equal to elastic limit.

Plasticity

Plasticity is the term used to express a metal's ability to be deformed beyond the range of elasticity without fracture, resulting in permanent change in shape. Characteristically the ratio of plastic-to-elastic deformation in metals is high, of the order of 100:1 or 1000:1.

A simple two-dimensional representation of a cubic crystal lattice in an unstrained condition is represented by *a* in Figure 2.32. If a shearing force is applied that is within the elastic range, the lattice is uniformly distorted as in *b*, the extent of the distortion being proportional to the applied force.

When the force is removed, the lattice springs back to its original shape *(a)*. When the force exceeds the elastic (or proportional) limit, however, a sudden change in the mode of deformation occurs; without further increase in the amount of elastic strain, the lattice shears along a crystallographic plane (or slip plane); one block of the lattice makes a long glide past the other and stops *(c)*. On release of load, the lattice in the two displaced blocks resumes its original shape *(d)*. If the applied force is continued, slip does not continue indefinitely along the original slip plane, which on the contrary appears to acquire resistance to further motion, but some parallel plane comes into action. Both the extent of slip per plane and the distance between active slip planes are large in comparison to the unit lattice dimensions. As slip shifts from one slip plane to another, progressively higher forces are required to accomplish it (i.e., the metal has been *work hardened*). At some stage, resistance to further slip along the primitive set of planes exceeds the resistance offered by some other set of differently directed slip planes, which then come into action. This process elaborates as plastic deformation progresses.

The actual strength of metals as ordinarily measured is but a small fraction of their theoretical strength. For pure copper, some significant comparisons are these:

- *Calculated (theoretical) tensile strength* = 1,300,000 psi.
- *Measured breaking strength* = 62,000 psi.

Similar relations exist for other pure metals.

Imperfections of many kinds may serve to localize and intensify stresses, such as flaws in the regularity of the crystal lattice, microcracks within a grain, shrinkage voids, nonmetallic inclusions, rough surfaces, and notches of all kinds. Many impurities owe their potency to a high degree of insolubility in the solid matrix coupled with high solubility in the fusion. This permits their freezing out relatively late in the solidification process, as concentrates or films between the grains, thus serving as effective internal notches. The great weakening effect of the graphite flakes in cast iron is an example.

Notches act not only as stress raisers but also as stress complicators and frequently induce stress in many directions. The deeper the notch and the sharper its root, the more effective it is in this respect. Notches are great weakeners, and practitioners do well to recognize their prevalence under many disguises (i.e., from either contouring instruments or grain boundaries).

STEEL AND ALUMINUM ALLOYS

Commercial name for metals

Before using the stress-strain diagram as a basis for comparing the properties of various metals, it is first necessary to discuss the types of steel and aluminum commercially available and used in orthotic and prosthetic applications.

The terms *surgical steel, stainless steel, tool steel*, and *heat treated* along with other general designations are freely used by manufacturers of orthotic and prosthetic components. It is misleading to think that the chemical content of these products is identical from vendor to vendor. The term *spring steel*, for example, used by many manufacturers, refers to a group of steels ranging in chemical composition from medium to high carbon steel and is used to designate some alloy steels. The term *tool steel* also covers a wide variety of steels that are capable of attaining a high degree of hardness after heat treatment. More care is exercised in manufacturing tool steel to insure maximum uniformity of desirable properties.

These general designations do not assure the orthotist or prosthetist of obtaining the exact material that he needs. Because the mechanical properties of a material and subsequent fabrication procedures depend on its chemical analysis and subsequent heat treatment or working, the practice of using general descriptions for metals is seriously inadequate. It is also unnecessary to rely on these categories because there already exist specific designations for each type of steel and processing treatment. The following sections give a clearer picture of the available steel and aluminum alloys and their specific properties.

Carbon steel

Iron as a pure metal does not possess sufficient strength or hardness to be useful for many applications. By adding as little as a fraction of 1% carbon by weight, however, the properties of the base metal are significantly altered. Iron with added carbon is called *carbon steel*. Within certain limits, strength and hardness of carbon steel is directly proportionate to the amount of carbon added. In addition to carbon, carbon steel contains manganese and traces of sulfur and phosphorus.

Alloy steel

To achieve desirable physical or chemical properties, other chemicals are added to carbon steel. The resultant product is known as *alloy steel*. In presenting some of the general characteristics distinguishing these alloys, it is necessary to define some of the terms commonly used to express them:

- *Toughness*—the ability to withstand shock force
- *Hardness*—the resistance to penetration and abrasion
- *Ductility*—the ability to undergo permanent changes of shape without rupturing
- *Corrosion resistance*—the resistance to chemical attack of a metal under the influence of a moist atmosphere

The addition of elements can also increase elasticity and tensile strength as well as improve surface finish and machinability.

Characteristics of specified alloys. Using some of these definitions, the important characteristics distinguishing some alloy steels are as follows. Nickel steels are characterized by improved toughness, simplified heat treating, less distortion in quenching, and improved corrosion resistance. Nickel chromium steels exhibit increased depth hardenability and improved abrasion resistance. Molybdenum steels rank with manganese and chromium as having the greatest hardenability, increased high temperature strength, and increased corrosion resistance. Chromium steels have increased hardening effect. (It is possible to decrease the amount of carbon content and obtain a steel with both high strength and satisfactory ductility.) Vanadium steels have increased refinement of the internal structure of the alloy, making them suitable for spring steels and construction steels. Silicon manganese steels possess increased strength and hardness. Double and triple alloys are a combination of two or more of these alloys and produce a steel having some of the characteristic properties of each. For example, chromium molybdenum steels have excellent hardenability and satisfactory ductility. Chromium nickel steels have good hardenability and satisfactory ductility. The effect of combining three alloys produces a material superior in quality to the sum of each alloy used separately.

Stainless steels. Steel alloys containing a large amount of chromium (> 3.99%) are called stainless steels. The American Iron and Steel Institute (AISI) uses a three-digit system to identify each type of stainless steel. The various grades are separated into three general categories according to their metallurgical structure and properties. These categories are austenitic, martinsitic, and ferritic.

Each category has special heat treatment and cold working properties. For example, the well-known "18-8" stainless steel used in orthopedic instruments are austenitic steels containing 18% chromium and 8% nickel. These chromium nickel stainless steels cannot be hardened by heat treatment and attain mechanical properties higher than the annealed (heat-treated) condition by cold working. Cold working refers to plastic deformation of a metal at temperatures that substantially increase its strength and hardness.

The tensile strength of the austenitic steel in the softened or annealed condition is more than that of mild steel. By cold working, ultimate strengths of 250,000 psi can be achieved. Because these steels rapidly work harden, it is necessary to use sharp drills and tools to work them quickly before they get too hard. These steels have the highest corrosion resistance of the stainless steel family.

Martinsitic stainless steel is the only category of the three subject to heat treatment. Ferritic stainless steel is nonhardenable by heat treatment and only slightly hardenable by cold working.

SAE number

The Society of Automotive Engineers has assigned a specific number known as an SAE number to identify each steel according to its chemical analysis. There is an equivalent American Iron and Steel Institute (AISI) number, but for simplicity one means of identification is sufficient. Four digits are used in the SAE description as follows.

Digit one refers to the type of steel. Digit two refers to the approximate percentage of the predominating alloy element in a simple alloy steel. Digits three and four refer to the approximate percentage of carbon by weight in 1/100 of a percent.

List of digit one is as follows:

    1XXX = carbon steel
    2XXX = nickel steel
    3XXX = nickel chromium
    4XXX = chromium molybdenum (cro-moly)
    5XXX = chromium
    6XXX = chromium vanadium
    7XXX = heat-resistant alloy steel castings
    8XXX = nickel cro-moly
    9XXX = silicon manganese

For example, SAE 1020 would be carbon steel (first digit 1) with no added element, (second digit 0) and with 0.20% carbon (third and fourth digits 20). SAE 4012, using the same method, would be chromium molybdenum steel with 0.12% carbon content. SAE 4130 identifies cro-moly steel with 1% chromium and 0.30% carbon. This is an airplane part alloy used in orthoses.

Comparison of steel and aluminum

Stress-strain diagram. Figure 2.33 is a comparative stress-stain diagram plotting one type of steel and one type of soft aluminum. The straight-line portion of both curves on the diagram indicates the elastic range and stiffness of the material. The dotted lines on the diagram indicate the increased stresses that the material can tolerate before reaching the yield and ultimate stress phase as the strength of the material is increased. In the case of steel, the modulus of elasticity is 30 million pounds per square inch. For aluminum it is 10 million pounds per square inch, one third that of steel.

Size, weight, and strength comparisons. Although for an equal amount of stress, steel strains (deflects) one third as much as aluminum (shown by ϵ and 3ϵ in Fig. 2.33), aluminum weighs only approximately one third as much as steel. This means that if a rectangular cross section of steel undergoing bending stresses is duplicated in aluminum, then to achieve the same stiffness (resistance to bending) one dimension

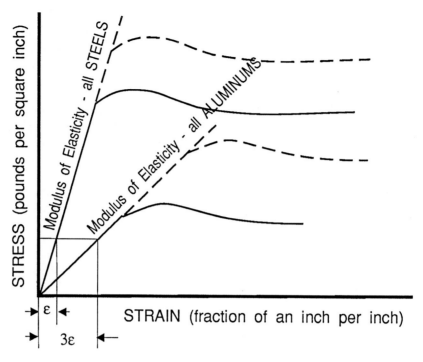

Fig. 2.33.   Comparative stress-strain diagram.

of the aluminum rectangle must be increased by 70%.

It is obvious that an aluminum orthosis must be made 70% larger in one dimension to be as rigid in this direction as a steel orthosis of the same general shape. Although bulkier, it is only 60% of the weight of the steel orthosis.

Aluminum has the advantage of being not only lighter in weight, but also easier to work with than steel. Where bulkiness is not critical, it is possible to construct an aluminum device just as rigid as steel and yet lighter in weight. However, the aluminum device is more subject to fatigue failure than steel.

STRENGTHENING ALUMINUM AND STEEL

Although the yield stress and ultimate stress of the aluminum alloy shown in Figure 2.33 is below that of the steel, all aluminums are not weaker than all steels. By the addition of certain alloying elements, proper heat treatment, or cold working, certain aluminums can be increased in strength to an ultimate stress tolerance of 90,000 lb per square inch (7178-T6), which is above the strength of some steels. However, the aluminum will still be more subject to fatigue failure than the steel. It is also possible to increase the strength of steel by similar processes. This section describes and discusses some of these methods.

Heat treatment

Purposes.   Chemical analysis of a metal indicates only its potential properties. Alloy steels from the rolling mills, for example, are still in a semiprocessed condition, and their mechanical properties are not realized until after heat treatment. Heat treatment can accomplish many purposes: increase or decrease hardness and tensile strength, relieve internal stresses because of hot or cold working, improve machinability, and increase toughness.

Techniques.   All of these qualities are desirable at different times and for different applications. They are achieved by varying techniques in the heat treatment processes as follows:

- If steel is heated above its critical temperature range, it undergoes definite internal changes.
- If the steel is slowly cooled from this elevated temperature, the internal changes have time to reverse themselves.
- If the steel is cooled more rapidly than the internal changes can reverse themselves, the structure of the steel is modified and its mechanical characteristics are altered.

Example.   A specimen of carbon steel (carbon content = 0.30%) is composed of microscopic grains of ferrite and pearlite. Ferrite is almost pure iron. Pearlite looks like mother-of-pearl and is composed of alternate layers of ferrite and cementite, which is an iron carbide or hard chemical combination of iron and carbon.

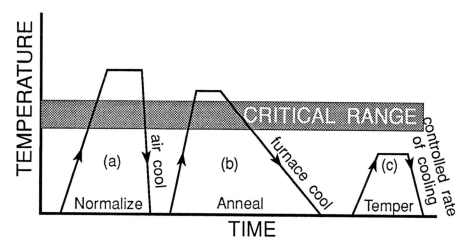

Fig. 2.34. Heat treat cycle.

As the steel is heated through its critical range, a transformation occurs. The iron changes its form and can no longer remain chemically combined with the carbon. The hard carbides are broken up and the carbon goes into solution in the iron. This is called a *solid solution* because the material is in a solid state (i.e., it is not molten). This material is now *austenite*.

When the steel is quenched, that is, rapidly cooled from above its critical range, the austenite does not have sufficient time to transform to ferrite and pearlite. Instead, *martinsite*, another iron carbide that is hard and brittle, is formed. If additional alloying elements are added, the formation of the martinsite is affected, and the resultant properties are changed.

Heat-treat cycle. To reduce residual stresses formed as a result of cold working or heating and cooling that were not uniform, two similar processes are used that achieve somewhat different results. The material is either *normalized* or *annealed*.

Normalizing the steel returns it to its original or normal internal structure. The metal is heated above its critical range (Fig. 2.34, *a*), which is slightly higher than in the annealing process, and then is cooled in air. A piece of normalized steel has higher strength and hardness but less ductility than the same piece of steel annealed.

Annealing the steel (Fig. 2.34, *b*) relieves internal stresses and lowers the yield point to obtain maximum ductility. As a result of this, the metal can be plastically deformed with minimum force. The steel is heated to a temperature above the critical range. Then it is slowly cooled in the furnace.

Tempering or drawing (Fig. 2.34, *c*) usually follows quenching. Steel that has been heat treated is fully hardened and is too brittle and hard for most applications. To make it softer, more ductile, and tougher, it is tempered. That means it is heated again to a point

below the critical range and then cooled at a controlled rate. The higher the temperature during the tempering process, the lower the strength and hardness are and the higher the ductility.

Heat treatment influencing shop practices

The mechanical properties of the metal are influenced by the rate of heating, the heat treatment temperature, the time held at this temperature, the atmosphere surrounding the work, and the rate of cooling. Obviously, this is a critical process and requires special skills and equipment. For this reason, it is usually done by the manufacturer. Improper shop practices influencing any of the above-mentioned conditions can nullify the desired results of the heat treatment and produce a substandard metal.

Most fabrication techniques call for as little heat as possible to be used on heat-treated alloys unless the material is to be heat-treated again.

Aluminum heat treatment

The tempering of an aluminum alloy is the major determinant of its strength, hardness, ductility, and other properties. Some aluminum alloys can be heat-treated to improve their properties; others must be strengthened and hardened by cold working. Aluminum alloys are assigned temper designations that are added to the end of the four identifying digits. These figures indicate the type of treatment undergone by the alloy as follows:

XXXX-0: Annealed condition of wrought alloys.
XXXX-T2: Annealed condition of cast alloys.
XXXX-F: For wrought alloys, no control is exercised over the temper of the alloy; For cast alloys, the term means as-cast (e.g., 43-F).
XXXX-T: (Followed by one or more numbers) indicates a heat-treated alloy, where the numbers refer to the type of heat treatment.

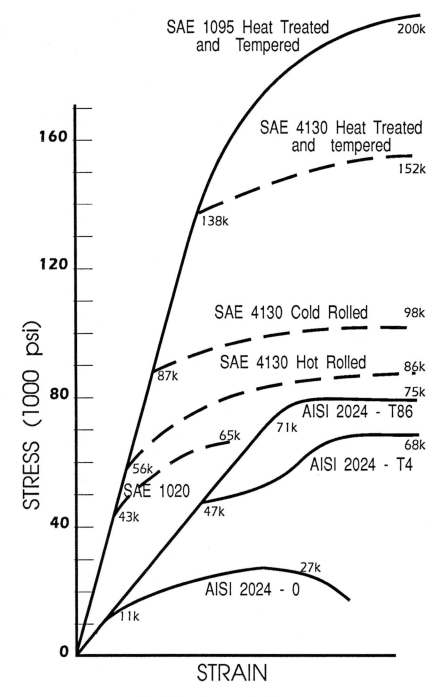

SAE 1095 Heat Treated and Tempered — 200k

SAE 4130 Heat Treated and tempered — 152k

138k

SAE 4130 Cold Rolled — 98k

SAE 4130 Hot Rolled — 86k

87k

75k

AISI 2024 - T86

71k

68k

AISI 2024 - T4

65k

56k

SAE 1020

47k

43k

27k

AISI 2024 - 0

11k

STRESS (1000 psi)

160

120

80

40

0

STRAIN

Fig. 2.35. Stress-strain diagram.

XXXX-H: Indicates cold work temper of a wrought alloy.

Example.   2024-T4 refers to aluminum of chemical composition defined by 2024, heat-treated and aged at room temperature to a stable condition.

Stress-strain diagram

The stress-strain diagram (Fig. 2.35) compares several steels and aluminums that have been heat treated and/or tempered in a variety of ways. Because all of the aluminums are of the same chemical composition (AISI 2024), the effect on the mechanical properties of differing types of heat treatment is clearly demonstrated by the aluminum curves. For instance, the yield and ultimate strength of the annealed alloy (2024-0) were raised from 11,000 psi and 27,000 psi to 71,000 psi and 75,000 psi, respectively, when heat treated (2024-T86).

The effect of hot and cold working on steel is shown by the SAE 4130 curves. The yield point and ultimate strength point of this alloy were raised from 87,000 psi

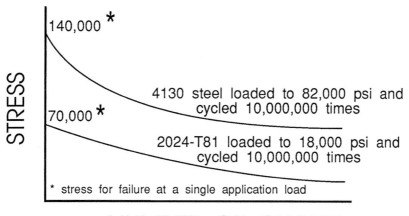

Fig. 2.36. Fatigue.

and 98,000 psi to 138,000 psi and 152,000 psi, respectively, demonstrating the increased strength obtained by heat treating this alloy.

The high carbon steel curve (SAE 1095) shows the effect of heat treatment on this material, raising it to 200,000 psi.

PREVENTING FAILURE

Fatigue

The range of elasticity, the yield and ultimate stress points are high enough in most metals to prevent orthosis failure. Fatigue stresses, which are the result of repeatedly applied small loads rather than application of a large load, are the main cause of breakage.

Fatigue stresses can be partially compared with the physiological stresses to which a normal individual is subjected to in walking. When a man is walking, the effort required for each step is only a fraction of his available energy. After a while, however, he reaches a point at which even the relatively small expenditure of energy necessary for lifting his limbs will require too much effort.

Fatigue stresses are fluctuating stresses of a magnitude less than the ultimate stress of the material. Although the ultimate stress would cause breakage immediately, fatigue stress causes failure after a number of cycles. In physiological stress, if the man rests for a period, the fatigue lessens or is completely alleviated. However, in fatigue stress, rest from stressing the material has no effect on the number of cycles before breakage occurs. Figure 2.36 illustrates the phenomenon of fatigue failure.

Steel and aluminum fatigue compared

By plotting the stresses on a material against the number of applications of such stress before breakage,

Table 2.4. Material strength (psi)*

ALLOY	YIELD STRENGTH	ULTIMATE STRENGTH	FATIGUE STRENGTH
2024-0	11,000	27,000	13,000
2024-T3	50,000	70,000	20,000
2024-T4	47,000	68,000	20,000
2024-T86	71,000	75,000	18,000
7075-T6	73,000	83,000	22,000

*Based on 50,000,000 cycles of completely reversed stress. Adapted from *Alcoa Aluminum Handbook*.

the curves in Figure 2.36 are obtained. In the case of steel, repeated stresses below a certain level do not cause fatigue failure. The steel curve levels off at a value of approximately 50% of its ultimate stress. Theoretically, this is the fatigue strength of the material, and any number of stresses at or below this level of 70,000 psi is not expected to cause fatigue failure.

The aluminum curve is quite different. Aluminum does not level off as steel does and is therefore more subject to fatigue failure. Although the addition of alloying elements raises the ultimate strength and yield point, it does not appreciably change the fatigue strength. Table 2.4 illustrates this point. Heat treatment also has only a small effect on aluminum fatigue.

Stress concentration

The average value of stress on a given object is obtained by dividing the amount of applied force by the size of the resisting area (Fig. 2.37). If there are nicks, notches, drilled holes, sharply bent corners, or name stampings, however, the stress is concentrated at these points and its value at them may be several

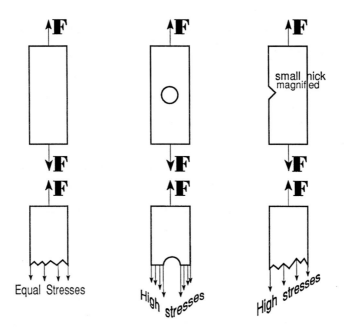

Fig. 2.37. Stress concentration.

times the average stress (Fig. 2.37). This increased stress lowers the resistance of the material to impact and fatigue loadings and is an important contributing factor in orthosis failures. It is easiest to see the effect of stress concentrations on a brittle material such as glass.

Example. A man wants to break a piece of glass in half. If he simply applies force to both ends and bends the glass, it shatters into a mass of splinters. If he scribes a line on the surface of the glass with a glazer's cutter, however, and then applies bending forces, the glass is neatly broken into two parts. The material is stressed the highest at the scribed line, concentrating the applied force at that location.

Although the effects of stress concentration on ductile materials, including some metals, are not as dramatic as with brittle materials, the same phenomenon occurs. With this in mind, it is possible to minimize the points of stress concentration and increase the strength of the material. This is done in orthoses by using certain fabrication procedures that minimize stress.

Minimizing stress concentration

The following recommendations help to minimize the points of stress concentration and thereby increase the strength of the orthoses:

1. Remove nicks and scratches from the material by polishing. (Here is an instance in which material is removed to distribute the stress equally and thereby strengthen the material.)
2. Cap the checkered jaws of the vise before clamping the work into the vise.

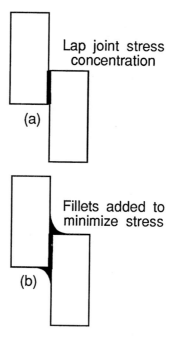

Fig. 2.38. Minimizing stress.

3. Make sure that contouring instruments have smooth, curved surfaces.
4. Do not shape the orthosis stirrups with a metal hammer.
5. Avoid abrupt changes in cross section. When two sections are being joined together, the stress may be concentrated on the joint area depending on the type of joint (Fig. 2.38). If extra material is added to form a fillet as in Figure 2.38, however, the stress concentration is minimized.

Table 2.5.   Approximate radii for 90-degree cold bend

ALUMINUM ALLOYS	RADII FOR VARIOUS THICKNESSES (INCH) EXPRESSED IN TERMS OF THICKNESS *T*					
	1/16	1/8	3/16	1/4	3/8	1/2
2024-0	0	0	0-1T	0-1T	1.5T-3T	3T-5T
2024-T3	3T-5T	4T-6T	4T-6T	5T-7T	6T-8T	6T-9T
2024-T36	4T-6T	5T-7T	5T-7T	6T-10T	7T-10T	8T-11T
2024-T4	3T-5T	4T-6T	4T-6T	5T-7T	6T-8T	6T-9T

Adapted from *Alcoa Aluminum Handbook*.

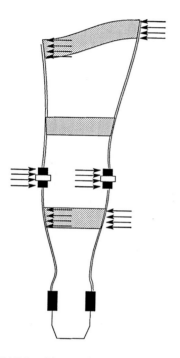

Fig. 2.39.   KAFO subject to bending stresses in mediolateral direction.

Minimizing stress concentration because of bending

Table 2.5 shows the minimum radii for bending aluminum alloys. The values given are for a 90-degree cold bend. Bending an orthosis part below this minimum radii causes excess stress concentration and increases the possibility of breakage at the bend.

Shape of orthotic parts

Many orthotic parts act in the same manner as beams. The upper side bars of an orthosis are subjected to lateral forces causing bending stresses (Fig. 2.39). Bending stresses on a member acting as a beam are not the same as pure tension, compression or shear stresses,

in which the strain depends on the amount of the area and not on the shape of the cross-sectional area. The magnitude of the bending stresses depends on the cross-sectional area of the member.

In the case of a beam, the top fibers of the beam are in maximum compression, whereas the bottom side is in maximum tension (Fig. 2.40, *a*). The stresses are in opposite directions and decrease towards the center of the area. In this location, called the neutral axis, the stress is 0. Distributing as much material as possible away from the neutral axis lowers the stress and therefore lowers the resulting strain on the member. Figure 2.40, *b*, illustrates this phenomenon.

Distribution of materials in beams

It is possible and advisable to distribute the same amount of material in different shapes to lower stresses. The familiar shape of a structural *I* beam illustrates this principle (Fig. 2.41).

Instead of rectangular cross sections, these beams are made in the shape of an I. The material in the rectangular beam, as represented by the hatched areas in the diagram, is removed from the sides and placed on the top and bottom. The rigidity of the beam is thus increased with reference to bending in this direction. Resistance to bending about the sides, however, is diminished. Proper design considers the anticipated direction of maximum bending and orients the structural member accordingly.

Designs in orthoses

In fabricating an orthosis, the Certified Orthotist positions the side bars of a lower limb orthosis having rectangular cross-sectional areas so that the long dimension of the rectangle is parallel to the anterior-posterior direction (Fig. 2.42). In this position, the bars are able to resist larger forces and are more rigid than in the mediolateral direction. This design and the attachment of cuffs are correct if the maximum anticipated forces

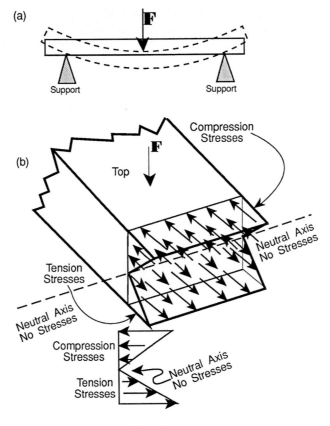

Fig. 2.40. Beam stresses.

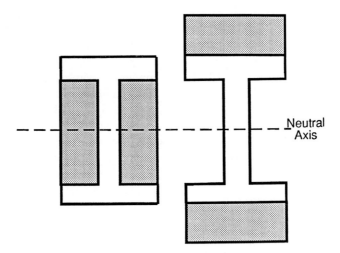

Fig. 2.41. Beam shape.

are generated by a knee lock preventing flexion in which increased rigidity is desirable with reference to mediolateral bending moments.

Other designing problems

Where the direction of maximum stress is not known, the material should be distributed in the form of a ring. The ring shape resists bending in all directions equally well (Fig. 2.43, *a*). Where there are significant moments in two known directions, and one is known to be larger than the other, tubular areas can be used to obtain effective resistance to bending (Fig. 2.43, *b*). The contouring of tubular cross sections is somewhat difficult. An example in orthoses is the case of a heavy individual who is bowlegged and therefore has large mediolateral bending moments and anterior-posterior bending moments as well.

European orthotists use a bar of the shape illustrated

in Figure 2.43, *c.* This shape increases resistance to bending about both directions with a minimum of material.

FASTENING COMPONENTS

Riveting aluminum

There are several advantages that cause riveting to be the most common method of joining aluminum. Welding, brazing, and soldering require the application of heat to the material. If this material depends on prior heat treatment for strength, this additional application of heat in fabrication may alter the desired mechanical properties that have been achieved. Rivets can be visually inspected, whereas it is usually necessary to obtain an X-ray film of a weld to determine its strength.

Rivet materials. The preferred material for fastening aluminum is aluminum. When dissimilar metals are in contact with each other in a moist atmosphere, galvanic corrosion takes place, which lowers the service life. In orthoses and certain other instances, however, stainless steel, hot-dipped aluminized or cadmium-plated steel rivets can be used. Because aluminum rivets must be larger than steel rivets to achieve the same strength, larger holes are needed to accommodate the aluminum rivets. In orthoses, the larger holes in

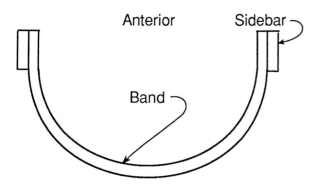

Fig. 2.42. Band design.

respect to the dimensions of the components weaken the material.

Size of rivet. The diameter of the rivet should not be less than the thickness of the thickest part through which the rivet is driven but should not be greater than three times the thickness of the thinnest part when joining different size members.

Spacing of rivets. The recommended minimum spacing between rivets is three times the nominal rivet diameter. As a general rule, the maximum distance should not be greater than two to four times the thickness of the thickest member.

Edge distance. The edge distance from the center of the hole to the end of the member should be at least twice the diameter of the rivet. This yields a joint with maximum bearing strength. Figure 2.44 illustrates these requirements.

Rivet holes. Recommended hole sizes for cold driven aluminum alloy rivets are listed in Table 2.6.

Rivet sets and bucking tools. Rivet sets should have smooth, polished surfaces to allow the metal to flow readily during the forming operation. The bucking tool should have sufficient mass and be of the shape illustrated in Figure 2.45.

Using the bucking-up set. The cup of the bucking-up set should be initially in contact with the top of the rivet so that the shank is not driven into the head during forming. Proper upsetting of the rivet fills the rivet hole and increases fatigue strength.

Length of rivet. Length of rivets necessary for proper forming of a head depend on the total thickness of metal through which the rivet is driven, the clearance between the rivet and the rivet hole, and the form of the head. The manufacturers recommend that because of the variation in driving conditions, various lengths should be tried to determine the optimum length. It is preferred to err on the long side. A short rivet may allow the rivet set to contact the member and damage it. Good practice with respect to countersunk rivets requires a unit length that leaves some material above the surface after the completion of riveting. This insures the complete filling of the countersunk hole and prevents

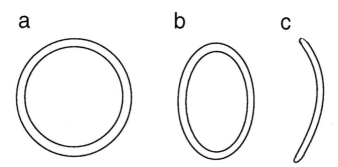

Fig. 2.43. Geometrical shapes.

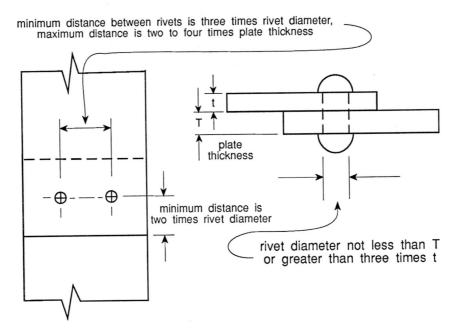

minimum distance between rivets is three times rivet diameter,
maximum distance is two to four times plate thickness

t

T

plate
thickness

minimum distance is
two times rivet diameter

rivet diameter not less than T
or greater than three times t

Fig. 2.44.   Edge distance.

Table 2.6. Rivet hole size					
NOMINAL RIVET DIAMETER (INCH)	1/8	5/32	3/16	1/4	5/16
Recommended hole diameter	0.1285	0.159	0.191	0.257	0.323
Drill size	30	21	11	F	P

Adapted from *Alcoa Structural Handbook.*

damage to the surrounding member. The excess can be ground off at a later time. For purposes of comparison, the strengths of some rivets are listed.

Aluminum rivet material.   Aluminum rivets are produced in the following alloys: 1100-H14, 2017-T4, 2117-T4, 6053-T61, and 7277-T4 (Table 2.7). All of these rivets can be driven cold in the condition received from the manufacturer with the exception of 2024-T4 and 7277-T4. Rivets 2024 and 7277 are strong but must be heated before driving.

It is not good practice to use a strong rivet in a weak plate because the plate may become distorted. Also, the strength of the rivet may be superfluous because the plate will fail before the rivet. For aluminum members made of 2024, 2017-T4 rivets can be used, whereas the 6000 series rivets are compatible with 3000 series members.

Riveting stainless steels

Advances in welding techniques have made this type of joining operation suitable for stainless steels.

Riveting, however, still offers many advantages. It is a quick method of joining and requires a minimum of accessory equipment. Also, as in the case of aluminum, cold riveting ends the hazards involved in the intense heat applications of the welding process. The possible loss of corrosion resistance and the danger of warping are also eliminated by riveting.

Recommended procedures

Rivet holes should be drilled and all burrs removed. For those steels that rapidly work harden, avoid center punching before drilling because the material will prove too hard to drill.

Rivet stock should be in the annealed condition. By work hardening the rivet in the forming operation, its physical properties are improved.

Austenitic rivets up to ¼-inch diameter can be driven cold. Because these work harden rapidly, however, the head should be formed with as few blows as possible.

Ferritic and martinsitic rivets up to ⅜-inch diam-

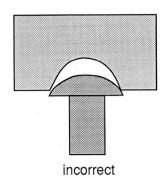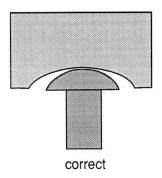

incorrect   correct

Fig. 2.45.   Rivet sets.

Table 2.7.   Aluminum alloys

ALLOY	SHEAR STRENGTH (PSI)
1100-H14	11,000
2017-T4	39,000
2024-T4	42,000
2117-T4	33,000
5056-H32	30,000
6053-T61	23,000
6061-T6	30,000
7244-T4	38,000

Adapted from Riveting Alcoa Aluminum.

Table 2.8.   Building blocks

ELEMENT	ATOMIC WEIGHT	ENERGY BONDS	
Hydrogen	1	—H	(1)
Carbon	12	—C—	(4)
Nitrogen	14	—N—	(3)
Oxygen	16	—O—	(2)
Fluorine	19	—F	(1)
Silicone	28	—Si—	(4)
Sulfur	32	—S—	(2)
Chlorine	35	—Cl	(1)

eter can be driven cold, preferably with a hydraulic riveter.

PLASTICS AND COMPOSITES

Plastics are the result of humankind's ability to innovate, to create new materials by combining organic building blocks—carbon, oxygen, hydrogen, nitrogen, chlorine, and other organic and inorganic elements—into new and useful forms (Table 2.8). A plastic is a solid in its finished state, but at some stage in its manufacture, it approaches a liquid condition and is formed into useful shapes. Forming is usually done through the application, either singly or together, of heat and pressure.

The number of permutations possible in combining the many chemical elements is virtually endless. This diversity has made plastics applicable to a broad range of consumer and industrial products. It has also made the job of selecting the best material from such a huge array of candidate plastics quite difficult.

Building polymers

Plastics are synthetic materials made from raw chemical materials called monomers. A monomer (one chemical unit) such as ethylene is reacted with other monomer molecules into long chains of repeating ethylene units, forming the polymer polyethylene (Table 2.9). In a similar manner, polystyrene is formed from styrene monomer, polypropylene from propylene monomer, and other thermoplastic polymers from their respective monomers.

The polymers consist of atoms of carbon in combination with other elements. Polymer chemists use only eight (see Table 2.8) of the more than 100 known elements to create thousands of different plastics.

Combining these atoms in various ways produces extremely large, complex molecules. Each atom has a limited capacity (energy bonds; see Table 2.8) for joining to other atoms, and every atom within a molecule must have all its energy bonds satisfied if the compound is to be stable. Hydrogen, for example, can bond to only one other atom, whereas carbon or silicon must attach to four other atoms to satisfy its four energy bonds. Thus, H — H and H — F are stable molecules, but C — H and Si — Cl are not stable.

As an illustration, consider the simple organic compound, methane (CH_4), the main component of natural gas. The carbon in methane is attached to four atoms of hydrogen, and each hydrogen atom is attached to the simple atom of carbon. The molecular weight of methane, 16, is the total of the individual atomic weights of its constituent atoms.

Table 2.9. Typical monomers and their repeating polymer units

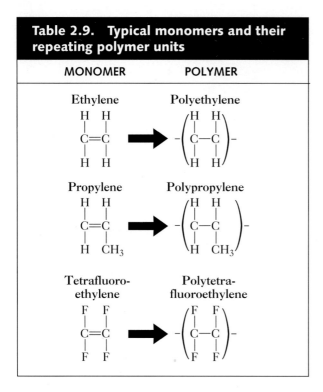

MONOMER	POLYMER
Ethylene	Polyethylene
Propylene	Polypropylene
Tetrafluoro-ethylene	Polytetra-fluoroethylene

Table 2.10. Building by adding CH_2 groups

COMMON NAME	CHEMICAL FORMULA	MOLECULAR WEIGHT
Methane	CH_4	16
Ethane	C_2H_6	30
Propane	C_3H_8	44
Butane	C_4H_{10}	58
Pentane	C_5H_{12}	72
Kerosene	$C_{17}H_{36}$	240
Paraffin	$C_{18}H_{38}$	254
Hard wax	$C_{50}H_{102}$	702
Polyethylene (LMW)*	$C_{100}H_{202}$	1402

*LMW, Low molecular weight.

Adding more carbon atoms in a chain and more hydrogen atoms to each new carbon creates heavier molecules. For example, ethane gas (C_2H_6) is heavier than methane because it contains an additional carbon and two additional hydrogen atoms. Its molecular weight is 30. In a similar manner, molecular weight can be increased in increments of 14 (1 C, 2 H) until the compound pentane (C_5H_{12}) is reached. Pentane is too heavy to be a gas and is, instead, a liquid at room temperature. Further addition of CH_2 groups makes progressively heavier liquids until $C_{18}H_{38}$ is reached. This is the solid, paraffin wax.

Thermoplastics

As molecules are made longer and become heavier, the polymer wax becomes harder and tougher. At approximately $C_{100}H_{202}$, the material, with a molecular weight of 1402, is tough enough to be useful as a plastic (Table 2.10). This is low-molecular-weight polyethylene, the simplest of the thermoplastics.

Continuing the addition of more CH_2 groups to the chain increases strength and toughness even more. The toughest polyethylene contains more than one quarter million CH_2 groups and is called ultra-high-molecular-weight polyethylene.

Although the example of polymer chain growth shown in Table 2.10 implies the addition of one CH_2 group at a time, in reality, a simple CH_2 group cannot be added easily because it does not exist as a stable compound. Instead, groups of organic compounds, called monomers, are used.

The structure of these monomers seems to conflict with the rule that carbon must be attached to four other atoms to be stable. But like all rules, there are exceptions. In certain cases, a double bond, which is stable, can be formed between atoms. As illustrated in Figure 2.46, ethylene monomer, $CH_2 = CH_2$ is made by removing (under heat and pressure) two hydrogens from ethane, $CH_3 - CH_3$. A redistribution of electrons occurs, and a double bond is formed. The double bond plus the two single bonds thus satisfy the four energy bonds of the carbon atom, forming a stable monomer.

Then, starting with billions of molecules of monomers in a reactor, heat and pressure are applied in the presence of catalysts, causing one of the monomer double bonds to rearrange into *half bonds*, one at each end (Fig. 2.47). These half bonds combine with half bonds of other rearranged monomer molecules, forming stable *whole bonds* between them. As each monomer joins (primary bonds) with others, the chain length grows until it meets a stray hydrogen, which combines with the reactive end, stopping chain growth at that point.

During the polymerization reaction, millions of separate polymer chains grow in length simultaneously, until all the monomers are exhausted. By adding predetermined amounts of hydrogen (or other chain stoppers), chemists can produce polymers having a fairly consistent average chain length. Chain length is important because it determines many properties of a plastic, and it also affects its processing characteristics. The major effects of increasing chain length are greater toughness, creep resistance, stress-crack resistance, melt temperature, melt viscosity, and processing difficulty.

All polymer molecules cannot be manufactured to an exact, specified length; however, each batch has an

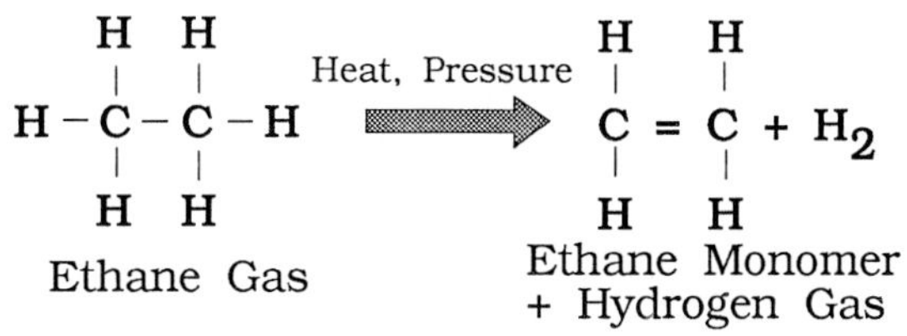

Fig. 2.46. Creating an ethane monomer.

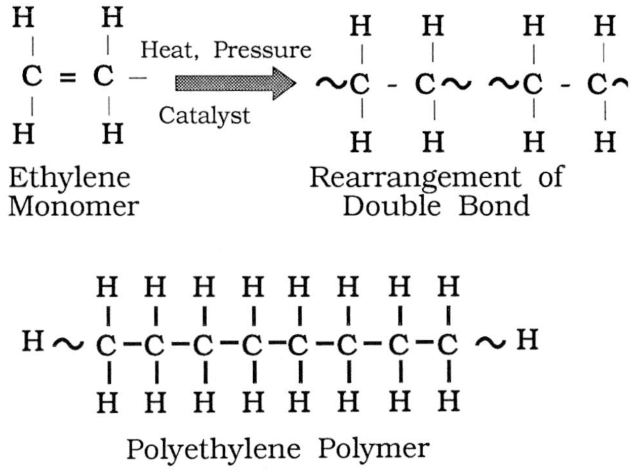

Fig. 2.47. Polymerization of polyethylene.

average molecular-weight distribution. There can be either a broad or a narrow spread between molecular weights of the largest and smallest molecules, and the polymer still could have the same average. A narrow distribution provides more uniform properties; a broad distribution makes a plastic easier to process.

After polymerization is completed, the finished polymer chains resemble long, intertwined bundles of spaghetti, with no physical connections between chains. Such a polymer is called a thermoplastic (heat-moldable) polymer.

Although there is no direct physical connection between individual thermoplastic chains, there is a weak electrostatic attraction (secondary bonds) between polymer chains that lie close together. This intermolecular force, which tends to prevent chain movement, is heat sensitive, becoming stronger when the plastic is cold and weaker when it is hot. Heating a thermoplastic, therefore, weakens the intermolecular forces of the secondary bonds, allowing the polymer molecules to slide over each other freely during the forming process. On cooling, the forces become strong again and "freeze" the molecules together in the new shape.

Forming a thermoplastic is similar to molding candle wax in this respect. If too much heat is applied or if the plastic is heated for too long a time, however, the molecular chains' primary bonds break, causing permanent damage, particularly material toughness. Continu-

ous bending or deforming stress on a formed part also causes the chains to slide over each other, resulting in creep, or cold-flow, which can seriously affect part shape.

Strength of the intermolecular attractive force (secondary bond) varies inversely with the sixth power of the distance between chains. Thus, as the distance is halved, the attractive force increases by a factor of 64. For this reason, chain shape is as important as chain length. If a polymer molecule has a symmetrical shape that can pack closely, the intermolecular forces are large compared with those of a nonsymmetrical shape.

Two kinds of polyethylene can have different physical properties because of the difference in their density, which depends on their ability to pack together (Fig. 2.48).

The molecules of high-density polyethylene have few side branches to upset their symmetry, so they can approach adjacent molecules quite closely, resulting in high intermolecular attractive forces (secondary bonds). Low-density polyethylene, on the other hand, contains many more side branches, which create asymmetrical areas of low density and, therefore, low intermolecular attraction.

Another consequence of denser molecular packing is higher crystallinity. As symmetric molecules approach within a critical distance, crystals begin to form in the areas of densest packing. A crystallized area is stiffer and stronger; a noncrystallized (amorphous)

Typical Chain Structure

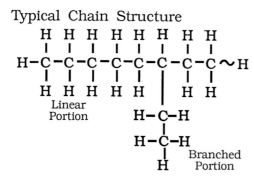

Linear Portion

Branched Portion

High-Density Polyethylene

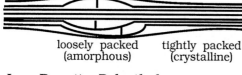

loosely packed   tightly packed
(amorphous)   (crystalline)

Low-Density Polyethylene

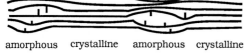

amorphous   crystalline   amorphous   crystalline

Fig. 2.48.   Polymer chain packaging.

area is tougher and more flexible. Other effects of increased crystallinity in a polyethylene polymer are increased resistance to creep, heat, stress cracking, and increased shrinkage after forming.

In general, crystalline polymers are more difficult to process, have higher forming temperatures and melt viscosities, and tend to shrink and warp more than the amorphous polymers. They have a relatively sharp melting point; that is, they do not soften gradually with an increase in temperature. Furthermore, they remain hard until a given quantity of heat is absorbed, then change rapidly into a low-viscosity liquid. Reinforcement of crystalline polymers with fibers of glass or other materials improves their load-bearing capabilities significantly.

Amorphous polymers soften gradually as they are heated, but they do not flow as easily (in forming) as do crystalline materials. Reinforcing fibers do not significantly improve the strength of amorphous materials at higher temperatures. Examples of amorphous thermoplastics are acrylonitrile-butadiene-styrene (ABS), polystyrene, polycarbonate, polysulfone, and polyetherimide. Crystalline plastics include polyethylene, polypropylene, and polyetheretherketone.

Another method for altering molecular symmetry is to combine two different monomers in the polymerization reaction so that each polymer chain is composed partly of monomer A and partly of monomer B. A polymer made from two different monomers is called a copolymer; one made from three different monomers is called a terpolymer.

All long repeating chains are polymers, regardless of how many monomers are used. But when a polymer family includes copolymers, the term *homopolymer* is used to identify the single monomer type. An example is the acetal family; acetal resins are available both in homopolymer and copolymer types. Final properties of a copolymer depend on the percentage of monomer A to monomer B, the properties of each, and on how they are arranged along the chain. As shown in Figure 2.49, the arrangement may alternate equally between the two monomers, producing a symmetric shape capable of a high degree of crystallization. Or the arrangement may be random, creating areas of high crystallinity separated by flexible, amorphous areas. Such a copolymer usually has good rigidity and impact strength.

Block copolymers have large areas of polymerized monomer A alternating with large areas of polymerized monomer B. In general, a block copolymer is similar to an alternating copolymer except that it has stronger crystalline areas and tougher amorphous areas. If both types of blocks are crystalline, or both amorphous, a wide variety of end properties is possible, having characteristics ranging from hard, brittle plastics to soft, flexible elastomers.

A graft copolymer is made by attaching side groups of monomer B to a main chain of monomer A. A copolymer having a flexible polymer for the main chain and grafted rigid side chains is stiff, yet has excellent resistance to impact, a combination of properties not usually found in the same plastic. Copolymers always have different properties from those of a homopolymer made from either monomer.

Compounds of plastics modify properties of a thermoplastic material by many other methods as well. For example, fibers are added to increase strength and stiffness, plasticizers for flexibility, lubricants for easier molding or for increasing lubricity of the molded parts, antioxidants for higher temperature stability, UV stabilizers for resistance to sunlight, and fillers for economy. Other additives, such as flame retardants, smoke suppressants, and conductive fibers or flakes, provide special properties for certain applications.

Thermosets

Thermoset plastics are made quite differently from thermoplastics. Polymerization (curing) of thermoset plastics is done in two stages, partly by the material supplier and partly by the molder. As illustrated in Figure 2.50, phenolic (a typical thermoset plastic) is first partially polymerized by reacting phenol with formaldehyde under heat and pressure. The reaction is stopped at the point at which mostly linear chains have been formed. The linear chains still contain unreacted

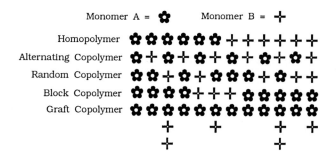

Fig. 2.49. Various copolymer arrangements.

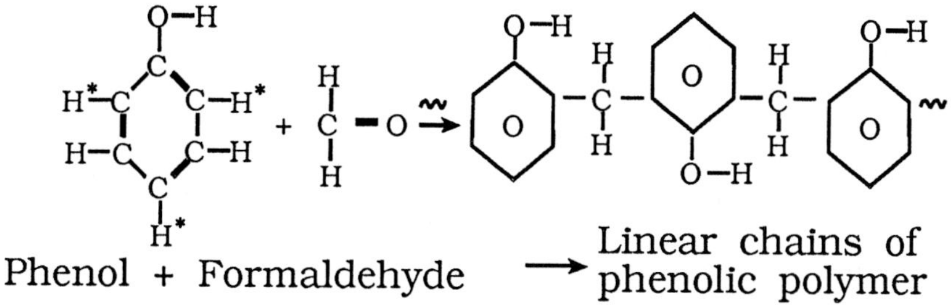

Phenol + Formaldehyde ⟶ **Linear chains of phenolic polymer**

Fig. 2.50. Condensation polymerization of phenolic.

portions, which are capable of flowing under heat and pressure. The chemical structure of phenol indicates three possible sites (see Fig. 2.50) for cross-linking. The hydrogens of two adjacent phenols are replaced by a CH_2 group from formaldehyde, and the remaining oxygen combines with the two replaced hydrogens to form water, which must be removed. The phenolic structure is shown in simplified form at the right. During molding, the CH_2 groups form cross-links in all planes, creating essentially a single, giant molecule.

The final stage of polymerization is completed in the molding press, where the partially reacted phenolic is liquefied under pressure, producing a cross-linking reaction between molecular chains. Unlike a thermoplastic monomer, which has only two reactive ends for linear chain growth, a thermoset monomer must have three or more reactive ends so that its molecular chains cross-link in three dimensions. Rigid thermosets have short chains with many cross-links; flexible thermosets have longer chains with fewer cross-links.

After it has been molded, a thermoset plastic has virtually all of its molecules interconnected with strong, permanent, physical bonds, which are not heat reversible. Theoretically the entire molded thermoset part could be a single giant molecule. In a sense, curing a thermoset is like cooking an egg. Once it is cooked, reheating does not cause remelting, so it cannot be remolded. But if a thermoset is heated too much or too long, the chains break and properties are degraded.

Besides the condensation thermosets wherein a byproduct (water for example) is created during the

reaction in the mold, there are *addition-cured* thermoset plastics. These include epoxy and polyester, which cure by an addition reaction, resulting in no volatile byproducts and fewer molding problems. Most addition-cured thermoset plastics are liquid at room temperature; the two ingredients can simply be mixed and poured into molds where they cross-link (cure) at room temperature into permanent form, much like casting concrete. Molds are often heated, however, to speed the curing process.

In general, thermoset plastics, because of their tightly cross-linked structure, resist higher temperatures and provide greater dimensional stability than do most thermoplastics.

Thermoplastic composites

Thermoplastics that are reinforced with high-strength, high-modulus fibers provide dramatic increases in strength and stiffness, toughness, or dimensional stability. The performance gain of the composites usually more than compensates for their higher cost. Processing usually involves the same methods used for unreinforced resins.

Molded products may contain as little as 5% and as much as 60% fiber by weight. Practically all thermoplastic resins are available in glass-reinforced compounds. Those used in largest volumes are nylon, polypropylene, and polystyrene. Glass-fiber reinforcement improves most mechanical properties of plastics by a factor of two or more. Tensile strength of nylon, for example, can be increased from about 10,000 psi to over

30,000 psi. A 40% glass-fortified acetal has a flexural modulus of 1.8×10^6 (up from 0.4×10^6) and a tensile strength of 21,500 psi (up from 8,800 psi). Reinforced polyester has double the tensile and impact strength and four times the flexural modulus of the unreinforced resin. Also improved in reinforced compounds are tensile modulus, dimensional stability, and fatigue endurance. Deformation under load of these stiffer materials is reduced significantly.

Carbon-fiber–reinforced compounds are available in a number of thermoplastics, including nylon 6/6, polysulfone, polyester, polyphenylene sulfide, polyetherimide, and polyetheretherketone. The carbon-fiber–reinforced material, at two to four times the cost of comparable glass-reinforced thermoplastics, offers the ultimate in tensile strength (to 35,000 psi), stiffness, and other mechanical properties.

It would seem that aramid fibers, with greater specific strengths than steel or aluminum, would be an ideal fiber reinforcement for thermoplastic resins. Chopped aramid fibers, however, do not compound as well as the conventional glass or carbon-fiber reinforcements.

Thermoset composites

Advanced thermoset composites consist of a resin-matrix material reinforced with high-strength, high-modulus fibers of glass, carbon, aramid, Kevlar, or even boron, and usually laid up in layers. An example is epoxy-resin-matrix materials reinforced with oriented, continuous fibers of carbon or a combination of carbon and glass fibers, laid up in multilayer fashion to form extremely rigid, strong structures.

Most of the thermoset composites are based on polyester and epoxy resins; of the two, polyester systems predominate. Polyesters can be molded by any process used for thermosetting resins. They can be cured at room temperature and atmospheric pressure. These resins offer a balance of low cost and ease of handling along with good mechanical properties and dimensional stability.

Epoxies are low-molecular-weight, syrup-like liquids that are cured with hardeners to cross-link thermoset structures that are hard and tough. Because the hardeners or curing agents become part of the finished structure, they are chosen to provide desired properties in the molding part. Epoxies can also be formulated for room-temperature curing, but heat curing produces higher properties.

Glass is the most widely used reinforcing material in thermoset composites. Glass fiber, with a tensile strength of 500,000 psi, accounts for almost 90% of the reinforcement in thermosetting resins. Other reinforcements used are carbon, graphite, boron, aramid, and Kevlar. Glass fibers are available in several forms: rov-ing (continuous strand), chopped strand, woven fabrics, continuous-strand mat, chopped-strand mat, and milled fibers. The longer fibers provide the greater strength; continuous fibers are the strongest.

Carbon fibers in thermosetting composites can be long and continuous, or short and fragmented, and can be directionally or randomly oriented. In general, short fibers cost less, and fabrication costs are lower; but, as with glass, properties of resulting composites are lower than those obtained with longer or continuous fibers. The outstanding design properties of carbon fiber/resin matrix composites are their high strength-to-weight and stiffness-to-weight ratios. With proper selection and placement of fibers, the composites can be stronger and stiffer than equivalent-thickness steel parts and weigh 40% to 70% less. Fatigue resistance of continuous-fiber composites is excellent. Similar to most rigid materials, however, carbon-fiber composites are relatively brittle. The composites have no yield behavior, and resistance to impact is low.

Mechanical properties

When forces are continuously applied, plastics are subjected to both elastic (spring-like) and viscous (slow-flow) behavior. This means that when forces are applied to a plastic, the total resulting deformation is not instantaneous but increases with time, and the deformation is most usually fully recoverable. Because the properties are time dependent, some of the most useful tests for deducing the mechanical behavior of plastics are creep tests. Creep tests are commonly performed by observing the deformation with time of tensile-type or bending specimens.

In the tensile type of creep test, a plastic specimen is clamped on its ends on the tensile tester, and the distance between gauge marks on the specimen is measured. A steady tensile force is applied to the specimen. The magnitude of the force divided by the original cross-sectional area of the specimen is the tensile stress in the material. After the load has been applied, the distance between the gauge marks is measured. The increase in length between the gauge marks divided by the original length is known as the strain. At the particular, constant, controlled, environmental condition of temperature, the strain is regularly observed over a long period of time for a given level of applied stress. The results are often plotted as shown in Figure 2.51.

The results typically show that the plastic immediately undergoes an elastic strain when the load is applied, then a period ensues in which further but retarded elastic strain occurs, and finally a period of steady viscous flow occurs (Fig. 2.52). The elastic portion of the deformation is deduced by removing the load from the specimen and observing its recovery. Usually the material contracts instantaneously and con-

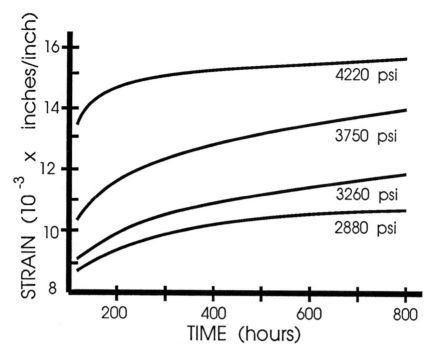

Fig. 2.51. Tensile creep of polycarbonate (at 73° F).

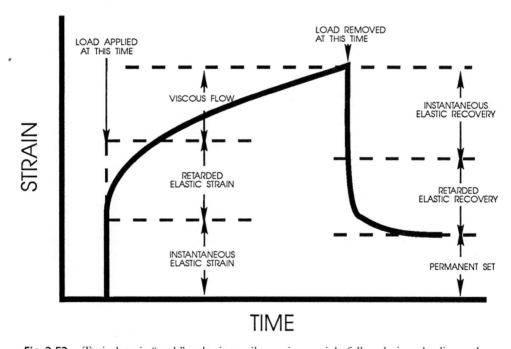

Fig. 2.52. Typical strain "path" a plastic tensile specimen might follow during a loading cycle.

tinues at a slowing rate, until it is clear that it will contract no longer and has suffered some permanent extension.

The various sections of the strain path shown in Figure 2.52 are associated with different types of atomic and molecular motions in the polymer. The instantaneous strain is the result of elastic action of interatomic bond angles and lengths; for all practical purposes, these deformations occur instantaneously. The retarded elastic strain region is thought to be accounted for by the cooperative motion of polymer chain segments that cannot occur instantaneously but need time for the necessary coiling or uncoiling and wriggling and jumping of mechanically entangled polymer chains to occur. The material flow of the polymer is associated with the slipping of one molecule past another.

A polypropylene AFO that has been designed and fabricated to restrain dorsiflexion, for example, yields into dorsiflexion as an anteriorly directed force is applied to the calf section with the foot section stabilized. The force required to collapse the AFO to a given angle gradually decreases over time. This *softening* illustrates the creep mechanism.

Changes in the individual polymer molecule's structure are likely to alter the ability of atoms and molecules to move relative to one another and therefore are changes that would alter the deformational characteristics of the plastic. Increasing the molecular weight of the polymer (by increasing the chain length) increases the viscosity of the polymer and the slope of the equilibrium flow region changes (Fig. 2.53). When all the chains are hooked together by cross-links and the molecular weight effectively reaches infinity, the chains cannot slip past one another so the viscous flow is eliminated. The amount of time any material takes to reach a particular level of strain depends on the applied

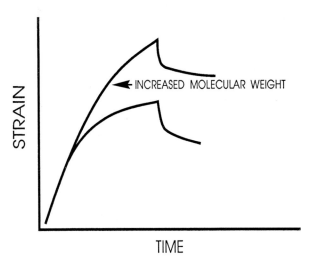

Fig. 2.53. Effect on strain "path" of molecular size.

stress and on the temperature, and increasing either causes the creeping to accelerate.

Short-term tensile tests

In the short-term tensile test, a specimen of plastic is elongated at a steady rate, and the force that has to be applied to the specimen to cause the steady elongation is recorded. From these observations, the plastic's short-term tensile stress-strain characteristic is deduced (Fig. 2.54).

For metallic materials, this stress-strain curve is extremely useful. The typical characteristic of a common ductile steel is illustrated in Fig. 2.55. Such materials are perfectly elastic if strained to the yield point even if the force applied remained for a long time before it were removed. The same is not true for plastics, which are viscoelastic in nature. However, because of the extremely common and appropriate usage of short-term tensile tests for metallic materials and because of their convenience, there has been a natural inclination to use those same type of tests for plastics. Typical characteristics results are shown in Figure 2.56. For these results to have any meaning at all, it must be known at what temperature and rate of elongation these tests were conducted.

Isochronous stress-strain curve

Isochronous stress-strain curves show the strain that would result if a particular stress were imposed for a particular period of time. The form of this plot is similar to that conventionally used to plot short-term tensile tests, but it must be remembered that the types of test are really quite different. If, however, the particular time chosen for isochronous stress-strain data is reasonably short (say, 100 seconds), then the form of the isochronous stress-strain curve will be very similar to short-term stress-strain data derived from constant-elongation-rate tests (Fig. 2.57).

These curves suggest that if a plastic is strained and

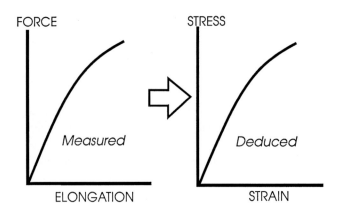

Fig. 2.54. Deduction of short-term stress-strain characteristics.

the strain is held constant with time, the stress in the plastic reduces with time. Thus, the viscoelastic nature of plastics can cause not only elongation creep under constant stress, but also stress relaxation at constant strain.

Stiffness and moduli

Elastic materials are most often used in situations where the stress levels imposed are lower than the material's yield point. The plastic's stiffness is measured by the stress that must be applied to cause strain. Graphically, this may be viewed on a short-term tensile stress-strain curve as the slope of the elastic portion of the curve. Stiffness for plastics is the same as the moduli of elasticity for metals. The results of short-term tensile tests are often presented in this way (Table 2.11). These nonreinforced plastics have stiffness and strengths much lower than metals. However, unlike moduli of simple elastic materials such as metals, the moduli of plastics are not single-valued constants but vary with time, temperature, and stress and strain. In general, plastics become less stiff with time and at unexpected rates (Fig. 2.58).

Strain recovery

Although all plastics creep, when the applied force is removed, the strain in the plastic decreases with time as though the material had a memory. When the loading on a plastic is intermittent, such as that during the stance phase of walking with a polypropylene AFO, there is not enough time in swing phase for the material's memory to return the plastic to its strain-free shape. When the plastic AFO is not worn, however, the creep strain set in during walking tends to disappear. The creep strain accumulates from loading cycle to cycle (Fig. 2.59).

Under the action of loads continuously applied for long periods of time, plastics may experience a variety of changes. The susceptibility of plastics to creep is obviously important. Strength of plastics, like creep, is also dependent on both time and temperature. Long-term strength data may be derived from creep-type tests in which tensile specimens are subject to steady loads at constant temperature. The tensile specimens eventually fail either by rupture or by the onset of necking (a phenomenon where the loaded tensile specimen begins to elongate rapidly because a local area of thinning-down occurs). The stress levels that cause failure by rupture or necking are presented as envelopes over creep data (Fig. 2.60). The fact that plastics weaken with age even under steady loads is called *static fatigue*.

Effects of temperature

Temperature has a major effect on the mechanical behavior of plastics. The effects of temperature on the

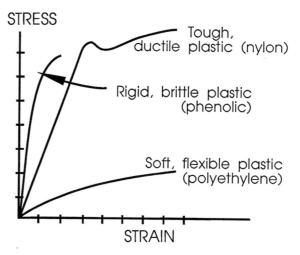

Fig. 2.56. Stress-strain curves for plastics.

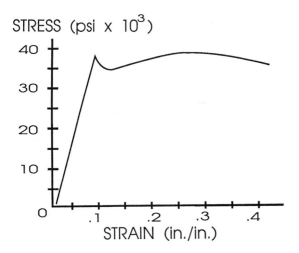

Fig. 2.55. Stress-strain curve for low carbon steel.

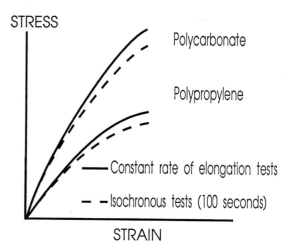

Fig. 2.57. Similarity of stress-strain curves at constant temperature.

Table 2.11.   Short-term mechanical properties of some plastics and metals

MATERIAL	SPECIFIC GRAVITY	TENSILE STRENGTH*	STIFFNESS IN TENSION*
Thermoplastics			
Nylon	1.09–1.14	8–12	200–400
Polyethylene	0.92–0.97	1–6	20–200
Polyester	1.31–1.38	8–10	—
Polypropylene	0.90–0.91	4–6	200
PVC	1.15–1.40	5–9	300–600
Thermosets			
Epoxy	1.11–1.40	4–13	300
Polyester	1.10–1.46	6–13	300–600
Metals			
Aluminum alloys	2.80	11–83	10,000
Steel alloys	7.85–7.92	73–230	28,000

*psi $\times 10^3$.

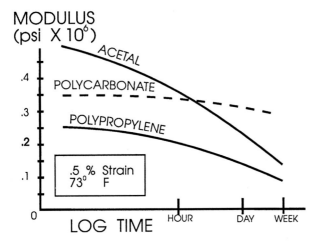

Fig. 2.58.   Variation of tensile creep with time.

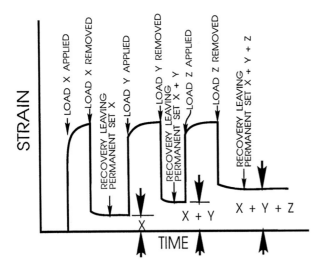

Fig. 2.59.   Deforming and recovery with intermittent loading.

creep of a thermoplastic are shown in Figure 2.61. Increasing temperature tends to cause softening of a plastic with consequent reduction in strength; lowering of temperature below the glass transition temperature can cause the plastic to become brittle.

Impact loading

The performance of plastics under impact loads may be compared by experimentally determining the amount of energy required to break specimens in impact, pendulum tests. In the Izod impact test, a cantilevered beam specimen of fixed dimensions with a carefully machined notch is placed in a clamp and a pendulum of known mass swung against it. The energy consumed in breaking the specimen is calculated by measurement of the pendulum swing-through height and comparison with the starting height. The impact strength of the plastic is then calculated as so many energy units per unit of specimen (ft.-lb./in.). The results of impact tests show that many plastics have high impact strengths and that some are sensitive to the sharpness of the notch radius and to the temperature of testing (Fig. 2.62).

In view of the inherent limitations of the Izod test caused by the specimen notch, other forms of impact tests have become more commonly used. One tensile type of test involves a tensile specimen mounted between a pendulum head and a cross-head clamp. When the pendulum is released and swings past a fixed anvil, the cross-head clamp is arrested, but the pendulum head continues forward, thus loading the specimen. The energy required to cause failure can then be measured without influence of the notch sensitivity.

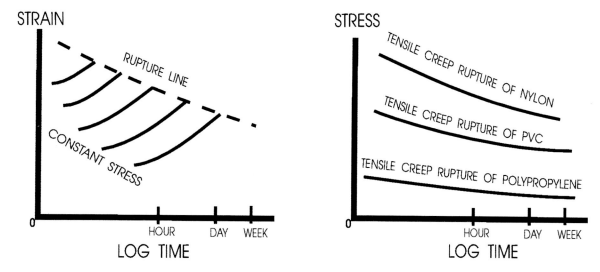

Fig. 2.60. Example of long-term strength data derived from tensile tests at constant loads and temperature.

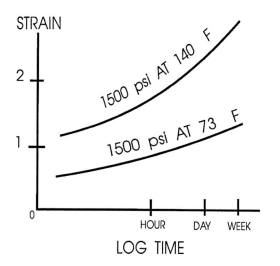

Fig. 2.61. Variation of tensile creep with temperature for a thermoplastic polyester.

Fig. 2.62. Effect of temperature on impact strength.

Hardness

Plastics are, in general, much softer than many other materials. The hardness of plastics is gauged by indentation tests of the Rockwell type. A steel ball under a minor load is applied to the surface of the specimen. This slightly indents and ensures good contact. The gauge is then set to 0. The major load is applied for 15 seconds and removed, leaving the minor load still applied. After 15 seconds, the diameter of the indentation remaining is measured and related to a hardness number. Rockwell hardness can differentiate relative hardness of different plastics, but because elastic recovery is involved as well as hardness, it is not valid to compare hardness of plastic entirely on the basis of this test.

THERMOSETTING PLASTICS

A thermosetting resin is a synthetic organic polymer that cures to a solid infusible mass by forming a three-dimensional network of covalent chemical bonds. In 1986, more than 5 billion pounds of thermosetting resins were manufactured in the United States. Phenolics accounted for about one third of the total production. Polyester resins were the next largest family, followed by epoxies.

Thermoset plastics compete with metals, ceramics, and thermoplastics. Compared to metals, they possess corrosion resistance, lighter weight, and insulating properties, and they can be processed at lower pressures and temperatures. The flow characteristics of uncured thermoset plastics can be used to form complex anatomic shapes, allowing low-cost production.

Compared to ceramics, thermoset plastics offer lighter weight, toughness, and easier processing. The principal advantage of ceramics is high-temperature performance. Thermosets offer advantages over thermoplastics in terms of reduced creep and improved crack resistance. The three-dimensional polymer network in thermosets also leads to improved machinability, low shrinkage, and improved high-temperature performance. The low initial viscosity of thermoset plastics permits incorporation of large amounts of fillers or fibers and has led to the development of many low-cost fabrication processes.

One limitation of many thermoset plastics is poor impact resistance. Consequently, devices requiring enhanced toughness are best served by thermoplastics.

Polyester thermoset plastics are popular because of their relative ease of fabrication. Epoxy thermoset plastics are only slightly more difficult to fabricate but are much higher in cost.

Thermoset plastics are made quite differently from thermal plastics. Polymerization (curing) of thermoset plastics is done in two stages, partly by the material supplier and partly by the practitioner. For example, phenolic is first partially polymerized by reacting phenol with formaldehyde under heat and pressure. The reaction is stopped at the point where mostly linear chains have been formed. The linear chains still contain unreacted portions, which are capable of flowing under heat and pressure. The final stage of polymerization is completed by the practitioner, where the partially reacted phenolic is liquefied under pressure, producing a cross-linking reaction between the chains. Unlike a thermal plastic monomer, rigid thermosets have short chains with many cross-links. After forming, a thermoset has virtually all of its molecules interconnected with strong, permanent, physical bonds, which are not reversible.

Epoxy and polyester thermosets cure by an "addition" reaction, resulting in no volatile byproducts and fewer fabrication problems. These plastics are liquid at room temperature; the two ingredients can simply be mixed and poured where they cross-link (cure) at room temperature into permanent form.

Most thermosetting plastics can be cured, or set, into shape permanently by the heat to which they are subjected during forming. Once thermosetting plastics have hardened, reheating does not soften them. A simplified comparison between the two classifications of plastics is to say that thermoplastic materials are softened by heat, and thermosetting materials are hardened by heat. Paraffin wax, in a sense, is a thermoplastic material that softens when heated and hardens or solidifies when cooled. The principle of the thermosetting material can be demonstrated by hard boiling an egg. The egg was originally soft and fluid but once hardened by heating it remains hard and no amount of reheating can return the egg to a fluid state.

Thermosetting plastics exhibit little cold flow and therefore can be subjected to continuous loads. Permissible loads must be determined from cold flow measurements, however, not from ultimate strengths.

Some thermosetting resins are cured, or hardened, by heat alone. Others are cured by the use of catalysts and promoters. Catalysts are materials that trigger the curing process. Promoters primarily control the rate of cure; an important factor is providing ample working time for the practitioner before hardening of the plastic takes place. Some plastics give off a heat of reaction once the cure has been started by a catalyst. The heat speeds the rate of hardening and must be taken into account when determining the amount of catalyst and promoter to be used.

The terms *thermoplastic* and *thermosetting* can be considered as chemical classifications of plastics. Plastics may also be divided into the following three physical classifications:

- *Rigid*—relatively nondeforming under loads.
- *Flexible*—deforming under loads.
- *Elastomeric*—compounds having high elongation.

Condensation reactions

Plastic resins are formed by condensation reactions in which two or more *unlike* molecules are combined to form a larger molecule, accompanied by the loss of water or a gas.

After condensation is complete, there is a noticeable separation between the resin and the water; this water must be removed. In certain condensation reactions, the byproduct is a gas, which is carried off while the reaction is taking place.

The raw materials for some of the plastic products show no disposition toward reacting when mixed with each other. It then becomes necessary to add a catalyst to start the reaction. Although the catalyst takes no part in the reaction, it has a direct influence on the outcome.

Polymerization

Polymerization is the stage or reaction that follows condensation. The resin formed in the condensation reaction, known as the monomer, is not suitable as a molding material but can be used as the base for lacquers. The monomer is converted into the polymer, and this usually takes place during molding or fabricating processes, when the monomer is subjected to the action of a catalyst and varying conditions of heat and pressure. The resin in the monomeric stage has a known molecular weight; the polymer is an unknown multiple of this weight.

By varying the amount of catalyst and the conditions of heat and pressure on a monomer, the degree of polymerization and the molecular weight of the resulting polymer can be increased or decreased. The higher the molecular weight, the harder the material becomes. Prolonged heating at a high temperature produces a polymer with a large molecular weight. High pressure causes the same result.

In general, a monomer is a liquid, whereas a polymer is a solid. Synthetic resins are usually amorphous—that is, noncrystalline—and have no definite melting point. They do, however, have a definite temperature range in which they soften. Because the transformation from monomer to polymer is the change from liquid to solid, there is an increase in viscosity during the polymerization process. Also, as polymerization progresses, the softening point, or temperature at which the material begins to soften, increases. The practitioner must keep all these factors in mind when choosing and using a thermosetting plastic.

It may seem strange that polymerized synthetic resins are found in both thermoplastic and thermosetting types of molding compounds. This can be explained by the fact that a synthetic resin in the thermoplastic class is fully polymerized when it is used as a molding compound, whereas a synthetic resin in a thermosetting molding material is only partially polymerized. The complete polymerization occurs in the actual molding or laminating operation.

Controlling rate of polymerization of thermosetting plastics

When fabricating plastics of the thermosetting type, it is usually necessary to adjust the rate of polymerization. The plastic may be polymerizing too fast, or it may not be polymerizing fast enough. The rate adjustment can be made by the addition of an accelerator or an inhibitor as the need dictates. An accelerator, or promoter, chemically activates the resin so that subsequent operation brings the resin to the desired polymerized state at a faster rate. The inhibitor holds back, or slows up, the rate of polymerization. The percentage of the promoter or inhibitor used depends on the storage temperature of the resin, the temperature of the working area, and the amount of working time required by the operator.

Laminated plastics

Laminates consist of base materials impregnated with a plastic resin, which is then allowed to harden under pressure. The plastic resins used are thermosetting and are hardened by polymerization. The base materials provide mechanical strength, and the resin provides rigidity and dimensional stability. Some of the base materials used are nylon, Dacron fabrics, fiberglass, boron, and Kevlar (aramid).

Laminated plastics are divided into three groups,

depending on the pressure used in their formation. The first group is *high-pressure laminates*. These laminates are formed from thermosetting materials under pressures ranging from 1000 to 2000 psi. They are strong, are light-weight, and have high-impact resistance. They are suitable for such uses as paneling, countertops, and safety helmets.

The second group, *low-pressure laminates*, use pressure ranging approximately from 15 to 1000 psi. Vacuum bag molding falls in this group. Layers of resin-impregnated, reinforcing fabric material is placed over the mold, and the layers are then covered with a flexible rubber sheeting or bag. The sheeting is sealed along the edges of the mold. Air is withdrawn between the mold and the sheeting, which causes atmospheric pressure (14.7 psi) to press the sheeting uniformly against the entire surface of the mold. With some changes in mold design, the same bag-molding principle can be used with positive air pressure considerably in excess of atmospheric pressure.

The third and final group, *contact pressure laminates*, are formed under as low as ¼ to 15 psi. This type of lamination is used in situations in which each piece has to be custom-made using hand pressure. Contact pressure laminates are usually made from thermosetting materials. They are economical, possess high strength, are lightweight, and can be formed in flat or three-dimensional shapes.

Cellular structures

Cellular plastics, or foamed plastics, consist of plastic resins that have been "foamed" or filled with bubbles of gas before the resin hardens. There are numerous ways of generating the gas bubbles in the resin, but a discussion of them goes beyond the scope of this book. It is sufficient to say that both thermoplastic and thermosetting resins can be used and that the foam structures resulting can be rigid, semirigid, or flexible as desired.

Sandwich constructions

Sandwich constructions are used where maximum stiffness is required for a given weight of material. They are made by laminating a cellular core between skins of metal or thin plastic-fabric laminates. The cellular cores may be resin-impregnated paper honeycombs, balsa wood, or cellular plastics.

Miscellaneous structures

Miscellaneous structures involving plastics that are of interest to the practitioner include glass and cotton fabrics coated with thermoplastic resins and fabrics of glass and plastic fibers woven together. After brief immersion in a solvent, these structures can be easily shaped to a form. When the solvent evaporates, a light, rigid formed article remains.

It is emphasized that the service success of any plastic article depends as much on the design and fabrication process as on the material itself. Frequently, good materials fail when the same material, if properly engineered, would have been quite satisfactory.

The type and amount of material (reinforcement) also plays a part in the service of the article. The practitioner must have a thorough understanding of the application for a device so that he or she can choose the proper plastic and the proper methods of fabrication.

Polyesters

Polyesters are versatile because they can be molded, cast, and laminated with contact pressure sleeves over inexpensive molds of plaster, rubber, or low-melting metals. Polyesters can range from rubber-like materials to hard, rigid substances. They are rapidly achieving great popularity for small-scale work. They do not liberate moisture in the curing process. Coloring possibilities are unlimited, and special grades are available that are flame-resistant or resistant to outdoor weathering. The chemical resistance of the different grades varies a great deal, but, in general, polyesters are swollen by ketones and esters and attacked by caustics. However, they are quite resistant to such common substances as gasoline, alcohol, acids, and moisture.

The unsaturated polyester resins range in color from clear water–white to light tan. Because of this, some are used in optical assemblies. However, one of their greatest uses is in fabric laminates, which, on a weight basis, are comparable to steel in strength and are extremely shock resistant as well. Using very low pressures, this fabric-resin combination can easily be formed into a large variety of shapes. The working time available before hardening can be controlled by adjusting temperature, catalyst, and promoter. The cured laminate is chemically stable and practically insoluble so that it forms a durable product.

Mixtures of polyesters and other resins are used in prostheses and orthoses to make laminated parts by contact lamination. A lamination made from 100% polyester resin is too brittle; therefore, mixtures of rigid and flexible resins are used. The flexible resins contain about 50% styrene by volume, the remainder being polyester. The composition of the mixtures ranges from 60% rigid and 40% flexible resin to 75% rigid and 25% flexible resin.

With special mixtures of resins, catalyst, and promoter, laminates can be formulated that bench cure without the use of external heating. The internal heat of reaction during polymerization is adequate to complete the cure. However, a toxic gas is given off during the curing process, and it is often recommended that all polyester laminates be heat cured to drive off all of the gas. It is felt that there is a risk of toxic reaction to the patient if any of the gas remains in the laminate. The toxic gases can originate from the use of certain plasticizers, such as tricresyl phosphate, which are vaporized by the heat given off during the curing process. Heat curing is usually done in an oven at a temperature of about 250° F.

Two types of polyester resin can be used for making laminates: the air-inhibited type and the non-air-inhibited type. Inhibition is the slowing down of polymerization or curing of the resin because of the presence of atmospheric oxygen. Usually a wax additive is used as a seal. It acts by migrating to the surface of the resin and forming a protective coating.

The air-inhibited resins require careful control of the air seal and manual mixing to control the flexibility. The flexibility range can be from 100% rigid to 100% flexible. The non-air-inhibited types have a preformulated flexibility. An air seal for these types is advisable but not required.

Uses for polyester laminates include sockets, cuffs, and artificial hands. Other devices used are mentioned in the instruction on lamination given later in this chapter.

Laminating plastic parts

Laminated plastic parts for orthoses and prostheses are best prepared over plaster of Paris forms. After the plaster has dried completely, it should be coated with a lubricant. In one method of laminating, the fabric is next placed in contact with the plaster form, and a thin coating of resin, sufficient to saturate the fabric, is applied to the exposed surface. Then a dry piece of fabric is smoothed into place in such a way as to provide intimate contact between the two layers of fabric and to force any excess resin to the surface. Another coat of resin and another piece of fabric are alternately added until the desired thickness is obtained. The whole assembly is then surrounded by a polyvinyl alcohol bag, excess resin is squeezed out, and the laminate is then oven cured.

In another plastic lamination method, tubular nylon or cotton stockinette is used as a resin reinforcement. Normally, three or four layers of the material are placed on the inner PVA bag on the cast to which has been applied a release agent. If there are indications of extra strength requirements, stronger materials, such as glass cloth or special metal reinforcements, may be used in particularly critical areas.

After the stockinette has been pulled over the plaster cast and tied, a snug-fitting PVA bag is pulled over the stockinette to form a tight and smooth outer surface. Prepared polyester resin is then poured into the outer PVA sleeve as shown in Figure 2.63 and made to impregnate the reinforcing stockinette. When the resin has been poured, the tapered, outer PVA sleeve is

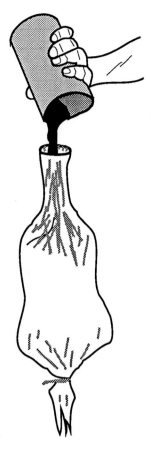

Fig. 2.63. Pouring polyester resin.

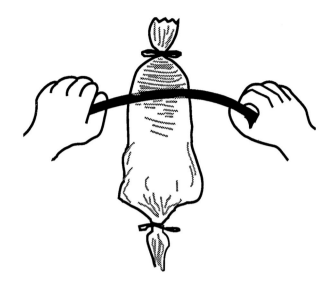

Fig. 2.64. Uniformly distributing resin.

Table 2.12. Gel times for Laminac 4128 (Lupersol ATC catalyst)		
GEL TIME (MINUTES)	PROMOTER*	CATALYST*
20	0.5	2.5
30	0.5	2.0
40	0.5	1.5
50	0.4	1.5
60	0.3	2.0
70	0.2	2.5
80	0.3	1.5
90	0.2	2.0

*Percent of resin by weight.

pulled down farther to increase the mold pressure and force the resin to impregnate the stockinette more effectively as well as to force air from the resin. The resin itself acts as a lubricant to facilitate the additional downward movement of the PVA sleeve. The sleeve provides a necessary airtight seal to insure airless cure of the polyester.

It is necessary to tie the end of the PVA bag and proceed with the *stringing* process using a light but strong cord. As shown in Figure 2.64, a length of this cord, held between the hands, is pressed against the outside PVA bag and moved up and down to distribute the resin uniformly and to eliminate air pockets.

The plastic laminate is then bench cured for about 45 minutes. Finally, an oven cure at 180 to 200° F for about 45 minutes is employed to complete the curing and solidification of the plastic. When curing has been completed, the PVA is stripped away, and excess cured plastic is removed.

Preparation of laminating resin

Some of the common polyesters used for lamination are Laminac 4110 (rigid), 4134 (flexible), and 4128 (general purpose). Another popular brand is Paraplex P43 (rigid) and Paraplex P13 (flexible).

The gel times for Laminac 4128 using Lupersol ATC catalyst (benzoyl peroxide paste in 50% tricresyl phosphate) and Naugatuck promoter No. 3 at room temperature (70° F) are given in Table 2.12.

Catalysts and promoters

The use of catalysts and promoters is an extremely important part of the technology of polyester resins. The conversion of the liquid resin to a solid infusible condition can be induced by the use of a catalyst, usually an organic peroxide, and the application of heat. Promoters are used to activate the catalyst to develop cure at room temperature or to accelerate heat cure.

Reaction is highly exothermic, and the total heat liberated during complete cure is a constant for any specific polyester resin. For a typical Laminac polyester resin of intermediate reactivity, the exotherm is in the order of 140 Btu per pound. Under strictly adiabatic conditions, this amount of heat would cause a temperature increase during the cure of about 280° F, so that if the cure is initiated at 180° F, the temperature would then rise to 460° F, whereas initiation at room temperature would give a peak temperature of about 350° F. Under practical conditions much of the heat is dissipated by radiation and conduction; consequently the actual temperature rise depends on the material of construction, mass of the cast and rate of cure as well as the initial temperature. If an excess of catalyst and promoter is used, the temperature may rise extremely fast toward the theoretical maximum causing adverse effects such as blistering or voids within the molded piece. A deficiency of catalyst may give such a slow exotherm that the cure is not self-propagating. Postcure would then be required.

Although the behavior during curing can be controlled to some extent by the resin manufacturer, the user can exercise far wider control by the judicious use of available catalysts and promoters. Both the rate of gelation and the rate of final cure can be controlled.

The most widely used peroxide catalysts are benzoyl peroxide, cumene hydroperoxide, and methylethyl ketone peroxide. Other peroxides available commercially and that may be of value under certain specific conditions include diteriary butylhydroperoxide, cyclohexanone peroxide, and chlorobenzoyl peroxide. They fall into two general classifications, high and low temperature types, but the former type can usually be activated at room temperatures by the use of the proper promoter.

Benzoyl peroxide is best suited for high temperature applications and methylethyl ketone peroxide for low temperatures. The former is a white granular solid sometimes used in the form of a 50% dispersion in tricresyl phosphate. Methylethyl ketone peroxide is available as a 60% solution in dimethyl phthalate. Cumene hydroperoxide is a liquid and is one of the lowest-priced catalysts now available. It is generally used at relatively high temperatures.

Cobalt naphthenate is the most widely used promoter for low temperature work. The commercial solutions usually contain 6% cobalt metal. From 0.66% to 0.3% of solution based on resin may be used, equivalent to a range of 0.004% to 0.18% cobalt. The effect on cure time increases rapidly with increasing concentrations up to 0.012% cobalt but almost levels off at 0.018% to 0.02%. The color introduced by cobalt is occasionally a disadvantage in some applications, particularly at the higher concentrations. Laminac resins 4102, 4110, 4116, 4128, and 4134 contain some cobalt as supplied and may require no further addition.

Laminac promoters 400 and 601 are available for use with Laminac resins for accelerating the effect of peroxides or for promoting their activity at low tem-

Table 2.13. Gel times for Laminac resin 4123

GEL TIME (MINUTES AT 77° F)	BENZOYL PEROXIDE (%)	LAMINAC PROMOTER (%)
110–130	0.5	0.5
40–60	1.0	1.0
20–30	1.0	2.0
4–8	2.0	4.0

peratures. Some general information is given here on the use of these materials, but technical representatives should be consulted about further details. The following information on catalysts is of a general nature. Reference should be made to the individual Laminac resin data sheets for further data.

Benzoyl peroxide. Benzoyl peroxide is the catalyst most often used for formulations to be cured above 170° F. From 0.25% to 1.5% may be used (0.5% to 3% of the 50% paste). The lower concentrations are desirable for thick cross sections. Cure times range from 1 to 15 minutes, depending on temperatures and catalyst concentration. Benzoyl peroxide in the absence of a promoter is relatively inactive at ordinary temperatures and catalyzed solutions may be held for days at room temperature. Stability is further extended below 60° F.

Laminac Promoter 400 may be used with benzoyl peroxide to reduce cure times at elevated temperatures or to induce gelation at low temperatures. The gel times shown in Table 2.13 can be obtained at 77° F with Laminac Resin 4123. Similar results are obtained with other styrene-type Laminac resins. Under certain conditions, the cure may not become complete at room temperature and a short period of heat cure may be necessary to gain maximum hardness.

Methylethyl ketone peroxide. Methylethyl ketone peroxide catalyst can be activated at room temperature by cobalt naphthenate or an organic promoter. Its activity at room temperature is low in the absence of a promoter. The rate of cure is sensitive to the amount of promoter used. This is particularly the case with cobalt in the range of 0.004% to 0.02% (Figure 2.65). The effect of increasing the cobalt concentration above 0.02% is not as pronounced.

Gel times at room temperatures of a few minutes can be obtained if a catalyst concentration above 1% is used with the cobalt naphthenate promoter. To develop a practical working life under these conditions, the dual-spray technique can be applied using the catalyst in one portion of the resin and cobalt in the other.

A combination of a low concentration of methylethyl ketone peroxide and promoter with the normal amount of benzoyl peroxide or cumene hydroperoxide provides

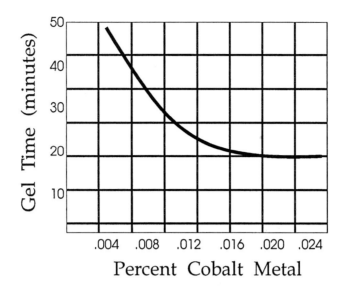

Fig. 2.65. Effect of cobalt content on gel time.

good working life, low temperature set, and good final cure. After the low-temperature catalyst starts to react, the exotherm gives a temperature increase to the range where the high-temperature catalysts are effective. Typical set times using methylethyl ketone peroxide 60% solution as catalyst and cobalt naphthenate as promoter with most styrene-type Laminac resins are shown in Table 2.14.

In formulating for white or pastel-colored laminates, cobalt should be kept to as low a concentration as possible to minimize effect on color.

Cumene hydroperoxide. The use of this material is suggested for intermediate temperatures within the range 150 to 200° F. Its cost is low, and it has a minimum tendency to bleach pigments or dyes. The use of a promoter is advisable. Laminac Promoter 601, used in a concentration of 0.05% to 0.10% with 0.5% to 1.5% cumene hydroperoxide, gives fast cure at 150° F. It may be desirable to add a small amount of benzoyl peroxide to insure complete final cure. The higher concentrations of catalyst and promoter give gelation at room temperature in 1 to 2 hours.

Other catalysts. In general, the fabricator is able to work out a formulation suitable for most applications using the aforementioned catalysts and promoters. Other catalysts such as cyclohexanone peroxide may be found useful under certain specific conditions. Tertiary butyl hydroperoxide has been reported as an excellent catalyst for the cure of parts designed for electrical applications.

Laminac promoters 400 and 601. Laminac Promoter 400 is effective in promoting room temperature cure with benzoyl peroxide catalyst. Concentrations of 1% to 2% are generally suggested with 0.5% to 2.0% benzoyl peroxide to give cure times ranging from 20 to

Table 2.14. Typical set times for methylethyl ketone peroxide*		
	PERCENT	
GEL TIME (MINUTES)	**MEK PEROXIDE 60% SOLUTION**	**COBALT (6%) NAPHTHENATE**
70–90	0.5	0.10
40–50	0.5	0.25
20–30	1.0	0.25
10–15	2.0	0.25

*60% solution with cobalt naphthenate as promoter.

180 minutes at normal room temperatures. Further data are available in the individual data sheets on Laminac. Dual spray gun technique is advisable when using the higher concentrations of catalyst and promoter. Laminac Promoter 601 is suggested for use with cumene hydroperoxide. As indicated previously under the description of the catalyst, it is effective in promoting gelation at room temperature or in promoting cure at 150° F or higher.

THERMOFORMING PLASTICS

Thermoplastic materials can be repeatedly softened by elevated heating and hardened by cooling. Thermoplastics make up 88% to 90% of all plastics processed.

Any thermoplastic resin that can be extruded or calendared into sheet or film can be thermoformed.

Those with low strength at forming temperature, however, may be difficult to form. Sheet and film are produced by extrusion, coextrusion, continuous casting, extrusion casting, calendaring, compression molding, autoclave, and press laminating. There are two types of thermoplastics.

Amorphous

Amorphous materials are devoid of crystallization (no definite order) and have a randomly ordered molecular structure. Their behavior is similar to a viscous, inelastic liquid. On heating, an amorphous sheet gradually softens and eventually acquires the characteristics of a liquid but without a definite point of transition from solid to liquid state. Amorphous materials normally have better hot strength characteristics than crystalline ones. Amorphous plastics are never as easy flowing as crystalline resins. When cooled, they do not reach a totally *non flowing* solid state. They do, therefore, have a tendency toward creep or movement with age when a load is applied. Such plastics as the following are amorphous: ABS, styrene, vinyl, acrylic, the celluosics, and polycarbonates.

Crystalline

Crystalline thermoplastic molecules are an orderly group of molecules and have a tendency to align in rigid, precise, highly ordered structures such as a chain link fence. This gives them good stiffness and low creep. Most of the crystalline materials used in thermoforming are also partly amorphous (e.g., polypropylene normally is about 65% crystalline and 35% amorphous). Unlike amorphous plastics, when crystalline sheet is heated, it remains stiff until it reaches the glass transition temperature (Tg). At the Tg, the crystalline material softens. In the case of HDPE, this temperature is above 257° F (at the Tg a natural HDPE sheet turns from translucent to transparent). This is also the minimum forming temperature of the sheet. As the sheet continues to become hotter, it rapidly becomes fluid. The next condition to occur is the ideal forming temperature. Unfortunately, with most crystalline materials, this is only a few degrees below the melt temperature. Consequently, much of this type of material is *cold formed* at the *orienting* temperature or slightly above. This can set up an excessive amount of internal stresses causing the lowering of the heat distortion point, increased warpage, and less impact strength. This is why some of the crystalline materials are difficult to thermoform. The polypropylene resin suppliers in particular have improved the behavior of this polymer only recently to correct these problems.

Crystalline materials require a greater amount of heat than amorphous plastics to reach the Tg. Once at this temperature, little additional heat is required to reach the forming temperature. Nylon, polypropylene,

polyethylene, and acetal are common examples of crystalline materials.

Commonly used materials
Polypropylene
- *Characteristics*—notch sensitive; edges must be smooth; surface easily marred when hot; may warp or distort if removed from the mold too rapidly (ideally leave overnight).
- *Common uses*—all orthoses where rigidity is required.
- *Typical shrink*—1.5% to 2%.
Co-polymer
- *Characteristics*—will cold flow (creep); not as rigid or brittle as polypropylene; blanching or crazing develops at areas of high or cyclic stress; moderately notch sensitive (polish edges to avoid crazing).
- *Common uses*—all orthoses where some flexibility is required; prosthetic check sockets.
- *Typical shrink*—1.5% to 2%.
Polyethylene
- *Characteristics*—flexible and easy to vacuum form; cold flow under pressure with sustained use; thinner gauges can be cut by hand; not particularly notch sensitive (however, edges should be polished).
- *Common uses*—spinal and upper limb orthoses; orthoses in which greater flexibility is required.
- *Typical shrink*—low density, 1.5% to 3%; high density, 3% to 3.5%.
Surlyn (Ionomer)
- *Characteristics*—transparent (for optimum clarity, material should be worked over a bare, wet, warm cast); not as rigid or brittle as polypropylene; very tough; cold flows; may be solvent bonded; not affected by cold; notch sensitive (tears rather than cracks); can be worked at a wide range of temperatures.
- *Common uses*—check sockets; all orthoses.
Co-polyester (Durr-Plex)
- *Characteristics*—very rigid and brittle; difficult to judge proper working temperature; for best results and to reduce brittleness work with a warm cast (140° F).
- *Common uses*—check sockets.
Polycarbonate
- *Characteristics*—hydrophilic (must be hydrated 48 hours at 275° F for 3/8-inch-thick material; rigid at proper working temperature; sensitive to acetone and other solvents.
- *Common uses*—check sockets.
Kydex
- *Characteristics*—abrasion resistance; dimensionally stable; rigid; can be drape formed without vacuum.

Table 2.15.   Thermoforming processing temperature (°F)

MATERIAL	CAST AND SET	LOWER LIMIT	NORMAL FORMING	UPPER LIMIT
Polypropylene	190	290	310–325	331
Co-polymer	190	290	310–325	331
High-density polyethylene	180	260	275	331
Low-density polyethylene	180	260	275	331
Surlyn	130	200	250	450
Co-polyester	170	250	300	330
Polycarbonate	280	335	375	400
Kydex	—	—	380–390	400

- *Common uses*—TLSO body jackets; cervical orthoses.

Thermoforming processing temperature

Cast and set.   The set temperature is the temperature at which the thermoplastic sheet hardens and can be safely taken from the cast (Table 2.15). This generally is defined as the heat distortion temperature at 66 psi (ASTM D 648). The closer the cast temperature is to the set temperature, without exceeding it, the less internal stress and warping.

Lower processing limit.   This is the lowest possible temperature for the sheet before it is completely formed (see Table 2.15). Material formed at or below this limit has severely increased internal stress that can cause warpage, lower impact strength, and other poor physical properties.

Normal forming.   This is the temperature at which the sheet should reach for proper forming conditions under normal circumstances (see Table 2.15). The core of the sheet should be at this temperature. The normal forming temperature is determined by heating the sheet to the highest temperature at which it still has enough hot strength or elasticity to be handled, yet below the degrading temperature.

Upper limit.   This is the temperature at which the thermoplastic sheet begins to degrade or decompose (see Table 2.15). It is crucial to ensure that the sheet temperature stays less than this amount. When using radiant heat, the sheet surface temperature should be carefully monitored to avoid degradation while waiting for the "core" of the material to reach forming temperature. These limits can be exceeded, for a short time only, with a minimum impairment to the sheet properties.

The least amount of internal stress is obtained by a hot cast, hot sheet, and a rapid vacuum.

Sheet selection

When selecting a sheet of plastic for forming, several factors have to be considered: (1) depth of draw, (2) desired finished thickness, (3) rigidity, and (4) shrink. The deeper the draw, the larger the sheet should be. By forcing a small sheet to stretch over a deep draw, shrink, additional stress, and uneven wall thickness can occur in the finished product.

A rule of thumb for forming sockets is the material sheet size should be twice as large as the depth of the draw to allow for the natural flow of material. An 8-inch draw would require a 16-inch piece of material. If the plastic is forced over a longer pull, it increases the stress in the plastic and increases the probability of increased shrink. This sizing has to be adjusted by considering the size of vacuum systems, finished wall thickness desired, available sheet sizes, and temperature of the cast.

Sheet heating considerations

Once the type of material and the sheet size have been selected, the next operation is to heat the plastic. The sheet of plastic should be supported in the center of the oven, allowing air to circulate on all sides. If the sheet is supported against the side of the oven, the air flow in that area is reduced and causes uneven heating.

To insure that the sheet is being heated evenly, the oven needs to be calibrated. To calibrate the oven, support a frame or grid inside the oven at the same position the plastic is to be heated. Using an accurate thermometer, take rapid readings every 4 to 6 inches, left to right and front to rear. Note any variations. If the variations are greater than 5° F, it is advisable to baffle or shadow the hot areas to as even a heat as possible.

During the heating of the plastic, minimize the number of times the doors of the oven are opened. This affects the heat cycles and may produce hot and cold spots throughout the sheet. When the plastic is completely heated and removed from the oven, avoid drafts from the doors, windows, or air conditioning vents, which can also cause cold spots in the sheet. Cold spots can cause uneven wall thickness, difficulties in forming, warping, and irregular surface finishes.

As the sheet is heated, the heat is transferred to the sheet by the circulating hot air. Also, heat is transferred to the sheet through the metal frames if the metal frame is clamped tightly to the sheet. The metal frame transfers heat to the sheet much faster than the air

Table 2.16. *K* factors (*K* = btu/hr-ft²-°F)		
MATERIAL	*K* FACTOR	HEAT TRANSFER RATE*
Air (ref.)	0.106	0.76
Wool felt	0.021	1.00
Spruce	0.052	2.50
Maple	0.094	4.50
Epoxy	0.131	6.20
Plaster of Paris	0.174	8.3
Alum-filled epoxy	0.50–0.99	24–47
Acrylic	1.4	67
Stainless steel	9.4	448
Bronze	20.5	976
Steel	26.0	1238
Kirksite	60.4	2876
Aluminum	115	5476

*Heat transfer rate factor—compared to wool felt.

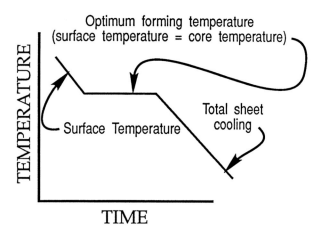

Optimum forming temperature (surface temperature = core temperature)

Fig. 2.66. Surface temperature.

around the plastic. This can be seen in increased thinning along the edges. To overcome this effect, insulate the plastic from the frame. See *K* factor (Table 2.16) for possible insulating materials.

The hot air comes in contact with the surface of the plastic, and heat transfer begins. The heat then migrates toward the center of the sheet increasing the total sheet temperature. In this process, however, there is uneven heating in the sheet because the outer surface is hotter than the internal core temperature (Fig. 2.66).

To heat a sheet more quickly, it is common to set the oven temperature higher than the upper limit temperature of the material. If excessive heat is absorbed by the plastic, the surface of the material begins to deteriorate.

If a sheet of polypropylene is heated with an oven set at 375 to 400° F, the plastic surface temperature is close to that temperature. The upper limit for polypropylene is 331° F. At the point that the material turns from milky to clear, it has reached the lower processing limit or the Tg point. The sheet now has a temperature gradient of 375° F at the surface to 290° F at the core. If the plastic is formed at this point, there are stresses, uneven forming, and uneven surface finishes. The sheet needs to reach equilibrium before it is formed.

A blast of cool air on the surface helps reduce the surface temperature and solidify the surface for a better finish. This procedure is tricky because the sheet is so close to the lower processing temperature. If the sheet cools too rapidly, it tends to warp from internal stresses. By referring back to the *K* factors table (see Table 2.16), it can be seen that plaster of Paris has a significantly greater *K* factor than air. When forming over a plaster cast, the plaster removes the heat much faster than the

outside air. The effects of this uneven cooling can be seen in body jackets. Body jacket plastic is formed directly on the plaster cast and has a tendency to curl inwardly after removal. Conversely, plastic that is formed against a foam liner has a tendency to curl outwardly after removal.

It is important to maintain the vacuum on the part until the entire plastic sheet reaches the set temperature of the plastic. With the low thermal conductivity of plastic, it takes several minutes for the core temperature to drop to the set temperature. It is not uncommon to maintain vacuum on a thick part for up to 1 hour.

Figure 2.67 shows the effect of removing the vacuum too soon. The memory of the sheet causes the return to its original flat shape.

Another effect that occurs is a thickening of material on the first surface contacted by the hot plastic (Fig. 2.68). The plaster cast chills the plastic and prevents it from being formed with uniform thickness over the entire cast.

Heating thermoplastics

The three methods of heating are convection, conduction, and radiation.

Convection. This is the slowest heating process. Convection heat transfer takes place when a material is exposed to a moving fluid (e.g., recirculating hot air) that is at a higher temperature.

Convection heating in the thermoforming industry is done with the use of a recirculating hot air oven. The oven temperature is carefully maintained at the thermoforming temperature of the particular material to be formed. Air is a greater insulator, and plastic materials absorb heat slowly, thus causing this method to be relatively slow. The specific heat of the particular material governs the heating cycle. When comparing convection heating with radiant heating, it is extremely slow. For example, a 0.125-inch-thick acrylic sheet has

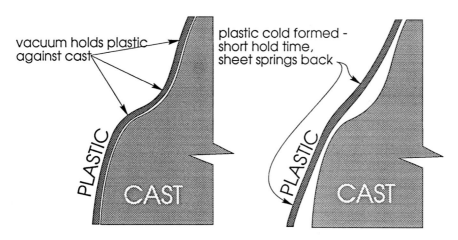

Fig. 2.67. Effect of inadequate vacuum hold time.

a specific heat of 0.35. In a well-baffled hot air recirculating oven running at the forming temperature of 360° F throughout, about 1 minute of heating is required for every 10 mils of sheet thickness. With radiant heat and using the proper wave length, 0.125-inch acrylic sheet can be brought to a core temperature of approximately 350 to 360° F in 2.1 minutes.

The main advantage of convection heat is its uniformity of heating and the ability to keep the sheet surfaces from getting hotter than the oven temperature. This method is recommended when heating (1) heavy-gauge foam sheet; (2) very thick, solid sheet; (3) sheet stock where the thickness is difficult to control accurately; (4) sheet where surfaces have been planished (heat-press polished); and (5) when surfaces might degrade easily if overheated. To hasten the cycle time, the oven can be run at a higher temperature than the normal forming range of the particular sheet. Care must be exercised when doing this to ensure that the surfaces of the sheet do not degrade. When a sheet heated in this manner is removed from the oven, it should be allowed to gain temperature equilibrium before it is formed.

The most accurate hot air recirculating ovens are electrically powered and for this reason are used whenever precise temperature control and heating is needed.

Conduction. This is a faster method than convection but slower than radiant. Heat transfer by conduction takes place when temperature gradients exist within a material.

Most conduction heater plates used in thermoforming are Teflon-coated aluminum plates that are electrically heated. Uniform heat can be maintained with electric heaters. The surface of the hot plate should have a uniform temperature and the same heat sink distribution throughout. As in convection heating, the contact plates are usually run at the same temperature as the forming temperature of the sheet. This prevents

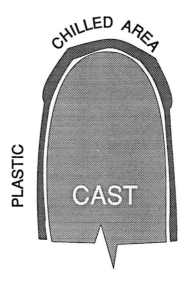

Fig. 2.68. Thickening effect.

degradation of the surface and gives extremely uniform heat even when sheet thickness varies.

Radiation. Radiation is the energy transmitted between two separated bodies (for thermoformers that is the sheet and the radiant heater surface) at different temperatures by means of electromagnetic waves. It is the most energy-efficient way of heating sheet material. Infrared wavelength radiation elements are the usual source of heat; the specific wavelength is related to a given temperature of a specific radiant heater.

All types of radiation have an important property in common: They all travel with the same velocity (the speed of light). This radiation can be considered as a transporter of energy. As the radiant emitter is directly exposed to the material to be processed, a high percentage of the electromagnetic waves are absorbed within the plastic sheet only if the emitter operates at the proper wavelength and the wavelength is determined strictly by the emitter-surface temperature. *Tuning* the radiant heater, to the particular material's best absorbing range, can be an advantage. Convection and conduction have to absorb and give up heat through contact of only the surface of the sheet and then transferred to the "core" by conduction, thus much slower and more inefficient than radiant heat.

Description of most popular heating elements

Small-Diameter Coiled Nichrome Wire
- *Efficiency*—new 16% to 18%; 6 months, 8% to 10%.
- *Average life*—1,500 hours.

Although the small-diameter coiled nichrome wire is least expensive, it is inefficient and heats nonuniformly with use.

Tubular Rods and Metal Panels
- *Efficiency*—new, 42%; 6 months, 21%.
- *Average life*—3,000 hours.

The tubular rods are also inexpensive, heat nonuniformly with use, and are difficult to screen or mask for profile heat.

Ceramic Panels and Quartz Panels
- Efficiency—new, 55% to 62%; 6 months, 48% to 55%.

- *Average life*—1200 to 1500 hours.

The ceramic and quartz panels are the most cost-efficient because they heat uniformly, are efficient, and are ideal for profile heating.

Gas Fired, Infrared Type
- *Efficiency*—new, 40% to 45%; 6 months, 25%.
- *Average life*—1000 to 6000 hours.

The gas-fired, infrared type of heating elements are inexpensive initially and inexpensive to operate but do not heat uniformly.

CONCLUSION

Successful orthotic management requires a clear understanding of the condition being treated and a realistic plan to address the biomechanical deficits presented. A thorough knowledge of the principles summarized in this chapter is the final prerequisite to insure that the orthosis provided is as durable, safe, and unobtrusive as possible. The engineering principles highlighted here are the fundamentals of modern orthotic design.

Appendix A begins on page 63.

A P P E N D I X   A

THERMAL STRESS

Example 1

A straight aluminum wire 100 feet long is subject to a tensile stress of 10,000 psi. Determine the total elongation of the wire. What temperature change would produce this same elongation? Take $E = 10^7$ psi and $\alpha = 12.5 \times 10^{-6}°$F. The total elongation is given by Eq 7:

$$\Delta L = \frac{FL_0}{AE} = \frac{(10,000)\,(100 \times 12)}{10^7}$$
$$\Delta L = 1.20 \text{ inches}$$

From Eq 6, it can be seen that a rise in temperature of ΔT would cause this same expansion if

$$1.20 = (12.5 \times 10^{-6})(100 \times 12)(\Delta T)$$
$$\Delta T = 78.2°\text{F}$$

CENTROIDS AND CENTER OF GRAVITY

Example 2

Calculate the centroid coordinates for a P-shaped object (Fig. 2.A1). This object can be divided into two rectangles (A_1 and A_2), one triangle (A_3), and a semicircle (A_4). Next draw a Cartesian coordinate system with the origin at the bottom left. The centroid is calculated from Eq 9 as follows:

$$\bar{x} = \frac{\bar{x}_1 A_1 + \bar{x}_2 A_2 + \bar{x}_3 A_3 + \bar{x}_4 A_4}{A_1 + A_2 + A_3 + A_4}$$

$$\bar{y} = \frac{\bar{y}_1 A_1 + \bar{y}_2 A_2 + \bar{y}_3 A_3 + \bar{y}_4 A_4}{A_1 + A_2 + A_3 + A_4}$$

MOMENT OF INERTIA AND PARALLEL AXIS THEOREM

Example 3

To increase mediolateral stability in a KAFO a standard ⅝ inch by ³⁄₁₆ inch sidebar on a KAFO is reinforced by welding ⅝ inch by ³⁄₁₆ inch reinforcing ribs perpendicular to the sidebar proximal to the mechanical knee joint (Fig. 2.A2). Calculate the moment of inertia of the sidebar proximally ($A - A$) and distally ($B - B$) to the mechanical knee joint. The proximal sidebar cross section at $A - A$ is more complicated and is determined first.

Proximal (Fig. 2.A3). The moment of inertia for the proximal ($A - A$) section about the centroidal axis must be calculated from the parallel axis theorem:

$$I_{cc} = I_{xx} - Ad^2 = \text{parallel axis theorem}$$

However, the moment of inertia about the base, I_{xx}, and vertical centroid, d, must be determined first. If section $A - A$ is divided into two rectangles (Fig. 2.A3), then

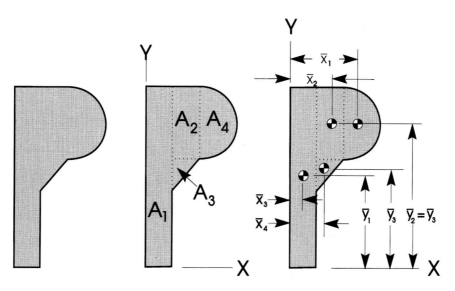

Fig. 2.A1.   Centroid analysis.

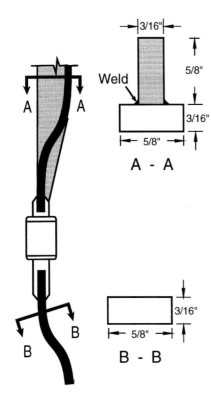

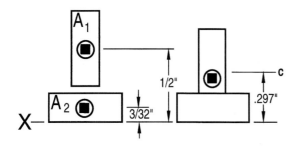

Fig. 2.A2.   Knee joint reinforcement.

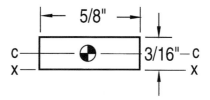

Fig. 2.A4.   Section *B-B* centroid.

$$d = \bar{y} = 0.297 \text{ in. (for section } A - A)$$

In general, $I = bh^3/12$ for a rectangle:

$$I_1 = \frac{(^3/_{16})(^5/_8)^3}{12} = 0.00381 \text{ in.}^4$$

$$I_2 = \frac{(^5/_8)(^3/_{16})^3}{12} = 0.00034 \text{ in.}^4$$

$$A_1 d^2 = (^5/_8)(^3/_{16})(^1/_2)^2 = 0.0293 \text{ in.}^4$$

$$A_2 d^2 = (^5/_8)(^3/_{16})(0.297)^2 = 0.00103 \text{ in.}^4$$

$I_{xx} = (0.00381 + 0.0293 + 0.00034 + 0.00103) \text{ in.}^4 = 0.0345$
in.^{4} = moment of inertia about base of section $A - A$

Solving for Ad^2:

$$A = (2)(^5/_8)(^3/_{16}) = 0.234 \text{ in.}^2 = d^2 = y^2 = (0.297)^2 = 0.0882 \text{ in.}^2$$

$$Ad^2 = (0.234 \text{ in.}^2)(0.0882 \text{ in.}^2) = 0.0207 \text{ in.}^4$$

Apply the parallel axis theorem:

$$I_{cc} = I_{xx} - Ad^2 = \text{parallel axis theorem}$$

$$I_{cc} = 0.0345 \text{ in.}^4 - 0.0207 \text{ in.}^4 = 0.0138 \text{ in.}^4$$

Distal.   (Fig. 2.A4, section $B - B$):

$$I_{cc} = \frac{(^5/_8)(^3/_{16})^3}{12} = I_{cc} = 0.00034 \text{ in.}^4$$

Note that I_{cc} (proximal)/I_{cc}(distal) = 40.6; that is, the proximal section of the sidebar is over 40 times as stiff as the distal section.

BEAM STRESS AND DEFLECTION

Example 4

The conventional AFO and KAFO contain sidebars that are subjected to bending stress in the mediolateral (coronal) and anterior-posterior (sagittal) planes. The

Fig. 2.A3.   Section *A-A* centroid.

total moment of inertia of the two rectangles about the base is

$$I_{xx} = (I_1 + A_1 d_1^2) + (I_2 + A_2 d_2^2)$$

$$d = \bar{y} = \frac{A_1 \bar{y}_1 + A_2 \bar{y}_2}{A_1 + A_2}$$

The variable d in the parallel axis theorem is, in this case, the same as the y-centroid. Given that $A_1 = A_2 = {}^5/_8$ inch $\times {}^3/_{16}$ inch = 0.117 in.^{2} and that $y_1 = {}^3/_{16} + {}^1/_2({}^5/_8)$ = 0.5 and $y_2 = {}^1/_2({}^3/_{16}) = 0.09375$ inch, the y-centroid of section A - A is

$$d = \bar{y} = \frac{(0.117)(0.5) + (0.117)(0.09375)}{0.234}$$

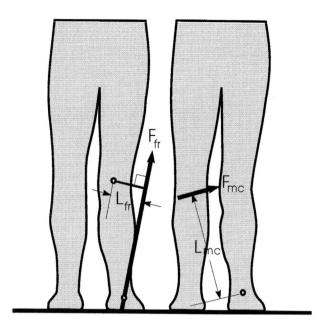

Fig. 2.A5. Valgum control.

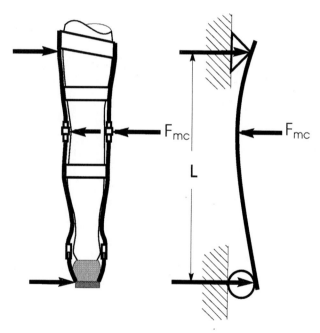

Fig. 2.A6. KAFO free body diagram.

sidebars may be treated as a freely supported beam with a midspan load. For example, consider the valgum condition illustrated in Figure 2.A5. The torque responsible for the valgum is given by:

$$T_{val} = F_{fr} \times L_{fr}$$

where

  F_{fr} = single limb stance floor reaction, pounds, and
  L_{fr} = floor reaction lever at knee joint, inches.

Assume that mediolateral flexibility in both the knee and the subtalar joints allows correction of the valgum deformity. A laterally directed force at the medial condyle, F_{mc}, restrains (or corrects) the valgum deformity. This force and its lever to the subtalar joint, L_{mc}, must produce at least as much torque as the deforming force and lever, or:

$$F_{mc} \times L_{mc} \geq F_{fr} \times L_{fr}$$

$$F_{mc} \geq (F_{mc} \times L_{fr}) \div L_{mc}$$

Typical values for the variables in the above equation are F_{fr} = body weight (assume 150 lb), L_{fr} = 4 inches, and L_{mc} = 17 inches. Under these circumstances, the medially directed force would be F_{mc} = 35.3 lb. The free body diagram of a KAFO that experiences this force is shown in Figure 2.A6.

The freely supported KAFO with medially directed valgum force (Fig. 2.A6) is replaced with two sidebars rigidly attached by way of the calf and distal thigh bands (Fig. 2.A6). This double-sidebar arrangement is replaced with a single beam composed of double-thickness sidebars (Fig. 2.A6). The medially directed valgum force is a distance $L/2$ from both the proximal and the distal ends. Recall from Eq 17 that the stress in a freely supported beam is given by

$$\sigma = \frac{3FL}{2bh^2} = 6025 \text{ psi}$$

where
$\quad F$ = 35.3 pounds,

L = 10 inches (assumed distance from distal thigh band to calf band),
$\quad b$ = ⅝ inch = AP thickness of sidebar, and
$\quad h$ = ⅜ inch = 2 × ³⁄₁₆ inch = ML thickness of two sidebars.

Recall from Eq 21 that the maximum deflection of a freely supported beam is given by

$$y_{\max} = -\frac{FL^3}{48EI} = -0.267 \text{ inch}$$

where E = Young's modulus = 10^7 psi, and

$$I = \frac{bh^3}{12} = \frac{(⅝)(⅜)^3}{12} = 2.75 \times 10^{-3} \text{ in.}^4$$

The stress in the sidebars is over 6000 psi, and the deflection is −0.267 inch (minus sign means inward).

Normal and Pathological Gait

Jacquelin Perry

Walking uses a complex interaction of hip, knee, ankle, and foot motions to advance the body in the desired line of progression. Forces with an ever-changing alignment are imposed on the supporting limb by the weight of the body. Selective muscle action controls these motions and forces for two essential functions: weight-bearing stability and progression over the supporting foot. In addition, the physical strain of walking is reduced by two accessory functions: shock absorption and energy conservation. Effectiveness of these gait mechanics is summarized by the individual's stride characteristics (e.g., velocity) and energetics.

NORMAL GAIT

Each limb blends the patterns of motion, passive force, and muscular control into a sequence of activity (called a *gait cycle* or a *stride*), which is repeated endlessly until the desired destination is reached. The two limbs perform in a reciprocal manner, offset by 50% of the gait cycle. The head, neck, trunk, and pelvis are self-contained passengers riding on the limb's locomotor system.[12]

Basic functions

The normal interactions of joint motion and muscle activity of walking serve four basic functions. Although each is described as a separate event, they occur in an overlapping fashion during the stride.

Weight-bearing stability. In a serial fashion, the extensor muscles maintain the limb's ability to support body weight. This begins with the hamstrings and quadriceps preparing the swinging limb for stance. Responding to the rapid drop of body weight onto the foot, the hip extensors and quadriceps stabilize the flexed hip and knee, while the hip abductors support the pelvis. As body weight progresses over the foot, the ankle plantar flexors restrain the tibia and provide indirect extensor stability of the hip and knee.

This pattern of muscle control is dictated by the changing alignment of the body weight line (vector) with the individual joints. As the vector moves away from the joint center, a rotational moment develops that must be controlled by opposing muscles to preserve postural stability.

Progression. To advance the weight-bearing limb over the supporting foot (i.e., stance limb progression), three rocker actions are used. A fourth rocker initiates swing limb advancement. The sites of progression are the heel, ankle, forefoot, and toe.

1. *Heel Rocker:* Following floor contact, the descent of body weight through the tibia plantar flexes the ankle while the pretibial muscles slow the rate of foot drop. This creates an unstable period of heel-only support, which rolls the limb forward on the rounded calcaneus.
2. *Ankle Rocker:* As momentum advances the body vector, ankle dorsiflexion allows the stance limb to roll forward over the stationary foot. Stance stability depends on graded restraint by the ankle plantar flexor muscles.
3. *Forefoot Rocker:* Heel rise moves body weight onto the forefoot. Both the foot and the limb roll forward over the unstable area of support provided by the rounded metatarsal heads.
4. *Toe Rocker:* Advancement of the body weight vector to the metatarsophalangeal (MP) joint allows the foot to dorsiflex rapidly about the base of the toes. The knee is unlocked and swing limb advancement initiated. Dorsiflexion availability at the ankle and MP joints is the critical factor.

The two forces stimulating progression are forward fall of body weight and momentum created by the swinging limb. From a quiet stance, forward fall is initiated by flexion of the swing limb and calf muscle relaxation, which allows the weight-bearing tibia to advance.

Shock absorption. The impact of rapid body weight transfer onto the limb is dissipated by knee flexion redirecting the force to the quadriceps. This action is initiated by the heel rocker.

Energy conservation. Selective relaxation of the muscles when momentum and passive positioning can substitute conserves energy. Cocontraction of antagonists is rare. The normal occurrences are hamstrings and quadriceps during limb loading and anterior and posterior tibialis for medial foot control.

Floor contact pattern

The simplest system for subdividing the continuum of activity that constitutes walking uses the timing of foot-floor contact as a frame of reference. The moment of initial floor contact has been designated as the start of the gait cycle. Within each cycle, the period of floor contact by any part of the foot is called *stance*. This is followed by an interval of midair limb advancement called *swing*. At the beginning and end of stance, there is an interval when both limbs are in contact with the floor for weight transfer. These intervals are called *initial* and *terminal double stance*. In between is a longer interval of *single-limb stance*, at which time the other foot is in the air. A more functional term is *single-limb support*. The limitation of this temporal classification system is that the divisions impart minimal indications of function.

Functional phases of gait

To understand the purpose of the individual joint motions and their modes of control, it is necessary to consider the action of the whole limb as the posture of each segment is influenced by the others. During a gait cycle, the limb moves through eight functionally distinct postural sequences, which are called phases of gait. Each has one or more events that is critical to accomplishing its purpose. These phases are combined into three primary tasks by the synergistic patterns of the muscles controlling the limb. Transitional actions between stance and swing create an offset in the phase sequence. Preparatory muscle action for stance starts in the final phase of swing (terminal swing), that is, before initial floor contact. Similarly, the preparatory events for swing begin in the final phase of stance (preswing) before the toe is lifted.

- **Task I: Weight Acceptance**
  Phase 1—Initial Contact: The way the foot contacts the floor is the first influence on the pattern of limb loading.
  Phase 2—Loading Response: There are three major functions: shock absorption to blunt the floor im-

pact force, limb stability to accept body weight, and preservation of progression.
- **Task II: Stance Limb Progression (Single-Limb Support)**
  Phase 3—Mid-Stance: The ankle serves as a rocker that allows the limb to advance over the stationary foot.
  Phase 4—Terminal stance: The forefoot provides a rocker that allows both the foot and the limb to roll forward.
- **Task III: Swing Limb Advancement**
  Phase 5—Pre-Swing: Actions at the ankle and hip of the unloaded limb initiate knee flexion in preparation for swing.
  Phase 6—Initial Swing: Muscle action at the hip, knee, and ankle lift the foot and advance the limb.
  Phase 7—Mid-Swing: The limb is advanced by continued hip flexion and early knee extension. With the tibia vertical, active foot support is required.
  Phase 8—Terminal Swing: Limb advancement is completed by knee extension, while further hip flexion is inhibited in preparation for stance.

INDIVIDUAL JOINT MOTION PATTERNS

Each joint makes a unique contribution to the functional demands of walking. This is reflected in the asynchronous nature of the motion patterns of the foot, ankle, knee, and hip.

Ankle and foot

During each stride, the ankle passes through four arcs of motion (Fig. 3.1). At the onset of stance, the ankle is in neutral dorsiflexion, and floor contact is by the heel. Loading the limb causes the ankle to plantar flex rapidly 10°. Following forefoot contact with the ground, ankle motion reverses to 10° dorsiflexion as the tibia advances over the stationary foot for stance limb progression. Then the ankle plantar flexes 20° during the final phase of stance (preswing). As toe-off starts swing, the foot again dorsiflexes under control of the pretibial muscles. Full elevation of the foot to neutral, however, is not completed until midswing.

The subtalar joint moves into eversion following initial floor contact by the heel. This unlocks the midtarsal joint, allowing it to dorsiflex slightly (arch flattens) following forefoot impact with the floor. Then the subtalar joint progressively inverts and locks the midtarsal joint through late midstance and terminal stance.

MP joint dorsiflexion is an essential component of heel rise. The foot rolls up over the base of the toes, particularly the great toe, as the trailing limb advances.[11]

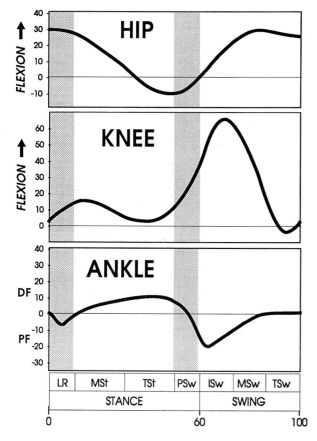

Fig. 3.1. Typical motion pattern of the limb during a gait cycle: Hip *(top)*, knee *(middle)*, and ankle *(bottom)*. *DF,* Dorsiflexion; *PF,* plantar flexion; *LR,* loading response; *MSt,* midstance; *TSt,* terminal stance; *PSw,* preswing; *ISw,* initial swing; *MSw,* midswing; *TSw,* terminal swing. *0,* Onset of gait cycle; *60,* end of stance; *100,* end of gait cycle.

Dorsiflexion control is provided by the pretibial muscles (tibialis anterior, extensor hallucis longus, and extensor digitorum) in swing and the loading response. The soleus and gastrocnemius control the tibia during stance limb progression and preswing.

Subtalar inversion control is available from the anterior tibialis, posterior tibialis, and soleus. Eversion restraint is provided by the peroneus brevis and peroneus longus muscles. Midtarsal restraint of the dorsiflexing forces created by body weight advancement is provided by the intrinsic flexor muscles as well as the subtalar muscles and the long toe flexors. The primary role of the flexor hallucis longus and flexor digitorum longus is to stabilize the MP joint during heel rise.

Knee

Within each gait cycle, the knee alternately flexes and extends both in stance and in swing (see Fig. 3.1). From a position of full extension at initial contact, the knee rapidly flexes 18° during weight acceptance. This is followed by progressive extension throughout the period of single stance, reaching a final position of 5° flexion. The knee then rapidly flexes to 40° during preswing and continues to 60° in initial swing. From this position, the knee then extends to neutral.

The quadriceps restrains knee flexion in stance and assists extension. All the vasti respond simultaneously. The gluteus maximus through its iliotibial band insertion also contributes to knee extensor stability. Brief and occasional action of the rectus femoris (and less frequently the vastus intermedius) restrains excessive preswing flexion. Knee flexion in swing is aided by the short head of the biceps femoris. Terminal swing knee extension is limited by the hamstring muscle group.

Hip

The major hip motions occur in the plane of progression (see Fig. 3.1). This consists of an arc of extension through stance, reaching 10° hyperextension in terminal stance. A similar arc of flexion occurs from preswing through midswing. The resulting 35° flexed posture is maintained in terminal swing and loading response. In the other planes, there are small (4-5°) arcs of postural accommodation, which are described as pelvic motions.

Hip extensor muscle action begins with the hamstrings in terminal swing and proceeds to the gluteus maximus and adductor magnus during the loading response. Lateral stability of the hip in stance is provided by the gluteus medius/minimus complex and the tensor fascia lata.

Hip flexion results from serial activation of several muscles: adductor longus (plus rectus femoris), iliacus, sartorius, and gracilis.

Pelvis

The pelvis moves through small (5°) arcs in each plane as it yields to body weight in stance and follows the advancing limb in swing. Stability is provided by the muscles of the weight-bearing hip.

Head and trunk

The basic function of the head and trunk is to maintain an upright posture. The small (5°) arcs of motion that occur reflect the uneven support provided by the reciprocal actions of the two limbs. Motion is greatest in the lumbar area and decreases at each higher segment. The spinal muscles act to preserve balance, absorb shock, and minimize head displacement.

INTEGRATED FUNCTION OF THE LIMB

Task I: weight acceptance

This is the first determinant of the ability to walk. Two objectives determine the events that occur during this task: the establishment of a stable limb for weight

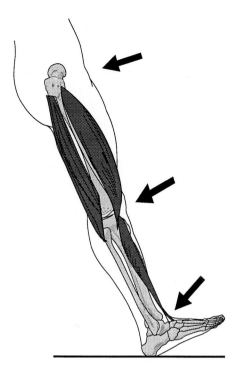

Fig. 3.2. Terminal swing pattern of muscle control. The limb is positioned for stance by synergistic action of the hamstrings (posterior thigh), quadriceps (anterior thigh), and tibialis anterior (anterior leg).

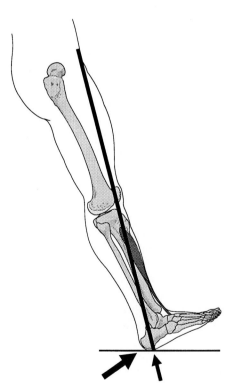

Fig. 3.3. Initial contact by the heel with pretibial muscle control (tibialis anterior shown) establishes the heel rocker. The vertical line represents the body weight vector. Both ground impact *(large arrow)* and base of the body weight vector *(small arrow)* are at the heel.

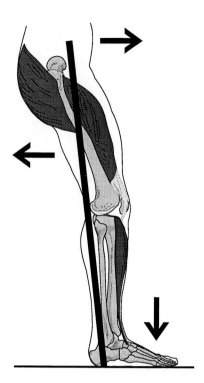

Fig. 3.4. Loading response vector *(vertical line)* is anterior to the hip (the flexor moment is restrained by the gluteus maximus), posterior to the knee (quadriceps restraint of the flexor moment), and posterior to the ankle (the plantar flexor moment is restrained by the tibialis anterior).

bearing and the minimization of the shock of floor impact. The last phase of swing and first two stance phases are dedicated to optimum weight acceptance.

Phase 8—terminal swing.   To prepare the swinging limb for stance, hip flexion is interrupted, the knee extends, and the ankle remains dorsiflexed (Fig. 3.2).

Rapid, intense action by the hamstring muscles (semimembranosus, semitendinosus, biceps femoris long head) stops hip flexion. These muscles then reduce their intensity and allow the quadriceps to extend the knee. The continuation of mild hamstring action prevents knee hyperextension from the residual tibial momentum. Pretibial muscle action supports the dorsiflexed foot.

Phase 1—initial contact.   Floor contact by the heel is the critical event (Fig. 3.3). Its purpose is to initiate the heel rocker. The significant postures are ankle dorsiflexion and full knee extension (see Fig. 3.3). Anterior tibialis control of the foot determines heel rocker effectiveness.

Phase 2—loading response (initial double stance).   This is a highly demanding phase of gait. The limb is destabilized by the heel rocker and then supported by strong extensor muscular response. There are three critical events (Fig. 3.4).

For both shock absorption and progression, the heel rocker drives the foot toward the floor as the limb is

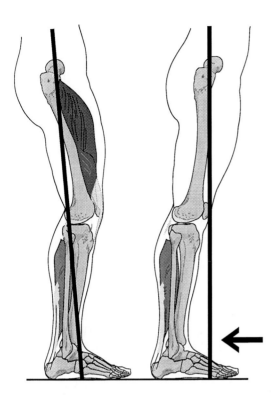

Fig. 3.5. Midstance progression of the limb over the stationary foot generates two patterns of muscle action. In early midstance *(left)*, the vector is behind the hip (no muscle action required) closer to the knee (less quadriceps) and anterior to the ankle (this dorsiflexor moment is retrained by the soleus). By late midstance *(right)*, the vector is anterior to the knee, and no quadriceps action is needed. The ankle dorsiflexor moment has increased.

loaded. Response of the pretibial muscles to decelerate the dropping foot pulls the tibia forward. This places the vector behind the knee, leading to rapid knee flexion for shock absorption. Prompt quadriceps response opposes the vector's flexor moment to preserve knee stability and absorb the shock of the initial floor impact.

Dorsiflexor muscle control is sufficiently incomplete to allow ankle plantar flexion of 10° for relatively early forefoot contact. This curtails the quadriceps demand. Knee extensor stability is aided by the femoral stability gained from the adductor magnus and gluteus maximus. Prompt relaxation of the hamstring muscles avoids an unnecessary flexor force.

At the hip, there is a rapid response by the abductor muscle group to stabilize the pelvis, which lost its contralateral support with the transfer of body weight to the forward limb.

Task II: stance limb progression

The basic function is advancement of the limb (and body) over the supporting foot. This is the second determinant of the ability to walk. Two phases of

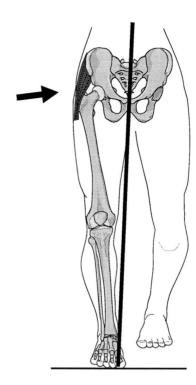

Fig. 3.6. Single-limb stance creates an adductor moment at the hip as the pelvis, with midline vector medial to hip, is unsupported. Gluteus medius action restrains the adductor moment.

single-limb support are involved as the means of progression differ.

Phase 3—midstance. The critical event is ankle dorsiflexion for progression of the stance limb over a stationary, flat foot (Fig. 3.5). As momentum from the contralateral swing limb moves the vector along the foot, the soleus (quickly assisted by the gastrocnemius) modulates the tibial advancement so it proceeds less rapidly than the femur. This provides passive extension of the hip and knee for weight-bearing stability. As a result, the hip extensor and quadriceps muscles rapidly relax.

At the hip, there also is a major adducting moment as lifting the other limb for swing removes the support for that side of the pelvis (Fig. 3.6). This creates a large medial vector, which is restrained by the gluteus medius.

Phase 4—terminal stance (late single stance). Heel rise is the critical event that continues progression (Fig. 3.7). Both the foot and the limb roll forward over the forefoot, which serves as a rocker. The large ankle dorsiflexion moment of the vector is opposed by strong soleus and gastrocnemius action. Passive hip and knee stability continues. There is no available force to restrain the foot's forward roll. By the end of this phase, body weight has moved ahead of the area of floor contact leading to free fall weight transfer to the other limb.

Task III: limb advancement

The ability to lift the foot is the third determinant of walking ability. Flexing the limb for floor clearance and swing advancement begins in the terminal double-support period of stance. Because the purpose is limb advancement rather than weight bearing, the phase has been titled *preswing*. The other actions occur throughout swing.

Phase 5—preswing.   Passive knee flexion to 40° is the critical event because this is the primary contributor to foot clearance of the floor in swing (Fig. 3.8).

Following floor contact by the other foot, body weight is rapidly transferred to that limb to catch the forward fall. This unloads the trailing limb, allowing several small forces to be effective. As the limb's trailing posture reduces the foot's floor contact to the anterior margins of the metatarsal heads and the toes (fourth rocker), there is no stabilizing force, so the foot as well as the leg is free to roll forward. This is accelerated by the rapid ankle plantar flexion stimulated by the release of the tension stored in the eccentrically stretched soleus and gastrocnemius. Passive knee flexion is initiated. Unloading the limb also releases the tension in the hip flexors. This force combined with adductor longus action initiates early hip flexion and assists knee flexion.

Phase 6—initial swing.   The critical event is knee flexion sufficient for the toe to clear the floor as the thigh advances. This involves total limb flexion (Fig. 3.9). Hip flexion may be a passive continuation of the preswing events or result from direct action by the iliacus, sartorius, and gracilis. Attainment of full knee flexion largely depends on the imbalance between the forward momentum of the femur generated by hip flexion and inertia of the tibia. Active assistance also is provided by the biceps femoris, short head. Brisk activation of the pretibial muscles initiates ankle dorsiflexion, but the arc is incomplete in initial swing.

Phase 7—midswing.   Ankle dorsiflexion to neutral is the critical event for floor clearance at this time (Fig. 3.10). Additional hip flexion and partial knee extension advance the limb. The relative vertical posture of the lower leg requires pretibial muscle support of the ankle.

Phase 8—terminal swing.   Forward swing of the limb for step length is accomplished by knee extension (see Fig. 3.2). The other actions relate to preparing the limb for stance as previously described.

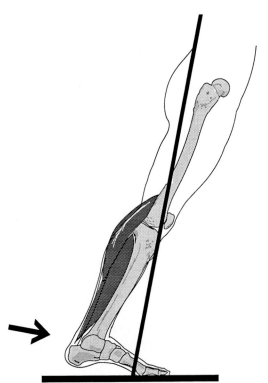

Fig. 3.7.   Terminal stance progression moves the vector to the forefoot, and the heel rises. The vector remains behind the hip and knee joints (knee hyperextension moment is restrained by the gastrocnemius). Vector alignment at the ankle creates a maximal dorsiflexion moment, which is restrained by the soleus and gastrocnemius.

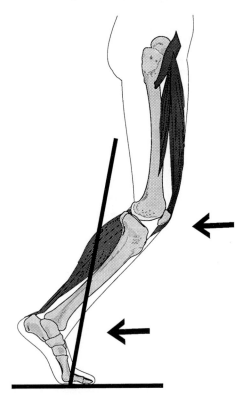

Fig. 3.8.   Preswing transfer of body weight to the other limb reduces the vector. The base of the vector now is at the metatarsophalangeal joint. The unloaded foot falls forward with the tibia as it follows the dorsiflexion moment. Gastro-soleus tension induces ankle plantar flexion. The knee flexes in response to the posterior moment, with rectus femoris restraint if needed. The posterior hip moment is opposed by the flexor component of the adductor longus and rectus femoris.

PATHOLOGICAL GAIT

Many types of disease and injury impair the patient's ability to walk. To the extent possible, patients accommodate their disability by altering the motion of adjacent joints or changing the timing and intensity of the controlling muscles. These substitutions increase the energy cost of walking. When the physiologic effort or pain exceeds the individual's tolerance, the disability becomes visible. To improve the patient's gait, the clinician must accurately identify the functional errors, differentiate the primary dysfunction from substitutive actions, correlate these events with the patient's pathology, and select the optimum corrective measures.

Pathological patterns

Systematic gait analysis can identify the specific modes of dysfunction. Interpretation of these findings for clinical management depends on an understanding of the functional penalties the different pathologies impose and the patient's ability to substitute.

To facilitate interpretation, the wide spectrum of causes that challenge the ability to walk has been grouped into five functional categories according to their anatomic and pathologic qualities.

Structural impairment. Although some lesions lead to hypermobility, restricted passive motion and malalignment are the more common problems. The contributing pathologies are contractures, skeletal deformity, and musculoskeletal pain.

Contractures. Freedom to move and attain optimal postures is readily impaired by fibrous connective tissue stiffness. Inactivity during the acute phase of illness, rigid immobilization for early healing, and stretch inhibition by spasticity are the major causes.

Fibrous tissue is present in every component of the musculoskeletal system (fascial sheaths, muscular aponeuroses, joint capsules, and ligaments). Stiffness is the inability of the strong, relatively inelastic collagen fibers to alter their alignment. Normally the collagen fibers move within the gel-like proteoglycan matrix that provides both support and lubrication.[1] With inactivity, the proteoglycan ground substance suffers chemical deterioration and loss of water. Measurable changes may occur within 2 weeks.[2]

Clinically, there are two levels of contracture: elastic and rigid. Both resist manual testing. The elastic contracture yields under body weight to allow near-normal function. A rigid contracture obstructs motion in both stance and swing. Walking can be significantly impaired by contractures. The most significant ones are ankle plantar flexion, knee flexion, and hip flexion.

Plantar flexion contractures of "mere" 15° can significantly impair stance limb progression. With the foot flat,

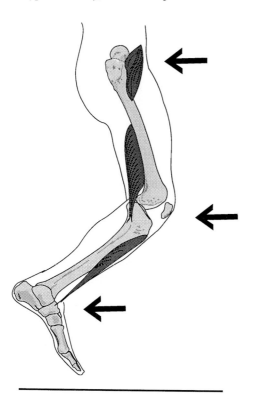

Fig. 3.9. Initial swing advancement of the limb by simultaneous active flexion at the hip (iliacus) and knee (biceps femoris, short head) and ankle dorsiflexion (tibialis anterior).

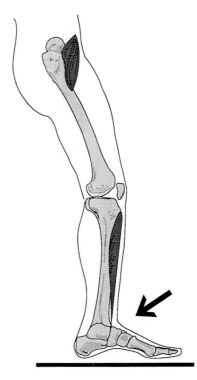

Fig. 3.10. Midswing limb advancement continues with residual active hip flexion, passive knee extension, and persistent ankle dorsiflexion to neutral by the pretibial muscles.

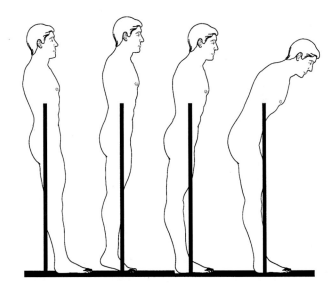

Fig. 3.11. A 15° plantar flexion contracture effects on standing balance and postural compensations. **A,** Flatfoot stance places the body vector behind the area of support, balance impossible. **B,** Heel rise shifts the vector over the forefoot, standing balance attained. Knee hyperextension (when available) **(C)** and forward trunk lean **(D)** move the vector over the flatfoot.

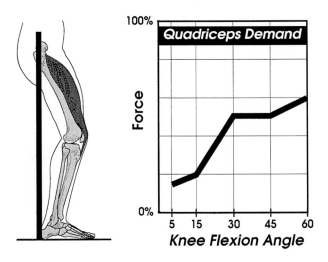

Fig. 3.12. Knee flexion contracture displacement of the vector behind the knee *(left).* Quadriceps demand is increased *(heavy line)* as the flexed posture becomes greater. The difference between 15° and 30° knee flexion is severe *(right).*

body weight cannot be balanced over the foot without substitutive posturing (Fig. 3.11). The vigorous walker substitutes a premature heel rise to roll on the forefoot. Less able persons use knee hyperextension or a forward trunk lean to advance their body vector over the stationary foot. These substitutions are only partially effective. Stride length is shortened.

Knee flexion contractures threaten stance stability. With the trunk erect, the body vector is behind the knee joint, leading to a greater demand on the quadriceps (Fig. 3.12). Based on a cadaver model, the inconspicuous 15° flexion angle requires a 20% quadriceps effort.[13] Increasing knee flexion to 30° raised the re-

quired quadriceps force to 50% of maximum. Patients with limited strength lose their ability to walk. Also, the quadriceps action created an equal compressive load on the joint, causing increased pain in arthritic patients.

Standing with a flexed knee requires increased ankle dorsiflexion. With limited ankle mobility, there is an early heel rise (Fig. 3.13). Inadequate knee alignment in terminal swing shortens stride length.

Hip flexion contractures threaten both stance stability and progression. The body vector becomes anterior to the supporting foot (Fig. 3.14). To stand erect, either the spine must provide excessive lordosis or the limb must be realigned by a flexed knee. Children com-

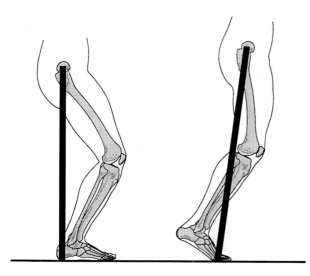

Fig. 3.13. Standing balance with a knee flexion contracture. Either excessive ankle dorsiflexion and hip flexion *(left)* or a proportional heel rise is necessary.

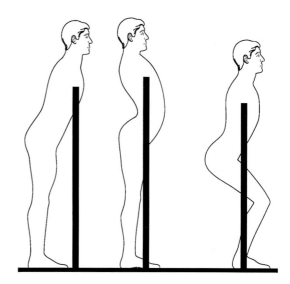

Fig. 3.14. Hip flexion contracture displacement of the vector anterior to the area of foot support *(left)*. Excessive trunk hyperextension *(center)* and knee flexion *(right)* are postures used to recover standing balance.

monly develop the needed spinal mobility, but few adults have sufficient flexibility. Then crutch support is needed.

Skeletal malalignment. Deformed joint surfaces and supporting shafts can be further impaired by continued weight bearing. Wolff observed, in 1892, that changes in one's weight-bearing pattern could alter the bones' internal architecture.[4] Children are most susceptible because their growing tissue accommodates to the abnormal stresses. Asymmetric forces discourage new growth on the compressed side while inducing overgrowth contralaterally.[9] Adults, lacking the adaptability of growing tissues, react with degenerative changes that lead to pain and loss of function. During walking, the malalignments are seen as motion errors.

Musculoskeletal pain. A common reaction to joint trauma or inflammation is swelling. The accumulated fluid makes the enveloping joint capsule tense and painful. In response, the swollen joints assume a resting position with minimal intra-articular pressure. For the ankle, it is 15° plantar flexion (Fig. 3.15, *A*), whereas the knee and hip approximate 30° flexion (Fig. 3.15, *B*).[7]

Swelling within the joint also inhibits muscle action, to avoid their compressive forces. Experimental testing of this response at the knee by progressive distention leads to quadriceps inhibition (Fig. 3.16).[6] The recovery of muscle action by intra-articular anesthesia confirmed the existence of a protective feedback mechanism. Secondary deformity and muscle weakness compromise the patient's ability to walk.

Motor unit insufficiency. Muscle weakness is the clinical penalty of having fewer motor units available to generate the forces needed for walking. Several different types of pathology (i.e., lower motor neuron diseases) can cause motor unit loss by selectively in-

vading one component of the motor unit. Although each disease has its unique characteristics, their common characteristic is that these patients have an excellent ability to substitute for the local weakness as normal sensation and control have been retained.

A motor unit has four major components (anterior horn cell, axon, myoneural junction, and muscle fibers) (Fig. 3.17). From the cell body lying within the anterior horn of the spinal cord, an axon extends to the muscle and then divides into multiple branches. Each axonal branch connects to a muscle fiber through a myoneural junction (end plate) that chemically transmits the activating signals from nerve to muscle. The multiple muscle fibers under that cell's control generate the force used to create or restrain motion. In the lower limb, the muscles contain about 500 motor units with 200 to 1000 muscle fibers in each.[8]

Poliomyelitis is an acute viral invasion of the anterior horn cells that causes a random pattern of paralysis. Anterior horn cell recovery averages 47% (range 12% to 91%).[5] Additional function is gained through axon sprouting to adopt orphaned muscle fibers,[14] enabling most patients to resume a normal lifestyle. Today, there is a second problem, the *postpolio syndrome.* Overuse of the subnormal neuromuscular system for 30 or more years has led to a significant loss of function. Affected adults now experience new muscle weakness, fatigue, and pain. Because of patients' substitutive expertise, careful gait analysis is required to identify their disability. Often the postural substitutions are the only signs of disability.

Strength is judged by the manual muscle test, but the examiner's maximum manual force does not equal

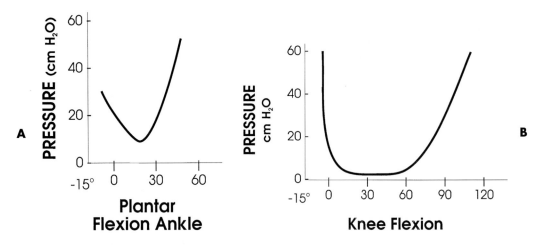

Fig. 3.15.   The influence of joint position on the intra-articular pressure created by joint swelling (experimental distention). **A,** Ankle joint pressure is minimal at 15° plantar flexion. **B,** Knee joint pressure is least at 30° flexion. Vertical axis is intra-articular pressure; horizontal axis is joint position. *(Modified from Eyring EJ, Murray WR: J Bone Joint Surg 46A:1235, 1965.)*

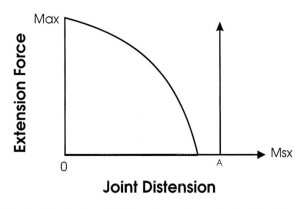

Fig. 3.16.   Reflex inhibition of quadriceps induced by joint distention. Anesthesia of the distended joint restored quadriceps action *(A)*. Vertical axis (extension force) represents quadriceps action. Horizontal axis is intensity of the joint distention. *(Modified from DeAndrade JR, et al: J Bone Joint Surg 47A:313, 1965.)*

the ability of the larger muscles.[3] Grade 5 (normal) for the quadriceps averaged 50%. Grade 4 (good) was only 40% of true normal (Table 3.1). Stationary dynamometry is indicated when the clinical strength and symptoms disagree.

Guillain-Barré syndrome is a self-limiting inflammatory disease of unknown origin that strikes the roots of the axons as they exit the spinal cord. Clinically the patients are similar to those with poliomyelitis except that the involvement is symmetrical and recovery is more rapid. If there is a sensory involvement, it is minor, mild dysesthesia.

Myasthenia gravis is an autoimmune disease that involves the neuromuscular junction. It is managed medically, rather than with orthoses. The disease was included merely to complete the picture of motor unit pathology.

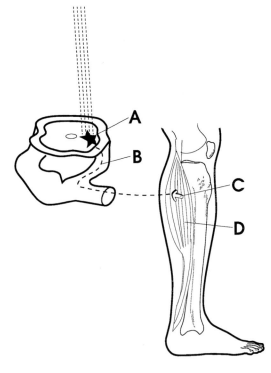

Fig. 3.17.   Motor unit components. *A,* Anterior horn cell; *B,* root of the axon; *C,* myoneural junction; *D,* muscle fibers. *(From Perry J, Hislop HJ: Lower extremity bracing, New York, 1967, American Physical Association.)*

Muscular dystrophy is a bilaterally symmetric, progressive degeneration of the muscle fibers. Among the differing patterns of involvement, Duchenne's pseudohypertrophic form is most common. Within the lower limbs, progressive weakness begins in the pelvic girdle and extends distally. Fatty connective tissue replace-

Table 3.1. Manual muscle test grades and Beasley equivalents		
TRUE NORMAL		**100%**
MANUAL GRADES (MRC)*		**BEASLEY**
Normal	5	75%
(quadriceps)		(50%)
Good	4	40%
Fair	3	20%
Poor	2	5%

From Medical Research Council (MRC): Aids to investigators of peripheral nerve lesion, Memorandum No. 7, ed 2, London, 1943, Her Majesty's Stationary Office.

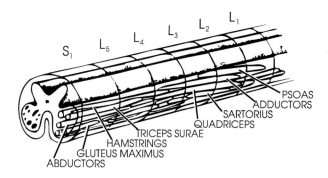

Fig. 3.18. Distribution of anterior horn cells within the spinal cord, indicating functional levels. Note the S1 cluster of triceps surae, hamstrings, and gluteals and the L2-3 cluster of quadriceps, hip flexors, and adductors. *(Modified from Sharrard WJW: J Bone Joint Surg 37B:540, 1955.)*

ment of the lost muscle fibers makes contracture formation a significant factor.

Peripheral sensory and motor impairment. The addition of a sensory loss to muscle paralysis reduces the patient's ability to substitute. One common cause is a cauda equina spinal cord injury. The cause may be congenital (spina bifida) or acute trauma. Impaired sensation occurs first on the soles of the feet. This delays awareness of floor contact. With complete foot and ankle paralysis, the patient must rely on the position sense within the flexed knee. Walking ability decreases with each higher level of spinal cord impairment (Fig. 3.18). Adults have less potential to walk than children.

Sacral (S1, S2) lesions primarily impair the posterior calf muscles (soleus and gastrocnemius). There also is early weakening of the hip extensor and abductor muscles.

Low lumbar (L5, L4) lesions increase the impairment extending the paralysis to include the hamstrings and most of the foot muscles. Excessive ankle dorsiflexion and knee flexion are the prominent postures in midstance. Heel contact persists through stance.

Upper lumbar (L3) lesions involve the quadriceps. Now the patient lacks the strength needed to independently support a flexed knee. Continued presence of L2 neural control preserves hip flexion for initiating a step.

The walking potential of each neurologic level is reduced by hip flexion contractures and bilateral involvement.

Central control dysfunction. Within the brain and spinal cord, there are several *upper motor neuron* pathways that control the anterior horn cells (Fig. 3.19). These central control systems determine what muscles are activated. Brain lesions such as a stroke, acute head

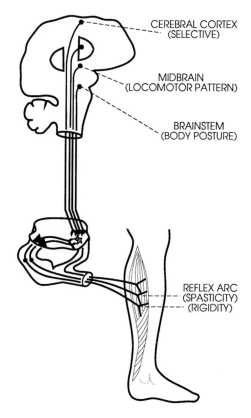

Fig. 3.19. Centers of upper neuron motor control. Levels below cortex (selective control) represent primitive control mechanism: midbrain (locomotion), brain stem (body position), intramuscular spindle (stretch reflex arc, spasticity, rigidity).

trauma, or cerebral palsy are the most common causes. Spinal cord injuries in the cervical and thoracic areas also create central control dysfunction. Spasticity is a universal characteristic. Beyond this, the nature of the resulting motion varies with the particular control pathways involved.

GAIT ANALYSIS: FULL BODY

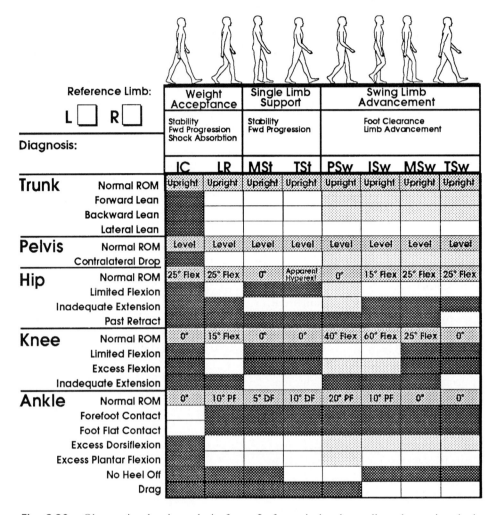

Reference Limb: L ☐ R ☐ / Diagnosis:	Weight Acceptance (Stability, Fwd Progression, Shock Absorbtion)		Single Limb Support (Stability, Fwd Progression)		Swing Limb Advancement (Foot Clearance, Limb Advancement)			
	IC	LR	MSt	TSt	PSw	ISw	MSw	TSw
Trunk Normal ROM	Upright	Upright	Upright	Upright	Upright	Upright	Upright	Upright
Forward Lean								
Backward Lean								
Lateral Lean								
Pelvis Normal ROM	Level	Level	Level	Level	Level	Level	Level	Level
Contralateral Drop								
Hip Normal ROM	25° Flex	25° Flex	0°	Apparent Hyperext	0°	15° Flex	25° Flex	25° Flex
Limited Flexion								
Inadequate Extension								
Past Retract								
Knee Normal ROM	0°	15° Flex	0°	0°	40° Flex	60° Flex	25° Flex	0°
Limited Flexion								
Excess Flexion								
Inadequate Extension								
Ankle Normal ROM	0°	10° PF	5° DF	10° DF	20° PF	10° PF	0°	0°
Forefoot Contact								
Foot Flat Contact								
Excess Dorsiflexion								
Excess Plantar Flexion								
No Heel Off								
Drag								

Fig. 3.20. Observational gait analysis form. Left vertical column lists the major deviations. Right group of eight columns identify the phases of gait. Horizontal rows designate the phases where each deviation has major significance *(white spaces)*, minor significance *(shaded)*, and no significance *(black area)*. *IC*, initial contact; *LR*, loading response; *MSt*, midstance; *TSt*, terminal stance; *PSw*, preswing; *ISw*, initial swing; *MSw*, midswing; *TSw*, terminal swing. *(Courtesy of Rancho Physical Therapy and Pathokinesiology Services: Observational Gait Analysis, 1993, LAREI.)*

Selective control allows independent movement of one joint or muscle relative to the direction, intensity, and duration of action. This determines the patient's ability to respond accurately to manual muscle testing. Walking relies on selective control for simultaneous action by the knee extensors and ankle dorsiflexors during weight acceptance, for quadriceps relaxation while the soleus increases its activity in stance progression, and for other sources of gait smoothness. Impaired selective control by itself results in muscle weakness.

Primitive control activates the muscles through basic synergies and reflex responses. Normally these are background actions that simplify function, but they become dominant when their suppressive pathways are damaged. There are three basic levels of primitive control: locomotor synergies, postural reflexes, and stretch reflexes.

The *locomotor synergies* provide two mass patterns of muscle action. An extensor pattern simultaneously activates the hip and knee extensors and the ankle plantar flexors. This meets the demand for early midstance but inhibits the ankle dorsiflexion needed for a heel rocker and obstructs the integration of knee flexion and ankle plantar flexion for preswing. The flexion pattern activates the ankle dorsiflexors in concert with the hip and knee flexor muscles. This is appropriate for initial swing but contradicts the needs of terminal swing. Although the limb synergies lie within the spinal cord, a locomotor center within the midbrain allows voluntary use of the patterns for walking.

Postural reflexes relate to both the body and the limb. A straight knee increases the tone in all of the extensor muscles, including the ankle plantar flexors. Conversely, limb flexion relaxes the extensors and augments the flexors. Being upright increases extensor tone compared to lying supine. Hence, limb and body posture modify the findings of a clinical examination.

Stretch reflexes vary with the intensity of the stimulus. Clonus is the usual response to a quick stretch. Sustained muscle action follows a slow stretch. This latter finding means one cannot differentiate contracture from spasticity by clinical examination unless the neural pathway has been inactivated by anesthesia.

Gait of an upper motor neuron lesion is typified by the relative stiffness of the action and only midrange mobility. Individual patients, however, differ considerably because of the variability in the severity of selective control impairment and relative emergence of the more primitive controls.

GAIT ANALYSIS PROCESS

The purpose of gait analysis is to identify the patient's walking disability. Observation, the basic clinical approach, is most effective when done systematically. In serial fashion, each joint is analyzed separately for its motion pattern throughout the gait cycle. Starting with the foot and ankle and advancing up the limb provides the easiest visualization of the activity. For each pertinent gait phase, the deviations from normal are identified. Interpretations to differentiate primary deficits from substitutive posturing are made by correlating the actions of all segments according to the gait phases (Fig. 3.20). The causes of the primary deviations are deduced from the clinical records of strength, range of motion, and, for spastic patients, upright spasticity and motor control. Laboratory analysis is indicated when problems remain. These data should be analyzed by the same format.

Gait motion errors represent either inadequate or excessive performance of the normal action. Their phasing has been emphasized because it facilitates visualization and interpretation. The functional significance of a gait error in one phase often becomes more evident when its development within the sequence of activity is noted. This relationship is displayed in many of the figures.

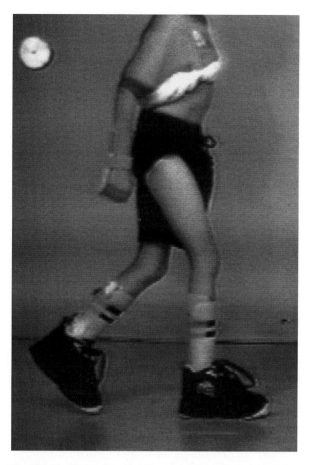

Fig. 3.21. Excessive dorsiflexion. Right limb in loading response with excessive ankle dorsiflexion, excessive knee flexion, and foot flat. Left limb in preswing with inadequate ankle plantar flexion. The patient's rigid ankle-foot orthosis prevents optimum function in both of these phases.

GAIT DEVIATIONS

Ankle

Because the ankle normally moves into selected arcs of dorsiflexion and plantar flexion, abnormal function could involve excessive or inadequate motion in either direction. To simplify the analysis, the term *excessive dorsiflexion* also relates to inadequate plantar flexion. Similarly, *excessive plantar flexion* includes inadequate dorsiflexion.

Excessive ankle dorsiflexion. Although occasionally present in swing, this is a functional problem only in stance. There are two distinct patterns of dysfunction.

Weight acceptance. Loss of passive ankle plantar flexion range causes a prolonged heel rocker. Following heel contact, forefoot drop to the floor is delayed until the tibia rolls forward to a vertical position (Fig. 3.21). The result is excessive knee flexion and prolonged quadriceps activity. The cause may be a solid shell

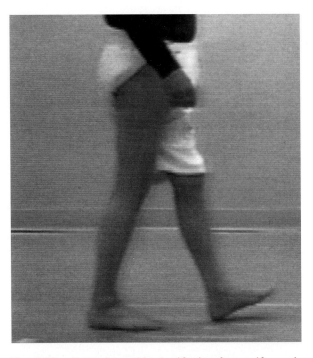

Fig. 3.22. Excessive ankle dorsiflexion from calf muscle weakness (right limb). Stance limb progression (terminal stance) with prolonged heel contact (foot flat), dorsiflexed ankle, and excessive knee flexion.

ankle-foot orthosis, prosthetic foot, or a combined fusion of the ankle and subtalar joints in neutral.

Stance limb progression.   The tibia advances over the foot in midstance or terminal stance either at an excessive rate or to an excessive dorsiflexion arc. Terminal stance heel rise is either delayed or absent. Weakness of the soleus and gastrocnemius is the most common cause. The secondary effect is persistent or excessive knee flexion. A weak elastic contracture becomes the final restraining force (Fig. 3.22). Posturing to approach foot flat support in the presence of fixed knee flexion is a secondary cause (Fig. 3.23, *B*).

Excessive ankle plantar flexion.   There are two basic patterns of dysfunction: paralytic passive drop foot (anterior insufficiency) and posterior restraint from contracture, spasticity, primitive extensor synergy, or deliberate posturing.

Passive drop foot.   Two gait tasks are involved.

Swing limb advancement.   The presence of a drop foot is most conspicuous in midswing. Also, this is the only phase in swing when the deviation is functionally significant. In initial swing, foot dorsiflexion is incomplete, and floor clearance is not dependent on the foot's position. With the tibia vertical in midswing, the passive drop at the ankle places the foot below horizontal

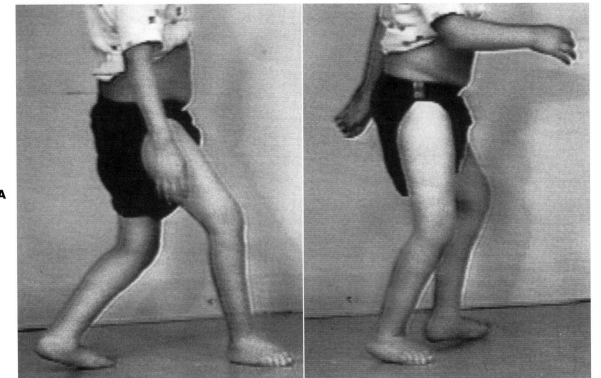

A   **B**

Fig. 3.23.   Excessive ankle dorsiflexion to accommodate excessive knee flexion. **A,** Weight acceptance with the limb reaching forward, the excessive knee flexion does not challenge the ankle or the flat foot contact. **B,** Stance limb progression (midstance): alignment of body weight over the supporting foot requires excessive ankle dorsiflexion and premature heel rise to accommodate the flexed knee.

(Fig. 3.24). The forefoot prematurely contacts the floor (foot drag) if there is no substitutive effort.

Weight acceptance. Initial contact generally is made with the forefoot, and the heel rocker is lost (Fig. 3.25, *B*). The loading response that follows forefoot contact is

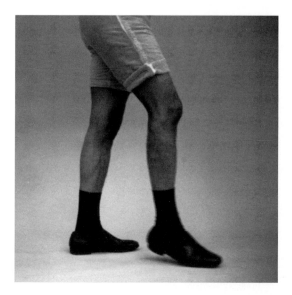

Fig. 3.24. Passive drop foot with drag (right limb). Swing limb advancement (midswing): Excessive ankle plantar flexion with normal flexion at the hip and knee causes premature forefoot floor contact. Further progression of limb is inhibited.

a passive drop of the limb. Ankle plantar flexion is reduced and foot flat contact initiated (Fig. 3.25, *C*). The lack of a heel rocker effect results in persistent knee extension. The subsequent stance phases are normal if a passive drop foot is the patient's only problem. Inadequate function of the tibialis anterior and long toe extensor muscles is the cause of a passive drop foot gait.

Plantar flexor rigidity. Excessive ankle plantar flexion caused by overly tense posterior structures (muscles or capsule) can begin in terminal swing (which positions the foot for initial contact) or any subsequent phase in stance depending on the severity and timing of the plantar flexor force.

Weight acceptance. Three associated factors determine the functional significance of excessive posterior restraint: knee position at initial contact, vigor (speed) of the patient's gait, and elasticity of the plantar flexor force. This results in several weight acceptance patterns.

Initial contact with an extended knee and only 15° plantar flexion allows a minimal heel strike (Fig. 3.26, *A*). Loading response includes a rapid forefoot contact (see Fig. 3.26, *B*) and a lack of knee flexion. More conspicuous evidence of plantar flexor restraint is the loss of ankle dorsiflexion in midstance (Fig. 3.26, *C*).

Initial contact with excessive ankle plantar flexion and a flexed knee is by the forefoot (Fig. 3.27). The subsequent loading response varies with the strength of

A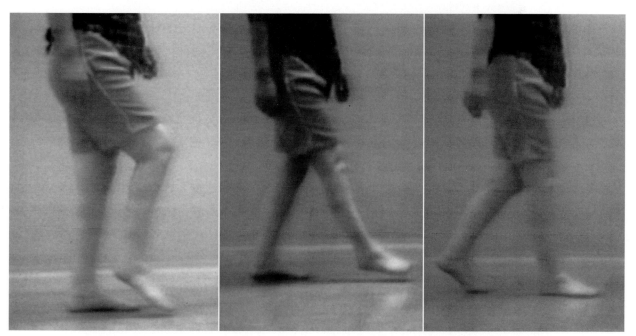**B, C**

Fig. 3.25. Passive drop foot with floor clearance (right limb). **A,** Midswing with excessive ankle plantar flexion and excessive knee and hip flexion provides toe clearance. **B,** Terminal swing with excessive ankle plantar flexion, fully extended knee, and flexed hip for forward reach positioning the foot for forefoot contact. **C,** Loading response with foot flat and less ankle plantar flexion. Shock-absorbing knee flexion is absent.

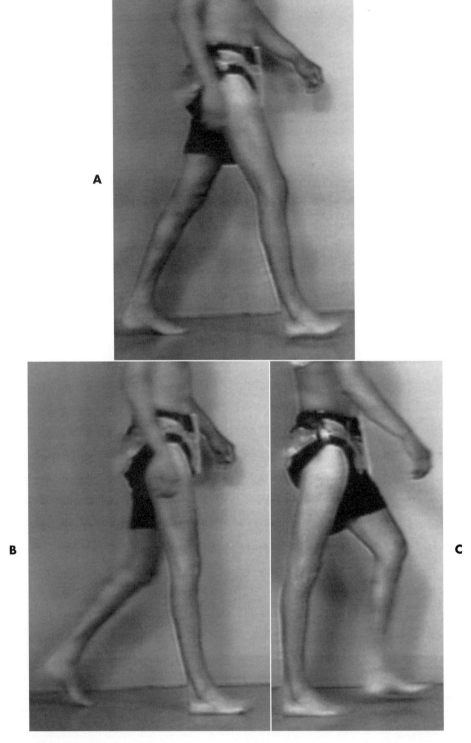

Fig. 3.26.   Mild rigid excessive ankle plantar flexion. **A,** Low heel strike (nearly foot flat) posturing of right ankle in terminal swing. **B,** Weight acceptance with a rapid foot flat contact and extension of the knee. Knee flexion for shock absorption absent. **C,** Stance limb progression (midstance) with foot flat contact, inadequate ankle dorsiflexion, and knee hyperextension.

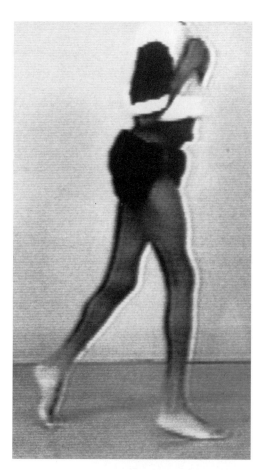

Fig. 3.27. Forefoot loading response with a rigid excessive ankle plantar flexion. Heel rocker lost and replaced with premature heel rise and mild forward lean (right limb).

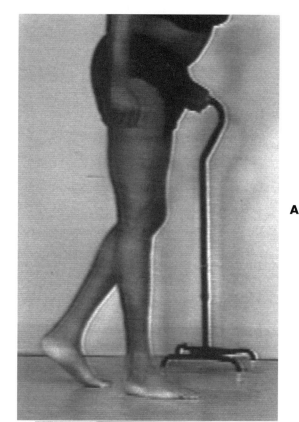

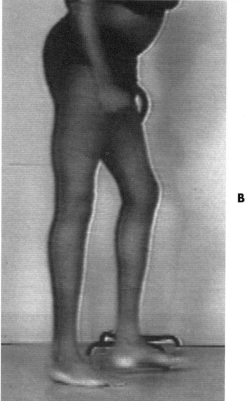

Fig. 3.28. Foot flat weight acceptance. **A,** Knee flexion absent. **B,** Stance limb progression with excessive ankle plantar flexion and premature heel rise.

the plantar flexor force and gait speed. With a slow gait and tissue elasticity, the heel drops to the floor and the knee extends (Fig. 3.28, *A*). Tibial advancement is delayed or obstructed relative to elasticity of the restraining tissues (see Fig. 3.28, *B*). Fast walkers with sufficient plantar flexor strength to support body weight maintain a heel-off, forefoot support posture (Fig. 3.29, *B*). Both the heel rocker and shock-absorbing knee flexion are inhibited.

Stance limb progression. The ankle rocker either is curtailed or lost (Fig. 3.26, *C*). Tibial advancement is inhibited unless there is a premature heel rise (Fig. 3.28, *C*). An early forefoot rocker makes metatarsal loading prolonged and excessive (Fig. 3.29, *B* and *C*). It also challenges the integrity of the midfoot plantar support (Figs. 3.28, *C*, and 3.29, *B*). Limitations in stance progression result in a short step by the other limb.

The obstructive forces generally are gastrocnemius-soleus contracture or spasticity. Persons with normal control and weak quadriceps may voluntarily mimic the pattern of a mild, elastic contracture.

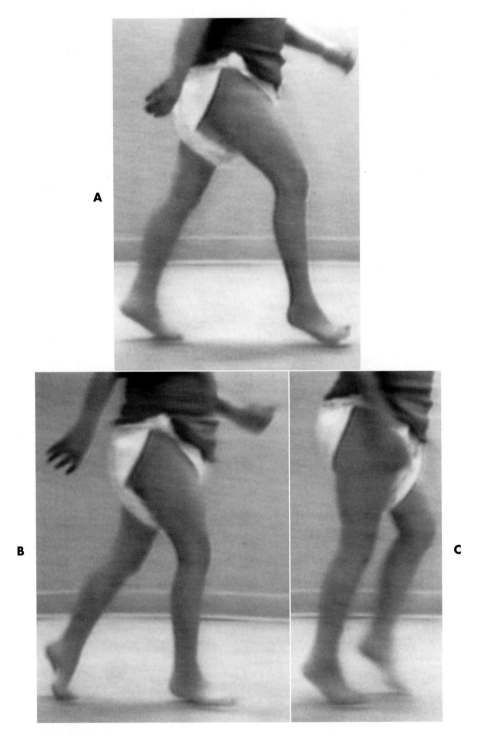

Fig. 3.29.   Excessive ankle plantar flexion and excessive knee flexion (right limb). **A,** Initial contact by the forefoot. **B,** Loading response weight bearing partially reduces the excessive plantar flexion, and posterior tibial thrust decreases the excessive knee flexion. Midfoot dorsiflexes under the forefoot load. **C,** Midstance forward alignment of body on foot redirects the ankle plantar flexion force to increase ankle posture and height of heel rise; excessive knee flexion is reduced.

Swing limb advancement.   Both midswing and terminal swing display excessive plantar flexion when the cause is a contracture. Elastic contractures that stretched under body weight in stance create a plantar

flexed posture in swing because the dorsiflexor muscles are a much weaker force. When the cause of the excessive ankle plantar flexion is primitive pattern control, ankle position differs in midswing and terminal

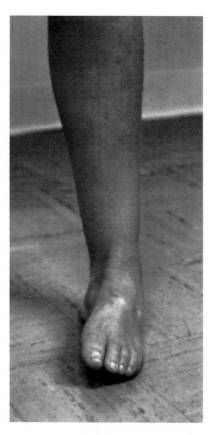

Fig. 3.30. Excessive inversion of the foot (varus). Floor contact has been shifted to the lateral side of the foot. The medial forefoot lacks floor contact. Overactivity of the anterior tibialis is apparent. Participation by the posterior tibialis cannot be assessed visually.

swing. Midswing is normal as the ankle is dorsiflexed as part of the flexor pattern. In terminal swing, the ankle actively plantar flexes in synergy with knee extension.

Foot

The loss of neutral foot alignment may occur in any gait phase. Functional significance, however, relates only to stance.

Excessive inversion (varus). Subtalar joint inversion displaces floor contact to the lateral side of the foot (Fig. 3.30). Continued inversion following heel rise leads to persistent forefoot weight bearing on the fifth metatarsal head. First metatarsal floor contact is delayed or absent. Unstable weight bearing is the result. The common causes are a soleus contracture; overactivity of the anterior tibialis, posterior tibialis, and soleus muscles; or primary bony malformation (clubfoot).

Excessive eversion (vagus). Subtalar joint eversion leads to medial heel weight bearing, a flat arch, and premature first metatarsal loading (Fig. 3.31). Generally the cause is invertor muscle weakness. Occasionally, there is peroneal muscle overactivity.

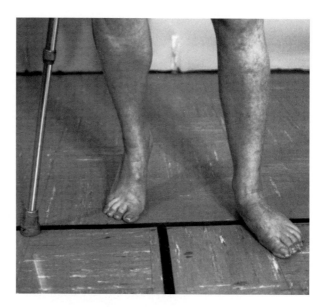

Fig. 3.31. Excessive eversion of the foot (valgus). Weight has been shifted towards the medial side of the foot, the arch is low, and the great toe is slightly rolled under.

Knee

Because the knee is in some degree of flexion throughout the gait cycle, function deviations relate to the magnitude of the motion in the individual phases. The significant deviations are excessive flexion, inadequate flexion, and excessive extension. Posturing at the knee may result from faulty ankle function as well as intrinsic knee dysfunction.

Excessive knee flexion. This is the most common knee dysfunction. Every phase of gait except initial swing can be impaired.

Weight acceptance. Weight-bearing stability is threatened by the added quadriceps demand of an overly flexed knee (see Fig. 3.23). Causes are a flexion contracture, overly intense hamstring muscle activity in spastic patients, or a lack of ankle plantar flexion.

Stance limb progression. Inability to extend the knee progressively from its initial flexed position prolongs the quadriceps demand (see Fig. 3.23, *B*). In addition, the flexed knee may obligate forefoot support and excessive ankle dorsiflexion, creating weight-bearing instability. Progression of the body over the supporting foot is inhibited by the lack of femoral advancement on the tibia.

Swing limb advancement. In midswing, increased knee flexion is a common voluntary effort to avoid a toe drag from a plantar flexed foot while the tibia is vertical (see Fig. 3.25, *A*). With premature and overly intense spastic hamstring action, as occurs in cerebral palsy diplegia (Fig. 3.32), tibial advancement is restricted. The result is persistent knee flexion in terminal swing with inadequate knee posturing for stance (Fig. 3.33).

Inadequate knee flexion

Weight acceptance. Without knee flexion, the shock-absorbing mechanism is absent, leading to greater joint impact. The most common cause is excessive ankle plantar flexion (passive or rigid; see Figs. 3.25 and 3.26). Persons also voluntarily avoid knee flexion to protect a weak quadriceps.

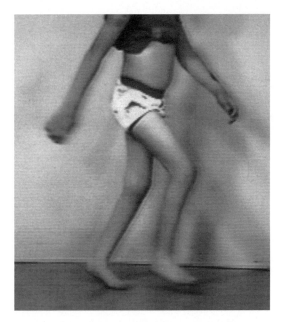

Fig. 3.32. Excessive knee flexion (bilateral). Swing limb advancement (right) knee flexion greater than hip flexion, which prevents tibia becoming vertical. Stance limb progression (left) knee does not attain full extension.

Swing limb advancement. In preswing, flexion less than 40° inadequately prepares the limb for swing. Likely causes are continued action of the vasti as part of a spastic extensor pattern or inadequate terminal stance rocker because of persistent heel contact and absent dorsiflexion.

During initial swing, inadequate knee flexion causes a toe drag unless the patient can substitute other motions (Fig. 3.34). The absence of a trailing foot posture reduces the need for knee flexion. There are several contributing factors. Out-of-phase quadriceps action is the most common. When the dynamic inhibition is limited to the rectus femoris, with or without vastus intermedius activity, surgical release can improve the patient's range (Fig. 3.35). Other situations that limit initial swing knee flexion are inadequate preswing flexion, hip flexor weakness, and premature hamstring action.

Excessive knee extension. This may be frank hyperextension (Fig. 3.36) or an extensor thrust (see Fig. 3.26, *C*). The latter term is used when the limb is rapidly driven backward but the knee lacks a passive range of hyperextension. Causes are rigid ankle plantar flexion (contracture or spasticity), spastic overactivity of the vasti, and voluntary premature soleus action to stabilize a knee with insufficient quadriceps strength. The time of knee hyperextension varies with its cause. It may follow forefoot contact or be delayed into midstance (see Fig. 3.35) or terminal stance.

Knee varus (adduction) and vagus (abduction). These are static knee postures related to the alignment of the joint surfaces or bony shafts.

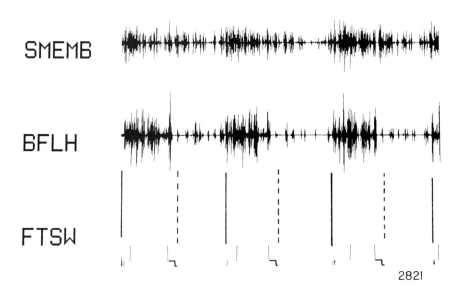

Fig. 3.33. Dynamic electromyography of hamstring muscles showing nearly continuous activity of semimembranosus (SMEMB) and biceps femoris, long head (BFLH) with most intense action in stance. Footswitch (FTSW) "staircase" indicates stance. *Vertical solid line* is onset of stance; *dotted line* is onset of swing.

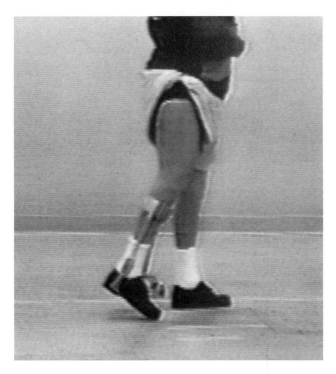

Fig. 3.34. Inadequate knee flexion (right limb). Swing limb advancement. Initial swing knee flexion is approximately 20° rather than the normal 60°. AFO support of ankle shows toe drag results from the limited posture of the knee, not the foot.

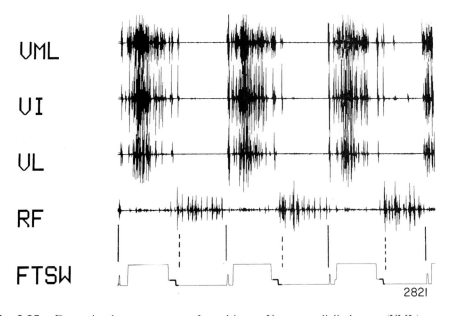

Fig. 3.35. Dynamic electromyogram of quadriceps. Vastus medialis longus (VML), vastus intermedius (VI), and vastus longus (VL) show intense and prolonged action in stance, which diminishes in preswing and is absent in swing. Rectus femoris (RF) overactivity (intensity and duration) throughout swing. *Solid vertical bar,* Onset of stance; *dashed vertical line,* onset of swing. FSW (footswitches) stair profile indicates sequence of floor contact: brief heel "scuff," return to baseline, support by heel and fifth metatarsal head, contact only by fifth metatarsal and toes.

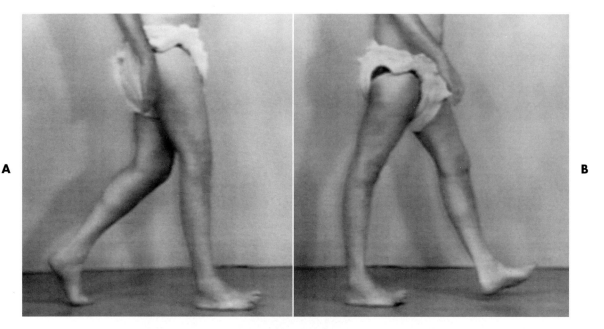

Fig. 3.36. Excessive knee extension (hyperextension) secondary to ankle plantar flexion contracture, right limb. **A,** Forward alignment of limb in weight acceptance allows a normal knee and ankle posture. **B,** Terminal stance advancement of thigh over the tibia restrained by the plantar flexion contracture and lack of heel rise results in knee hyperextension.

Hip

Dysfunction at the hip relates to both thigh and pelvis postures. Inappropriate thigh posturing is reflected as inadequate flexion in swing and inadequate extension in stance. Excessive adduction and abduction are infrequent findings.

Inadequate hip flexion

Swing limb advancement. The critical time is initial swing. Primary hip flexor weakness is infrequent because grade 2+ is sufficient in flaccid paralysis. In spastic patients, inadequate hip flexion most often is caused by premature hamstring action or represents inhibition by a stiff knee gait (Fig. 3.37).

Weight acceptance. Inadequate hip flexion that continues into terminal swing limits the limb's forward reach for stance (Fig. 3.38).

Inadequate hip extension. Stance limb progression is the only task that is impaired. Without hip extension, the patient is denied a trailing limb position in late midstance and terminal stance (see Fig. 3.23, *B*). Stride length is shortened. Direct causes are the avoidance of stretching a painful joint capsule, a hip flexion contracture, or spasticity. Common indirect causes are postural adaptations for balance over a plantar flexed ankle or a flexed knee (see Fig. 3.37, *B*).

Hip past-retract. In terminal swing, a voluntary substitution is used to gain knee extension when the quadriceps muscle is paralyzed. Rapid, excessive hip flexion advances both the thigh and the tibia. Then, rapid hip extension retracts the thigh while inertia sustains the forward tibia.

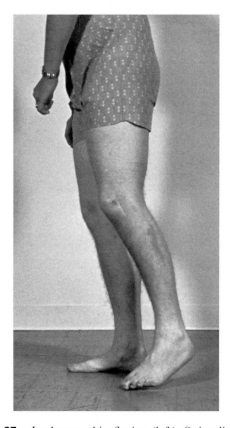

Fig. 3.37. Inadequate hip flexion (left). Swing limb advancement with inadequate flexion and hip, knee and ankle dorsiflexion. Right lateral lean for floor clearance.

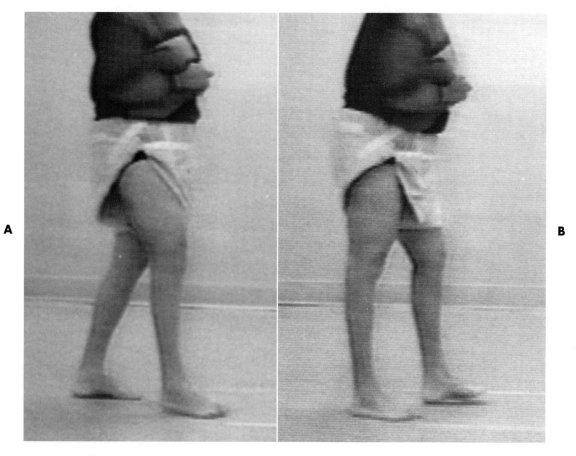

Fig. 3.38.   Inadequate hip flexion (right). **A,** Weight acceptance with trunk erect, short forward reach, excessive ankle plantar flexion, and forefoot contact. **B,** Stance limb advancement with forward trunk for balance over plantar flexed ankle.

Pelvis

Malalignments of the pelvis are secondary reactions to demands at the hip.

Contralateral pelvic drop

Weight acceptance.   Transfer of body weight to the stance limb in preparation for swing removes the support of the opposite side. Hip abductor muscle weakness (gluteus medius, gluteus minimus, and upper gluteus maximus) allows the unsupported contralateral pelvis to drop (Fig. 3.39). The demand on the abductor muscle complex is aggravated by a long leg. Protection is provided by a tight iliotibial band or prepositioning into adduction by a short leg.

Pelvic hike

Swing limb advancement.   Elevation of the ipsilateral side of the pelvis is used for foot clearance when hip and/or knee flexion is inadequate (Fig. 3.40).

Excessive rotation

Swing limb advancement.   Anterior pelvic motion substitutes the trunk muscles for weak hip flexors to assist limb advancement.

Stance limb progression.   Posterior rotation and drop in terminal stance provide mild leg lengthening to accommodate persistent heel contact.

Trunk

Normal trunk motions are so small (5°) that any visible deviation from the upright posture is abnormal. Patients with intrinsic spine deformity (scoliosis, lordosis, kyphosis) or paralysis have a constant posture abnormality that may increase the demand on the lower limbs to preserve standing balance.

Variable postural deviations of the trunk (*trunk leans*) are used to preserve standing balance by displacing the body vector or to assist limb advancement. Each deviation has a functional significance.

Forward trunk lean

Weight acceptance.   The quadriceps demand is reduced by moving the vector anterior to the knee. The indications are muscle weakness.

Stance progression.   Anterior displacement of the body vector is used to restore standing balance over a plantar flexed ankle or flexed knee (see Fig. 3.38). Excessive hip flexion that lacks compensatory lordosis also creates a forward trunk lean.

Backward trunk lean

Weight acceptance and stance progression.   Posterior displacement of the body vector reduces the demand on weak hip extensor muscles (Fig. 3.41). The

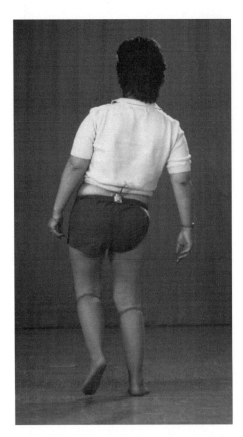

Fig. 3.39. Contralateral pelvic drop and ipsilateral trunk lean indicate abductor muscle weakness.

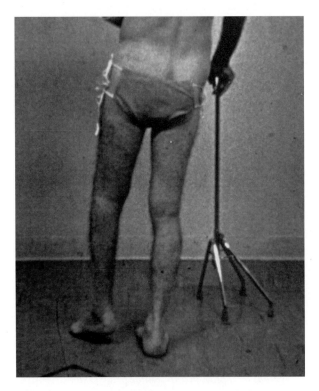

Fig. 3.40. Ipsilateral pelvic hike for floor clearance with inadequate hip and knee flexion.

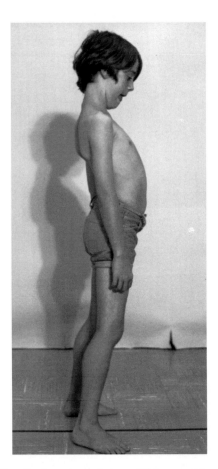

Fig. 3.41. Backward trunk lean. With poor hip extensor muscles and a hip flexion contracture, standing balance gained by trunk lordosis and both arms slightly posterior to substitute for weak hip extensors. Note the ankle dorsiflexion used to align the body mass center over the foot.

protective alignment begins with floor contact. A hip flexion contracture increases the amount of backward lean required to preserve standing balance. Bilateral posterior arm position adds further balance protection.

Swing limb advancement. In initial swing, a backward lean accompanied by anterior pelvic tilt assists limb advancement when the hip flexors are weak.

Lateral trunk lean

Weight acceptance through stance progression. An ipsilateral lean is used to reduce the demand on the hip abductor muscles (see Fig. 3.39). The amount of lateral trunk lean is proportional to the severity of the weakness.

Swing limb advancement. Combined contralateral lateral lean of the trunk and ipsilateral pelvic hike is another substitution to assist limb advancement (see Fig. 3.40).

REFERENCES

1. Akeson WH, et al: The connective tissue response to immobility: Biochemical changes in periarticular connective tissue of the immobilized rabbit knee, Clin Orthop Rel Res 93:356–362, 1973.

2. Akeson WH, et al: Biomedical and biochemical changes in the periarticular connective tissue during contracture development in the immobilized rabbit knee, Connect Tissue Res 2:315–323, 1974.

3. Beasley WC: Quantitative muscle testing: Principles and applications to research and clinical services, Arch Phys Med Rehabil 42:398–425, 1961.

4. Bick EM: Source book of orthopedics, New York, 1968, Hofner Publishing.

5. Bodian D: Motoneuron disease and recovery in experimental poliomyelitis. In Halstead LS, Weichers DO, editors: Late effects of poliomyelitis. Miami, 1985, Symposia Foundation.

6. deAndrade MS, Grant C, Dixon A: Joint distension and reflex muscle inhibition in the knee, J Bone Joint Surg 47A:313–322, 1965.

7. Eyring EJ, Murray WR: The effect of joint position on the pressure of intra-articular effusion, J Bone Joint Surg 46A:1235–1241, 1964.

8. Feinstein B, et al: Morphological studies of motor units in normal human muscles, Acta Anat 23:127, 1955.

9. Haas SL: Retardation of bone growth by wire loop, J Bone Joint Surg 27A:25, 1945.

10. Medical Research Council: Aids to investigators of peripheral nerve lesions, Memorandum No. 7, ed 2, London, 1943, Her Majesty's Stationary Office.

11. Murray MP, Clarkson BH: The vertical pathways of the foot during level walking: I. Range of variability in normal men, Phys Ther 46:585–589, 1966.

12. Perry J: Gait analysis, normal and pathological function, Thorofare, NJ, 1992, Charles B. Slack.

13. Perry J, Antonelli D, Ford W: Analysis of knee-joint forces during flexed-knee stance, J Bone Joint Surg 57A:961–967, 1975.

14. Weiss P, Edds MV: Spontaneous recovery of muscle following partial denervation, Am J Physiol 145:587–607, 1946.

Biomechanics of the Spine

Melvin D. Law, Jr.
Augustus A. White III
Manohar M. Panjabi

The human spine consists of 7 cervical, 12 thoracic, 5 lumbar, and 5 fused sacral vertebrae. The spine articulates with the pelvis through the sacroiliac joints. The vertebrae with their articulations and supporting structures maintain proper alignment of the spine. The spine has three fundamental biomechanical functions: (1) it transfers weights and the resultant bending moments of the head, trunk, and any weights being lifted to the pelvis; (2) it allows physiologic motions between these three body parts and within itself; and (3) it protects the spinal cord from potentially damaging motions and forces produced by physiologic movements and trauma.[81] Motion is described in terms relative to the subjacent vertebra. The right-handed orthogonal (90-degree angle) coordinate system has been recommended for precise orientation about the human body (Fig. 4.1).[55,82]

KINEMATICS

Terms and definitions

Kinematics. *Kinematics* involves the study of motion of rigid bodies without consideration of the forces involved.

Kinetics. *Kinetics* is concerned with the study of motion and the weights, moments, and muscle forces acting on the spine.

Degrees of freedom. Vertebrae have six *degrees of freedom*, translation along, and rotation about each of the three orthogonal axes. Translation is expressed in meters or inches, and rotation is expressed in degrees.

Neutral zone. Spinal displacement from the neutral position to the initiation of spinal resistance to physiologic motion is the *neutral zone*. Translational and rotatory neutral zones are expressed in meters and degrees. The neutral zone can be expressed for each of the six degrees of freedom (Fig. 4.2).

Elastic zone. Spinal displacement between the end of the neutral zone and the end of the range of motion is the *elastic zone*. Translational and rotatory elastic zones are expressed in meters and degrees. The elastic zone can be expressed for each of the six degrees of freedom (see Fig. 4.2).

Range of motion. *Range of motion* (ROM) can be expressed for each of the six degrees of freedom and is measured from the neutral position to the end of the ROM. Displacement between the end of the neutral zone and the end of the ROM is the elastic zone where higher forces occur. ROM can also be expressed as the sum of the neutral and elastic zones. Forces that exceed the elastic zone may produce injury to spinal elements.

Coupling. *Coupling* refers to motion (translation or rotation) about one axis on the coordinate being consistently associated with motion about another axis.

Instantaneous axis of rotation. For a body in plane motion, there is a point in the body in which a line can be extended perpendicular to the plane of motion. The point where this extended line at the start of motion bisects the analogous line at the end of motion is the *instantaneous axis of rotation* (IAR) (Fig. 4.3).

SPINAL MOTION

The motion segment or functional spinal unit (FSU) is composed of two adjacent vertebrae and their intervening soft tissues. The most representative values for rotatory ROM at different levels of the spine are presented in Fig. 4.4.[11,19,49,58,60,62,81,85]

The muscles are located anterior, posterior, and lateral to the spine. They provide for motion and stabilize the spine to carry physiologic loads. The anterior muscles flex the spine. If an anterior muscle runs a little obliquely and contracts independently of the corresponding muscle on the opposite side, it

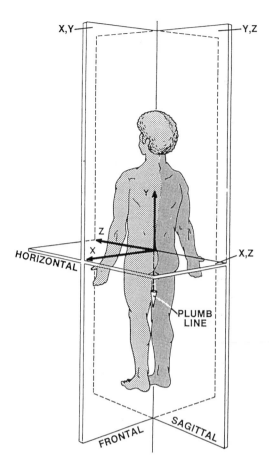

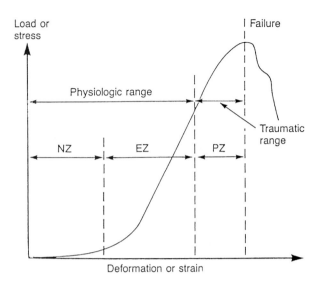

Fig. 4.2. Typical load-deformation curve of a ligament, obtained from a materials testing machine. One end of the ligament is displaced with respect to the other, while the load and deformation of the ligament are continuously recorded. The deformation, being the independent parameter, is plotted on the horizontal axis. This load-deformation curve may be divided into physiologic and traumatic ranges. The physiologic range may be further divided into two parts. A ligament deformation around the neutral position where little effort is required to deform the ligament is called the *neutral zone* (NZ). In the second part, a more substantial effort is required to deform the ligament; this is called the *elastic zone* (EZ). In the trauma range, there is microtrauma with increasing load eventually leading to failure. This has been designated as the *plastic zone* (PZ).

Fig. 4.1. Suggested central coordinate system with origin between the cornua of the sacrum. Its orientation is as follows. The −*y*-axis is described by the plumb line dropped from the origin, and the +*x*-axis points to the left at a 90-degree angle to the *y*-axis. The +*z*-axis points forward at a 90-degree angle to both the *y*-axis and the *x*-axis. The human body is shown in the anatomic position. Some basic conventions are observed that make the system useful. The sagittal plane is the *y,z* plane; the frontal or coronal plane is the *x,y* plane; the horizontal plane is the *x,z* plane. Movements are described in relation to the origin of the coordinate system. The *arrows* indicate the positive direction of each axis. The origin is the zero point, and the direction opposite to the arrows is negative. Thus, direct forward translation is +*z*; up is +*y*; to the left is +*x*; to the right is −*x*; down is −*y*; and backward is −*z*. The convention for rotations is determined by imagining oneself at the origin of the coordinate system looking in the positive direction of the axis. Clockwise rotations are +θ, and counterclockwise rotations are −θ. Thus, θ*x* is roughly analogous to flexion; +θ*z* is analogous to right lateral bending; +θ*y* is axial rotation toward the left. A coordinate system may be set up at any defined point parallel to the master system described above. The location of the coordinate system should be clearly indicated for precise, accurate communications. In spinal kinematics, the motion is usually described in terms of the subjacent vertebra. The secondary coordinate system may be established in the body of the subjacent vertebra. For in vivo measurements, the tip of the spinous process may be used. *(From Panjabi MM, White AA, Brand RA: J Biomech 7:385, 1974.)*

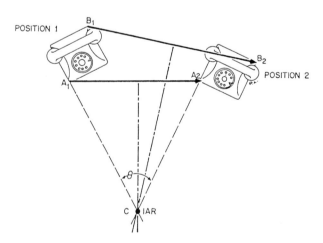

Fig. 4.3. In uniplanar motion, the *instantaneous axis of rotation* (IAR) is determined by the intersection of the perpendicular bisectors of the two lines A_1A_2 and B_1B_2. The angle θ formed at the IAR by points A_1A_2 and B_1B_2 is the angle of rotation. *(From White AA, Panjabi MM: Spinal kinematics: The research status of spinal manipulative therapy, NINCDS Monograph 15:93, Washington, D.C., 1975, U.S. Department of Health, Education, and Welfare.)*

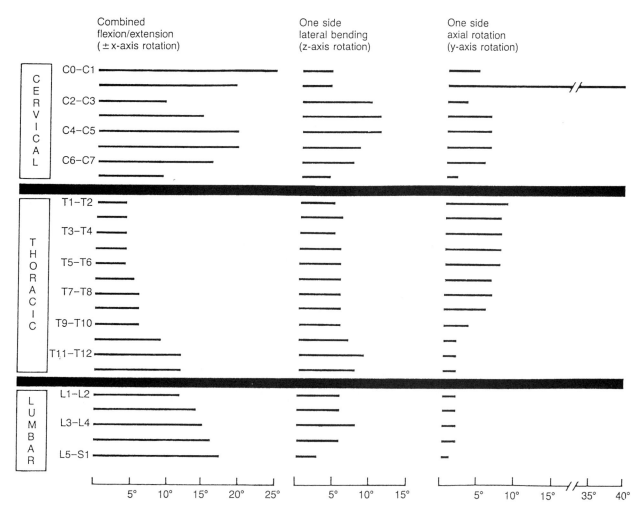

Fig. 4.4. A composite of what the authors consider, based on careful review of the literature, to be the most representative values for rotatory ranges of motion at different levels of the spine in the traditional planes of motion. *(From White AA, Panjabi MM: Clinical biomechanics of the spine, ed 2, Philadelphia, 1990, JB Lippincott.)*

rotates and bends the spine laterally as well as flexes it. The muscles posterior to the spine provide extension. If a posterior muscle runs a little obliquely and contracts independently of the corresponding muscle on the opposite side, it rotates and bends the spine laterally as well as extends it. The muscles on the side bend the spine laterally.§

Anterior Muscles

Longus colli*	Obliquus internus
Longus capitis	abdominis*
Rectus capitis anterior	Psoas major†
Rectus capitis lateralis†	Psoas minor†
Obliquus externus	Iliacus
abdominus*	Quadratus lumborum

§The list below is from White AA, Panjabi MM: Clinical biomechanics of the spine, ed 2, Philadelphia, 1990, JB Lippincott; with permission.

Posterior Muscles

Superficial stratum	*Deep stratum*
Splenius capitis*†	Semispinalis thoracis*
Splenius cervicis†	Semispinalis cervicis*
Erector spinae	Semispinalis capitis*
(sacrospinalis)	Multifidi*
Iliocostalis*†	Rotatores*
Longissimis*†	Interspinales
Spinalis*†	Intertransversarii†

Lateral Muscles

Trapezius	Scalenus anterior*
Sternocleidomastoid*	Scalenus medial*
Quadratus lumborum	Scalenus posterior*

*Muscles with axial rotation function
†Muscles with lateral bending function

The coordinated action of the muscles stabilizes the spine to resist compressive loads.[46,48] These muscle actions are important, because the normal loads on the

Regional Coupling Patterns

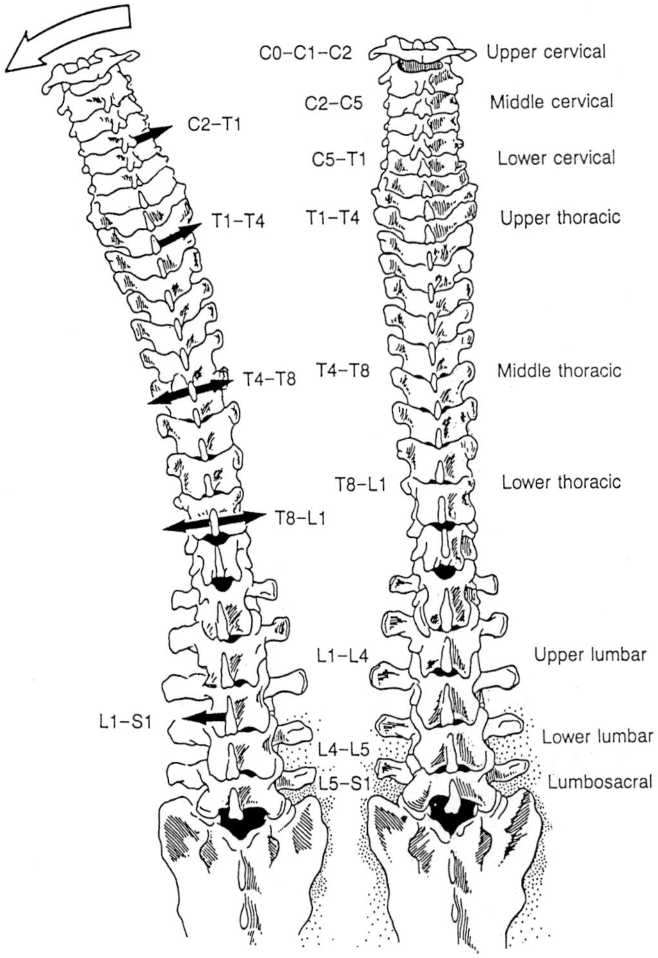

C0–C1–C2 — Upper cervical
C2–C5 — Middle cervical
C5–T1 — Lower cervical
T1–T4 — Upper thoracic
T4–T8 — Middle thoracic
T8–L1 — Lower thoracic
L1–L4 — Upper lumbar
L4–L5 — Lower lumbar
L5–S1 — Lumbosacral

C2–T1
T1–T4
T4–T8
T8–L1
L1–S1

Fig. 4.5. Summary of the coupling of lateral bending and axial rotation in the various biomechanical subdivisions of the spine. The actual coupling is between ±z-axis rotation and ±y-axis rotation. It can also be thought of in terms of the direction of movement of the spinous process with left lateral bending. Note that in the *middle* and *lower* cervical spine as well as the *upper* thoracic spine, the same coupling pattern exists. In the *middle* and *lower* thoracic spine, the axial rotation, which is coupled with lateral bending, can be in either direction; that is, it can be ±y-axis rotation. The direction of this axial rotation varies between different specimens. In the *lumbar spine*, there is –y-axis rotation associated with z-axis rotation. That is, the spinous processes go to the left with left lateral bending. The same pattern is also present at the lumbar spine FSU. (*From White AA, Panjabi MM: Clinical biomechanics of the spine, ed 2, Philadelphia, 1990, JB Lippincott.*)

spine by body mass alone in standing are about two to three times body weight (140 to 210 kg).[40,48]

Motion and load-bearing capabilities are directed by the contours, dimensions, and relationships of the vertebrae, discs, and facet joints. The ligaments, joint capsules, and discs provide constraints to motion in a checkrein manner. In general, for flexion/extension (±θx)* movements, ligaments that are located posterior and the bony structures located anterior to the IAR resist flexion. Ligaments located anterior and bony structures located posterior to the IAR resist extension.

*See Fig. 4.1 and legend for explanation.

In lateral bending (±θz) and axial rotation (±θy), the ligament functions are often more complex. Coupling patterns vary for different parts of the spine. The coupling of axial rotation with lateral bending is shown in Fig. 4.5.

UPPER CERVICAL SPINE (OCCIPITAL-ATLANTO-AXIAL COMPLEX)

Both joints of this complex (C0-C1 and C1-C2) significantly contribute to the total motion of this area. The amount of flexion and extension at the two joints is

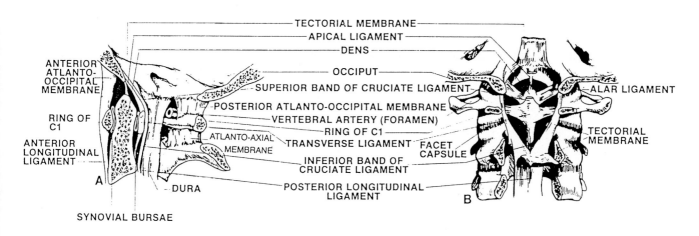

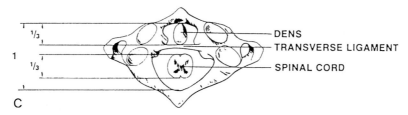

Fig. 4.6. Three anatomic perspectives of the ring of C1. **A,** Lateral view. **B,** View from behind with anterior bone and tectorial membrane removed. **C,** Transverse view emphasizing Steele's rule of thirds. The dens, spinal cord, and free space each make up one third of the anteroposterior diameter of the ring of C1. *(From White AA, Panjabi MM: Clinical biomechanics of the spine, ed 2, Philadelphia, 1990, JB Lippincott.)*

Table 4.1. Atlanto-occipital range of motion (C0-C1)

TYPE OF MOTION	PASSIVE CONSTRAINTS	MUSCLES RESPONSIBLE FOR ACTION
Flexion ($+\Theta x$)	Tectorial membrane Posterior atlanto-occipital membrane Articular capsule between occipital condyles and superior atlantal facets (posterior) Ligamentum nuchae Anterior margin of the foramen magnum and the tip of the dens*	Longus capitis Rectus capitis anterior
Extension ($-\Theta x$)	Anterior atlanto-occipital membrane Articular capsule between occipital condyles and superior atlantal facets (anterior) Anterior longitudinal ligament Apical dental ligament	Rectus capitis posterior major Rectus capitis posterior minor Obliquus capitis superior (both acting simultaneously) Splenius capitis Semispinalis capitis
Lateral bending (Θz) (one side)	Lateral atlanto-occipital ligament Alar ligaments Occipital condyle and atlantal facet*	Obliquus capitis superior Splenius capitis Sternocleidomastoid Trapezius
Axial rotation (Θy) (one side)	Alar ligaments Articular capsule between occipital condyles and superior atlantal facets	Sternocleidomastoid Semispinalis capitis Splenius capitis

*Skeletal (nonligamentous) constraint.

Table 4.2. Atlantoaxial range of motion (C1-C2)

TYPE OF MOTION	PASSIVE CONSTRAINTS	MUSCLES RESPONSIBLE FOR ACTION
Flexion ($+\Theta x$)	Transverse ligament of the atlas Atlantoaxial articular capsules Ligamentum flavum Ligamentum nuchae Tectorial membrane	Longus colli Rectus capitis anterior Longus capitis
Extension ($-\Theta x$)	Median atlantoaxial joint* Atlantoaxial ligament Anterior longitudinal ligament Capsule of lateral atlantoaxial joint	Rectus capitis posterior major Rectus capitis posterior minor Obliquus capitis superior (both acting simultaneously) Splenius capitis Splenius cervicis Semispinalis capitis Semispinalis cervicis
Lateral bending (Θz) (one side)	Capsule of lateral atlantoaxial joint Alar ligaments Lateral atlantoaxial joints*	Obliquus capitis superior Obliquus capitis inferior Splenius capitis
Axial rotation (Θy) (one side)	Alar ligaments Capsule of lateral atlantoaxial joint Deep (accessory) portion of tectorial membrane	Obliquus capitis superior Obliquus capitis inferior Rectus capitis posterior major Rectus capitis posterior minor Sternocleidomastoid Semispinalis capitis Splenius capitis

*Skeletal (nonligamentous) constraint.

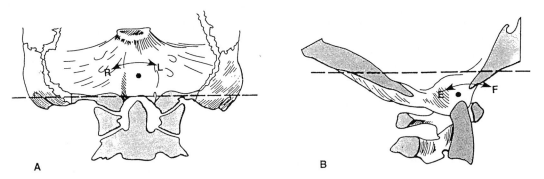

A   B

Fig. 4.7.   A, Approximate location of IAR for the atlanto-occipital joint in the frontal plane. Lateral bending *(R,L)* of the occiput on C1 is thought to take place around the indicated *dot.* The *broken line* indicates the IAR for flexion/extension *(F,E)* motion. **B,** The converse is true in the sagittal plane. The *broken line* indicates the IAR for lateral bending; the *dot* shows the axes for flexion/extension. *(From White AA, Panjabi MM: Clinical biomechanics of the spine, ed 2, Philadelphia, 1990, JB Lippincott.)*

roughly equal,[77,81] and most of the rotation occurs at C1-C2.[12,13,49,62,77] The cogent anatomy of this complex is shown in Fig. 4.6. The ligament and muscle stabilizers for C0-C1 and C1-C2 are given in Tables 4.1 and 4.2.

For the C0-C1 articulation, the IAR in flexion/ extension (x-axis) passes through the centers of the mastoid processes (Fig. 4.7, *B*). Flexion movement is checked by skeletal contact between the anterior margin of the foramen magnum and the tip of the dens. Extension is checked by the tectorial membrane. With

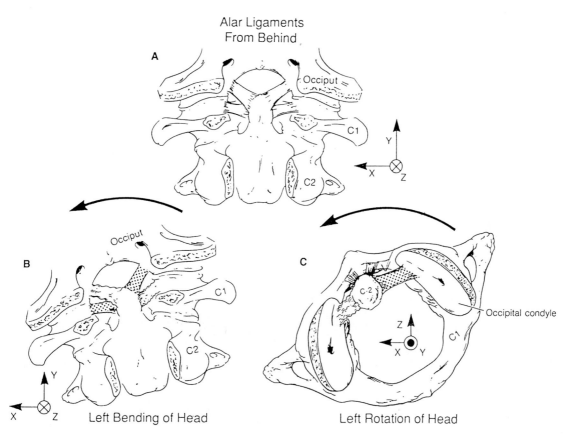

Fig. 4.8. Role of alar ligaments in lateral bending and axial rotation. **A,** View of the alar ligaments from behind with C0-C1-C2 complex in neutral position. **B,** Left lateral bending (−*z*-axis rotation) of the head and neck. This motion is restrained by a taut right upper and left lower alar ligament. **C,** Left axial rotation (+*y*-axis rotation) of the head and neck. This is checked by a taut right alar ligament. *(From Jofe MH, White AA, Panjabi MM: In The Cervical Spine Research Society: The cervical spine, ed 2, Philadelphia, 1989, JB Lippincott.)*

flexion of the C0-C1 joint beyond neutral, the tectorial membrane becomes taut and limits forward flexion at the C1-C2 joint. Similarly, with extension of the C0-C1 joint, the tectorial membrane again becomes taut and limits extension between C1 and C2.[77,81]

In lateral bending (*z*-axis rotation), the IAR is located at a point 2 to 3 cm above the tip of the dens (see Fig. 4.7, *A*). The motion involves 5 degrees to one side at C0-C1 and C1-C2 and is controlled by both components of the alar ligaments (Fig. 4.8, *B*). During left lateral bending, the right upper portion of the alar ligament, which is connected to the occiput, and the left lower component, which is connected to the ring of C1, check the motion. The opposite is true for right lateral bending.

Axial rotation at C0-C1 involves about 5° to one side and is limited by the ligaments and osseous anatomy of the C0-C1-C2 complex (see Fig. 4.8, *A*). The joint surfaces are cup-shaped, with the arcuate occipital articulation fitting into the cup of C1. At C1-C2, roughly 40° of axial rotation to one side occurs, and the IAR is located in the dens. During left axial rotation, motion is

checked by the right alar ligament (Fig. 4.8, *C*); the opposite is true for right axial rotation. The C1-C2 articulation is biconvex and has been described as a "double-threaded screw" joint.[81] This biconvexity gives rise to a coupling pattern of motion where there is translation along the axis of the dens so that alternating rotations produce a pistonlike cephalocaudal movement. Radiographic evaluation may reveal apparent translation because of a shift in the projection of the lateral masses of C1 in relation to the dens (Fig. 4.9).[68] Kinematic studies, however, confirm that there is insignificant lateral translation (*x*-axis) of the C1-C2 joint because of the snug fit of the anterior ring of C1 and transverse ligament around the dens.[24,68,77]

MIDDLE AND LOWER CERVICAL SPINE (C2-T1)

Rotation ranges for the middle and lower cervical spine are shown in Table 4.3. The C5-C6 FSU has the largest range.[31] There may be a causal relationship

FROM ABOVE

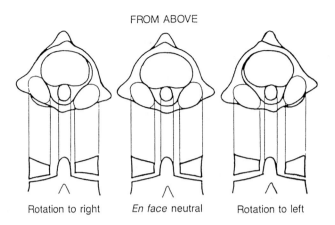

Rotation to right   *En face* neutral   Rotation to left

Fig. 4.9. When C1 rotates (±θ*y*), the concomitant movement of the lateral mass causes an apparent increase in the distance between the lateral mass and the dens on the anteroposterior radiograph. *(From Shapiro R, Youngberg AS, Rothman SLG: Radiol Clin North Am 11:505, 1973.)*

Table 4.3. Middle and lower cervical spine range-of-motion limits and representative values (C2-T1)

	COMBINED FLEXION/ EXTENSION (+Θ*x*)		LATERAL BENDING (ONE SIDE) (Θ*z*)		AXIAL ROTATION (ONE SIDE) (Θ*y*)	
	LIMITS OF RANGES (DEG)	REPRESENTATIVE ANGLE (DEG)	LIMITS OF RANGES (DEG)	REPRESENTATIVE ANGLE (DEG)	LIMITS OF RANGES (DEG)	REPRESENTATIVE ANGLE (DEG)
Interspace						
Middle						
C2-3	5–16	10	11–20	10	0–10	3
C3-4	7–26	15	9–15	11	3–10	7
C4-5	13–29	20	0–16	11	1–12	7
Lower						
C5-6	13–29	20	0–16	8	2–12	7
C6-7	6–26	17	0–17	7	2–10	6
C7-T1	4–7	9	0–17	4	0–7	2

From White AA, Panjabi MM: Clinical biomechanics of the spine, ed 2, Philadelphia, 1990, JB Lippincott.

between this relative increased range and the higher incidence of cervical spondylosis at this interspace.[80] In lateral bending and axial rotation, there is a smaller range in the more caudal segments.

Flexion and extension motion involves a strong coupling of rotation (*x*-axis) and translation (*z*-axis).[15,31,36] The uncovertebral joints guide flexion and extension and prevent lateral (*x*-axis) translation.[7] In extension, the cervical vertebrae are positioned in series and form a smooth curve. As flexion occurs, the vertebrae translate forward (+θ*z*) in a slight stair-step pattern of motion. The anterior vertebral disk heights decrease, and the posterior heights increase. The facet joints glide anteriorly and superiorly, and the posterior interspinous space widens. The upper limit of normal translation radiographically is 3.5 mm, which takes into account a 25% magnification.[81] The same motion pattern occurs in reverse when going from flexion to extension. Lysell[31] coined the term *top angle* to indicate the steepness of the arch that was described by the vertebra while moving from full extension to full flexion. The arches were almost flat at C2 and the steepest at C6 (Fig. 4.10). The cephalocaudal decrease in the top angle (decrease in the arch) indicates a greater amount of translation occurs in the middle cervical spine than in the lower, where more tilting motion of the vertebral body occurs.[31] The anatomic constraints for motions of the middle and lower cervical spine are given in

Upper

C2

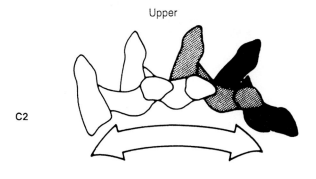

Middle

C4

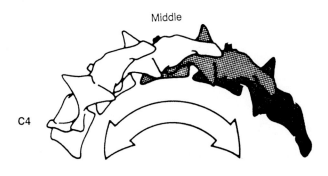

Lower

C7

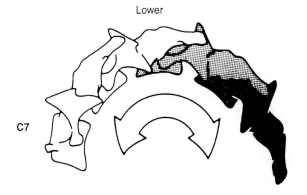

Fig. 4.10. Diagrammatic approximation of relative regional cephalocaudal variations in radii of curvature of the arches defined by the cervical vertebrae as they rotate and translate in the sagittal plane. The diagram depicts the patterns of motion of C2, C4, and C7, moving back and forth between full flexion and full extension. *(From White AA, Panjabi MM: Clinical biomechanics of the spine, ed 2, Philadelphia, 1990, JB Lippincott.)*

Table 4.4; the ligamentous structures are diagramed in Fig. 4.11.

Lateral bending (z-axis rotation) is coupled with axial rotation (y-axis) such that the spinous processes go in the opposite direction of the lateral bending ($-z$-axis is coupled with $+y$-axis, and $+z$-axis is coupled with $-y$-axis) (Fig. 4.12). About 50% of head rotation occurs through the middle and lower cervical spine. The annulus and facet joints are the major limiting structures to axial rotation. The amount of axial rotation coupled with lateral bending varies by level. At C2, there are 2 degrees of coupled axial rotation for every 3

degrees of lateral bending, a ratio of 2:3 or 0.67. At C7, lateral bending of around 7.5 degrees is coupled with 1 degree of axial rotation, a ratio of 1:7.5 or 0.13. Between C2 and C7, there is a gradual cephalocaudal decrease in the amount of axial rotation that is associated with lateral bending, which may be related to the orientation of the facet joints in the frontal plane. Left lateral bending in this region of 0.75 degree is associated with 1 degree of axial rotation for a ratio of 0.75.[50]

THORACIC SPINE

The thoracic spine is the least mobile portion of the spinal column mainly because of the anatomically restrictive rib cage. The ranges of rotation for the thoracic spine are given in Table 4.5. The median figure for sagittal plane rotation is 4 degrees in the upper, 6 degrees in the middle, and 12 degrees in the lower two segments. In lateral bending, there are 6 degrees in the upper and 2 degrees in the lower three segments. In axial rotation, there are 8 to 9 degrees of motion in the upper half and 2 degrees for each interspace in the lower three segments.[17]

Flexion and extension motion (sagittal plane rotation) is coupled with translation. There is not as much translation in the thoracic spine as there is in the cervical spine, and this is indicated by the relatively flat arch. There is no pattern of cephalocaudal variation. The *top angle* can also be employed to indicate the acuity of the arch.[78]

Coupling of lateral bending (z-axis rotation) with axial rotation (y-axis) occurs such that the spinous processes go toward the convexity of the curve as in the cervical spine. The cephalocaudal variability in this coupling pattern within the thoracic spine is of considerable interest. Biomechanically the thoracic spine is separated into three distinct regions.[51] In the upper portion of the thoracic spine, the coupling pattern is strong. In the middle and lower portions, the coupling pattern is not as strong. This makes the pattern of motion inconsistent, and the spinous processes may rotate toward the concavity of the lateral curve.

The anatomic constraints for motions of the thoracic spine are given in Table 4.6, the ligamentous structures are diagramed in Fig. 4.13.

LUMBAR SPINE

The representative ranges of motion are given in Table 4.7. In sagittal plane motion, there is a gradual cephalocaudal increase in motion. In flexion and extension motions, there is no coupling pattern seen; however, up to 2.8 mm of translation on flexion-extension

Table 4.4. Middle and lower cervical motion (C2-T1)

TYPE OF MOTION	PASSIVE CONSTRAINTS	MUSCLES RESPONSIBLE FOR ACTION
Flexion $(+\Theta x)$	Supraspinous ligament Interspinous ligament Ligamentum flavum Facet joint capsules Posterior longitudinal ligament Posterior annulus	Longus colli Rectus capitis anterior Longus capitis
Extension $(-\Theta x)$	Anterior longitudinal ligament Anterior annulus Facet joints*	Rectus capitis posterior major Rectus capitis posterior minor Obliquus capitis superior (both acting simultaneously) Splenius capitis Splenius cervicis Semispinalis capitis Semispinalis cervicis
Lateral bending (Θz) (one side)	Facet joint capsules (tension side) Facet joints* (compression side) Uncovertebral joints* Intertransverse ligament	Obliquus capitis superior Obliquus capitis inferior Splenius capitis
Axial rotation (Θy) (one side)	Annulus fibrosus Facet joint capsules Interspinous and supraspinous ligaments	Obliquus capitis superior Obliquus capitis inferior Rectus capitis posterior major Rectus capitis posterior minor Sternocleidomastoid Semispinalis capitis Splenius capitis

*Skeletal (nonligamentous) constraint.

may be seen normally.[10,57,63] Lateral bending is strongly coupled to axial rotation such that the spinous processes point in the same direction as the lateral bending (see Fig. 4.5).[10,34,52,53,56,59] Axial rotation and lateral bending are associated with flexion when the spine is in the extended posture and extension when the spine is in the flexed posture.[53]

The IAR is shown in Fig. 4.14. The IAR for sagittal plane motion in the normal disc is located at the posterior aspect of the disc.[8,65] In the degenerated disc, the IAR for sagittal plane motion varies and can occur outside the spine.[9,61,65] In lateral bending, the IAR in the normal disc falls in the region of the lateral aspect of the disc on the same side as bending occurs. In the degenerated disc, the IAR has a larger dispersion (see Fig. 4.14).[9,65,67]

The anatomic constraints for motions of the lumbar spine are given in Table 4.8; the ligamentous structures are diagrammed in Fig. 4.15.

SACROILIAC JOINT

The lumbosacral and sacroiliac joints transmit the weight of the body to the pelvis. The sacroiliac joint is partly synovial and partly syndesmotic. It may be ankylosed in as many as 76% of subjects over 50 years old.[5] The geometry of the sacroiliac joint anatomy and the ligaments confers stability to the joint. The posterior sacroiliac ligaments are the strongest ligaments and are oriented to provide stability with increasing vertical loading (Fig. 4.16).[71] Further ligamentous stability is provided by the sacroiliac joint capsule, the interosseous ligament, the sacrospinous ligament, the sacrotuberous ligament, and the ventral sacroiliac ligaments. The sacroiliac joint is also stabilized to the lumbar spine by the iliolumbar ligament, which is a strong ligament that passes from the transverse process of L5 to the posterior part of the iliac crest. Bony stability is achieved because of the coarse irregular

Text continued on p. 107.

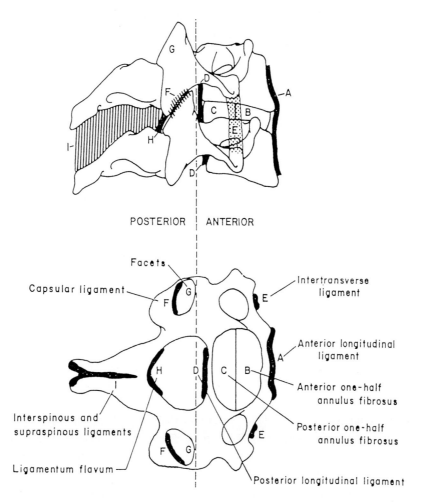

POSTERIOR | ANTERIOR

Facets

Capsular ligament

Intertransverse ligament

Anterior longitudinal ligament

Anterior one-half annulus fibrosus

Posterior one-half annulus fibrosus

Interspinous and supraspinous ligaments

Ligamentum flavum

Posterior longitudinal ligament

Fig. 4.11. Lateral and transverse views of the ligamentous and bony anatomy of a vertebra from the middle and lower cervical spine. In the experiments on clinical stability, ligaments were cut in alphabetical order from anterior to posterior and in reverse alphabetical order from posterior to anterior. *(From White AA, Panjabi MM: Clinical biomechanics of the spine, ed 2, Philadelphia, 1990, JB Lippincott.)*

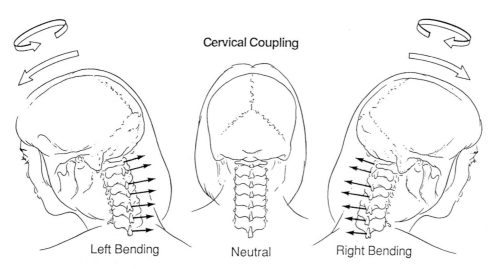

Cervical Coupling

Left Bending   Neutral   Right Bending

Fig. 4.12. The cervical coupling pattern is such that with lateral bending, the spinous processes rotate in the opposite direction. (See also Fig. 4.5). *(From White AA, Panjabi MM: Clinical biomechanics of the spine, ed 2, Philadelphia, 1990, JB Lippincott.)*

Table 4.5. Thoracic spine range-of-motion limits and representative values

Interspace	COMBINED FLEXION/ EXTENSION ($+\Theta x$)		LATERAL BENDING (ONE SIDE) (Θz)		AXIAL ROTATION (ONE SIDE) (Θy)	
	LIMITS OF RANGES (DEG)	REPRESENTATIVE ANGLE (DEG)	LIMITS OF RANGES (DEG)	REPRESENTATIVE ANGLE (DEG)	LIMITS OF RANGES (DEG)	REPRESENTATIVE ANGLE (DEG)
T1-2	3–5	4	5	5	14	9
T2-3	3–5	4	5–7	6	4–12	8
T3-4	2–5	4	3–7	5	5–11	8
T4-5	2–5	4	5–6	6	5–11	8
T5-6	3–5	4	5–6	6	5–11	8
T6-7	2–7	5	6	6	4–11	7
T7-8	3–8	6	3–8	6	4–11	7
T8-9	3–8	6	4–7	6	6–7	6
T9-10	3–8	6	4–7	6	3–5	4
T10-11	4–14	9	3–10	7	2–3	2
T11-12	6–20	12	4–13	9	2–3	2
T12-L1	6–20	12	5–10	8	2–3	2

From White AA, Panjabi MM: Clinical biomechanics of the spine, ed 2, Philadelphia, 1990, JB Lippincott.

Table 4.6. Thoracic motion (T1-L1)

TYPE OF MOTION	PASSIVE CONSTRAINTS	MUSCLES RESPONSIBLE FOR ACTION
Flexion ($+\Theta x$)	Supraspinous ligament Interspinous ligament Ligamentum flavum Facet joint capsules Posterior longitudinal ligament Posterior annulus Radiate ligaments of head of rib Intertransverse ligament	Obliquus externus abdominis Obliquus internus abdominis
Extension ($-\Theta x$)	Anterior longitudinal ligament Anterior annulus Facet joints*	Iliocostalis thoracis Longissimus thoracis Spinalis thoracis Semispinalis thoracis Multifidis Rotatores longus thoracis Rotatores brevis thoracis
Lateral bending (Θz) (one side)	Facet joint capsules (tension side) Superior costotransverse ligaments Intertransverse ligament Costotransverse ligament	Iliocostalis thoracis Longissimus thoracis Trapezius
Axial rotation (Θy) (one side)	Annulus fibrosus Facet joint capsules Interspinous and supraspinous ligaments Ribs	Rotatores longus thoracis Rotatores brevis thoracis Serratus posterior inferior Serratus posterior superior Multifidi

*Skeletal (nonligamentous) constraint.

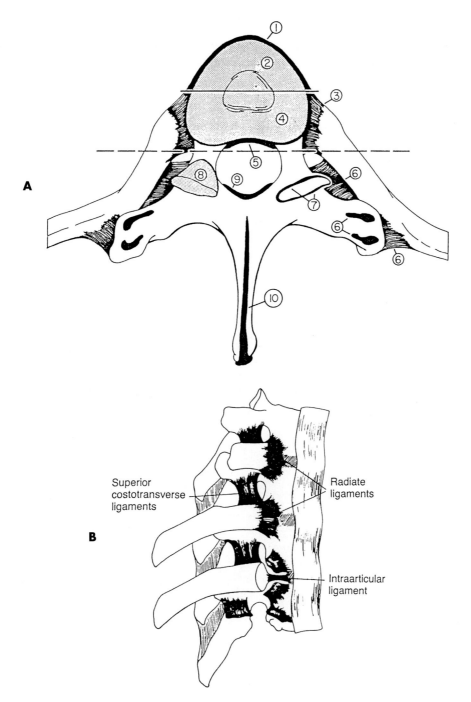

Fig. 4.13. Schematic representation of the major ligaments involved in stabilization of the thoracic spine. **A,** The *solid line* separates the anterior half of the disk from the posterior half. The *broken line* separates the anterior from the posterior elements of the thoracic spine. *1,* Anterior longitudinal ligament; *2,* anterior half of the annulus fibrosus; *3,* radiate and costovertebral ligaments; *4,* posterior half of the annulus fibrosus; *5,* posterior longitudinal ligament; *6,* costotransverse and intertransverse ligaments; *7,* capsular ligaments; *8,* facet articulation; *9,* ligamentum flavum; *10,* interspinous ligaments. **B,** The costovertebral articulation makes some contribution to the clinical stability of the thoracic spine. Note the radiate ligaments attaching to the head of the rib and to *both* vertebral bodies. The costotransverse ligaments may offer some secondary stability. *(From White AA, Panjabi MM: Clinical biomechanics of the spine, ed 2, Philadelphia, 1990, JB Lippincott.)*

Table 4.7.   Lumbar spine range-of-motion limits and representative values

	COMBINED FLEXION/ EXTENSION ($+\Theta x$)		LATERAL BENDING (ONE SIDE) (Θz)		AXIAL ROTATION (ONE SIDE) (Θy)	
	LIMITS OF RANGES (DEG)	REPRESENTATIVE ANGLE (DEG)	LIMITS OF RANGES (DEG)	REPRESENTATIVE ANGLE (DEG)	LIMITS OF RANGES (DEG)	REPRESENTATIVE ANGLE (DEG)
Interspace						
L1-2	5–16	12	3–8	6	1–3	2
L2-3	8–18	14	3–10	6	1–3	2
L3-4	6–17	15	4–12	8	1–3	2
L4-5	9–21	16	3–9	6	1–3	2
L5-S1	10–24	17	2–6	3	0–2	1

From White AA, Panjabi MM: Clinical biomechanics of the spine, ed 2, Philadelphia, 1990, JB Lippincott.

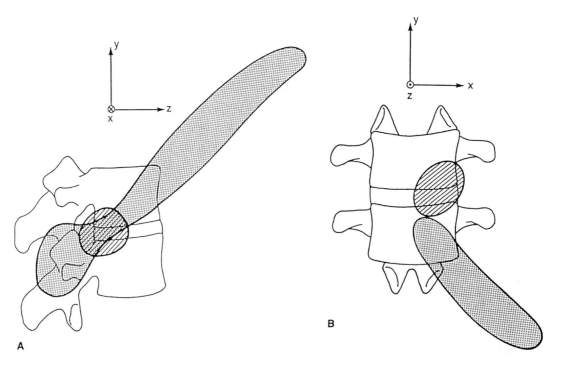

Fig. 4.14.   Changes in location of IAR in the lumbar spine motion segment with and without degenerative disc disease. The axes for the normal discs are shown in the dark areas with longitudinal lines, and those for the degenerated discs are shown in the lighter gray areas. **A,** Flexion. **B,** Right lateral bending. *(From White AA, Panjabi MM: Clinical biomechanics of the spine, ed 2, Philadelphia, 1990, JB Lippincott.)*

Table 4.8. Lumbar motion (L1-S1)

TYPE OF MOTION	PASSIVE CONSTRAINTS	MUSCLES RESPONSIBLE FOR ACTION
Flexion ($+\Theta x$)	Supraspinous ligament Interspinous ligament Ligamentum flavum Facet joint capsules Posterior longitudinal ligament Posterior annulus	Obliquus externus abdominis Obliquus internus abdominis Quadratus lumborum Iliopsoas
Extension ($-\Theta x$)	Anterior longitudinal ligament Anterior annulus Facet joints	Erector spinae (sacrospinalis) Multifidis Rotatores longus thoracis Rotatores brevis thoracis Interspinalis Intertransversarii
Lateral bending (Θz) (one side)	Facet joints and capsules Lateral annulus	Erector spinae Quadratus lumborum Intertransversarii
Axial rotation (Θy) (one side)	Annulus fibrosus Facet joints and capsules Supraspinous ligament	Rotatores longus Rotatores brevis Multifidi

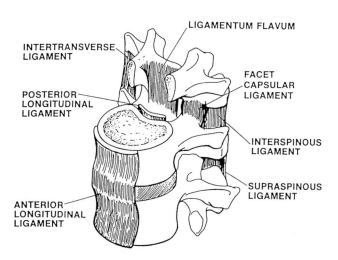

Fig. 4.15. Ligaments of the lumbar spine. Besides the disc, there are seven ligaments that connect one vertebra to the next. Contribution to spine stability by an individual ligament is dependent upon its cross section, distance from IAR, and orientation in space. The anatomy of the ligaments is such to collectively provide stability to the spine in its various physiologic motions. *(From White AA, Panjabi MM: Clinical biomechanics of the spine, ed 2, Philadelphia, 1990, JB Lippincott.)*

surface of the syndesmotic portion of the joint and the shape of the sacrum.[71] The shape of the sacrum is analogous to the keystone in that it wedges under compression loading and causes tensile loading in the ligaments. Thus, the articulating surfaces and the sacroiliac ligaments work together to provide a shock-absorbing mechanism for the base of the spine. Movements of the sacroiliac joint are small and involve 1 to 2 degrees of rotation and 0.5 to 1.0 mm of translation.[35,72,75]

BIOMECHANICS OF THE SPINE

Terms and definitions

Clinical instability. *Clinical instability* has been defined by White and Panjabi[81,83] as "the loss of the ability of the spine under physiologic loads to maintain its pattern of displacement so that there is no initial or additional neurologic deficit, no major deformity, and no incapacitating pain."

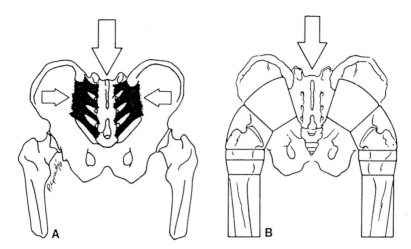

Fig. 4.16. A, The posterior sacroiliac ligaments are oriented to provide increased stability to the sacroiliac articulation with increased loading. **B,** The sacrum functions like the keystone in that it wedges in under compressive loading and causes tensile loading of the sacroiliac ligaments. *(From White AA, Panjabi MM: Clinical biomechanics of the spine, ed 2, Philadelphia, 1990, JB Lippincott.)*

Stress.   *Stress* is the force per unit area of a structure and a measurement of the intensity of this force.

Strain.   *Strain* is the change in unit length or angle in a material subjected to load.

Viscoelasticity.   *Viscoelasticity* is the time-dependent property of a material to show sensitivity to the rate of loading or deformation. For example, a constant load is applied to the disc, and over time deformation of the disk occurs such that the disk narrows (creep). If the ligaments of the spine are placed on stretch as in distraction instrumentation, over time the amount of force required to maintain this fixed distraction diminishes (stress relaxation).

Anatomy

The spine is generally straight in the frontal plane, although in some individuals there may be a slight right thoracic curve. In the sagittal plane, there are four curves. The cervical and lumbar spines are lordotic, and the thoracic spine and sacrum are kyphotic. The lordosis that occurs in the cervical and lumbar spines is due mostly to the wedge shape of the intervertebral disc.[76] The kyphosis that occurs in the thoracic spine is due mostly to the trapezoidal shape of the vertebral body,[51] and the vertebral end-plates are relatively parallel. Consequently, distraction forces placed on the spine cause greater loss of cervical or lumbar lordosis as compared with thoracic kyphosis. The more trapezoidal-shaped disc combined with anterior compressive forces causes disc degeneration to have a greater effect on the loss of lordosis in the cervical and lumbar spine.

The intervertebral disc constitutes 20% to 33% of the entire height of the vertebral column. Compressive loads placed on the spine are transferred through the trabecular bone and cortical shell of the vertebral body.

The compressive forces between adjacent end-plates are transmitted through the disc. The viscoelastic properties of the disc allow dampening of compression and shock stresses.

INTERVERTEBRAL DISC

The intervertebral disc has three parts: nucleus pulposus, annulus fibrosus, and cartilaginous end-plates.[26]

The *nucleus pulposus* is a three-dimensional lattice-gel structure composed of an interlacing fine network of collagen fibers that lie in a mucoprotein gel containing various mucopolysaccharides. The imbibition pressure exerted by the mucoprotein-mucopolysaccharide gel gives the nucleus its hydrophilic property. The water content ranges from 70% to 90%, being highest at birth and decreasing with age.[45] The ability of the nucleus to accept compressive loading and generate pressure is related to its water-binding capacity. The nucleus is usually central except in the lumbar spine, where it is located at the junction between the middle and posterior thirds of the disc. The size of the nucleus and the capacity to swell are greater in the cervical and lumbar regions.

The *annulus fibrosus* is composed of fibrous tissue in concentric laminated bands. The fibers in each band run in the same direction but run in the opposite direction of the next adjacent band. The fibers are oriented at 30 degrees to the vertebral body and 120 degrees to each other (Fig. 4.17). The outer layers are attached to the vertebra through Sharpey's fibers; the inner layers are attached to the cartilaginous end plate.

The *cartilaginous end-plate* is composed of hyaline

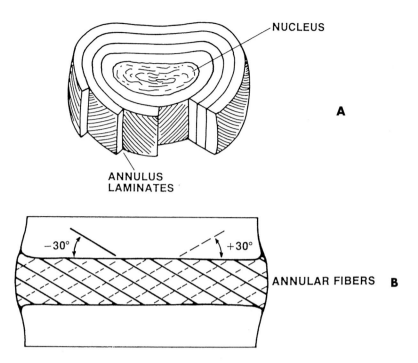

Fig. 4.17. The intervertebral disc. **A,** The disc consists of a nucleus pulposus surrounded by the annulus, made of concentric laminated bands of collagen fibers. In any two adjacent bands, the fibers are oriented in opposite directions. **B,** The fibers are oriented at about ±30° with respect to the placement of the disc. *(From White AA, Panjabi MM: Clinical biomechanics of the spine, ed 2, Philadelphia, 1990, JB Lippincott.)*

cartilage and separates the annulus and nucleus from the vertebral bony end plate. The cartilaginous end plate also degenerates with age resulting in irregularly arranged growth cartilage that over time disappears and is replaced by bone.[2]

Physical properties

The intervertebral disc is a viscoelastic structure. This causes the disc to behave differently when subjected to physiologic loads (slow loading rate) and traumatic loads. The disc may undergo creep or relaxation under various loading conditions.[23,32,65] In neutral standing, the normal nucleus is subjected to compressive stresses, whereas the normal annulus is subjected to tensile stresses.[6,14,20,21,23,32,74] In flexion, because the IAR passes through the midportion of the disk, the posterior annulus is subjected to tensile forces. Tensile stress is present in the anterior annulus during extension. In lateral bending, the tensile stresses are produced on the convex side of the bend. In axial rotation, the tensile stresses develop at about 45 degrees to the plane of the disc.[6]

Compressive loading of the normal disc produces pressure in the nucleus. This pressure pushes the annulus outward causing physiologic bulging of the annulus[4,6,64] and pushes the end plates to deform them axially.[3,66] Axial, circumferential, and radial compres-

sive stresses are present in the inner layers of the annulus. The fiber stress in the outer annulus is larger and tensile (Fig. 4.18).[69] Intradiscal pressures were studied by Nachemson[41–43] in healthy volunteers using pressure-sensitive needles placed into the L3 disk, and pressure associated with a variety of activities was recorded (Fig. 4.19). Intradiscal pressures, which are an indicator of the compressive loads being carried, are rather large. Lying supine gave the lowest pressure readings; sitting upright and standing in 20 degrees of flexion revealed compressive forces roughly 200% of body weight.

Pathologic changes of the disc

Disc degeneration begins around 20 years of age and is characterized by a gradual decrease in the water content of the nucleus. There is progressive fibrosis with increasing cellular degeneration, nuclear fissuring with cavitation, and focal deposition of calcium salts. Disc degeneration or injury (traumatic or surgical) may alter the load-transferring mechanism of the disc such that the nucleus pulposus is not capable of building sufficient fluid pressure. As a result, the end-plates are subjected to less pressure at the center, and the loads are distributed more around the periphery.

The annulus, which is normally subjected to alternating tension and compression, is then subjected to

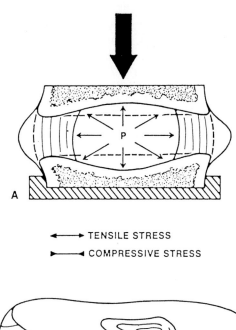

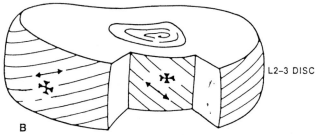

Fig. 4.18.   The normal intervertebral disc under compression. **A,** Pressure within the nucleus is produced because of compression. This pressure pushes the disc annulus and the end plates outward. The disc bulges out in the horizontal plane, and the end-plates deflect in the axial direction. **B,** In the outer layers of the annulus, the stresses are small. Axial, circumferential, and radial stresses are compressive, whereas annular fiber stresses are tensile. In the inner layers of the annulus, the axial, circumferential, and radial stresses are still compressive, but their magnitude is larger. The fiber stress is larger and still tensile. *(From White AA, Panjabi MM: Clinical biomechanics of the spine, ed 2, Philadelphia, 1990, JB Lippincott.)*

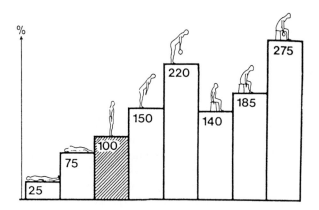

Fig. 4.19.   Diagrammatic comparison of in vivo loads (disc pressures) at L3 during various activities. Note that sitting pressures are greater than standing pressures. *(From Nachemson AL: Spine 1:59, 1976.)*

continuous compressive forces. The annulus develops swelling of the lamellae with areas of mucinous degeneration between the lamellae. This gives rise to concentric fissures between the bands of the annulus that enlarge with age. The collagen fibers of the annulus degenerate with continuous compression disrupting the fibrous structure, which may become fragmented leading to radial fissures. Clinically, increasing annular bulging and disc narrowing result. It has been suggested by Hirsch et al[22,23] that if the nucleus loses its ability to produce an even distribution of pressure, the annulus is no longer capable of even meeting physiologic demands placed on it. Nachemson[38] has determined that the stress on the annulus in the pathologic disc is roughly four times that of the normal disc, and the weight-bearing capacity of the normal disc is 50% greater than that of the degenerated disc.

The cartilaginous end-plates become thinner, and degeneration and decreased cellularity occur. Fibrillation, tears, and Schmorl's nodes increase in frequency.

The nucleus has no blood or neural supply and relies on diffusion for oxygen and glucose.[25,33] This provides for no direct cellular repair of the disc once the degenerative process starts. Circuitous repair may occur by granulation tissue ingrowth through the fissures in the annulus, which transforms the disc into a modified fibrous ankylosis between the two vertebrae. When this occurs, if pain has been present, it often decreases or disappears.[37]

INSTABILITY

Tension on the spinal ligaments from the imbibition pressure of the nucleus confers stability to the spine. When the ingrowth of granulation tissue into the disc is insufficient to withstand the stresses applied, instability occurs. The degenerative process leads to the loss of disc height, which causes ligamentous laxity and caudal subluxation of the facet joints. In flexion, the upper vertebra displaces anteriorly and in extension displaces posteriorly. Because the lower lumbar discs are not parallel to the horizontal plane, shear stresses occur, which increase the loads on the facet joints causing facet arthrosis, and may produce degenerative spondylolisthesis. This abnormal mobility[47] causes further ligamentous injury, and the annular fibers may become elevated off the periosteum. Bone growth in these recesses between the elevated periosteum and bone forms osteophytes.[14,18,27] These osteophytes may decrease the laxity in the ligament and enhance the stability of the spine. When translation becomes greater than 3.5 mm in the cervical spine[83] or 4.5 mm in the lumbar spine[63,81] on radiographs, this is abnormal. Abnormal motion of the FSU may cause pain and nerve or spinal cord injury from impingement, stretching, and irritation.[30,39,84] An increased incidence of disc herniation is also seen at the unstable segment.[81] Narrowing of the foramen from loss of disc height may also cause nerve root irritation.[54,80] Practical checklists for the diagnosis of clinical instability in the cervical, thoracic, and lumbar spine have been suggested by White and Panjabi.[63,81,83]

Osteophytes may develop circumferentially around the vertebral body under the annulus at various points.[27] These vertebral osteophytes occasionally may coalesce to form a bony ankylosis. More commonly, deterring of abnormal motion of the FSU occurs through osteophytic overgrowth around the vertebral body and the facet joints.[14,18,27] The facet joint capsules and ligaments (especially the ligamentum flavum) may thicken and calcify. This process to deter abnormal motion at the involved FSU combined with bulging of the annulus may cause encroachment on the spinal nerves and produce spinal stenosis.[27,44]

Panjabi[48] has offered a novel hypothesis of the stabilizing system of the spine in which there are three subsystems. The vertebrae, discs, and ligaments constitute the passive subsystem. All muscles and tendons surrounding the spinal column that can apply forces to the spinal column constitute the active subsystem. The nerves and central nervous system constitute the neural subsystem. The neural subsystem monitors various transducer signals from the structures making up the passive subsystem and directs the active subsystem to provide the needed stability. A dysfunction of any one of the subsystems may lead to one or more of the following three possibilities: (1) an immediate response from other subsystems to successfully compensate, (2) a long-term adaptation response of one or more subsystems, and (3) an injury to one or more components of the subsystem. Conceptually, the first response results in normal function, the second results in normal function with an altered spinal stabilizing system, and the third leads to overall system dysfunction.

In cases where adaptation for insufficiencies in the spinal column (disc injury, degeneration, or surgical trauma), muscle weakness (aging, atrophy, or surgical trauma), or lack of neural control for proper muscle action (brain, spinal cord, or nerve injury) is not adequate, spinal pain, nerve irritation, instability, and deformity may occur. Adequate compensation of these deficiencies may be achieved with exercise, bracing, or surgical fusion.

SPINAL DEFORMITY

Spinal deformity may be caused by congenital anomalies, idiopathic scoliosis, or alterations in spinal anatomy (bone, ligaments, muscles, and neural control):*

Alterations of the osseous structures

Trauma	Radiation
Neoplasm	Metabolic bone disease
Infection	Intrinsic bone disease
Asymmetrical growth	

Alterations of the ligaments or disc

Disk degeneration	Arthrogryposis
Trauma	Collagen disorders
Surgery	Mucopolysaccharidoses

Alterations in neuromuscular balance

Head injury	Ataxia
Spinal cord injury	Cerebral palsy
Stroke	Polio

*The list below is adapted with permission from White AA, Panjabi MM: Clinical biomechanics of the spine, ed 2, Philadelphia, 1990, JB Lippincott.

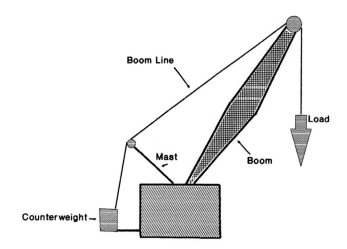

Fig. 4.20.   Loading of the spine in the sagittal plane is analogous to the crane. The vertebral column is analogous to the boom. The erector spine muscles are analogous to the counterweight with the boom lines. The spinous processes supply the lever arms to improve efficiency similar to the mast. Anterior loads (compressive forces) must be counterbalanced by posterior tensile forces for proper functioning. *(Inspired by Jurgen Harms, M.D., Karlsbad-Langensteinbach, Germany.)*

Alterations in muscular function
Surgical trauma
Muscular dystrophy

Dynamic alterations in postural balance
Vestibular abnormalities
Visual abnormalities
Torticollis

Static alterations in postural balance

Klippel-Feil	Transitional vertebra
Surgical fusion of the spine	Ankylosing spondylitis
Surgical fusion of the hip	Leg-length discrepancy
Spinal deformity	Pelvic deformity

A spinal deformity causes a compensatory deformity to occur in the otherwise normal spinal segments. A right lateral curvature in one area of the spine causes a compensatory left lateral curvature over the neighboring segments. If there are enough segments to compensate and enough flexibility, compensation in one or two planes may be complete and restore some of the balance to the spine. Because lateral bending is coupled with axial rotation, and the amount of this coupling varies for different regions of the spine, it is unlikely that more than one plane of motion is able to be fully compensated. In idiopathic scoliosis deformity, the coupling of the lateral bending and axial rotation is such that the spinous processes rotate into the concavity of the curve (the normal spine is usually the opposite); however, sometimes the normal spine follows this coupling pattern. This abnormal coupling adds further complexity to the understanding of scoliosis and has been suggested as a possible component in the cause of

idiopathic scoliosis by White.[79,81] Scoliosis is also associated with sagittal plane deformity; therefore, it must be studied functionally and three dimensionally rather than as a combination of three snapshots for better understanding.

The biomechanics of kyphosis involves a balance of the compressive forces borne by the anterior elements and the tensile forces resisted by the posterior elements (Fig. 4.20). Kyphosis of one or more spinal segments in the cervical and lumbar spine causes compensatory lordosis in adjacent segments. Because of the limited sagittal plane motion in the thoracic spine, compensation of thoracic kyphosis in the upper portion of the thoracic spine usually affects the cervical spine, and the lower portion of the thoracic spine usually affects the lumbar spine. If compensation is incomplete in the cervical spine, there is difficulty with extending the head. If compensation is incomplete in the lumbar spine, standing upright becomes difficult.[28,70]

Biomechanical consequences of uncompensated deformities affecting the spine include a shifting of the center of gravity. The normal center of gravity in neutral standing lies in the midsagittal plane approximately 3 to 4 cm anterior to the S1 vertebral body. Kyphosis shifts the center of gravity anteriorly, which causes an increase in compressive forces on the spine. The increased moment increases the compressive forces on the anterior column and tensile forces on the posterior column. Compensatory increased lordosis in the cervical and lumbar spine increases the intradiscal pressures and facet joint stresses and accelerates the degenerative process.[1,16,29] The asymmetric loading of the disc and facets in the coronal plane that occur with scoliosis also accelerate the degenerative process. Another possible consequence of spinal deformity and the compensatory deformity that occurs is the change in the resting length of the muscles and the lever arm length, which may place the muscle at a mechanical disadvantage.[73] This mechanical disadvantage of the muscles may produce inadequate compensation, fatigue, and pain.

SUMMARY

The human spine is a three-dimensional structure that exhibits nonlinear viscoelastic mechanical behavior.[52] When function is normal, it transfers the loads of the body parts, allows physiologic motions between the body parts, and protects the spinal cord and nerves. The nervous system controls the muscles to provide a delicate, complex balance of the forces exerted on the spine to carry out these functions. Dysfunction in one or more of the components of the spine may be compensated by various complex mechanisms of adaptation. Failure of these mechanisms to compensate causes spinal dysfunction.

ACKNOWLEDGMENTS
The authors thank the Daniel E. Hogan Spine Fellowship, Beth Israel Hospital, Harvard Medical School, Boston, Massachusetts.

REFERENCES

1. Baba H, et al: Late radiographic findings after anterior cervical fusion for spondylotic myeloradiculopathy, Spine 18:2167–2173, 1993.
2. Bernick S, Cailliet R: Vertebral end-plate changes with aging of the human vertebrae, Spine 7:97, 1982.
3. Brinkmann P, Frobin W, Hierholzer E, et al: Deformation of the vertebral end-plate under axial loading of the spine, Spine 8:851, 1983.
4. Brinkmann P, Horst M: The influence of vertebral body fracture, intradiscal injection, and partial discectomy on the radial bulge and height of human lumbar discs, Spine 10:138, 1983.
5. Brooke R: The sacroiliac joint, J Anat 58:297, 1924.
6. Brown T, Hanson R, Yorra A: Some mechanical tests on the lumbo-sacral spine with particular reference to the intervertebral discs, J Bone Joint Surg 39A:1135, 1957.
7. Compere EL, Tachdjian M, Kernakan WT: The Lushka joints—their anatomy, physiology and pathology, Orthopedics 1:159, 1958/59.
8. Cosette JW, et al: The instantaneous center of rotation of the third lumbar intervertebral joint, J Biomech 4:149, 1971.
9. Dimnet J, et al: Radiographic studies of lateral flexion in the lumbar spine, J Biomech 11:143–150, 1978.
10. Dvorak J, et al: Functional radiographic diagnosis of the lumbar spine: Flexion-extension and lateral bending, Spine 16:562–571, 1991.
11. Dvorak J, et al: Functional radiographic diagnosis of the cervical spine: Flexion/extension, Spine 13:748–755, 1988.
12. Dvorak J, Hayek J, Zehnder R: CT-functional diagnostics of the rotatory instability of the upper cervical spine: Part 2. An evaluation on healthy adults and patients with suspected instability, Spine 12:726, 1987.
13. Dvorak J, Panjabi MM, Gerber M: CT-Functional diagnostics of the rotatory instability of the upper cervical spine: An experimental study in cadavers, Spine 12:197, 1987.
14. Farfan HF: Mechanical disorders of the low back, Philadelphia, 1973, Lea & Febiger.
15. Fielding JW: Cineroentgenography of the normal cervical spine, J Bone Joint Surg 39A:1280, 1957.
16. Goto S, et al: Anterior surgery in four consecutive technical phases for cervical spondylotic myelopathy, Spine 18:1968–1973, 1993.
17. Gregersen GG, Lucas DB: An in vivo study of the axial rotation of the human thoracolumbar spine, J Bone Joint Surg 49A:247, 1967.
18. Harris RI, Mcnab I: Structural changes in the lumbar intervertebral discs: Their relationship to low back pain and sciatica, J Bone Joint Surg 36B:304–322, 1954.
19. Hayes MA, et al: Roentgenographic evaluation of lumbar spine flexion-extension in asymptomatic individuals, Spine 14:327–331, 1989.
20. Hirsch C: The reaction of intervertebral discs to compression forces, J Bone Joint Surg 37A:1188, 1955.
21. Hirsch C: The mechanical response in normal and degenerated lumbar discs, J Bone Joint Surg 38A:242, 1956.
22. Hirsch C, Ingelmark B, Miller M: The anatomical basis for low back pain: Studies on the presence of sensory nerve endings in ligamentous, capsular, and intervertebral disc structures in the human lumbar spine, Acta Orthop Scand 33:1–17, 1963.
23. Hirsch C, Nachemson A: New observations on the mechanical behavior of lumbar discs, Acta Orthop Scand 23:254–283, 1954.
24. Hohl M, Bajer HR: The atlanto-axial joint, J Bone Joint Surg 46A:1739, 1964.
25. Holm S, et al: Nutrition of the intervertebral disc, Connect Tissue Res 8:101–119, 1981.
26. Inoue H: Three-dimensional architecture of lumbar intervertebral discs, Spine 6:139, 1981.
27. Kirkaldy-Willis WH: Managing low back pain, New York, 1983, Churchill Livingstone.
28. Lagrone MD, et al: Treatment of symptomatic flatback after spinal fusion. J Bone Joint Surg 70A:569, 1988.
29. Law MD, et al: Deterioration of outcome after two years in patients treated with posterolateral lumbar spine fusion with and without pedicle screw instrumentation, Presented at North American Spine Society, Eighth Annual Meeting, San Diego, 1993.
30. Lehman T, Brand R: Instability of the lower lumbar spine, Proceedings of the International Society for the Study of the Lumbar Spine, Toronto, 1982.
31. Lysell E: Motion in the cervical spine, Acta Orthop Scand Suppl 123, 1969.
32. Markolf KL, Morris JM: The structural components of the intervertebral disc: A study of their contributions to the ability of the disc to withstand compressive forces, J Bone Joint Surg 56A:675–687, 1974.
33. Maroudas A, et al: Factors involved in the nutrition of human lumbar intervertebral disc: Cellularity and diffusion of glucose in vitro, J Anat 120:113–130, 1975.
34. Miles M, Sullivan WE: Lateral bending at the lumbar and the lumbosacral joints, Anat Rec 139:387, 1961.
35. Miller JA, Schultz AB, Anderson GB: Load displacement behavior of sacroiliac joints, J Orthop Res 5:92, 1987.
36. Moroney SP, et al: Load displacement properties of lower cervical spine motion segments, J Biomech 21:769, 1988.
37. Morris JM, Markolf KL: Biomechanics of the lumbosacral spine. In American Academy of Orthopaedic Surgeons: Atlas of orthotics: Biomechanical principles and application, St Louis, 1975, CV Mosby.

38. Nachemson A: Lumbar intradiscal pressure: Experimental studies on postmortem material, Acta Orthop Scand Suppl 43:9–104, 1960.

39. Nachemson A: Lumbar spine instability: A critical update and symposium summary, Spine 10:290–291, 1985.

40. Nachemson A, Evans J: Some mechanical properties of the third human lumbar interlaminar ligament (ligamentum flavum), J Biomech 1:211–220, 1968.

41. Nachemson AL: The influence of spinal movement on the lumbar intradiscal pressure and on the tensile stresses in the annulus fibrosus, Acta Orthop Scand 33:183, 1963.

42. Nachemson AL: In vivo discometry in lumbar discs with irregular radiograms, Acta Orthop Scand 36:418, 1965.

43. Nachemson AL: A critical look at the treatment for low back pain: The research status of spinal manipulative therapy, DHEW Publication No. (NIH) 76-998:21B, Bethesda, MD, 1975.

44. Paine KWE, Huang PWH: Lumbar disc syndrome, J Neurosurg 37:75, 1972.

45. Panagiotacopulos ND, et al: Water content in human intervertebral discs: Part II. Viscoelastic behavior, Spine 12:918, 1987.

46. Panjabi M, et al: Spinal stability and intersegmental muscle forces: A biomechanical model, Spine 14:194–200, 1989.

47. Panjabi M, Goel V: Relationship between chronic instability and disc degeneration, International Society for the Study of the Lumbar Spine, Toronto, 1982.

48. Panjabi MM: The stabilizing system of the spine: Part I. Function, dysfunction, adaptation, and enhancement, J Spinal Disord 5:383–389, 1992.

49. Panjabi MM, et al: Three-dimensional movements of the upper cervical spine, Spine 13:726–730, 1988.

50. Panjabi MM, et al: Three-dimensional load displacement curves of the cervical spine, J Orthop Res 4:152, 1986.

51. Panjabi MM, et al: Thoracic human vertebrae, quantitative three-dimensional anatomy, Spine 16:888–901, 1991.

52. Panjabi MM, et al: Mechanical behavior of the human lumbar spine as shown by three-dimensional load-displacement curves, J Bone Joint Surg 76A:413–424, 1994.

53. Panjabi MM, et al: How does posture affect coupling? Spine 14:1002, 1989.

54. Panjabi MM, Takata K, Goel VK: Kinematics of lumbar intervertebral foramen, Spine 8:348, 1983.

55. Panjabi MM, White AA, Brand RA: A note on defining body parts configurations, J Biomech 7:385, 1974.

56. Parnianpour M, et al: The triaxial coupling of torque generation of trunk muscles during isometric exertions and the effect of fatiguing isoinertial movements on the motor output and movement patterns: 1988 Volvo Award in Biomechanics, Spine 13:982–992, 1988.

57. Pearcy MJ: Stereo radiography of lumbar spine motion, Acta Orthop Scand Suppl 56:212, 1985.

58. Pearcy MJ, Portek I, Sheperd J: Three dimensional x-ray analysis of normal movement in the lumbar spine, Spine 9:294–297, 1984.

59. Pearcy MJ, Portek I, Sheperd J: The effect of low-back pain on lumbar spinal movements measured by three dimensional x-ray analysis, Spine 10:150–153, 1985.

60. Pearcy MJ, Tibrewal SB: Axial rotation and lateral bending in the normal lumbar spine measured by three-dimensional radiography, Spine 9:582–587, 1984.

61. Pennal GF, et al: Motion studies of the lumbar spine: A preliminary report, J Bone Joint Surg 54B:442, 1972.

62. Penning L: Normal movements of the cervical spine, AJR Am J Roentgenol 130:317, 1979.

63. Posner I, et al: A biomechanical analysis of the clinical stability of the lumbar and lumbosacral spine, Spine 7:374–389, 1982.

64. Reuber M, Schultz A, Denis F: Bulging of lumbar intervertebral discs, J Biomech Eng 104:187, 1982.

65. Rolander SD: Motion of the lumbar spine with special reference to the stabilizing effect of posterior fusion [thesis], Acta Orthop Scand Suppl 90:1–186, 1966.

66. Rolander SD, Blair WE: Deformation and fracture of the lumbar vertebral end-plate, Orthop Clin North Am 6:75, 1975.

67. Seligman J, et al: Computer analysis of spinal segment motion in degenerative disc disease with and without axial loading: 1984 Volvo Award in Basic Science, Spine 9:566–573, 1984.

68. Shapiro R, Youngberg AS, Rothman SLG: The differential diagnosis of traumatic lesions of the occipito-atlanto-axial segment, Radiol Clin North Am 11:505, 1973.

69. Shirazi-Adl SA, Shrivastava SC, Ahmed AM: Stress analysis of the lumbar disc-body unit in compression: A three dimensional nonlinear finite element study, Spine 9:120, 1984.

70. Shufflebarger HL, Clark CE: Thoracolumbar osteotomy for sagittal imbalance, Spine 17:S287–S290, 1992.

71. Solonen KA: The sacroiliac joint in the light of anatomical, roentgenographical and clinical studies, Acta Orthop Scand Suppl 26, 1957.

72. Sturesson B, Selvik G, Uden A: Movements of the sacroiliac joints: A roentgen stereophotogrammetric analysis, Spine 14:162–165, 1989.

73. Tveit P, et al: Erector spinae lever arm length variations with changes in spinal curvature, Spine 19:199–204, 1994.

74. Virgin W: Experimental investigations into physical properties of intervertebral disc, J Bone Joint Surg 33B:607, 1951.

75. Walheim GG, Olerud S: Chronic pelvic instability: New diagnostic techniques, Trans Orthop Res Soc 4:248, 1979.

76. Wambolt A, Spencer DL: A segmental analysis of the distribution of lumbar lordosis in the normal spine, Orthop Trans 11:92–93, 1987.

77. Werne S: Studies in spontaneous atlas dislocation, Acta Orthop Scand Suppl 23, 1957.

78. White AA: Analysis of the mechanics of the thoracic spine in man [thesis], Acta Orthop Scand Suppl 127, 1969.

79. White AA: Kinematics of the normal spine as related to scoliosis. J Biomech 4:405, 1971.

80. White AA, et al: Relief of pain by anterior cervical spine fusion for spondylosis. J Bone Joint Surg 55A:525, 1973.

81. White AA, Panjabi MM: Clinical biomechanics of the spine, ed 2, Philadelphia, 1990, JB Lippincott.

82. White AA, Panjabi MM, Brand RA: A system for defining position and motion of the human body parts, Med Biol Eng 13:261, 1975.

83. White AA, Southwick WO, Panjabi MM: Clinical instability in the lower cervical spine, a review of past and current concepts, Spine 1:15–27, 1976.

84. Wyke B: The neurological basis of thoracic spine pain, Rheumatol Phys Med 10:356, 1970.

85. Yamamoto I, et al: Three-dimensional movements of the whole lumbar spine and lumbosacral joint, Trans Int Soc for Study of Lumbar Spine, Kyoto, Japan, 1989.

Biomechanics of the Upper Extremity

Marjorie E. Johnson
Kai-Nan An

Upper extremity function allows for complex task accomplishment in reaching, prehension, and manipulation. The upper extremity can be examined as a linkage system. The main effector of the upper extremity is the hand; the wrist, elbow, and shoulder act to place the hand in space. The description and analysis of function can be assisted by study using biomechanical principles. Application of this information is especially relevant for orthotic design and prescription. This chapter discusses upper extremity biomechanics according to the main joint functions of motion, stability, and strength.

MOTION

Description of motion

Biomechanically, anatomic joints are described according to joint axes and degrees of freedom. For example, the interphalangeal joint is considered to be a uniaxial joint with 1 degree of freedom, allowing motion in the one plane. The type and range of movement of a joint is dependent on passive constraint provided by the shape and contour of the joint surfaces, ligaments, and soft tissue as well as active facilitation by the neuromuscular system.

Definition of rotation

The description of motion becomes detailed when multiaxial joints, as is the glenohumeral joint, are studied. The Eulerian angle system is a method that has utility in describing three-dimensional rotation.[2,3] This method decomposes a single rotation into three separate rotations about orthogonal axes. The axes are fixed in the moving body, making the resulting motion dependent on the sequence. A useful rotation sequence at the shoulder joint is the x-z'-x'' sequence. For

example, with the arm hanging at the side of the body, the z axis is defined to be perpendicular to the scapular plane. The y axis points out laterally, and the x axis points distally along the humeral shaft axis. The rotational sequence for the Eulerian description of the humerus relative to the scapula is as follows: First, ϕ about x axis defines the plane of elevation. Then, rotation of the arm around the rotated z (z') axis by an amount θ represents arm elevation. Finally, the third rotation around the rotated x (x'') axis by an amount of ψ represents axial humeral rotation.

During circumduction motion of the humerus, for example, the corresponding Eulerian angles can be measured as shown in Fig. 5.1. This description can be applied clinically in describing the range of joint motion as well as in specifying joint position in orthotic prescription.

Normal range of motion arcs versus functional motion requirements

When studying upper extremity motion, it is important to delineate between the normal arc of movement standards for specific joints and the functional arc of motion required for most daily activities. For example, although the elbow has a normal arc of flexion-extension of 0 to 150 degrees and pronation and supination of 75 to 85 degrees, respectively,[11] the full arc of motion is not generally used for most activities of daily living. A study of the functional elbow arc of motion conducted by Morrey et al[30] revealed that 15 activities of daily living can be carried out with an arc of motion of 30 to 130 degrees of flexion-extension (Fig. 5.2). Furthermore, these same activities required an equal amount of 50 degrees of pronation and 50 degrees of supination. Those activities that use an arc of motion require that it be roughly equally centered between pronation and supination. Note that the activities stud-

1 – 3′ – 1″ Rotation Sequence
[Left Shoulder (PA View)]

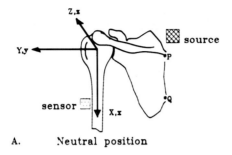

A.   Neutral position

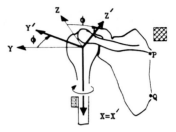

B.   1st Rotation φ about X axis
defines the plane of elevation.

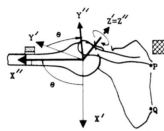

C. 2nd Rotation θ about z′ axis
represents arm elevation.

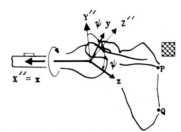

D. 3rd Rotation ψ about x″ axis
represents axial humeral rotation.

Fig. 5.1.   Three-dimensional rotation around each of the orthogonal axes is most accurately described using the Eulerian angle system. Glenohumeral motion is defined by the sequence-dependent Eulerian angles. *(From Morrey BF, An KN: In Rockwood CA, Matsen FA III, editors: The shoulder, Philadelphia, 1990, WB Saunders.)*

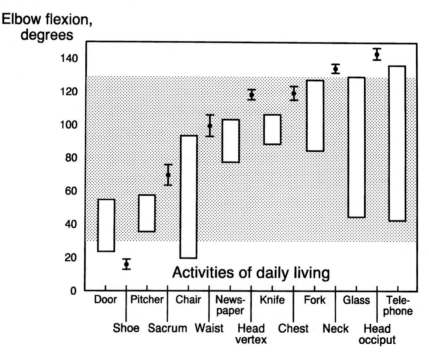

Fig. 5.2.   Functional arc of elbow motion for activities of daily living is approximately 100 degrees, between 30 and 130 degrees. *(From An KN, Morrey BF: In Morrey BF, editor: Joint replacement arthroplasty, New York, 1991, Churchill Livingstone.)*

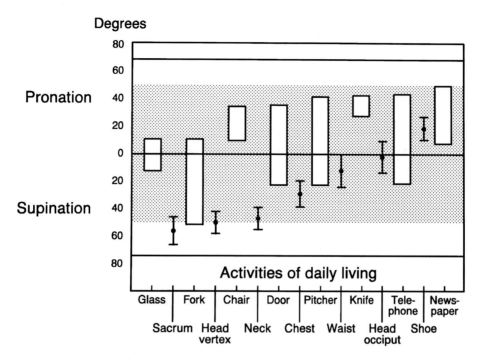

Fig. 5.3. Functional arc of forearm rotation is approximately 50 degrees of pronation and 50 degrees of supination for most activities of daily living. *(From An KN, Morrey BF: In Morrey BF, editor, Joint replacement arthroplasty, New York, 1991, Churchill Livingstone. Reprinted with permission by Mayo Foundation.)*

ied were related to activities of daily living. Special requirements for other activities, including occupational tasks, have not been clearly elucidated. Figure 5.3 illustrates the importance of forearm supination and pronation in positioning the upper extremity for feeding and dressing tasks.

Similarly the wrist has a normal arc of flexion of 80 to 85 degrees, approximately 70 degrees of extension, 20 degrees of radial deviation, and 30 degrees of ulnar deviation.[1] Ryu et al[40] examined 40 normal subjects (20 men and 20 women) to determine the range of motion (ROM) required to perform activities of daily living. The amount of wrist flexion and extension, as well as radial and ulnar deviation, were measured simultaneously by means of a biaxial wrist electrogoniometer. The entire battery of evaluated tasks could be accomplished with 60 degrees of extension, 54 degrees of flexion, 40 degrees of ulnar deviation, and 17 degrees of radial deviation. The majority of the hand placement and ROM tasks that were studied in this project could be accomplished with 70% of the maximal range of wrist motion (Fig. 5.4). This converts to 40 degrees each of wrist flexion and extension and 40 degrees of combined radial-ulnar deviation (30 degrees of ulnar deviation, 10 degrees of radial deviation). The knowledge of functional ROM requirements for activities of daily living can act as a guide when developing orthotic assistive devices. It should be an objective to provide

devices that allow motion to perform functional tasks and, ideally, occupational tasks.

Compensatory motion in the upper extremity

The primary functions of the shoulder complex and elbow are mutually exclusive contrary to accepted thought. It has been observed clinically that patients can tolerate elbow flexion contractures of about 30 degrees without much functional impairment. On the other hand, it is also well recognized that when a motion loss of greater than 30 degrees occurs, patients readily complain of functional impairment. To better understand the implications of this loss of motion, it should be recognized that the shoulder functions as a ball-and-socket joint, allowing the hand to move in a spherical boundary in space.[29] As the elbow moves into a more extended position, a new sphere surface may be described. Thus, the effective sphere of influence of the hand extends from the patient to as far in space as the link at the elbow allows (Fig. 5.5).

A study by O'Neill and associates[38] analyzed compensatory motion in the upper extremity after simulated elbow arthrodesis. The 3Space Tracker System (Polhemus, Inc., Colchester, Vermont) was used to measure shoulder motion; a biaxial wrist goniometer was used to measure wrist compensation; and all subjects were videotaped to observe qualitatively other compensatory motion. Ten healthy male subjects were

Personal Care/Hygiene

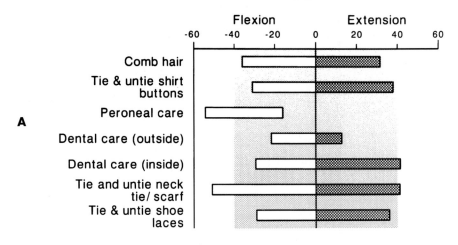

Personal Care/Hygiene

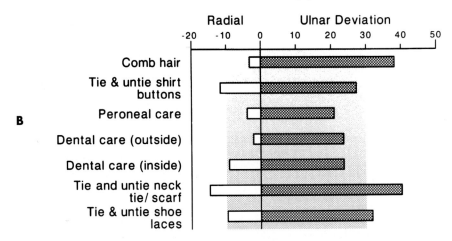

Fig. 5.4. Range of wrist motion required during personal care and hygiene activities. **A,** Extension-flexion. **B,** Ulnar-radial deviation. The gray-striped area represents 70% of the maximum motion (40 degrees extension, 40 degrees flexion, 10 degrees radial deviation, and 30 degrees ulnar deviation). *(From Ryu J, et al: J Hand Surg 16A:409–419, 1991.)*

asked to complete a series of tasks that represented use of the elbow in functional tasks. They were fitted with a custom adjustable brace that simulated elbow arthrodesis at 50, 70, 90, and 100 degrees of flexion and asked to repeat the tasks. Unlike other joints, elbow arthrodesis at any angle resulted in a significant impairment, since the adjacent shoulder and wrist joints could not compensate to allow completion of activities. In upper extremity orthotic design, it is important to apply this information to understand the role and limits compensatory motion of adjacent joints can have in providing function after injury or disease.

Synergistic motion of wrist and hand

Awareness of the relationship between wrist joint position and tendon excursion is essential for under-

standing motor control of the fingers and hand. Positioning the wrist in the direction opposite that of the fingers alters the functional length of the digital tendons so that synergistic finger movement can be attained. Wrist extension is synergistic to finger flexion and increases the length of the finger flexor muscles, allowing increased flexion with stretch.[44] In contrast, wrist flexion is synergistic to finger extension, with wrist flexion placing tension on the long extensors, facilitating finger extension. This relationship has application in tendon-splinting techniques with respect to affecting tendon excursion through positioning. The potential benefits of synergistic wrist motion and MP joint motion in promoting flexor tendon gliding after repair need further study. Also, synergistic wrist motion principles are the basis for many orthotic de-

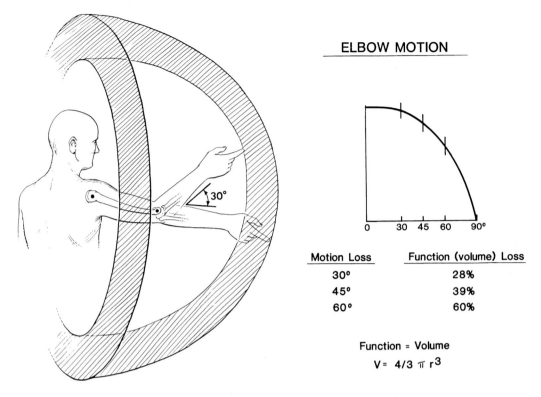

ELBOW MOTION

Motion Loss	Function (volume) Loss
30°	28%
45°	39%
60°	60%

Function = Volume

$$V = 4/3 \, \pi \, r^3$$

Fig. 5.5. Restricted elbow motion limits the sphere of influence of the hand in space. Flexion contractures over 30 degrees are associated with a rapid loss of effective reach area. *(From An KN, Morrey BF: In Morrey BF, editor: Joint replacement arthroplasty. New York, 1991, Churchill Livingstone, 1991. Reprinted with permission by Mayo Foundation.)*

signs in providing assistive function of the hand with quadriplegia.

In a study by Horii et al,[22] the efficacy of a new technique that used synergistic wrist motion (S-splint) was compared with traditional dorsal splinting methods used for mobilization of the flexor tendon after repair: the Kleinert splint (K-splint) and the Brooke Army Hospital/Walter Reed modified Kleinert splint with a palmar bar (P-splint). The results of this study question the anticipated tendon excursion associated with postoperative splinting. They demonstrated that the measured tendon excursion under a condition of low tendon tension was almost half that of theoretically predicted values. In zone II, the magnitude of excursion introduced by the three mobilization methods were in descending order: S-splint, P-splint, K-splint ($p < 0.05$). Differential tendon excursion between the flexor digitorum profundus and the flexor digitorum superficialis had a mean value of 3 mm and was not significantly different among the three methods. Passive proximal interphalangeal joint motion was the most effective means of providing increased amplitude of tendon gliding in zone II. Passive distal interphalangeal joint motion did not increase excursion in zone II as much as had been predicted. Further study is needed to test new designs of splints in vivo.

STABILITY

It is believed that any joint constraint, in part, consists of static and dynamic elements. The static factors may be divided into articular, capsular, ligamentous, and intra-articular pressure components. Dynamic stability originates from muscle activity.

Shoulder

In the normal shoulder, the articulating surfaces of the humerus and glenoid provide minimal stability to the shoulder.[7] The contact area between the two articulating surfaces is relatively small, with only 25% to 30% of the humeral head being in contact with the glenoid surface in any anatomical location. Because the glenohumeral joint does not possess inherent bony stability, it relies to a greater extent on capsular, ligamentous, and dynamic muscular activity for constraint.

The capsule and ligamentous structures of the shoulder function in a coordinated manner to resist joint translation. Primarily this occurs by resisting displacement, but secondarily it occurs by the soft tissue constraints imparting an increased joint contact pressure opposite the direction of the displacement. The relationship between increased joint contact pressure and resistance to translation has been studied and described by Dempster.[16] The influence of atmospheric pressure or the intra-articular pressure on stability of the shoulder has been assessed by Browne et al[14] and Itoi et al[26] in experimental and analytic investigations. The shoulder was seen to subluxate inferiorly by as much as 2 cm after capsular puncture, with marked alteration in joint constraint while performing passive motion. Venting of the capsule in cadaveric specimens was found to have a significant effect on the position of the humeral head. The mean intra-articular pressure was −76 cm H_2O without load, and values decreased in a linear fashion with increased load.

Dynamic shoulder stability during activity is achieved by the shoulder musculature.[41] The role of the rotator cuff in shoulder joint stability has been well recognized. It has been demonstrated in a cadaveric study by Howell et al[24] that the humeral head is positioned in the center of the glenoid in the horizontal plane by a centering mechanism provided by the active rotator cuff. It should be noted even in an unbalanced situation, without equal simulated muscle contraction from the anterior or the posterior cuff components, the activity of the remaining cuff centers the humerus on the glenoid surface. Thus, it is believed that compression of the articular surfaces and the centering effect are accomplished by secondary tightening of the ligaments. The central role of the deltoid muscle to elevate the arm is also known to be countered by depressive action of the anterior and posterior rotator cuff musculature. Thus, the shoulder rotators stabilize the joint by increasing the compressive force between the glenohumeral articular surfaces.

Joint stability can also be enhanced by what has been described as the barrier effect of the contracted muscle. The subscapularis has been shown to be an important dynamic stabilizer as an anterior barrier to resist anterior-inferior humeral head displacement with abduction and external rotation. Because the cross-sectional areas of the rotator cuff musculature anteriorly and posteriorly are essentially equal, the torque generated by these groups is balanced with respect to a force couple that resists both anterior and posterior humeral head translation.

The stabilizing effect of the long head of the biceps (LHB) and short head of the biceps (SHB) muscle has been investigated in a study by Itoi et al.[25] Anterior stability was analyzed in 13 cadaver shoulders. The LHB and SHB were replaced by spring devices, and translation tests at 90 degrees abduction of the arm were performed by applying a 1.5-kg anterior force. The position of the humeral head was monitored by an electromagnetic tracking device with or without an anterior translational force; with 0-kg, 1.5-kg, or 3-kg loads applied on either LHB or SHB tendons in 60, 90, or 120 degrees of external rotation; and with the capsule intact, vented, or damaged by a simulated Bankart lesion.

The authors concluded that the LHB and SHB have similar functions as anterior stabilizers of the glenohumeral joint with the arm in abduction and external rotation and that their role increases as shoulder stability decreases. Both heads of the biceps, if contracted, have a stabilizing function in resisting anterior head displacement.

Elbow

The anterior bundle of the medial collateral ligament (MCL) has been implicated as the primary valgus stabilizer of the elbow with the radial head serving as a secondary joint stabilizer.[6,28] Hotchkiss and Weiland[23] reported that all elbows became unstable after this structure was sectioned. Morrey et al,[31] in an unconstrained kinematic study using an electromagnetic tracking device, demonstrated moderate joint laxity after sectioning of the anterior bundle of the MCL, even with an intact radial head. Sojbjerg et al[43] also confirmed the importance of the anterior bundle of the MCL in a cadaveric model. Clinically, both Schwab et al[42] and Conway et al[15] have emphasized the functional importance of the ligament reconstructions for patients with a deficiency of this structure.

Recent studies by O'Driscoll et al[36] have suggested that the lateral ulnar collateral ligament is a major stabilizing structure for both rotational and varus instability. Injury to this ligament results in posterolateral rotatory subluxation of the elbow, as demonstrated by feelings of instability and a positive pivot shift test. Reconstruction of this ligament has been shown to restore stability to the elbow both clinically and experimentally.[33,35]

An et al,[8] in a cadaveric study, addressed the importance of the proximal ulna articular surface in providing joint stability. In this study, progressive excision of the proximal ulna resulted in a progressive decrease in the stability of the elbow. Valgus stress was in large measure (80%) resisted by the proximal portion of the greater sigmoid notch, whereas varus stress was primarily resisted by the distal portion of the joint surface (65%).

The coronoid process of the ulnar is also an important stabilizer of the elbow. A failure to reconstitute this structure after fractures occur has been correlated with elbow instability and a poor functional outcome.[39] The coronoid process appears to be an essential osseous block to prevent posterior subluxation of the elbow joint, especially with the elbow in extension.

Wrist

In the wrist, the complex system of ligamentous constraints and the articulations of the joint surfaces contribute to stability. This complex ligament system can be divided into extrinsic and intrinsic components. The palmar intrinsic ligaments of the distal row appear to be strongly connected to the carpal bones, as demonstrated by the studies of Garcia-Elias et al.[17,18]

The scapholunate (SL) and lunotriquetral (LT) ligaments are thought to be the most critical ligaments of the wrist, and they accept the greatest load and strain before failure.[32] Biplanar x-ray studies of normal and abnormal kinematics after sectioning of these ligaments have elucidated their importance in providing stability to the scaphoid and lunate.[21] The ultimate strength behavior, stress strain curves, and joint kinematic pattern descriptions may be of value in developing repair or reconstruction techniques for the SL and LT ligaments.

Hand

Primary joint instability is related to muscle and tendon responses to sustained pinch and grasp forces.[4,10] In contrast, the ligaments and capsules appear to play the role of initial stabilizer against instantaneous joint load and provide a second line of defense in maintaining joint stability.

The collateral ligaments of all joints in the hand are important soft tissues. Depending on the orientation of the fibers, various portions of the collateral ligaments play different roles in joint stability. Understanding the anatomic characteristics and function of the capsuloligamentous structures is important for orthotic design when ligamentous structures are impaired.

STRENGTH

Muscle mechanics

Three parameters have commonly been used to describe the size and morphology of the muscle.[5,13] Muscle fiber length (FL) is related to the potential for tendon excursion. The physiological cross-sectional area (PCSA) of a muscle is proportional to the maximum tension of the muscle. Because work equals force times distance, the muscle mass or volume is proportional to total work capacity.

The arrangement of the muscle fiber architecture further influences the characteristics of the muscle contraction. It has been demonstrated that parallel muscle fibers produce a length-tension curve with maintained force throughout a greater distance than the sharply peaked length-tension curve of shorter fiber pennate muscles.[27,46] The muscle architecture has been defined based on the pennation angle. More recently, the concept of muscle index of architecture, i_a, has been adopted to describe the muscle architecture and the length-tension relationship. As shown in the schematic representation of the muscle (Fig. 5.6), the muscle fibers lie at an angle to the direction of induced motion. Two measurements can be taken at muscle optimum length, the muscle fiber length and the muscle belly length. The ratio of the mean fiber length to the muscle belly length is defined as the index of architecture.[46] A typical length-tension relationship of muscles as a function of different architecture indices is shown in Fig. 5.7.

Muscle moment arms around the joint determine the efficiency of the muscle in generating motion and torque; the larger the moment arm, the higher the torque and rotation angle generated for the same amount of muscle force and excursion. The determination of the potential moment arm contributions of muscles can provide insight into the balance of forces at a joint for planning tendon transfers or for designing orthoses to assist in providing mobility or stability with loss of function. A good example is looking at the tendon excursion and moment arms of the wrist muscles. Numerous investigators have examined tendon excursion and moment arm relationships at the wrist.[9,12,20,37] In a study by Horii et al,[22] tendon excursion and joint rotation angles were measured using an electric potentiometer and an electromagnetic tracking device. Instantaneous moment arms of each tendon could then be calculated on the basis of the slope of the curve between tendon excursion and joint angular displacement. Five prime wrist motor tendons were studied on freshly frozen cadavers. Calculated tendon moment arms were found to be consistent throughout a full range of flexion-extension wrist motion and radioulnar deviation and corresponded closely to the anatomic location and orientation of the tendons. The flexor carpi ulnaris tendon provided the largest moment contribution to the wrist joint. Forearm rotation did not affect the function of the wrist tendon except for the extensor carpi ulnaris. During flexion-extension motion, the excursion of the extensor carpi ulnaris decreased significantly from 10 to 4 mm, with the forearm in neutral and pronated positions. During radioulnar deviation, the excursion of the extensor carpi ulnaris increased from 14 to 17 mm, with the forearm in supinated and pronated positions. When a tendon transfer is planned, the entire tendon balance must be considered case by case. For example, the FCU tendon is recommended for reconstruction with radial nerve palsy.[19] However, the moment contribution of this muscle is large,[45] and one might predict that an imbalance of the wrist may result from the FCU transfer.

The maximum muscle tension that can be developed is directly related to the length of the muscle at contraction, which is dependent on the position of the joint. This concept is well illustrated by O'Driscoll et al[34] in a study that analyzed the relationship between wrist position and grip strength. In their study, the

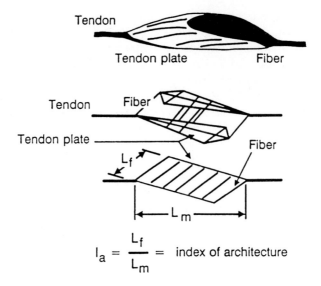

Fig. 5.6.   Schematic representation of muscle fiber arrangement and architecture. Important architectural parameters of muscle fiber length (L_f) and muscle belly length (L_m) define the index of architecture (i_a). *(From An KN, Horii E, Ryu J: In An KN, Berger RA, Cooney WP III, editors: Biomechanics of the wrist joint, New York, 1991, Springer-Verlag.)*

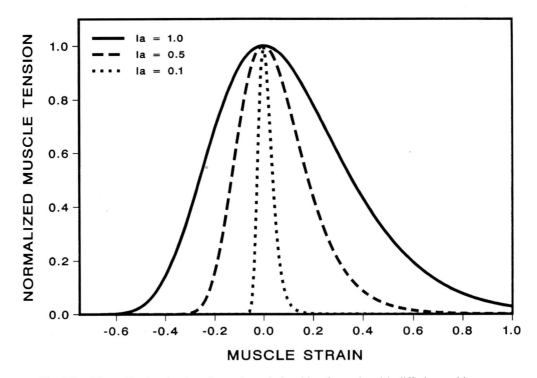

Fig. 5.7.   Normalized active length-tension relationship of muscle with differing architecture. Index of architecture is indicated. *(From An KN, Horii E, Ryu J: In An KN, Berger RA, Cooney WP III, editors: Biomechanics of the wrist joint. New York, 1991, Springer-Verlag.)*

position assumed by a normal wrist during unconstrained maximal grip and the relationship between wrist position and grip strength were investigated in 20 healthy subjects using a biaxial electrogoniometer and grip dynamometer. Grip strength and wrist position were recorded in the self-selected position and then again while the subjects voluntarily deviated the wrist randomly into flexion, extension, or radial or ulnar deviation of 10 to 15 degrees. The self-selected position was 35 degrees of extension and 7 degrees of ulnar deviation (Fig. 5.8). Grip strength was significantly less in any position of deviation from this self-selected

Grip Strength vs. Wrist Position

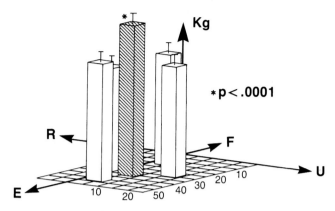

Fig. 5.8. Mean (±1 SE) grip strengths in self-selected positions (*hatched bar*) and positions of deviation (*shown in degrees*) into flexion (*F*), extension (*E*), and radial (*R*), and ulnar (*U*) deviation. Grip strengths were significantly lower in each of the deviated positions than in the self-selected position. *(From O'Driscoll SW, et al: J Hand Surg 17A:169–177, 1992.)*

position, even after accounting for fatigue. With the wrist in only 15 degrees of extension or in neutral radial-ulnar deviation, grip strength was reduced to two thirds to three fourths of normal. Gender did not affect wrist position. The dominant wrists were within 5 degrees of the nondominant wrists but were relatively less extended and in more ulnar deviation. Grip strength is significantly reduced when wrist position deviates from this self-selected optimal position. It has been hypothesized that as the wrist moves into ulnar deviation, the length/tension relationship affords a more effective functional length of the finger flexors, resulting in an increased level of force.

CONCLUSION

Orthotic design and prescription can be aided by understanding upper extremity biomechanical principles. Knowledge of the ROM arcs required to perform functional tasks and the degree to which compensatory motion at adjacent joints can provide task accomplishment is especially relevant. For example, the wrist and shoulder cannot effectively compensate for the loss of elbow motion.

One also needs to consider, however, the importance of joint stability requirements for rehabilitation considerations in use of orthoses, as illustrated by the shoulder. Shoulder motion is complex, allowing movement in a sphere of motion placing the humerus at a fixed angle. Because of the multiaxial nature of this joint, it has been difficult to provide effective orthotic management when there is a lack of dynamic stability of the rotator cuff muscles and long head of the biceps.

Strength parameters based on muscle mechanics can also guide orthotic development based on consider-

ations of tendon excursion, physiological cross-sectional area, moment arm determination, and the muscle-length tension relationship. The use of synergistic wrist motion in orthotic design and the application of the muscle-length tension relationship in optimally positioning the wrist for force production are two illustrations of the importance of understanding biomechanical principles. Further collaborative studies are needed between clinicians and biomechanicians to continue in the advancement of orthotic assistive devices.

REFERENCES

1. American Academy of Orthopaedic Surgeons, Joint Motion: Methods of measuring and recording, American Academy of Orthopaedic Surgeons, 1965, Chicago.
2. An KN, et al: Three-dimensional kinematics of glenohumeral elevation, J Orthop Res 9:143–149, 1991.
3. An KN, Chao EY: Kinematic analysis of human movement, Ann Biomed Eng 12:585–597, 1984.
4. An KN, Cooney WP III: Biomechanics: Section II. The hand and wrist. In Morrey BF, editor: Joint replacement arthroplasty, New York, 1991, Churchill Livingstone.
5. An KN, et al: Muscle across the elbow joint: A biomechanical analysis, J Biomech 14:659–669, 1981.
6. An KN, Morrey BF: Biomechanics: Section III. The elbow. In Morrey BF, editor: Joint replacement arthroplasty, New York, 1991, Churchill Livingstone.
7. An KN, Morrey BF: Biomechanics—Section IV: The shoulder. In Morrey BF, editor: Joint replacement arthroplasty, New York, 1991, Churchill Livingstone.
8. An KN, Morrey BF, Chao EYS: The effect of partial removal of proximal ulna on elbow constraint, Clin Orthop 209:270–279, 1986.
9. Armstrong TJ, Chaffin DB: An investigation of the relationship between displacements of the finger and wrist joint and the extrinsic finger flexor tendons, J Biomech 11:119–128, 1977.
10. Basmajian JV: Muscles alive, Baltimore, 1962, Williams & Wilkins.
11. Boone DC, Azen SP: Normal range of motion of joints in male subjects, J Bone Joint Surg 61A:756, 1979.

12. Brand PW: Clinical mechanics of the hand, St. Louis, 1985, CV Mosby.

13. Brand PW, Beach RB, Thompson DE: Relative tension and potential excursion of muscles in the forearm and hand, J Hand Surg 6:209–219, 1981.

14. Browne AO, et al: The influence of atmospheric pressure on shoulder stability, Presented at the 6th Open Meeting of the American Shoulder and Elbow Surgeons, New Orleans, February 11, 1990.

15. Conway JE, et al: Medial instability of the elbow in throwing athletes, J Bone Joint Surg 74A:67–83, 1992.

16. Dempster WT: Mechanisms of shoulder movement, Arch Phys Med Rehabil 46A:49–70, 1965.

17. Garcia-Elias M, et al: Stability of the transverse carpal arch: An experimental study, J Hand Surg 14A:277–282, 1989.

18. Garcia-Elias M, et al: Transverse stability of the carpus: An analytical study, J Orthop Res 7:738–743, 1989.

19. Green DP: Radial nerve palsy. In Green DP, editor: Operative hand surgery, New York, 1988, Churchill Livingstone.

20. Horii E, An KN, Linscheid RL: Excursion of prime wrist tendons, J Hand Surg 18A:83–90, 1993.

21. Horii E, et al: A kinematic study of lunotriquetral dissociations, J Hand Surg 16:355–362, 1991.

22. Horii E, et al: Comparative flexor tendon excursion after passive mobilization: An in vitro study, J Hand Surg 17:559–566, 1992.

23. Hotchkiss RN, Weiland AJ: Valgus stability of the elbow, J Orthop Res 5:372–377, 1987.

24. Howell SM, et al: Normal and abnormal mechanics of the glenohumeral joint in the horizontal plane, J Bone Joint Surg 70A:227–232, 1988.

25. Itoi E, et al: Stabilising function of the biceps in stable and unstable shoulder, J Bone Joint Surg 75-B:546–550, 1993.

26. Itoi E, et al: Intraarticular pressure of the shoulder, J Arth Rel Surg 9:406–413, 1993.

27. Kaufman KR, An KN, Chao EYS: Incorporation of muscle architecture into muscle length-tension relationship, J Biomech 22:943–948, 1989.

28. King GJW, Morrey BF, An KN: Stabilizers of the elbow: Review article, J Shoulder Elbow Surg 2:165–174, 1993.

29. Morrey BF: Applied anatomy and biomechanics of the elbow joint. In American Academy of Orthopaedic Surgeons Instructional Course Lectures (Vol 35), St. Louis, 1986, CV Mosby.

30. Morrey BF, et al: A biomechanical study of functional elbow motion, J Bone Joint Surg 63A:872–877, 1981.

31. Morrey BF, Tanaka S and An KN: Valgus stability of the elbow: A definition of primary and secondary constraints, Clin Orthop 265:187–195, 1991.

32. Nowak MD, Logan SE: Ultimate strength patterns of 10 clinically significant human wrist ligaments, IEEE Eng in Med and Biol Soc 10th Ann Int Conf, 1988.

33. O'Driscoll SW, Bell DF, Morrey BF: Posterolateral rotatory instability of the elbow, J Bone Joint Surg 73A:440–446, 1991.

34. O'Driscoll SW, et al: The relationship between wrist position, grasp size, and grip strength, J Hand Surg 17:169–177, 1992.

35. O'Driscoll SW, Morrey BF, Bell DF: Posterolateral rotatory instability of the elbow: Clinical, pathoanatomic, and radiographic features, J Bone Joint Surg 72B:543, 1990.

36. O'Driscoll SW, Morrey BF, Korinek SL: The pathoanatomy and kinematics of posterolateral rotatory instability (pivot-shift) of the elbow, Trans ORS 15:6, 1990.

37. Ohnishi N, et al: Tendon excursion and moment arm of wrist motors and extrinsic finger motors at the wrist, Presented at the Annual Meeting of the American Society for Surgery of the Hand, Toronto, September 24-27, 1990.

38. O'Neill OR, et al: Compensatory motion in the upper extremity after elbow arthrodesis, Clin Orthop Rel Res 281:89–96, 1992.

39. Regan WD, Morrey BF: Fractures of the coronoid process of the ulna, J Bone Joint Surg 71A:1348–1354, 1989.

40. Ryu J, et al: Functional ranges of motion of the wrist joint, J Hand Surg 16A:409–419, 1991.

41. Saha AK: Dynamic stability of the glenohumeral joint, Acta Orthop Scand 42:491–505, 1971.

42. Schwab GH, et al: Biomechanics of elbow instability: The role of the medial collateral ligament, Clin Orthop 146:42–52, 1980.

43. Sojbjerg JO, Ovesen J, Nielsen S: Experimental elbow instability after transection of the medial collateral ligament. Clin Orthop 218:186–190, 1987.

44. Tubiana R: Architecture and functions of the hand. In Tubiana R, Thomine J-M, Mackin E, editors: Examination of the hand and upper limb, Philadelphia, 1984, WB Saunders.

45. Volz RG, Lieb M, Benjamin J: Biomechanics of the wrist, Clin Orthop 149:112–117, 1980.

46. Woittiez RD, et al: A three-dimensional muscle model: A quantified relation between form and function of skeletal muscles. J Morph 182:95–113, 1984.

Biomechanics of the Hand

William W. Eversmann, Jr.
James C. Johns

The hand is an extremely complex anatomic structure with a myriad of moving parts interacting in smooth coordination to provide an amazing functional capability. From concert pianist to carpenter, this functional capacity seems endless. The hand's beautiful array of complex interactions is often overlooked until injury disturbs the process and interferes with needed function. Many times, it is only after hand injury that the user realizes how dependent daily living is on function of the hand. The bones, ligaments, fascial tethers, and muscle-tendon units that provide function are dependent on each other to continue mechanical function. When these structures are removed through amputation, prosthetics must try to provide the same biomechanical functions previously present. It is naturally necessary to understand the unique anatomy of the hand to grasp the biomechanical principles that the Certified Orthotist must simulate.

BONY ANATOMY

The bony skeleton of the hand provides the stability and framework for suspension of the remaining soft tissue structures. The two bones of the forearm, the *radius* and *ulna*, position the hand and provide rotation of the wrist as the radius rotates around the ulna. Eight bones make up the carpus itself, usually classified into proximal and distal rows of four each. The proximal row consists of the *scaphoid* (boat-shaped), *lunate* (crescent-shaped), *triquetrum* (pyramidal-shaped), and *pisiform*. The *trapezium, trapezoid, capitate* (largest or chief carpal bone), and *hamate* make up the distal carpal row. Articulating with this distal row are the five metacarpals. The thumb has a proximal phalanx and a distal phalanx, whereas the index through small fingers have three phalanges each (Fig. 6.1).

WRIST ARTICULATIONS

The forearm bones actually articulate with three joints: *distal radioulnar joint, radiocarpal joint*, and *ulnocarpal joint* (Fig. 6.2). Rotation is the principal motion component of the distal radioulnar joint, although translation in the AP plane is present. Pronation and supination occur primarily as the distal radius rotates around the more stationary ulna, with an average arc of 80 degrees in each direction. This joint is inherently unstable because of the differing radii of curvature between the sigmoid notch of the radius and the ulnar head, allowing a significant amount of motion. The distal radius articulates with the scaphoid and lunate of the proximal carpal row, and a small bony ridge divides the radial surface into scaphoid and lunate concavities called facets. A shock-absorbing soft tissue complex of cartilage, ligament, and tendon sheath is interposed between the distal ulna and the two carpal bones just distal to the ulna (lunate and triquetrum). This complex has been labeled the *triangular fibrocartilaginous complex* (TFCC).

The entire wrist joint is actually a triaxial joint, allowing flexion and extension, radial and ulnar deviation, and a small degree of pronation and supination. The scaphoid is primarily coated with articular cartilage because of its numerous articulations. Joint surfaces are linked with the trapezium, trapezoid, capitate, lunate, and distal radius. Intracarpal joints between the scaphoid and lunate and between the lunate and triquetrum are highly dependent on their ligamentous constraints. A semilunar joint exists between the convex proximal surface of the capitate and the distal concave surface of the lunate. Minimal motion occurs between the hamate and capitate in a joint that allows no more than 5 degrees of motion.[1] The pisiform is actually a sesamoid bone lying within the fibers of the

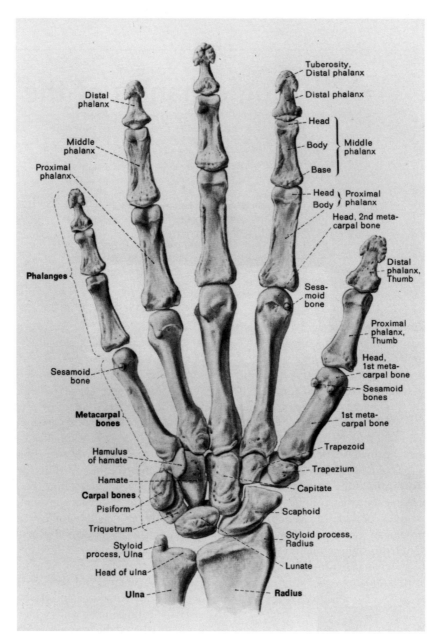

Fig. 6.1. Bones of the right wrist and hand (palmar view) showing the attachments of muscles. *(From Clemente CD: Anatomy: A regional atlas of the human body, ed 3, Baltimore, 1987, Urban & Schwarzenberg.)*

flexor carpi ulnaris tendon. It does have a cartilage-covered joint with the triquetrum.

WRIST KINEMATICS

Kinematic studies have shown that 63% of wrist flexion occurs through the radiocarpal joint, whereas 37% occurs through the midcarpal joint. The percentages for wrist extension are 53% from the radiocarpal joint and 47% from the M-C joint. Forty-four percent of radial deviation and 45% of ulnar deviation occur through the R-C joint, with the remainder of those two directions occurring through the M-C joint. Studies have attempted to measure the amount of motion required for an individual to be able to perform most activities of daily living. Results indicated that 5 degrees flexion, 30 degrees of extension, 10 degrees of radial deviation, and 15 degrees of ulnar deviation were the minimal amounts of motion needed to accomplish those tasks. Electronic goniometers used to measure these motions also indicated that the average individual has a flexion/extension arc of 133 degrees and 40.5 degrees of radioulnar deviation.[13]

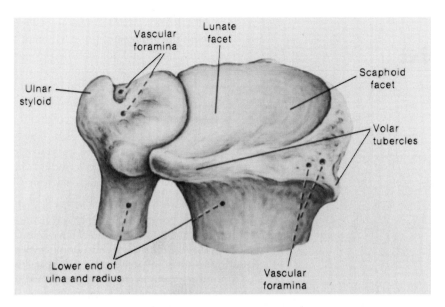

Fig. 6-2. Anterior distal end of the radius and the ulna to demonstrate constant vascular foramina at the base of the styloid process of the ulna and over the anterior ridge of the distal end of the radius (right forearm). *(From Spinner M: Kaplan's functional and surgical anatomy of the hand, Philadelphia, 1984, JB Lippincott.)*

HAND ARTICULATIONS

The thumb *carpometacarpal* (CMC) joint is the most mobile of the CMC articulations. This saddle-shaped joint allows flexion and extension, abduction and adduction, and a high degree of rotation so that the thumb can be opposed to the other digits. The index and long finger CMC joints are much more constrained and allow little motion, around 2 degrees each. This results from the joint geometry as well as from the surrounding soft tissues. The index metacarpal base is fork-shaped, allowing it to lock into the trapezium and trapezoid, whereas the long finger metacarpal base has facets that link it to the adjacent CMC joints.[9] The CMC joints of the ring and small fingers are somewhat more mobile, allowing up to 15 and 40 degrees, respectively, which gives the hand the capacity to grip and cup objects.[9]

Metacarpophalangeal (MCP) joints are shaped to allow considerable flexion and extension in the anteroposterior plane of motion as well as motion in lateral and rotatory planes. The metacarpal head has a cam shape around which the base of the proximal phalanx rotates. *Interphalangeal* (IP) joints are similarly constructed, with two convex condyles separated by a central depression on the distal aspect of the proximal and middle phalanges. These articulate with a concave base of the next more distal bone, which has a central ridge that fits into the corresponding central depression of the proximal bone. Cartilage surfaces extend dorsally to allow some degree of hyperextension. Flexion to 80 degrees is possible in the distal interphalangeal (DIP) joints, with approximately 100 degrees in the proximal inter-

phalangeal (PIP) joints. The PIP joint is not a simple hinge joint and has been compared to the knee joint because it allows some degree of multidirectional stability. The index finger PIP joint, for example, allows 5 degrees of adduction and 9 degrees of supination during normal flexion.[12]

ROTATIONAL AXES

Efforts have been made to determine the axis of rotation for upper extremity joints, which can be of help in designing and prescribing orthoses or prostheses. The elbow has a flexion/extension axis that passes anterior and just distal to the epicondyles, whereas the proximal forearm rotational axis passes through the radial head.[11] The wrist joint is multidirectional, with the main axis of rotation through the capitate. The thumb ray is made up of the IP, MCP, and CMC joints, with the last two having two axes of rotation as shown in Fig. 6.3. In the fingers, MCP joints are multiaxial with the main flexion-extension axis passing transversely through the metacarpal head. PIP joints have a flexion-extension axis that passes through the head of the proximal phalanx just volar to the origin of the collateral ligaments.

LIGAMENTS

In addition to the inherent stability provided by the geometry or shape of the individual joints, stability is

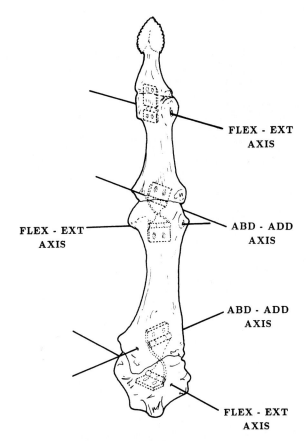

FLEX - EXT
AXIS

FLEX - EXT
AXIS

ABD - ADD
AXIS

ABD - ADD
AXIS

FLEX - EXT
AXIS

Fig. 6.3. The thumb has three joints, the carpometacarpal, the metacarpophalangeal, and the interphalangeal joints. The carpometacarpal and metacarpophalangeal joints both have two axes of rotation, shown here by the *linked, offset pairs of hinges*. The interphalangeal joint has one axis or hinge. None of the hinges are perpendicular to the bones or to one another, so there are conjunct rotations with flexion-extension at all of the joints and with abduction-adduction at the carpometacarpal and metacarpophalangeal joints. *(From Brand PW, Hollister A: Clinical mechanics of the hand, St. Louis, 1993, Mosby-Year Book.)*

also highly dependent on the supporting ligamentous structures. The previously mentioned TFCC helps provide this type of stability to the distal radioulnar joint and is the main intrinsic stabilizer of that joint (Fig. 6.4). The TFCC is made up of an articular disk, a meniscus homologue that blends into the ulnar collateral ligament, the ulnolunate and ulnotriquetral ligaments, the volar and dorsal radioulnar ligaments, and the sheath of the extensor carpi ulnaris tendon. In addition to the restraining force it provides, the TFCC also absorbs some of the load transmission traveling proximally up the wrist. The wrist joint itself is highly dependent on a wide array of ligaments. In general, the volar wrist ligaments are somewhat stronger and thicker than those on the dorsal side (Fig. 6.5). CMC joints are constrained by fairly thick and rigid intermetacarpal ligaments as well as by dorsal and volar CMC ligaments. The highly mobile thumb CMC joint is primarily

stabilized by the volar and dorsal metacarpal ligaments, with the anterior oblique ligament felt to be the single most important for stability.[8] Wear or injury to those ligaments leads to predictable patterns of degeneration.

MCP joints have a complex surrounding soft tissue envelope that includes the joint capsule, a thick capsular volar plate, and both collateral and accessory ligaments on each side. The collateral ligaments are stretched in flexion and more relaxed when the joint is in extension. The accessory ligaments attach firmly to the volar plate (Fig. 6.6). PIP and DIP joint envelopes are similar with a strong volar plate connected to accessory collateral ligaments on each side. Collateral ligaments again run from proximal-dorsal to volar-distal, and a relatively thin dorsal capsule lies under the extensor mechanism. At the PIP joint, the main collateral ligament has been found to be the primary stabilizer for lateral deviation. It has a dorsal portion that is relaxed in extension and tight in flexion, and a volar portion relaxed in flexion and tight in extension.[5] If the collateral ligament is completely cut, maximal deviation is less than 20 degrees unless other secondary restraints (e.g., volar plate, accessory collateral) are also cut. If only one half of the main collateral remains after sectioning of all other primary and secondary restraints, lateral stability is still maintained.[12]

MUSCLE-TENDON UNITS

The extrinsic muscle-tendon units that power the wrist and hand are loosely divided into volar and dorsal groups. Those muscles lying on the volar surface of the extremity provide forearm pronation and flexion of the wrist and digits, whereas those on the dorsal side allow forearm supination and extension of the wrist and digits. The volar forearm muscles can be grouped into deep and superficial muscles, with the five superficial muscles originating primarily from the medial epicondyle. The *pronator teres* inserts on the radius; the *flexor carpi radialis* on the bases of the index and long finger metacarpals; the *palmaris longus* into the palmar fascia; the *flexor carpi ulnaris* into the bones of the pisiform, hamate, and small finger metacarpal; and finally the *flexor digitorum superficialis* into the middle phalanges of the index through small fingers. There are three muscles in the deep volar group. The *flexor digitorum profundus* originates from the proximal ulna and interosseous membrane and inserts on the distal phalanges of the four fingers. The profundus tendons are interconnected at their origin, which significantly limits independent motion of these tendons, an effect termed *quadriga*. The index profundus is the most independent of the four profundi. The *flexor pollicis longus* travels from the radius and interosseous mem-

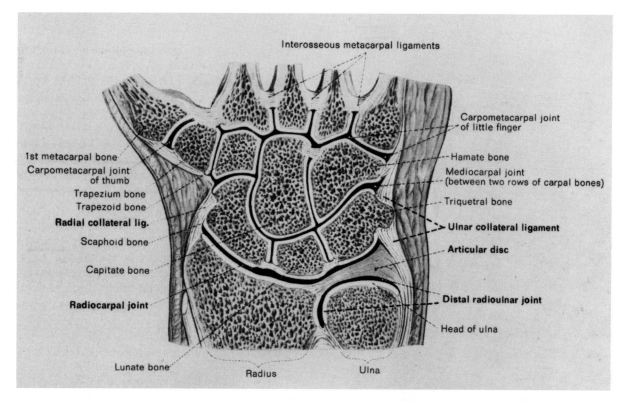

Fig. 6.4. Coronal (frontal) section through the left wrist joints. *(From Spinner M: Kaplan's functional and surgical anatomy of the hand, Philadelphia, 1984, JB Lippincott.)*

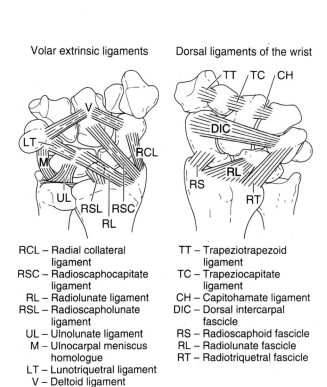

RCL – Radial collateral
    ligament
RSC – Radioscaphocapitate
    ligament
RL – Radiolunate ligament
RSL – Radioscapholunate
    ligament
UL – Ulnolunate ligament
M – Ulnocarpal meniscus
    homologue
LT – Lunotriquetral ligament
V – Deltoid ligament

TT – Trapeziotrapezoid
    ligament
TC – Trapeziocapitate
    ligament
CH – Capitohamate ligament
DIC – Dorsal intercarpal
    fascicle
RS – Radioscaphoid fascicle
RL – Radiolunate fascicle
RT – Radiotriquetral fascicle

Fig. 6.5. Radiocarpal articulation. *(From Tountas CP, Bergman RA: Anatomic variations of the upper extremity, New York, 1993, Churchill Livingstone.)*

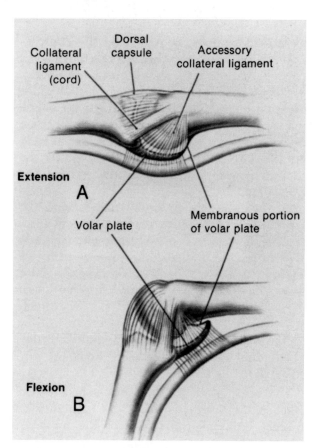

Fig. 6.6. Metacarpophalangeal joint. Note the relationships of the collateral ligaments, volar plate, and dorsal capsule in extension (**A**) and flexion (**B**). *(From Spinner M: Kaplan's functional and surgical anatomy of the hand, Philadelphia, 1984, JB Lippincott.)*

longus and *brevis*, which insert on the base of the index and long finger metacarpals, respectively; the *extensor digitorum communis* (EDC), which divides into the complicated finger extensor mechanism with bony insertions into the bases of the middle and distal phalanges of the fingers; the *extensor digiti minimi* to the small finger extensor mechanism; and the *extensor carpi ulnaris*, which inserts on the base of the small finger metacarpal. The deep group of muscles includes the *supinator*, which travels from the lateral epicondyle and proximal ulna to the radius; the *abductor pollicis longus* (which is more of a radial deviator of the carpus and thumb extender than it is a thumb abductor), from the radius and interosseous membrane to the base of thumb metacarpal; the *extensor pollicis brevis*, from the radius and interosseous membrane to the thumb proximal phalanx base; the *extensor pollicis longus*, from the ulna to the distal phalanx of the thumb; and the *extensor indicis*, which originates from the ulna and interosseous membrane and inserts into the extensor mechanism of the index finger. The EDC tendons are connected at the dorsal hand through tendinous bands termed *juncturae tendinae*, which limits independent function to some extent. Because of the independent EIP and EDQ muscle tendon units, the index and small fingers have more independent extension at the MCP joints.

INTRINSIC MUSCLES

Intrinsic muscles are those muscles that have their origin and insertion in the hand. There are three thenar muscles that act to oppose, flex, and abduct the thumb. The *abductor pollicis brevis* comes off the scaphoid and trapezium and inserts on the lateral aspect of the thumb proximal phalanx. The *opponens pollicis* and *flexor pollicis brevis* originate off the flexor retinaculum and trapezium, and both insert into the lateral aspect of the thumb. On the other side of the palm are the three hypothenar muscles, which have similar functions of abduction, flexion, and opposition of the small finger (cupping the palm). The *abductor digiti minimi*, the *flexor digiti minimi*, and the *opponens digiti minimi* originate off the areas of the hamate, pisiform, and FCU while they insert on the ulnar aspect of the small finger metacarpal and proximal phalanx. There is a *palmaris brevis* muscle on the ulnar side of the palm, which comes off the flexor retinaculum and inserts into the ulnar border of the palmar skin. The *adductor pollicis* originates from the capitate and long finger metacarpal to insert on the ulnar aspect of the thumb metacarpal, adducting the thumb. There are four *lumbrical muscles*, with the radial-most two originating off the radial aspect of the index and long FDP tendons (Fig. 6.8). The ulnar two lumbricals originate from adjoining sides of the long through small

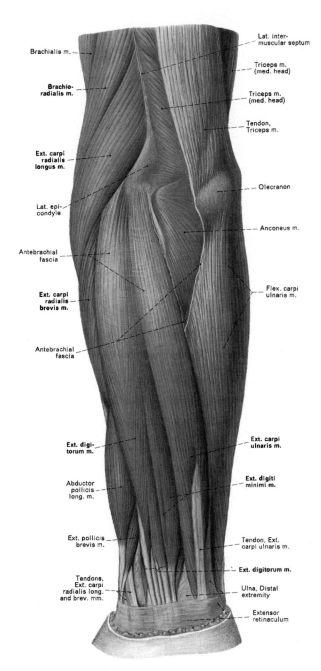

Fig. 6.7. Posterior muscles of the left forearm, superficial group. *(From Clemente CD: Anatomy: A regional atlas of the human body, ed 3, Baltimore, 1987, Urban & Schwarzenberg.)*

brane to the base of the thumb distal phalanx. The *pronator quadratus* is the third muscle of the deep group and originates from the distal part of the ulna, traveling transversely to insert on the distal part of the radius.

The muscles of the dorsal forearm can also be grouped into deep and superficial groups (Fig. 6.7). The superficial group primarily originates off the lateral epicondyle and include the *brachioradialis*, which inserts on the radial styloid; the *extensor carpi radialis*

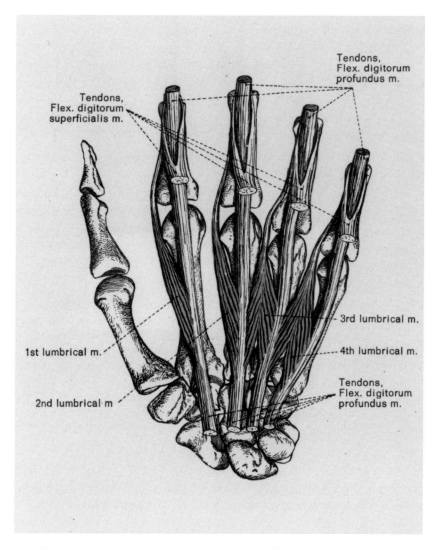

Fig. 6.8. The four lumbrical muscles (left, palmar view). *(From Clemente CD: Anatomy: A regional atlas of the human body, ed 3, Baltimore, 1987, Urban & Schwarzenberg.)*

flexor profundus tendons. All four lumbricals insert on the radial aspect of the EDC tendons, one to each of the four fingers. The remaining intrinsic muscles are the *interossei*, with three muscles on the palmar aspect and four dorsally (Fig. 6.9). The index palmar interosseous comes off the ulnar aspect of the index metacarpal and inserts into the ulnar aspect of the index proximal phalangeal base and partly into the EDC tendon. The ring and small interossei originate off the radial aspect of the ring and small finger metacarpals to insert into the radial aspect of the proximal phalanx and EDC tendons. These three palmar interossei all act to adduct the fingers as well as flex the MCP joints and extend the more distal IP joints. On the dorsal aspect, the four interossei come off adjacent sides of the metacarpals and insert again into the bone of the proximal phalangeal base as well as partly into the EDC tendon. The radial two dorsal interossei insert into the radial

aspect of the index and long fingers, whereas the ulnar two interossei insert into the ulnar aspect of the ring and small fingers. These four dorsal interossei also flex the MCP joint and extend the IP joints, whereas they abduct the fingers.

TENDON PULLEYS

Mechanical advantage is increased for most of these muscle-tendon units through the use of pulleys. For the wrist tendons, the *extensor retinaculum* is divided into six compartments and acts as the pulley for each of those tendon compartments. On the volar side, the *transverse carpal ligament* acts as a pulley for the nine tendons that pass through the carpal tunnel. Other tendons, such as the FCR, have their own tendon sheath that serves as a pulley. Agee has noted that wrist motions cause carpal

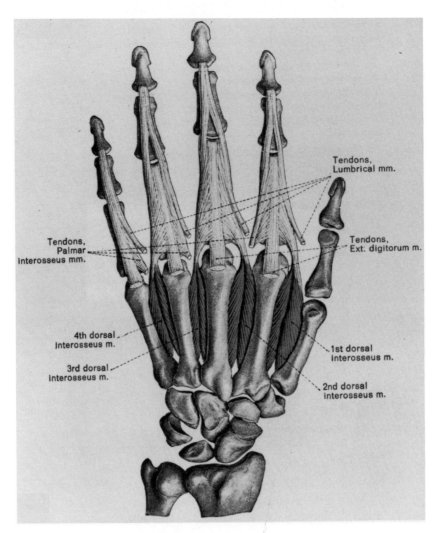

Fig. 6.9. The four dorsal interosseus muscles (left, dorsal view). *(From Clemente CD: Anatomy: A regional atlas of the human body, ed 3, Baltimore, 1987, Urban & Schwarzenberg.)*

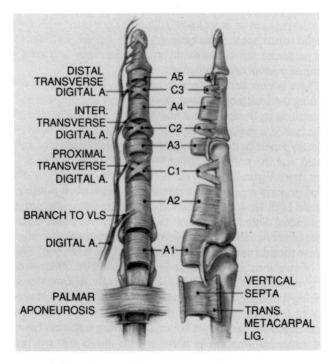

Fig. 6.10. The fibrous retinacular sheath starts at the neck of the metacarpal and ends at the distal phalanx. It can be divided into five heavier annular bands and three filmy cruciform ligaments. Note the palmar aponeurosis pulley proximal to A1. *(From Green DP, editor: Operative hand surgery, ed 3, New York, 1992, Churchill Livingstone.)*

Table 6.1. Architectural properties measured*

MUSCLE	MUSCLE MASS (G)	MUSCLE LENGTH (MM)	FIBER LENGTH (MM)	PENNATION ANGLE (DEGREES)	CROSS-SECTIONAL AREA (CM²)	FL/ML RATIO
BR (n = 8)	17 ± 2.8	175 ± 8.3	121 ± 8.3	2 ± 0.6	1.33 ± 0.22	0.69 ± 0.062
PT (n = 8)	16 ± 1.7	130 ± 4.7	36 ± 1.3	10 ± 0.8	4.13 ± 0.52	0.28 ± 0.012
PQ (n = 8)	5 ± 1.0	39.3 ± 2.3	23 ± 2.0	10 ± 0.3	2.07 ± 0.33	0.58 ± 0.021
EDC I (n = 8)	3 ± .45	114 ± 3.4	57 ± 3.6	3 ± 0.5	0.52 ± 0.08	0.49 ± 0.024
EDC M (n = 5)	6 ± 1.2	112 ± 4.7	59 ± 3.5	3 ± 1.0	1.02 ± 0.20	0.50 ± 0.014
EDC R (n = 7)	5 ± .75	125 ± 10.7	51 ± 1.8	3 ± 0.5	0.86 ± 0.13	0.42 ± 0.023
EDC S (n = 6)	2 ± .32	121 ± 8.0	53 ± 5.2	2 ± 0.7	0.40 ± 0.06	0.43 ± 0.029
EDQ (n = 7)	4 ± .70	152 ± 9.2	55 ± 3.7	3 ± 0.6	0.64 ± 0.10	0.36 ± 0.012
EIP (n = 6)	3 ± .61	105 ± 6.6	48 ± 2.3	6 ± 0.8	0.56 ± 0.11	0.46 ± 0.023
EPL (n = 7)	5 ± .68	138 ± 7.2	44 ± 2.6	6 ± 1.3	0.98 ± 0.13	0.31 ± 0.020
PL (n = 6)	4 ± .82	134 ± 11.5	52 ± 3.1	4 ± 1.2	0.69 ± 0.17	0.40 ± 0.032
FDS I(P) (n = 6)	6 ± 1.1	93 ± 8.4	32 ± 3.0	5 ± 0.2	1.81 ± 0.83	0.34 ± 0.022
FDS I(D) (n = 9)	7 ± 0.8	119 ± 6.1	38 ± 3.0	7 ± 0.3	1.63 ± .22	0.32 ± 0.013
FDS I(C) (n = 6)	12 ± 2.1	207 ± 10.7	68 ± 2.8	6 ± 0.2	1.71 ± .28	0.33 ± 0.025
FDS M (n = 9)	16 ± 2.2	183 ± 11.5	61 ± 3.9	7 ± 0.7	2.53 ± .34	0.34 ± 0.014
FDS R (n = 9)	10 ± 1.1	155 ± 7.7	60 ± 2.7	4 ± 0.6	1.61 ± .18	0.39 ± 0.023
FDS S (n = 9)	2 ± 0.3	103 ± 6.3	42 ± 2.2	5 ± 0.7	0.40 ± .05	0.42 ± 0.014
FDP I (n = 9)	12 ± 1.2	149 ± 3.8	61 ± 2.4	7 ± 0.7	1.77 ± .16	0.41 ± 0.018
FDP M (n = 9)	16 ± 1.7	200 ± 8.2	68 ± 2.7	6 ± 0.3	2.23 ± .22	0.34 ± 0.011
FDP R (n = 9)	12 ± 1.4	194 ± 7.0	65 ± 2.6	7 ± 0.5	1.72 ± .18	0.33 ± 0.009
FDP S (n = 9)	14 ± 1.5	150 ± 4.7	61 ± 3.9	8 ± 0.9	2.20 ± .30	0.40 ± 0.015
FPL (n = 9)	10 ± 1.1	168 ± 10.0	45 ± 2.1	7 ± 0.2	2.08 ± .22	0.24 ± 0.010

From Lieber RL, et al: J Hand Surg 17A:787–798, 1992.
*FDS I(P) and FDS (I/D) refer to the proximal and distal bellies of the FDS I. FDS I(C) represents the combined properties of the two bellies as if they were a single muscle.

bone movements that alter extrinsic tendon courses, increasing moment arms to stabilize the wrist. For example, in wrist extension, the EDC tendons bowstring, while the scaphoid pushes the FCR tendon away from the wrist central axis to increase the moment arm.[2]

The digital flexor tendons have a tendon sheath with annular and cruciform thickenings that serve as a unique pulley system (Fig. 6.10). Three of the five *annular pulleys*—A1, A3, and A5—derive from the volar plate of the MCP, PIP, and DIP joints respectively. The other two—*A2* and *A4*—are attached to bone of the proximal and middle phalanges and are the thickest and strongest of the flexor tendon pulleys. These five annular pulleys control the moment arm of the flexor tendons by keeping them close to the joints they are flexing. The three cruciform pulleys help approximate the sheath during flexion of the digit. There is also a palmar aponeurosis that functions as a pulley proximal to the A1 pulley.[4]

BIOMECHANICS

Load transmission studies have been performed for the wrist and isolated parts of the hand. Cooney's study from the Mayo Clinic indicates 93% of load is normally transmitted across the radiocarpal joint, with only 7% across the ulnocarpal joint. The radiocarpal joint transmitted load is divided into the scaphoid fossa (48%) and the lunate fossa (45%). Other studies have indicated that the ratio of scaphoid fossa load to lunate fossa load is 1.47% and that contact areas move from the volar aspect of the joint to a more dorsal location as the wrist goes into extension. Scapholunate instabilities cause the lunate to shift out of contact with the distal radius and place more load transmission across the radioscaphoid joint. Palmar's study[13] found 80% of load transmission across the radiocarpal joint with 20% occurring through the ulnocarpal joint. The shock-absorbing TFCC can be injured and affect that 20%. With loss of the articular disk portion of the TFCC, only 5% is transmitted through this part of the wrist, whereas no load is transmitted this way if the distal ulna is resected as in a Darrach procedure.

The result of a muscle moving a joint is called *torque* (or *moment*). The measurement of torque can be calculated through the formula

$$\text{Torque} = \text{Force} \times \text{Moment arm}$$

Moment arm is a linear measurement between the joint central axis and the tendon along a perpendicular line drawn as the tendon crosses that particular joint.

Many studies have attempted to measure upper extremity muscles and their output. Generally, muscle force reflects the pressure a muscle exerts on its insertion and is a direct reflection of the cross-sectional area of the muscle. The physiologic (not anatomic) cross-sectional area should be used for calculation of maximum muscle tension. Excursion potential is also important in work calculations and has been measured through muscle fiber length for these muscle/tendon units.[10] The work capacity of a muscle is calculated by multiplying force times distance, where distance re-

flects the length of the muscle. This leads to work being a direct reflection of the total volume of a muscle. Physiologic cross-sectional area and volume of individual muscles have been calculated by different investigators (Table 6.1). These investigations have made it easier for surgeons or engineers to replace lost function through tendon transfers or prosthetic use.

CONCLUSION

Anatomic study of the hand reveals the amazing complexity that exists as well as the interdependence of skeletal elements, ligamentous structures, and muscle-tendon units. Detailed studies have derived biomechanic principles that aid understanding of the hand and its function. It is the goal of the prosthetic team to preserve as much of this function as possible and simulate that which is lost.

REFERENCES

1. Almquist EA: Capitate shortening in the treatment of Kienbock's disease, Hand Clin 9:505–512, 1993.
2. Brand PW, Hollister A: Clinical mechanics of the hand, St. Louis, 1993, Mosby-Year Book.
3. Clemente CD: Anatomy: A regional atlas of the human body, ed 3, Baltimore, 1987, Urban & Schwarzenberg.
4. Doyle JR: Anatomy of the finger flexor tendon sheath and pulley system, J Hand Surg 13A:473–484, 1988.
5. Eaton RG: Joint injuries of the hand, Springfield, IL, 1971, Charles C Thomas.
6. Elliot BG: Abductor pollicis longus: A case of mistaken identity. J Hand Surg 17B:476–478, 1992.
7. Green DP, editor: Operative hand surgery, ed 3, New York, 1992, Churchill Livingstone.
8. Imaeda T, Cooney WP, Linscheid R: Anatomy of trapeziometa-carpal ligaments, J Hand Surg 18A:226–231, 1993.
9. Jebson PJL, Engber WD, Lange RH: Dislocation and fracture-dislocation of the carpometacarpal joints, Orthop Rev 19–28, 1994.
10. Lieber RL, et al: Architecture of selected muscles of the arm and forearm: Anatomy and implications for tendon transfer. J Hand Surg 17A:787–798, 1992.
11. London JT: Kinematics of the elbow, J Bone Joint Surg 63A:529–535, 1981.
12. Minamikawa Y, et al: Stability and constraint of the proximal interphalangeal joint, J Hand Surg 18A:198–204, 1993.
13. Palmer AK, et al: Functional wrist motion: A biomechanical study, J Hand Surg 10:39–46, 1985.
14. Pansky B, House EL: Review of gross anatomy, ed 3, New York, 1975, Macmillan.
15. Smith RJ: Tendon transfers of the hand and forearm, Boston, 1987, Little, Brown.
16. Spinner M: Kaplan's functional and surgical anatomy of the hand, Philadelphia, 1984, JB Lippincott.
17. Tountas CP, Bergman RA: Anatomic variations of the upper extremity, New York, 1993, Churchill Livingstone.
18. Viegas SF, et al: Evaluation of the biomechanical efficacy of limited intercarpal fusions for the treatment of scapho-lunate dissociation, J Hand Surg 15A:120–128, 1990.

Biomechanics of the Foot

Roger A. Mann
Jeffrey A. Mann

The subject of the biomechanics of the foot and ankle during gait is a complex one. It is important for the orthopedic surgeon to have an intimate knowledge of this subject because most of the clinical problems affecting the foot and ankle are at least in part a function of abnormal biomechanics. The functional biomechanics influence decision making about the placement of the ankle after an arthrodesis or the foot when carrying out a triple arthrodesis. It is also reflected in basic thinking when using a shoe lift or an arch support for various other clinical problems.

The foot is a unique structure that is flexible at initial ground contact and is converted to a rigid lever arm at lift-off. The biomechanics of the foot and ankle describes the mechanics by which the foot is converted from a flexible to a rigid structure. The main function of the foot at initial ground contact is to absorb impact and adapt to the ground. This is a passive mechanism that is limited by the shape of the joints and the integrity of the supporting ligamentous tissue. Lift-off, on the other hand, is an active mechanism by which the foot is converted from a flexible to a rigid structure. When one of these mechanisms in the foot fails to function properly, it results in an alteration of the relationship of the foot to the ground, which increases stress on one or more of the joints in the foot and ankle or in the leg or pelvis more proximally.

This chapter discusses the mechanics by which energy is absorbed at the time of initial ground contact and the mechanisms by which the foot is converted to a rigid lever at the time of lift-off. The biomechanical implications of various surgical procedures on the foot are also discussed.

NOMENCLATURE

When reading the literature pertaining to the biomechanics of the foot and ankle, nomenclature at times can become quite confusing. Several terms are used to describe separately the hindfoot and forefoot, and some terms represent motions in more than one joint.

In this discussion, the motion at the ankle is described as *dorsiflexion* and *plantar flexion. Subtalar motion* is described as inversion (varus) and eversion (valgus). *Transverse tarsal motion* is adduction and abduction and is carried out with the foot parallel to the ground with the hindfoot being held in neutral position. The posture of the forefoot is described as forefoot varus or forefoot valgus, depending upon whether the lateral (varus) or medial (valgus) border of the foot is in a more plantar flexed position.

The terms *pronation* and *supination* represent a combination of movements of the foot. When the foot is pronated, there is dorsiflexion of the ankle, eversion of the subtalar joint, and abduction of the transverse tarsal joint. When the foot is supinated, there is plantar flexion of the ankle joint, inversion of the subtalar joint, and adduction of the transverse tarsal joint.

WALKING CYCLE

The walking cycle is used to describe the various phases of gait. It is divided into a stance phase, in which the foot is on the ground, and a swing phase, in which the foot is off the ground and swinging forward. Normally, stance phase consumes approximately 60% of

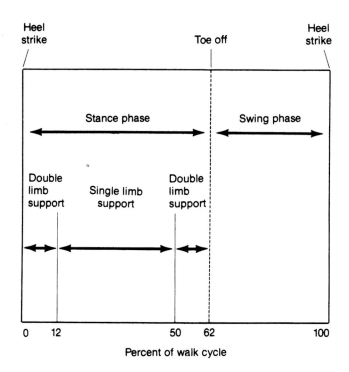

Fig. 7.1. Walking cycle.

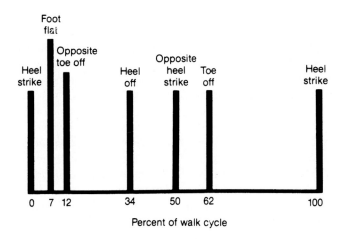

Fig. 7.2. Events of walking cycle.

the walking cycle and swing phase 40% (Fig. 7.1). The stance phase is further subdivided into two periods of double-limb support and one period of single-limb support. The initial period of double-limb support begins with initial ground contact and ends with toe-off of the opposite limb at 12% of the cycle. Single-limb support then occurs until 50% of the cycle, when the opposite foot strikes the ground, entering the second period of double-limb support. This is shortly followed by lift-off, which initiates swing phase. The stance phase can be further divided into various events that occur during a normal walking cycle (Fig. 7.2). Following initial ground contact at 0%, the foot flat is achieved by 7%, and opposite toe-off occurs at 12%. Heel rise of the stance foot begins at 34% of the cycle, which is when the swing leg passes by the stance leg. Opposite heel strike occurs at 50% of the cycle and lift-off of the stance leg at 62%, which initiates swing phase.

From a clinical standpoint, the events of a walking cycle are important. When a patient is observed walking, the initial ground contact should be noted because at times in a patient with spasticity (or tight heel cords) the initial ground contact is with the toe rather than the heel. Foot flat should occur by 7% of the cycle, but if there is an equinus contracture or severe spasticity, this may be delayed or might not occur. The event of heel rise, which occurs as the opposite leg swings by the stance leg, should also be carefully noted. If a patient

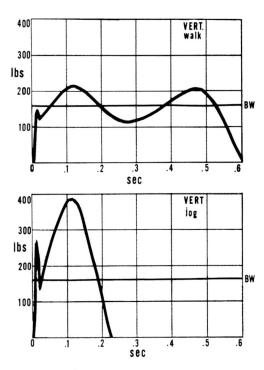

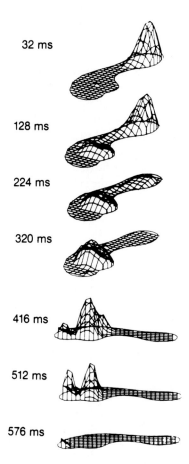

32 ms

128 ms

224 ms

320 ms

416 ms

512 ms

576 ms

Fig. 7.4. Force plate analysis by Clarke.

Fig. 7.3. Vertical force curve for walking compared with that for jogging. Note the markedly increased loading that occurs during jogging.

has spasticity, early heel rise may occur, or if there is weakness in the calf (or an elongated Achilles' tendon), delayed heel rise may result. Occasionally the entire stance phase is prolonged because of significant dysfunction of the lower extremity.

WEIGHT-BEARING FORCES

As we walk, forces are created against the ground. A force plate can be used to measure the forces, which consist of a vertical force, a fore and aft shear, a medial-lateral shear, and torque. The vertical force demonstrates that the initial impact against the ground is approximately 80% of body weight, following which the initial peak is approximately 115% of body weight (Fig. 7.3). There is then a dip in the force curve to approximately 80% of body weight, following which there is a second peak of about 110% of body weight, after which the force against the ground rapidly falls to zero at the time of lift-off. The initial spike of 80% of body weight is the result of the foot striking the ground. The initial peak is brought about by the upward acceleration of the center of gravity. The valley between the two peaks is caused by the fact that as the center of gravity is accelerated upward, the foot is unloaded, resulting in less than body weight against the ground, after which the second peak results from the falling of the center of gravity and opposite ground contact. The

magnitude of the force against the ground can vary. A person walking slowly exerts less force than a person who is jogging or running.

When a computerized force analysis is carried out, one observes a large initial force against the heel, which rapidly passes from the heel to the metatarsal area (Fig. 7.4).[1] The foot is usually on the ground for approximately 620 msec, and by approximately 300 msec all of the force is concentrated in the metatarsal region, after which it is transferred distally to the toes, particularly the hallux. This transfer of force from the metatarsals to the toes is an important one and is a direct reflection of the mechanism by which the plantar aponeurosis functions.

JOINTS OF THE FOOT AND ANKLE

Ankle joint

The axis of the ankle joint passes just distal to the tip of each malleolus and may be estimated by placing one finger on each malleolus. Anthropometric studies demonstrate that although the tibial plafond is parallel to the floor, the angle between the axis of the ankle joint and that of the long axis of the tibia is tilted medially about

80 degrees (Fig. 7.5).[5] Comparing the long axis of the foot with the ankle axis, the foot is slightly internally rotated. In relation to the axis of the knee, the ankle axis is externally rotated approximately 20 to 30 degrees. These axes vary slightly from person to person, and this fact makes it imperative that when carrying out an ankle arthrodesis the rotation of the operated extremity should always match that of the opposite side.

The motion that occurs at the ankle joint is that of dorsiflexion and plantar flexion. Dorsiflexion is most accurately assessed when the calcaneus is placed in line with the tibia, and the head of the talus is covered by the navicular. This places the foot in neutral position (Fig. 7.6). Passively, dorsiflexion is approximately 20 degrees and plantar flexion 50 degrees, although there is a great deal of variation from individual to individual. Figure 7.7 demonstrates the normal motion rotation that occurs at the ankle joint during walking.

Subtalar joint

The axis of rotation of the subtalar joint is oblique, deviating approximately 23 degrees medially from the

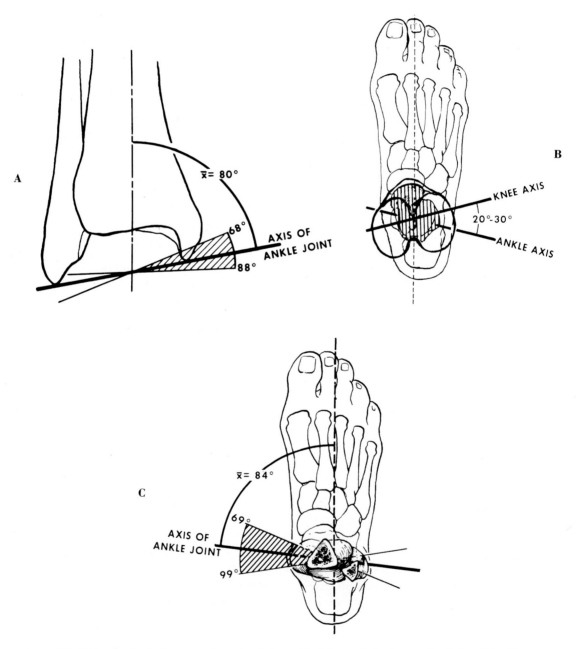

Fig. 7.5. **A,** Angle between the axis of the ankle joint and the long axis of the tibia. **B,** Relationship of the knee, ankle, and foot axes. **C,** Relationship of the ankle axis to the longitudinal axis of the foot.

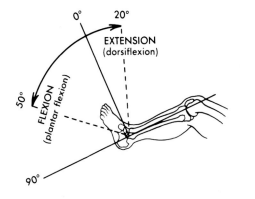

Fig. 7.6.   Range and type of motion in the ankle joint.

long axis of the foot in the transverse plane from medial to lateral and in the sagittal plane approximately 40 degrees to the horizontal plane (Fig. 7.8).[2,6] There is a significant degree of variation in the axis of the subtalar joint. Inman[5] believed that the axis of the subtalar joint permitted it to function as an oblique hinge-type mechanism. As noted in Fig. 7.9, this oblique hinge mechanism permits rotatory motion to be passed back and forth between the lower extremity and foot. In this way, rotation that occurs in the subtalar joint can be imparted proximally across the ankle joint into the tibia and distally into the transverse tarsal joint. If this rotation does not occur, a certain amount of the trans-

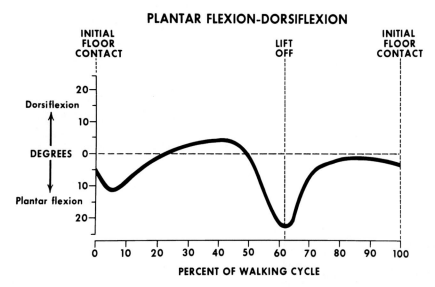

Fig. 7.7.   Normal rotation of the ankle joint during one walking cycle.

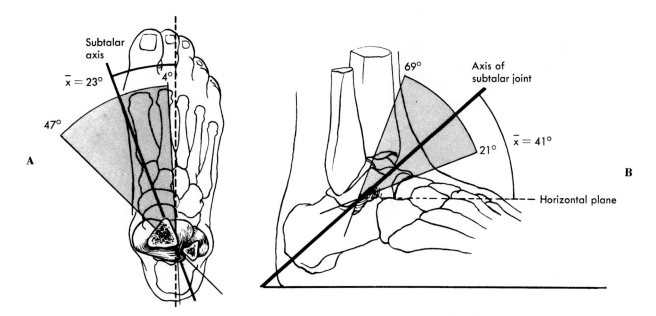

Fig. 7.8.   Subtalar axis in the transverse plane (**A**) and the horizontal plane (**B**).

verse plane rotation is absorbed in the ankle joint, which if long-standing may result in degenerative arthrosis or a ball-and-socket ankle joint (Fig. 7.10). Distally, one may observe changes in the talonavicular joint because of increased stress as well (Fig. 7.11).

The motion that occurs in the subtalar joint is that of inversion and eversion. Inversion is movement of the heel in an inward direction, and eversion is movement outward (Fig. 7.12). The range of motion of the subtalar joint includes inversion of approximately 30 degrees and eversion about 10 degrees, although there is significant variation from individual to individual. During normal walking, the magnitude of inversion during the stance phase is about 8 degrees in individuals with a normal foot and 12 degrees in individuals with flat foot (Fig. 7.13).[13] In individuals with a cavus foot, the degree of subtalar motion is less than that observed in normal feet. During normal walking, eversion occurs at

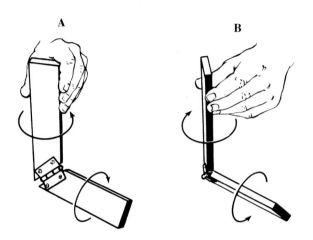

Fig. 7.9. Analogy of the subtalar axes to an oblique hinge. **A,** Outward rotation of the upper stick results in inward rotation of the lower stick. **B,** Inward rotation of the upper stick results in outward rotation of the lower stick.

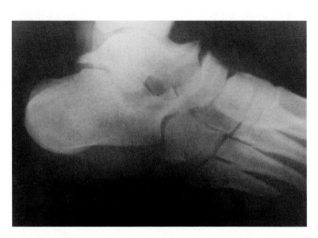

Fig. 7.11. Beaking and alteration of the head of the talus secondary to loss of normal function in the transverse tarsal joint area. This, in turn, was secondary to a calcaneonavicular coalition.

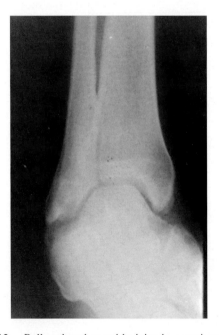

Fig. 7.10. Ball-and-socket ankle joint in a patient with a congenital abnormality of the subtalar joint that did not permit subtalar motion to occur. The resulting transverse rotation, which normally would be absorbed in the subtalar joint, was passed to the ankle joint, which, in turn, adopted an abnormal configuration to compensate for the loss of subtalar joint motion.

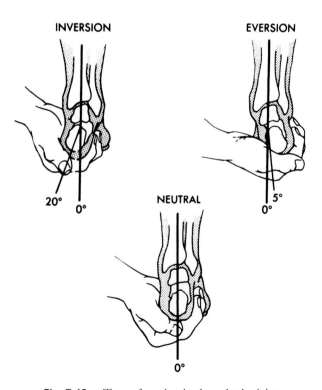

Fig. 7.12. Type of motion in the subtalar joint.

the time of initial ground contact until about 15% of the stance phase, after which progressive inversion occurs until the time of toe-off.

Normal function of the subtalar joint is related to normal function of the talonavicular and calcaneocuboid joints. If normal motion cannot occur in either of these joints, the motion in the subtalar joint is significantly restricted, because for subtalar joint motion to occur, rotation must occur about the talonavicular and calcaneocuboid joints. When subtalar joint motion cannot occur, increased stress is placed on the ankle joint proximally and the talonavicular joint distally.

Transverse tarsal joint

The transverse tarsal joint consists of the talonavicular and calcaneocuboid joints. The transverse tarsal joint should be looked on as an integral part of the subtalar joint because for normal motion to occur in the transverse tarsal and subtalar joints, all three joints must be functioning in a normal manner. The transverse tarsal joint motion has been studied by Elftman,[3] who demonstrated that when the axes of the talonavicular and calcaneocuboid joints are parallel to one another, there is flexibility in the transverse tarsal joint, but when the axes are nonparallel, there is rigidity (Fig. 7.14). When the subtalar joint is in an everted position, the transverse tarsal joint axes are parallel, and the transverse tarsal joint is flexible. This is what is observed at the time of initial ground contact when impact absorption is occurring. In the last half of stance phase, there is progressive inversion occurring in the subtalar joint, which results in the axes being nonparallel, and this results in rigidity of the transverse tarsal joint and hence the forefoot.

Metatarsophalangeal joints

The motion that occurs in the metatarsophalangeal joints is that of dorsiflexion and plantar flexion. The degree of this motion is extremely variable from individual to individual, but normally there is approximately 60 degrees of dorsiflexion and 20 degrees of plantar flexion. During normal gait, dorsiflexion of the metatarsophalangeal joints is a rather passive mechanism that results from the body moving forward over the fixed foot. Plantar flexion during the gait cycle usually does not occur. The main function of the dorsiflexion during the last half of the stance phase is to activate the mechanism of the plantar aponeurosis by which the metatarsal heads are depressed and the longitudinal arch is elevated.

Metatarsal break

The metatarsal break is the oblique axis that overlies the four lateral metatarsophalangeal joints. As noted in Fig. 7.15, this axis passes from medial to lateral at an angle at about 62 degrees to the longitudinal axis of the foot.[6] The importance of this axis is that as we rise up onto the metatarsal heads, the obliquity of this axis results in enhancing the external rotation of the lower extremity, which secondarily brings about inversion of the subtalar joint.

Plantar aponeurosis

The plantar aponeurosis, which arises from the tubercle of the calcaneus, passes distally to insert into the proximal phalanx of each of the toes. When inserting into the great toe, it surrounds the sesamoid bones (Fig. 7.16). The mechanism of action of the plantar aponeurosis during gait results in stabilization

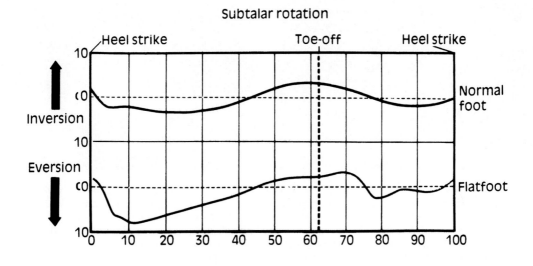

Fig. 7.13. Subtalar joint rotation.

of the longitudinal arch of the foot.[4] In fact, it is probably the main stabilizer of the longitudinal arch. As the body passes forward across the foot during the gait cycle, the metatarsophalangeal joints are passively dorsiflexed. The plantar aponeurosis, which is attached to the base of the proximal phalanges, is drawn forward over the metatarsal heads and at the same time depresses them. This results in elevation of the longitudinal arch, which also secondarily brings about inversion of the calcaneus. This powerful mechanism is most functional at the level of the first metatarsophalangeal joint and becomes less functional as one moves laterally toward the fifth metatarsophalangeal joint. If this mechanism is destabilized by loss of the metatarsal head or base of the proximal phalanx of the great toe, significant weakness results in the foot, and the stabilization of the longitudinal arch is significantly impaired.

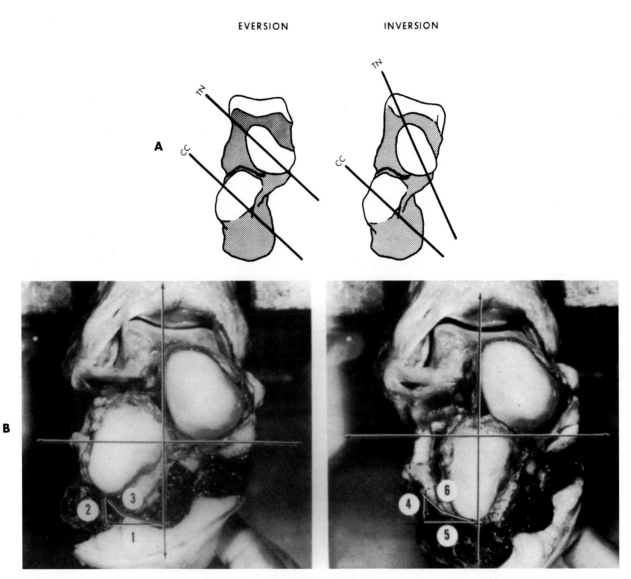

Fig. 7.14.   **A,** Axes of rotation in the talonavicular *(TN)* and calcaneocuboid *(CC)* joints. When the hindfoot is everted, these axes are parallel, so relatively free motion in the transverse tarsal joint is permitted. When the hindfoot is inverted, the axes are divergent, so there is restriction of motion in the transverse tarsal joint and hence greater stability. **B,** Anatomic model of hindfoot, demonstrating relationship between talus and calcaneus. *Left,* Valgus position of os calcis involving abduction *(1),* extension *(2),* and pronation *(3). Right,* Varus position of calcaneus involving flexion *(4),* adduction *(5),* and supination *(6).* When calcaneus is in valgus position, transverse tarsal joint is mobile. When calcaneus is in varus position, transverse tarsal joint is locked. *(From Sarrafian SK: Anatomy of the foot and ankle, Philadelphia, 1993, JB Lippincott, p 513.)*

Talonavicular joint

The articulating surface of the talonavicular joint is not shaped like a simple ball-and-socket but rather is shaped like an elliptical paraboloid with differing radii of curvatures in the transverse and sagittal planes. As a result of this, as force is applied across the joint, during the last half of stance phase, the joint becomes increasingly stable. Conversely, when there is diminished force across the joint, such as observed at initial ground contact, there is flexibility within this joint (Fig. 7.17).

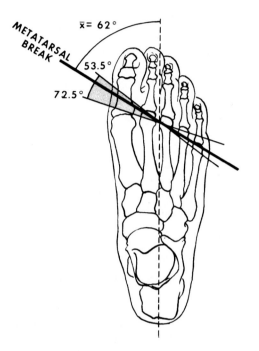

Fig. 7.15. Metatarsal break in relation to the longitudinal axes of the foot.

TRANSVERSE PLANE ROTATION

During gait, the entire lower segment, which consists of the pelvis, femur, and tibia, undergoes a rotation in the transverse plane.[11] After initial ground contact, the transverse plane motion passes from the foot proximally and is part of the impact absorption mechanism of the lower extremity. Following initial ground contact, inward rotation occurs in the tibia, femur, and pelvis (Fig. 7.18). This motion is probably initiated by heel strike, which results in eversion of the calcaneus. The eversion that occurs in the calcaneus is then transmitted proximally across the ankle joint and results in internal rotation of the remainder of the lower segment. In the last half of stance phase, there is progressive external rotation occurring in the lower extremity, which is initiated by the external rotation of the pelvis as the swing leg is moved forward ahead of the stance leg. The external rotation is transmitted distally to the femur, tibia, and across the ankle joint and is then translated by the subtalar joint into inversion. Subtalar joint inversion helps to bring about stabilization of the longitudinal arch via the transverse tarsal joint. The function of the plantar aponeurosis and the functional axis of the metatarsal break help to bring about maximum external rotation. The magnitude of the rotation that occurs increases as one proceeds distally from the pelvis to the tibia.

MUSCLE FUNCTION VERSUS JOINT AXES

The muscles of the lower extremity play a vital role in function. The function of a muscle is related to its

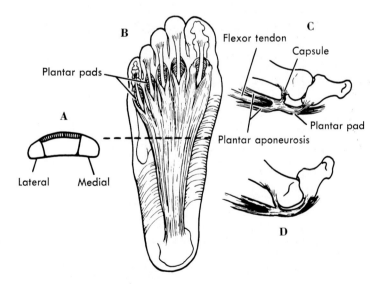

Fig. 7.16. Plantar aponeurosis. **A,** Cross section. **B,** Division of the aponeurosis around the flexor tendons. **C,** Components of the plantar pad and its insertion into the base of the proximal phalanx. **D,** Toes in extension with the plantar pad drawn over the metatarsal head.

relative position in relation to the axis across which it exerts a force. The greater distance a muscle is from the axis of rotation, the greater its leverage, and conversely, the closer, the lesser its leverage (Fig. 7.19). The axes of the subtalar and ankle joints are presented in Fig. 7.20. Those muscles posterior to the ankle axis result in plantar flexion, and those anterior to it result in dorsiflexion. The muscles lateral to the subtalar joint axis bring about eversion, and those medial to it bring about inversion. Looking at the figure, one notes that the muscles of the posterior calf are significantly greater in number and in mass than those anterior to it. This apparent imbalance is kept in check by the proper function of the central nervous system that enables coordinated function of these muscles to occur. One is well aware that following a head injury, stroke, or neuromuscular disorder, a significant deformity about

the foot and ankle can occur because of the resultant muscle imbalance.

The main function of the anterior calf muscles, the tibialis anterior and to a lesser extent the extensors of the toes, is to control plantar flexion, which occurs following initial ground contact by an eccentric contraction (Fig. 7.21). If these muscles are not functioning or are weak, a foot slap results. Following foot flat, the anterior compartment muscles cease to function until about the time of lift-off, when they once again become functional. This time, through a concentric or shortening contraction, dorsiflexion of the ankle joint is brought about, which provides clearance of the foot during the swing phase of gait. If the anterior tibial group fails to function, a foot drop occurs that results in a steppage type of gait. A steppage gait is one in which there is increased flexion of hip and knee to provide adequate toe clearance because of lack of dorsiflexion at the ankle joint.

The posterior calf muscles function during the stance phase of gait. These muscles become active basically as a group, following foot flat. The calf muscles then undergo an eccentric contraction until approximately 40% of the gait cycle, when plantar flexion of the ankle joint begins (see Fig. 7.21). The muscle then undergoes a concentric or shortening contraction, bringing about plantar flexion of the ankle joint, which ceases just before toe-off. The main function of the posterior calf in the first half of stance phase is to control the forward movement of the tibia over the fixed foot.[9,10] If this muscle group fails to function, the support of the stance limb is inadequate, and this results in a shortened step length on the contralateral limb.

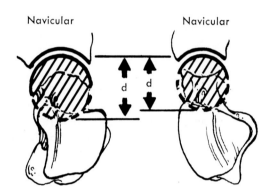

Fig. 7.17. Relationship of the head of the talus to the navicular, left superior and right lateral views. Note the differing diameters of the head of the talus.

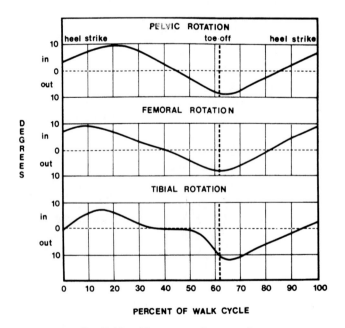

Fig. 7.18. Transverse plane rotation.

The intrinsic muscles of the foot are active during the stance phase of gait and continue their activity until the time of toe-off.[7] These small muscles probably help with the functioning of the plantar aponeurosis and the stabilization of the metatarsophalangeal joints and toes, but by nature of their small size probably do not play a significant role when compared to the plantar aponeurosis in the stability of the longitudinal arch.

MECHANICS OF WALKING

Thus far in this chapter, the forces against the ground and the function of the various joints of the foot and ankle have been discussed. This section correlates the various isolated facts and describes the function of the foot and ankle through a complete walking cycle.

It was pointed out that the forces exerted against the ground exceed body weight during normal walking. If

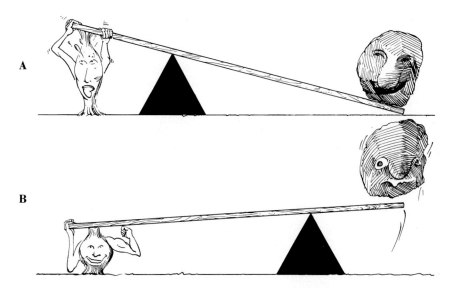

Fig. 7.19. **A,** The closer the muscle is to the axis of rotation, the less leverage it has to effect rotation about the axis. **B,** A muscle far from the rotation has a longer arm and hence can exert greater movement across the axis.

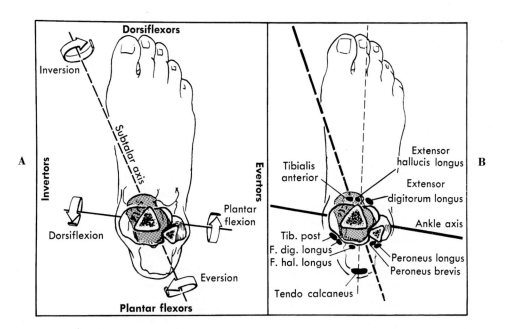

Fig. 7.20. **A,** Rotation about the subtalar and ankle axes. **B,** Relationship of the various muscles about the subtalar and ankle axes.

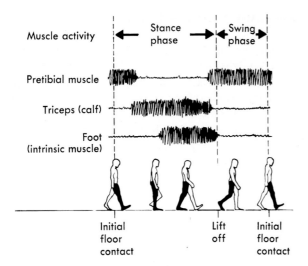

Fig. 7.21. Phasic activity of the leg and foot muscles during normal gait.

one were to extrapolate this for a 150-lb individual walking a mile, approximately 63 tons of force needs to be dissipated per foot per mile. This gives one an appreciation for the amount of force that is dissipated at ground contact. Ground contact is basically an impact absorption type of mechanism and is passive in nature. The only functioning muscles at the time of initial ground contact below the knee are the anterior compartment muscles, which are functioning to control the plantar flexion of the ankle joint, thus again helping to absorb energy. The foot, on striking the ground, literally collapses and is restrained only by the shape of its articulations and their ligamentous support.

The passive events that occur at initial ground contact are:

1. Heel pad striking the ground.
2. Controlled ankle joint plantar flexion.
3. Eversion of the calcaneus, which results distally in parallel axes of the transverse tarsal joint, thereby making it flexible, and proximally enhancing the internal rotation of the lower extremity.

All of these mechanisms result in absorption of the impact against the ground. This impact absorption can be further enhanced by soft shoe material, as opposed to hard leather heels and soles.

The events that occur at the time of toe-off are all dynamic in nature. These consist of the following:

1. Progressive external rotation of the tibia.
2. Subtalar joint inversion.
3. Transverse tarsal joint axes made nonparallel, resulting in locking of the joint.
4. Dorsiflexion of the metatarsophalangeal joints, resulting in the plantar aponeurosis elevating the longitudinal arch.
5. Locking of the talonavicular joint.

To appreciate better the mechanisms that occur, one may look at the function of the foot in the sagittal plane and the transverse plane.

Sagittal plane activities include:

1. Ankle joint motion.
2. Metatarsophalangeal joint motion.
3. Plantar aponeurosis function.
4. Intrinsic muscle function.
5. Configuration of the talonavicular joint.

Following initial ground contact, there is rapid plantar flexion of the ankle joint, which is mediated by the eccentric contraction of the anterior compartment muscles. This muscle function initially controls the plantar flexion of the ankle joint and then probably helps to propel the tibia forward over the fixed foot. Progressive dorsiflexion of the ankle joint begins following foot flat until approximately 40% of the gait cycle. As this dorsiflexion occurs, it is controlled by an eccentric contraction of the posterior calf muscles. At 40% of the gait cycle when the force across the ankle joint is maximal,[12] plantar flexion of the ankle joint begins as a result of a concentric contraction of the posterior calf musculature (Fig. 7.22). This muscle function ceases at approximately 50% of the gait cycle, following which the remainder of the plantar flexion becomes progressively passive until the time of lift-off. During the swing phase, the anterior compartment muscles become active bringing about dorsiflexion at the ankle joint.

The metatarsophalangeal joints play a passive role until the body moves across the fixed foot and plantar flexion of the ankle joint begins. Following this, there is progressive dorsiflexion of the metatarsophalangeal joints until the time of lift-off. The main function of the dorsiflexion is to activate the mechanism of the plantar aponeurosis, which results in plantar flexion of the metatarsal heads and elevation of the longitudinal arch. The intrinsic muscles of the foot are functioning during this same period of time to stabilize the metatarsophalangeal joints and then cease functioning after toe-off. The force analysis in Fig. 7.4 demonstrates this weight transfer from the metatarsal area to the toes.

The talonavicular joint at initial ground contact is somewhat unstable, but the stability of the joint is progressively increased as increasing force is placed across the joint in the last half of stance phase. The elliptical paraboloid shape of the joint aids in the progressive stability of the joint.

Transverse plane mechanisms include:

1. Rotation of the lower extremity, particularly the tibia.
2. Subtalar joint motion.
3. Transverse tarsal joint motion.
4. Function of the metatarsal break.

FUNCTIONAL ANATOMY OF THE FOOT AND ANKLE

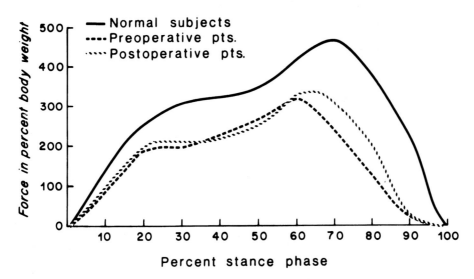

Fig. 7.22. Forces across the ankle joint.

At the time of initial ground contact, internal rotation occurs in the lower extremity. This is a passive event, the magnitude of which is controlled by the degree of rotation permitted by the joints of the foot and their ligamentous support. The inward rotation reaches a maximum at the time of foot flat, following which progressive external rotation begins, which reaches its peak at the time of toe-off. The rotation at the time of initial ground contact begins with the collapse of the subtalar joint into eversion, which relays an internal rotation force proximally up the lower extremity. Subsequent external rotation is probably mediated from proximal to distal, starting at the pelvis with the rotation transmitted through the femur, across the knee and ankle joints to the subtalar joint. The progressive external rotation of the lower extremity helps to bring about inversion of the subtalar joint.

The rotation of the subtalar joint at the time of initial ground contact is one of eversion, which is a passive motion brought about by the loading of the hindfoot by the body. The magnitude of this rotation is mediated by the joints and the ligamentous support of the foot. An individual with a flat foot generally has a greater degree of eversion following ground contact than a person with a normal foot or cavus foot. There is then progressive inversion of the subtalar joint, which reaches a maximum at the time of toe-off. The progressive inversion is brought about by the progressive external rotation that is occurring in the leg above, but it is significantly enhanced by the function of the plantar aponeurosis and the metatarsal break. The plantar aponeurosis, as it becomes more functional in depressing the metatarsal heads, also brings about inversion of the calcaneus, and this is further enhanced by the obliquity of the meta-

tarsal break. Precisely what percent of the internal rotation can be attributed to the external rotation of the tibia, plantar aponeurosis, and metatarsal break has not been determined, but these three mechanisms work in concert to bring about the final stabilization of the longitudinal arch.

The transverse tarsal joint functions in association with the subtalar joint.[8] At the time of initial ground contact, when the subtalar joint is everted, the joint axes of the calcaneocuboid and talonavicular jonts are parallel to one another, and this results in unlocking of the transverse tarsal joint. In the last half of the stance phase, the subtalar joint is inverting, and the joint axes are nonparallel, producing marked stability of the joint. The stability of the transverse tarsal joint is further enhanced by the seating of the talus into the navicular, the complete inversion of the subtalar joint, and the function of the plantar aponeurosis and the intrinsic muscles.

The model presented in Fig. 7.23 points out these various mechanisms, all of which are functioning simultaneously but have been described individually thus far.

During a full gait cycle, at the time of initial ground contact the foot is loaded, which results in plantar flexion of the ankle joint, eversion of the subtalar joint, internal rotation of the tibia, and unlocking of the transverse tarsal joint. This mechanism provides for maximum absorption. In the last half of stance phase, there is increasing stability of the foot, brought about by the external rotation of the lower extremity, progressive inversion of the subtalar joint, locking of the transverse tarsal joint, and the function of the plantar aponeurosis mediated by dorsiflexion of the metatar-

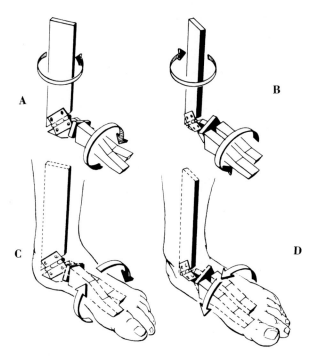

Fig. 7.23. Mechanism by which rotation of the tibia is transmitted through the subtalar joint into the foot. **A,** Outward rotation of the upper stick results in inward rotation of the lower stick. Thus, as seen in **C,** outward rotation of the tibia causes inward rotation of the calcaneus with elevation of the medial border of the foot and depression of the lateral border. **B,** Inward rotation of the upper stick results in outward rotation of the lower stick. Thus, as seen in **D,** inward rotation of the tibia causes outward rotation of the calcaneus with depression of the medial side of the foot and elevation of the lateral side.

sophalangeal joints. This mechanism produces a rigid foot for the time of toe-off (Fig. 7.24).

SURGICAL IMPLICATIONS OF THE BIOMECHANICS OF THE FOOT

When carrying out operative procedures around the foot and ankle, the biomechanics of the foot must always be considered. In particular, when an arthrodesis is carried out, increased stress on an adjacent joint results. This has long-term implications and needs to be carefully considered in the surgical decision making. As a general rule, if an arthrodesis can be avoided by carrying out a corrective osteotomy or tendon transfer, this is preferable to avoid the added stress on adjacent joints. The use of an orthotic device, likewise, should always be considered when feasible.

Ankle joint

An ankle arthrodesis is commonly carried out for a painful affliction of the ankle joint. Following an ankle arthrodesis with elimination of dorsiflexion and plantar flexion, increased stress is placed on the subtalar and transverse tarsal joints. In an in vitro analysis following ankle fusions, it was observed that approximately 50% of dorsiflexion and 70% of plantar flexion were eliminated. This means that the 50% of dorsiflexion and 30% of plantar flexion that still remain occur at other joints (Fig. 7.25). If arthrosis is present in the subtalar or transverse tarsal joints following an ankle fusion, there is a possibility of persistent pain. This concept needs to be taken into account when considering a fusion.

The alignment of the ankle fusion is extremely important because if the foot is not placed into a plantigrade position, abnormal stresses are applied to the foot and knee, resulting in patient dissatisfaction. When fusing an ankle, it should be placed into neutral position as far as dorsiflexion–plantar flexion, into 3 to 5 degrees of valgus, and the degree of external rotation should be equal to that of the opposite side. Shortening should be kept to a minimum.

Plantar flexion of 5 to 10 degrees should be considered if the patient requires knee stability because of loss of quadriceps muscle function. With the foot fixed in equinus, it provides a back knee thrust, thereby helping to stabilize the knee joint. In the absence of this condition, however, it is important that the joint not be placed into equinus to prevent pressure against the posterior portion of the knee joint. If the ankle joint is placed into excessive dorsiflexion, increased stress is placed on the heel, which may be a problem particularly in the patient with an insensate foot. When carrying out a pan-talar arthrodesis, however, slight dorsiflexion is probably beneficial because it permits the individual to roll over the foot more easily than when it is placed in neutral. The varus-valgus alignment is critical because if the ankle is placed into too much varus, instability of the subtalar joint results because the weight-bearing line is passing lateral to the axis of the subtalar joint. The varus alignment also results in locking of the transverse tarsal joint producing a rigid foot and a vaulting type of gait pattern. If the ankle is placed into excessive valgus, this results in stress being applied along the medial side of the knee joint.

Subtalar joint

When arthrodesis of a subtalar joint is performed, the biomechanical principle is that it be placed in 5 to 7 degrees of valgus. In this way, the transverse tarsal joint is kept parallel, which permits increased flexibility through the midtarsal area. If the subtalar joint is placed into varus, the joints are nonparallel, resulting in increased rigidity of the forefoot. A rigid forefoot results in a vaulting gait pattern or external rotation of the leg to compensate for it. The varus position also results in increased stress along the lateral aspect of the foot, and

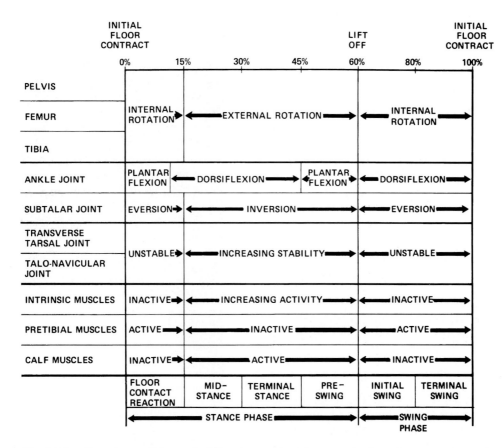

	INITIAL FLOOR CONTRACT				LIFT OFF		INITIAL FLOOR CONTRACT
	0%	15%	30%	45%	60%	80%	100%
PELVIS							
FEMUR	INTERNAL ROTATION	←—— EXTERNAL ROTATION ——→			←— INTERNAL ROTATION —→		
TIBIA							
ANKLE JOINT	PLANTAR FLEXION	←— DORSIFLEXION —→		PLANTAR FLEXION	←— DORSIFLEXION —→		
SUBTALAR JOINT	EVERSION→	←——— INVERSION ———→			←— EVERSION —→		
TRANSVERSE TARSAL JOINT	UNSTABLE→	←—INCREASING STABILITY—→			←—UNSTABLE—→		
TALO-NAVICULAR JOINT							
INTRINSIC MUSCLES	INACTIVE→	←—INCREASING ACTIVITY—→			←—INACTIVE—→		
PRETIBIAL MUSCLES	ACTIVE→	←——— INACTIVE ———→			←—ACTIVE—→		
CALF MUSCLES	INACTIVE→	←——— ACTIVE ———→			←—INACTIVE—→		
	FLOOR CONTACT REACTION	MID-STANCE	TERMINAL STANCE	PRE-SWING	INITIAL SWING	TERMINAL SWING	
	←——————— STANCE PHASE ———————→				←— SWING PHASE —→		

Fig. 7.24. Complete walking cycle. Note the rotations that occur in the various segments and joints as well as activity in the foot and leg musculature.

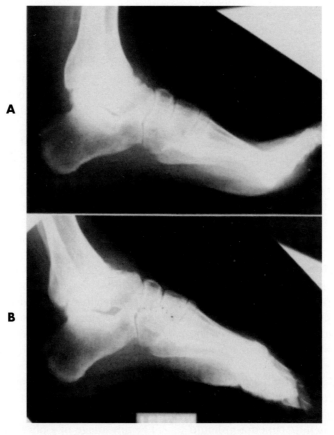

Fig. 7.25. Compensatory motion in the transverse tarsal and subtalar joints after an ankle arthrodesis. **A,** Full dorsiflexion. **B,** Full plantar flexion. Note the motion occurring in the joints distal to the ankle joint to compensate for loss of ankle motion.

a diffuse callus may develop beneath the fifth metatarsal area.

Transverse tarsal joint arthrodesis

Arthrodesis of the talonavicular joint or calcaneocuboid joint often significantly eliminates pain caused by arthrosis or deformity. It does, however, also result in loss of motion of the subtalar joint. This loss of motion is due to the fact that the subtalar joint complex, which includes the subtalar and transverse tarsal joints, requires motion in each of the joints for full motion to occur. With elimination of motion at the talonavicular joint, essentially all of the subtalar joint motion is eliminated. Likewise, if the calcaneocuboid joint is arthrodesed, the majority of subtalar and talonavicular joint motion is eliminated. It is therefore essential that when carrying out a fusion through the transverse tarsal joint, the hindfoot be placed into 5 to 7 degrees of valgus so a plantigrade foot results.

Triple arthrodesis

The triple arthrodesis combines the fusion of the subtalar and transverse tarsal joints. This is an excellent procedure and one that is used to create a plantigrade foot. Following this fusion, approximately 13 degrees of dorsiflexion and 16 degrees of plantar flexion are eliminated. It also must be kept in mind that the normal function of the subtalar joint, torque conversion from the tibia above into the calcaneus below, is eliminated, which places increased rotational stress on the ankle joint. Several studies have demonstrated that in years following a triple arthrodesis, in a certain percentage of cases, arthrosis occurs at the ankle joint as an unfortunate sequela of this procedure (Fig. 7.26). The alignment of the triple arthrodesis is critical and follows the principles that have already been stated for the subtalar and transverse tarsal joint. Two other factors, however, must be considered. The forefoot abduction-adduction must be corrected back to neutral through the transverse tarsal joint as well as correcting any varus or valgus deformity of the forefoot. In essence, the joints have to be aligned to create a plantigrade foot.

Tarsal and metatarsal fusions

Fusions involving the tarsal and metatarsal joints one, two, and three result in a certain degree of stiffness of the forefoot, which usually does not result in any significant problem for the patient. This stiffness can be a factor if one of the metatarsals is fused in a plantar flexed position, which might result in a plantar callosity beneath the plantar flexed metatarsal head. If the fusion mass includes the fourth and fifth metatarsocuboid articulation, if possible, the articulation between the cuboid and lateral or third cuneiform should

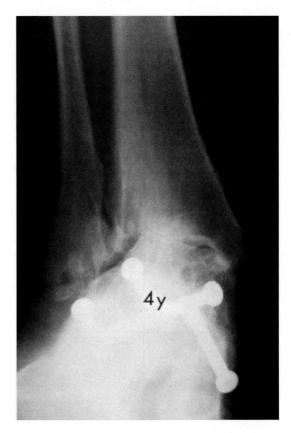

Fig. 7.26. Degeneration of the ankle joint.

be spared because dorsiflexion–plantar flexion motion occurs in this joint.

Metatarsophalangeal joint arthrodesis

When carrying out a first metatarsophalangeal joint arthrodesis, the joint should be placed into approximately 15 degrees of valgus and 10 to 15 degrees of dorsiflexion in relation to the ground. This is approximately 25 to 30 degrees of dorsiflexion in relation to the first metatarsal shaft, which is inclined plantarward about 15 degrees. The rotation of the great toe must also be taken into account to be sure that the pad is placed flat on the ground and the toenails are all aligned in the same plane. Proper alignment diminishes the stress placed on the interphalangeal joint.

In the patient whose first metatarsophalangeal joint has undergone arthrodesis, high-speed motion picture gait studies have demonstrated that as pressure is exerted against the great toe, the foot comes off the ground sooner than in the foot that has full dorsiflexion of the metatarsophalangeal joints.

Tendon transfers

The main consideration for a tendon transfer about the foot and ankle is to attempt to use a muscle that is working in the same phase as the nonfunctional one. The advantage of a phasic transfer is that the muscle

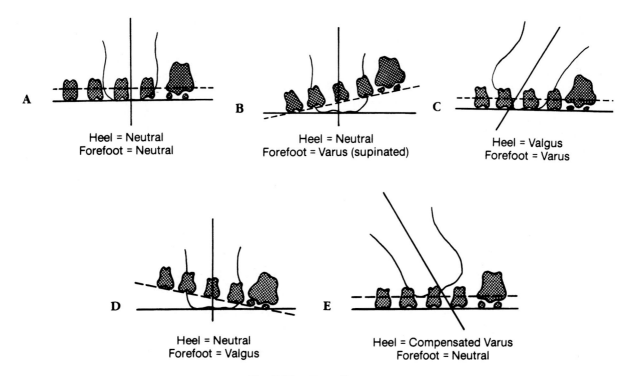

A   Heel = Neutral
Forefoot = Neutral

B   Heel = Neutral
Forefoot = Varus (supinated)

C   Heel = Valgus
Forefoot = Varus

D   Heel = Neutral
Forefoot = Valgus

E   Heel = Compensated Varus
Forefoot = Neutral

Fig. 7.27. Foot alignment.

naturally contracts at the same time of the walking cycle as the one it is being substituted for. A nonphasic transfer is one in which a muscle that normally works in the stance phase is transferred anteriorly to function as a swing phase muscle. Although muscles involved in nonphasic transfers can be trained, most of the literature indicates that in time these procedures tend to function more as a tenodesis and do not actually provide active motor function.

The other main principle in carrying out a tendon transfer is that for a tendon transfer to work successfully, the joint over which the tendon acts should have a normal or near-normal range of motion. If a joint contracture exists, the tendon transfer is unable to function.

Plantigrade foot

A plantigrade foot is one in which the foot is placed on the ground in such a way that the center of gravity passes along the plantar aspect of the foot in a normal manner. There are times, however, in which the foot posture may be altered either because of a congenital abnormality or because of an acquired problem. An example of a congenital abnormality is an untreated clubfoot, and an acquired problem might be in the patient with a ruptured posterior tibial tendon or post-traumatic condition in which there has been significant distortion of the bony architecture. For the foot to function efficiently, it should be placed flat on the ground in near-normal alignment. Proper alignment at

the time of surgery has been discussed previously, particularly when carrying out an arthrodesis.

To observe whether the foot is in a normal planti-grade position, the foot must be placed into what is termed neutral alignment. This is carried out by placing the calcaneus in line with the long axis of the tibia, or in up to 5 degrees of valgus; centering the navicular over the head of the talus; and placing the metatarsal heads so that they are perpendicular to the long axis of the tibia. In this manner, the foot is in neutral alignment and is plantigrade. A malalignment of the foot can occur because of an abnormal posture of the hindfoot, forefoot, or both.

When the calcaneus is in neutral position and the medial side of the forefoot is more plantar flexed than the lateral, it is stated that the forefoot is in a valgus position (Fig. 7.27). In this situation, the first metatarsal is more plantar flexed than the fifth metatarsal. From a clinical standpoint, this most frequently occurs in the patient with Charcot-Marie-Tooth disease or a cavus foot deformity. When an individual with a fixed forefoot valgus configuration takes a step, for the foot to remain plantigrade the calcaneus must rotate into a varus position. Conversely, if the lateral border of the foot is more plantar flexed than the medial border, it is called forefoot varus. Under these circumstances, the calcaneus moves into a position of valgus with weight bearing. This is most frequently seen in the patient with a long-standing rupture of the posterior tibial tendon.

When a deformity is flexible, an orthotic device can be used to support and realign the foot, holding it in a plantigrade position. If the heel is in a neutral position, the orthotic device needs to support the forefoot either on the medial side for a varus deformity or on the lateral side for a valgus deformity so that the foot presents as plantigrade a posture to the ground as possible. There are times, however, in which the deformity may involve mainly the hindfoot, in which excessive varus or valgus is present. Under these circumstances, some type of medial or lateral heel support to realign the hindfoot is required along with possibly a forefoot post (support), if necessary, to obtain as plantigrade a foot as possible. As a general rule, the orthotic device should be made out of a semiflexible material that has adequate padding to help with absorption of forces at the time of initial ground contact.

REFERENCES

1. Clarke TE: The pressure distribution under the foot during barefoot walking (doctoral dissertation), University Park, PA, 1980, Pennsylvania State University.
2. Close JR, Inman VT: The action of the subtalar joint, Univ Calif Prosthet Devices Res Rep, Series 11, Issue 24, May 1953.
3. Elftman H: The transverse tarsal joint and its control, Clin Orthop 16:41, 1960.
4. Hicks JH: The mechanics of the foot: II. The plantar aponeurosis and the arch, J Anat 88:25, 1954.
5. Inman VT: The joints of the ankle, Baltimore, 1976, Williams & Wilkins.
6. Isman RE, Inman VT: Anthropometric studies of the human foot and ankle, Bull Prosthet Res 10:11, 1969.
7. Mann R, Inman VT: Phasic activity of intrinsic muscles of the foot, J Bone Joint Surg 46A:469, 1964.
8. Manter JT: Movements of the subtalar and transverse tarsal joints, Anat Rec 80:397, 1941.
9. Simon SR, et al: Role of the posterior calf muscles in normal gait, J Bone Joint Surg 60A:465, 1978.
10. Sutherland DH: An electromyographic study of the plantar flexors of the ankle in normal walking on the level, J Bone Joint Surg 48A:66, 1966.
11. Sutherland DH, Hagy JL: Measurement of gait of movements from motion picture films, J Bone Joint Surg 54:787, 1972.
12. Stauffer RN, Chao EY, Brewster RC: Force and motion analysis of the normal, diseased, and prosthetic ankle joint, Clin Orthop 127:189–196, 1977.
13. Wright DG, Desai ME, Henderson BS: Action of the subtalar and ankle-joint complex during the stance phase of walking, J Bone Joint Surg 46A:361, 1964.

PRINCIPLES, MATERIALS, AND COMPONENTS

INTRODUCTION
John W. Michael

Section Two provides a conceptual overview of the fundamental elements of orthotic practice. This will be of special interest to the practicing and aspiring Certified Orthotist as well as to the general reader who wishes to understand the rationale behind the specific orthotic management of various pathologies reviewed in subsequent chapters.

Nonoperative management of spinal deformities, particularly idiopathic scoliosis, is one of the most extensively studied fields of orthotic practice. Chapter Eight reviews the available data in detail, illustrating the effectiveness of clearly defined treatment parameters—which can be developed only when the natural history of the disorder has been thoroughly documented. Key principles for orthotic management of fractures and postoperative applications are also reviewed. Important concepts such as the three columns of the spine and the biomechanical functions of various orthotic elements are highlighted.

Preliminary initial data are also presented in an effort to build a rational foundation for the selective orthotic treatment of back pain. The emphasis throughout Chapter Eight is to encourage the development of increasingly objective measures of the effect of spinal orthoses to help clinicians more clearly define the advantages and disadvantages of specific orthotic devices.

Chapter Nine provides a concise overview of the specialized area of upper limb orthoses. Illustrative examples of typical orthoses for each level of complexity are provided, divided into static and dynamic designs. Specific applications are given for both therapeutic and functional applications.

The significant contribution of occupational therapy training is highlighted to illustrate the importance of team management when dealing with upper limb pathologies. Patient acceptance of upper limb orthoses is often contingent on developing a well-defined therapeutic or functional purpose that the orthosis provides—which cannot be accomplished by any other means, including substitution.

The principles of the ubiquitous lower limb orthoses are highlighted in Chapter Ten. From the simplest accommodative foot orthosis to the most complicated reciprocating gait orthosis, typical examples from each level of lower limb management are described and illustrated, along with the desired functional goals.

A brief overview of component options available summarizes the biomechanical control choices the orthotist must make when designing a specific device. Advantages and disadvantages of typical materials are also reviewed.

The importance of functional prescription and functional justification, based on the biomechanical goals desired, is stressed throughout Chapter Ten. More detailed applications for specific orthoses are given in the subsequent chapters dealing with particular pathologies.

Finally, Chapter Eleven summarizes the key functions of a variety of specialized shoes, for sports and therapeutic applications. Sports-specific designs are highlighted, and modifications commonly used for biomechanically deficient feet are reviewed.

Collectively the chapters in Section Two provide a concise overview of the fundamental principles that determine rational orthotic management for a variety of pathologies, highlighting typical materials and components available to provide effective biomechanical control.

Principles and Components of Spinal Orthoses

Thomas M. Gavin
Avinash G. Patwardhan
Wilton H. Bunch
Donna Q. Gavin
Phyllis D. Levine
Laura Fenwick

Orthoses are the oldest recorded methods of treatment of spinal injury and deformity. Galen (c. 129 to c. 200), who coined the words we still use to describe spinal deformity, used dynamic orthoses for treatment. Crude lumbar supports fashioned from tree bark have been recovered from the cliff dwellings of the pre-Columbian Indians.[1] Pare (1510–1590) and Andre (1658–1742) wrote extensively about spinal supports for stability and correction of deformity. The eponyms applied to various thoracolumbosacral orthoses (TLSOs) such as Taylor, Knight, and Williams remind us of the widespread use of orthoses by more recent professionals.

Throughout history, external devices have been used to correct deformities and immobilize the spine. Although current scientific analysis has yielded a more thorough understanding of the mechanism of action of these devices, the function has always remained the same. All spinal orthoses reduce gross spinal motion (limiting bending and twisting of the torso), stabilize individual motion segments (thus reducing the planar range of motion of one vertebra relative to those above and below), and apply forces to correct or prevent progression of vertebral column deformities.

Orthotic treatment for low back pain, spinal injury, or deformity requires a solid knowledge of biomechanical mechanisms of action combined with sound clinical procedure, adequate follow-up, proper patient instruction, and physical therapy to ensure the best result. This chapter covers biomechanical mecha-

nisms, orthoses, and physical therapy as an adjunct to orthotic treatment for back pain, spinal injury, and spinal deformity.

LOW BACK PAIN

Biomechanics

It is generally agreed that mechanical loading of the spine is one important factor in the cause of the low back pain syndrome. Mechanical loading of the spine also plays an important role in affecting the treatment outcome for spinal disorders. This has prompted many investigators to study the contributions of various elements of a spinal segment in resisting the external load and providing stability to the lumbar spine. The findings of these studies are summarized in this section.

Physiologic loads on the lumbar spine

Loads on the lumbar spine are produced by body weight, muscle tension, and external forces. Several studies have been performed to estimate the forces generated in the lumbar spine and spinal musculature. Lumbar intradiscal pressure has been used as an indirect measure of loads on the spine.[2,64] Studies of the third lumbar disk have shown that higher loads are placed on the disk in an unsupported sitting posture as compared to standing. Loads calculated from the measured intradiscal pressures ranged from 100 to 175 kg in the seated position and from 90 to 120 kg in the standing

Table 8.1. Average range of motion in degrees at individual lumbar motion segments

MOTION SEGMENT	FLEXION	EXTENSION	LATERAL BENDING	AXIAL ROTATION
L1-2	8	5	6	1
L2-3	10	3	6	1
L3-4	12	1	6	2
L4-5	13	2	3	2
L5-S1	9	5	1	1

From Schultz AB, Ashton-Miller JA: Biomechanics of the human spine. In: Mow VC, Hayes WC, editors: Basic orthopaedic biomechanics, New York, 1991, Raven Press.

position. The disk is loaded the least in the relaxed supine position.

Two factors are at work here. One is external load alignment of the lumbar spine. In the unsupported sitting or standing postures, the weight of the trunk above the disk level increases the load on the disk. In addition to the gravitational load of the trunk, lifting a weight further increases the disk load. Not only is the weight of an object being lifted important, but also the moment arm of the weight relative to the lumbar spine acts to amplify the load on the spine. An object being lifted in an outstretched arm in front of the body causes a significantly larger flexion load on the lumbar spine as compared with the same object lifted closer to the body.

The second factor is the alignment of a lumbar segment, which influences the load sharing between the disk and the facet joint. The proportion of the total load shared by the disk increases with increasing flexion. Conversely, in extension, the facets share a portion of the total load, thereby reducing the load on the disk. Thus, maintenance of lumbar lordosis helps reduce the loads on the disk, whereas flexion exacerbates the disk loading.

Loads on the lumbar spine are shared by the disk, facets, ligaments, and muscles of the lumbar spine. The problem of load sharing between the ligamentous spine and the muscles is complex because of the large number of muscles that may be involved (active) in stabilizing the spine in a given task. Assumptions concerning which muscles are actively sharing the external load can be made to simplify the task of estimating spinal loads. Studies of muscle activity during various tasks using electromyography are helpful in identifying the most important muscles to be considered in the analysis. A more detailed discussion of this method of estimating lumbar spine loads is beyond the scope of this chapter but can be found in the literature.[31,81]

Range of motion

Forward bending of the trunk involves combined spine and hip flexion. The first 60 degrees of flexion takes place in the lumbar spine. An additional 25 degrees of flexion can be achieved from a forward tilting of the pelvis (hip flexion).[71,89] In forward bending, it is necessary to shift the buttocks posteriorly to keep the center of gravity over the base of support. The combined motion of the pelvis and the lumbar spine is reversed from full flexion to a vertical trunk position; the pelvis rotates backward followed by the extension of the lumbar spine. It should be noted that forward bending can be achieved by hip flexion alone, without flexing the spine. The hip extensors control hip flexion by providing a counterbalancing force to support the trunk against gravity. To stand upright with the pelvis tilted forward, the lumbar spine must assume a lordotic configuration.

Measurement of intersegmental motion using three-dimensional radiographic techniques has yielded more reliable data on lumbar segment motions than was possible before.[5,6,81] Intersegmental motion data are listed in Table 8.1. The lumbar segments are most mobile in flexion-extension as compared to lateral bending. There is more motion in flexion than in extension. The orientation of the articular facets limits the allowable axial rotation at lumbar segments. In the upper lumbar vertebrae, the superior facets are oriented approximately in the sagittal plane, whereas more caudally they are nearly aligned with the frontal plane. This characteristic orientation of facets allows only 1 to 2 degrees of axial rotation at lumbar segments.

Load-bearing characteristics

A spinal segment consisting of two vertebral bodies interconnected by an intervertebral disk, facet joints, and ligaments acts as a unit of the ligamentous spine in transmitting loads imparted to the trunk. Although the disk is a major structural component of the spinal column, a spinal segment is often viewed as a three-joint complex consisting of the disk and the two facets.

The disk carries substantial loads because of gravitational and muscle forces. The external loads applied to a disk are resisted by both the nucleus pulposus and the annulus fibrosis. In a healthy disk, the abundance of proteoglycans in the nucleus pulposus increases its osmotic pressure and attracts water. The resultant swelling pressure enables the nucleus to support an applied load similar to the way air pressure in a tire supports the weight of a car.[38] The osmotic swelling pressure developed in the nucleus balances the applied load. If the applied load is increased (or decreased), water is forced out of the disk (or the disk rehydrates) until a new balance is reached.

The collagen fibers in the individual layers of the annulus fibrosus are organized in much the same way as fibers in the tendons and are therefore well suited to resisting tension along the fiber directions. The pressure in the nucleus pulposus stretches the fibers in the annulus, and the resistance of the fibers to tensile loading allows the annulus to contribute to load sharing. The annulus fibrosis is particularly well suited to resisting torsional loads applied to a spinal segment because of the characteristic orientation of fibers in each layer.

Although the disk is the major anterior load-bearing structure, the facet joints provide a posterior load pad. Biochemical studies show that facets carry 10% to 20% of the compressive load in an upright standing posture and more than 50% of the anterior shear load on the spine. In torsion, the facet under compression is loaded significantly. Torsion combined with axial compression and flexion appears to load the facets significantly. In extension, the load is transmitted through the pedicles, laminae, and articular facets processes. Load transmission through the articular facet surfaces as well as through the tips of the interior facets (of the cephalad vertabrae) in extension can relieve some of the load on the intervertebral disk.

Pathologic changes, injuries, and surgical procedures can potentially alter the normal load-bearing characteristics of the three-joint complex.[31,81] Degenerative changes in a disk are associated with a loss of proteoglycans in the nucleus, which, in turn, leads to a decrease in the ability of the nucleus to attract water. Thus, disk degeneration has a detrimental effect on the ability of the nucleus to carry load. Loss of normal alignment between the two vertebrae can also influence the facet loads. Loss of disk height secondary to degeneration can increase the facet loads. Experimental removal of the nucleus pulposus in animals has been found to cause a significant loss of disk height and increase in disk flexibility in bending and torsion.

Changes in facet joint cartilage have been demonstrated following removal of the nucleus material. Disruption of the ligamentum flavum and posterolateral annular integrity and removal of the nucleus material simulating partial diskectomy has been shown to induce segmental instability manifested by significantly increased primary motions in flexion, rotation, and side bending.

Orthotic treatment

Eighty percent of the population experiences low back pain at some time in their lives.[32] Traditionally, many different types of orthoses have been used to treat low back pain. The most common choices currently are the lumbosacral corset and the rigid, thermoplastic TLSO.

The primary expectation when wearing an orthosis is a decrease in pain. This end is achieved by decreasing motion in the lumbar spine and increasing abdominal support.[77]

Currently, lumbosacral corsets are the most frequently prescribed orthosis for low back pain. If pain relief is not achieved with this device, orthotic treatment is often abandoned. Corsets do provide a degree of immobilization of the spine and an increase in intra-abdominal cavitary pressure. Being a soft canvas or dacron garment fortified with both rigid and flexible stays, they are not capable of the same degree of immobilization of the spine as a rigid TLSO.[23] They may be useful in the treatment of acute low back pain but rarely for chronic low back pain.

Optimal lumbar posture has also been found to play a role in pain reduction.[24,28] Micheli and coworkers[60] reported patients being treated for low back or leg pain secondary to spondylolysis or spondylolisthesis experienced good-to-excellent results in a TLSO fitted in lumbar flexion. In other studies, lumbar extension seems to be effective in reducing discogenic pain; exclusive of discogenic pain at the L5-S1 junction, near complete symptomatic relief was demonstrated in the bay cast spica.[28] All of these findings suggest that an orthosis may sometimes be an effective, conservative treatment modality for low back pain. Willner,[92] however, reported that using a rigid orthosis to treat low back pain, when prescribed randomly and independent of diagnosis, was effective about half the time. In a later study, using a test instrument, Willner[93] was able to predict the success of a rigid orthosis for low back pain with reasonable accuracy.

Using Willner's instrument for spinal stabilization (WISS), a program has been devised for the treatment of chronic low back pain. The WISS (Fig. 8.1) consists of an adjustable lumbosacral orthosis that can either flex or extend the lumbar spine.[28,93] The posterior pad may be set in flexion, neutral, or extension as determined on

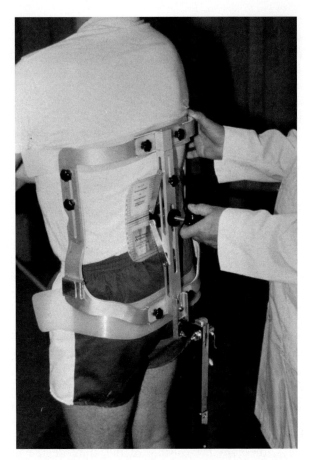

Fig. 8.1. Willner's instrument for spinal stabilization (WISS). Test orthosis for chronic low back pain.

the initial fitting. An adjustable anterior panel provides abdominal support and helps keep the orthosis in place.

Gavin and colleagues[28] conducted a prospective study to test the hypothesis that a 5-day trial wearing the WISS would be a good prediction of the outcome of orthotic treatment for chronic low back pain. The criteria for patient selection in this study included a report of low back pain for 6 months or more, unrelieved after conventional forms of treatment.

For treatment of discogenic pathologies, including disk herniation, multiple level disk bulging, degenerative disk disease, and combinations of the previously mentioned but exclusive of discogenic pathologies at the L5-S1 level and those with lumbar instability, the lumbar sagittal geometry was set in maximum extension. The patients who presented with spondylolisthesis, lumbar stenosis, or facet syndrome were fitted with the test instrument for 5 days in maximum lumbar flexion. Preliminary results suggested that if a patient has low back pain and has exhausted all conventional treatment modalities short of spinal fusion, orthotic treatment provides acceptable results when prescribed after a 5-day trial wear with the test instrument of Willner.

Traditional metal orthoses

Traditional metal spinal orthoses are recommended for three basic goals: abdominal support, motion control, or pain management. Trunk support is indicated when patients have weakened spinal or abdominal musculature. Motion control is necessitated when fracture or other pathology would be aggravated by motion. When spinal pain impedes functional capabilities, a spinal orthosis may be tried to reduce the intensity of the pain.[28,60,79,83,85,92]

Orthoses are best described using generic names referring to the anatomic levels they are capable of treating. Whenever possible, popular eponym adjectives are mentioned. For a complete catalogue of eponymic orthoses, the reader is referred to the text *Orthotics Etcetera.*[52,54]

Fabric sacroiliac orthoses, lumbosacral corsets, and dorsolumbar corsets primarily reduce gross motion. In addition, when a nonelastic lumbosacral or dorsolumbar corset is worn snugly, there is an increase in intracavitary pressure, which contributes to abdominal support and to the reduction in axial load on the vertebral bodies. Fabric corsets function in part by compressing the fluid and tissue of the abdomen.[36,59,62,77]

The great variety in corset design is based on only a few details: area of the body controlled, size, and amount of control necessary (Fig. 8.2). Corsets can be effective for management of pain caused by muscle strain because the activity of spinal and abdominal muscles is reduced while they are worn. When a corset is used long-term, however, these muscles can atrophy and increase the chance of reinjury. The corset should therefore be used only as long as necessary.

Corsets are typically fabricated with vertical stay channels, fabric "tunnels" that contain spring steel stays to increase the rigidity of the cloth garment. Stays may be contoured to accommodate a deformity or left straight to encourage postural correction. Many authors have recommended an effort to reduce lordosis to manage lumbosacral muscle strain.[54,79,88,92] Theoretically the flexed spine allows vertical transmission of the body weight through the vertebra and reduces the necessity for muscle activity. This alteration in posture combined with increased intracavitary pressure is believed to relieve pain caused by lumbosacral muscle strain.

In contrast, research has shown that patients with disk herniation may be more comfortable with lumbosacral orthoses that maintain or even increase lumbosacral lordosis.[28] An orthosis fabricated to increase lordosis tends to open the intervertebral body spaces and close the facet joints. This postural alteration is helpful for pathologies such as herniated nucleus pulposa.[35] In general, spinal orthoses should be fabricated with the posture that reduces pain most effectively or best

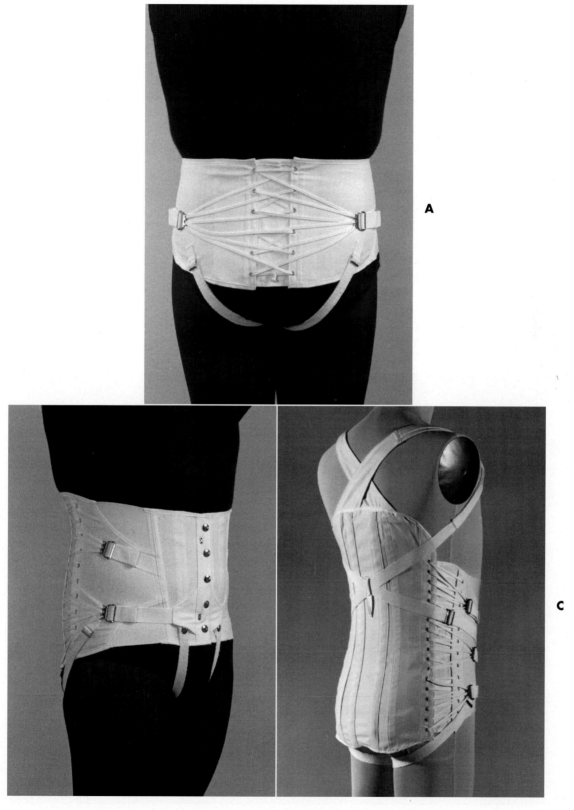

Fig. 8.2.   Commercially available corsets. **A,** Sacroiliac. **B,** Lumbosacral. **C,** Thoracolumbosacral (dorsolumbar).

accommodates a rigid deformity. Most spinal orthoses reduce gross and intersegmental motion of the vertebral column,[18,23,30,47,55,68,69,70,77] which has been shown to be effective for pain management as well as fracture healing and postoperative immobilization.[15,28,80]

Sacroiliac corsets are meant to provide assistance to the pelvis only. These garments encompass the pelvis with end points inferior to the waist and superior to the pubis. These corsets offer minimal support to the spine and are typically used to effect a slight increase in abdominal circumferential pressure for mild conditions.

Lumbosacral corsets encompass the pelvis and abdomen. In exerting circumferential pressure, they increase intracavitary pressure in the abdomen and transmit a three-point pressure system on the lumbar spine. The trimlines of the lumbosacral corset are inferior to the xiphoid process and superior to the pubic symphysis anteriorly and extend between the inferior angle of the scapula and the sacrococcygeal junction posteriorly. On female styles, the posterior trimline may extend to the gluteal fold posteriorly to reduce migration when there is significant hip development.

Thoracolumbosacral corsets increase the leverage of the corset system. The trimlines of this style are the same as the lumbosacral garments except that the superior edge terminates inferior to the scapular spine. Further, shoulder straps on this garment provide a posteriorly directed force meant to extend the thoracic spine. The thoracolumbosacral corset serves mostly as a kinesthetic reminder to control motion in the thoracic spine but does not provide a rigid lever to prevent such motion. For this reason, thoracolumbosacral corsets have been discussed as providing trunk support but not motion control.

The following components are used to construct most common metal spinal orthoses. Ideally, they are custom-fabricated to fit specific landmarks so that the orthosis provides adequate motion control through the best possible leverage. The components are typically aluminum alloys that are radiolucent and malleable yet of sufficient strength to hold their shape.

The *thoracic band* is fitted as follows. The superior edge rests 24 mm inferior to the most inferior angle of the scapulae. The band may be horizontal across the back or may be convex superiorly to provide the great-

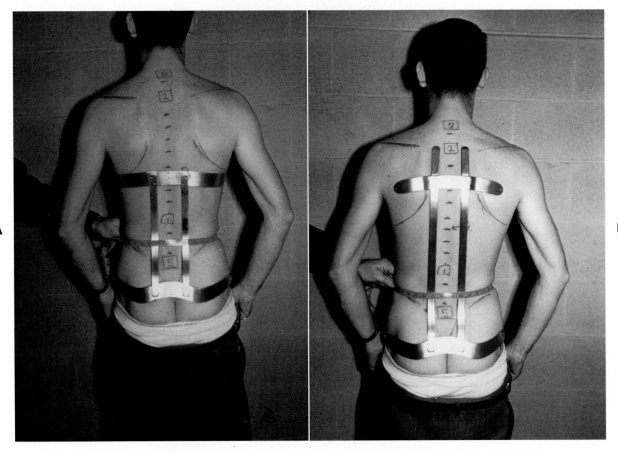

Fig. 8.3. These custom-fabricated orthoses show the appropriate location for some common spinal orthotic components such as the thoracic band, pelvic band, paraspinal bars, lumbosacral length, thoracolumbosacral length, and interscapular band.

est height in the midline while allowing for relief of the scapulae. Lateral to the scapula, the component dips inferiorly to relieve for the axilla. The component ends just anterior to the lateral midline of the body, or the midaxillary trochanteric line, a line defined by a bisection of the body at the axilla and trochanter.

The *pelvic band* is fitted as follows. At the midline, the pelvic band's inferior edge rests at the sacrococcygeal junction. Lateral to the midline, the component usually dips inferiorly to contain the gluteal musculature. The rationale for this curve is to provide the greatest leverage for the orthosis. This component also ends just anterior to the midaxillary trochanteric line. Norton and Brown[69] described an alteration to this pelvic band design to increase motion control at the lumbosacral junction. The pelvic section that they described has inferior projections from the lateral bars that terminate in disks resting over the trochanters. A strap that fastens anteriorly is connected to these disks and thus offers additional leverage in the sagittal plane, and the disks increase the leverage for coronal plane motion control as well.

The *paraspinal bars* are fitted to follow the paraspinal musculature. On lumbosacral orthoses (LSOs), the bars may appear vertical and pass from the pelvic band to the thoracic band. For thoracolumbar styles, the space between the paraspinal bars often narrows toward the superior end to follow the reduction in coronal diameter of the vertebrae. In TLSOs, the paraspinal bars terminate inferior to the spine of the scapula.

The *lateral bars* follow the midaxillary trochanteric line from the superior edge of the thoracic band to the inferior edge of the pelvic band.

The *interscapular band* is contained within the lateral borders of the scapulae with its inferior edge superior to the inferior borders of the scapulae. All metal orthoses may be worn with a corset or with an anterior panel of corset material.

Common examples

LSO: Sagittal control.   This orthosis (also known as LSO: chairback style) consists of a thoracic band, pelvic band, and two paraspinal bars (Fig. 8.3, *A*). Fitting parameters are as described previously for each

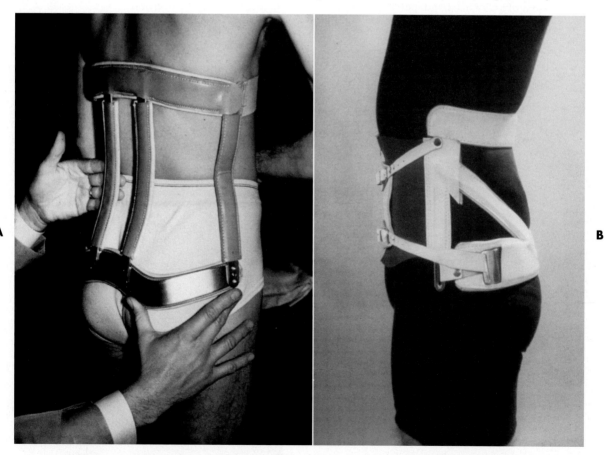

Fig. 8.4.   A, LSO: Sagittal-coronal control. Note the location of the lateral bar. The lateral bars follow the midaxillary-trochanteric line, an imaginary line that connects the lateral midline at axilla level with the lateral midline at the trochanter level. **B,** LSO: Extension-coronal control. The oblique bars follow the body contour. The oblique bars provide structural integrity for the orthosis but do not contribute control of motion.

of the components. It is indicated to reduce gross motion in the sagittal plane, including both flexion and extension. The mechanism is through two 3-point pressure systems. For flexion control, there are two posteriorly directed forces (at the xiphoid level and pubic level on the corset panel) and one anteriorly directed force at the midpoint of the paraspinal bars. For extension control, there are two anteriorly directed forces (arising from the thoracic and pelvic bands) and one posteriorly directed force from the midpoint of the corset panel.

LSO: Sagittal-coronal control. This orthosis adds a component of coronal control by the addition of lateral bars. The eponym for this orthosis, LSO: Knight style, refers to Knight, who described a version of the orthosis in *Orthopaedia* in 1884.[4] The present form of this orthosis consists of a thoracic band, pelvic band, paraspinal bars, and lateral bars. In addition to the three-point pressure systems described for sagittal plane hold of motion, this orthosis adds three-point pressure systems in the coronal plane to limit lateral flexion (Fig. 8.4, *A*).

LSO: Extension-coronal control. This dynamic orthosis consists of a thoracic band, pelvic band, lateral bars, and oblique bars as seen in Fig. 8.4, *B*. The oblique bars provide structural integrity. The attachments at the thoracic band and lateral bars are mobile. This orthosis then articulates to allow motion in the sagittal plane. As it is worn, an inelastic pelvic strap is tightened so that there is free flexion, but extension is stopped. Williams originally described this orthosis in 1937 as a treatment for spondylolisthesis,[91] and it may still be prescribed for this pathology today.[28,45,56]

TLSO: Flexion control. This orthosis (Fig. 8.5) is commercially available in various styles and sizes from a number of manufacturers. One style consists of an aluminum frame with pads at the pubis, sternum, and lateral midline of the trunk. This Jewett style is named for Jewett, who described it in 1937.[40] Other styles provide similar motion control. Control is achieved through one 3-point pressure system. There are two posteriorly directed forces, one at the sternal pad and one at the pubic pad. There is an equal but opposite anteriorly directed force from the lumbar pad. When the orthosis is worn, it prevents the patient from flexing but allows extension.

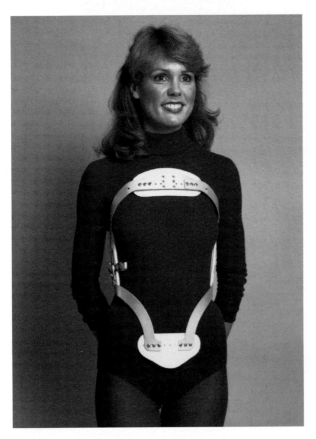

Fig. 8.5. TLSO: Flexion control. Jewett style. *(Courtesy Ben Moss, Florida Brace Corp.)*

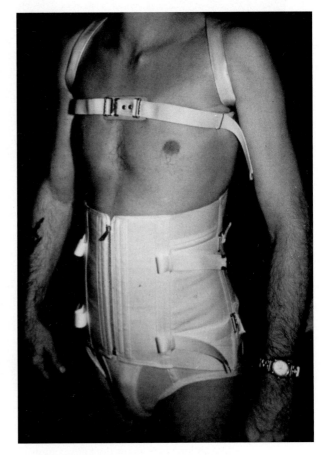

Fig. 8.6. TLSO: Sagittal control. Taylor style.

TLSO: Sagittal control. The eponym TLSO: Taylor style is for Taylor, the New York orthopedist who described it in 1863.[84] The orthosis consists of a pelvic band, paraspinal bars, an interscapular band, and axillary straps (Fig. 8.6). This orthosis provides two 3-point pressure systems in flexion and extension for the thoracic and lumbar spine. The interscapular band provides one of the anteriorly directed forces to limit extension, and the axillary straps provide one of the posteriorly directed forces to reduce the range of flexion.

TLSO: Sagittal-coronal control. This combination orthosis has the apt eponym TLSO: Knight-Taylor style. It is fabricated with a thoracic band, pelvic band, paraspinal bars, lateral bars, interscapular band, and axillary straps. Through the use of these components, the orthosis limits flexion, extension, and lateral flexion of the thoracic and lumbar spine. The three-point pressure systems in the sagittal plane for the TLSO: sagittal-coronal control are illustrated in Fig. 8.7.

TLSO: Triplanar control. This orthosis consists of thoracic band with subclavicular extensions, pelvic band, paraspinal bars, and lateral bars. The addition of the subclavicular extensions, which are colloquially referred to as cowhorn projections, adds transverse plane control to this orthosis. As an individual attempts right or left rotation of the thoracic spine, counterforces are encountered from the thoracic band and subclavicular extension that limit motion (Fig. 8.8).

Cervical orthoses

Prefabricated cervical orthoses can be generally categorized as hard and soft (Fig. 8.9). A comparison of the control provided by various styles of cervical orthoses is outlined in Table 8.2 and summarized in the following comments. The most commonly used soft cervical orthosis is the foam collar style. This orthosis functions primarily as a kinesthetic reminder for the individual to reduce excessive motion. The hard cervical collar styles are available in a great variety of prefabricated styles. As a group, these orthoses reduce cervical motion somewhat better in the sagittal plane than foam collars but still provide little control of lateral flexion and rotation. More control of the cervical spine can be provided by the poster-style orthoses. Pictured (Figs. 8.10 and 8.11) are the two-poster and four-poster types of cervical orthoses. These orthoses offer more rigid immobilization of the cervical spine because of the occipital pad, mandibular pad, and sternal and thoracic pads. Any of the aforementioned orthoses can be modified with a thoracic extension to provide more effective leverage for motion control of the lower cervical spine.[16]

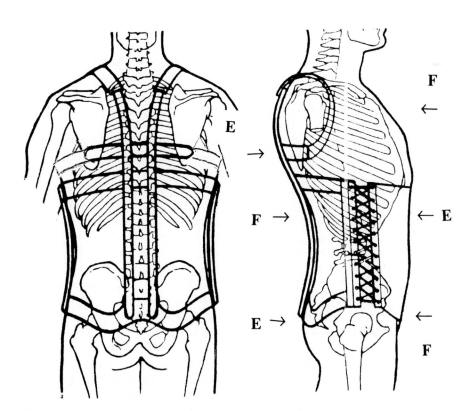

Fig. 8.7. TLSO: Sagittal-coronal control with three-point pressure systems delineated. *F,* Flexion control; *E,* extension control. *(From American Academy of Orthopaedic Surgeons: Atlas of Orthotics, ed 2, St. Louis, 1985, CV Mosby.)*

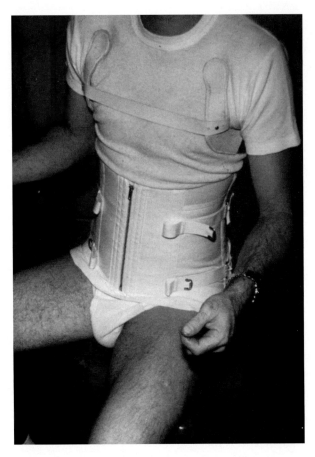

Fig. 8.8. Subclavicular extensions of the TLSO: Triplanar control.

A commercially available cervicothoracic orthosis that is frequently used for motion control is the sternal occipital mandibular immobilizer (SOMI) (Fig. 8.12). This orthosis consists of a sternal plate with shoulder components, mandibular pad and bar, and occipital pad and bars. It provides good motion control of flexion, especially in the lower cervical segments, but actually allows some extension motion because of a swivel-type occipital pad.[42]

The Halo cervicothoracic orthosis provides triplanar motion control in the cervical spine (Fig. 8.13). This orthosis consists of a halo ring fixed to the skull with pins, a chest jacket, and superstructure that connects the ring and jacket. This orthosis provides the best end point control of the cervical spine but because of its lack of total contact allows a phenomenon called intersegmental snaking to occur. A total contact cervicothoracic orthosis such as a Minerva style might provide better intersegmental immobilization of the cervical spine.[7,57] Despite the intersegmental motion, however, Halo fixation is usually best for fracture healing.[37,43,87]

Spinal orthotic recommendation can be difficult because of the variety of orthoses available to achieve a given goal and the variety of pathologies involved.

Viewing the orthotic recommendation as a method of matching functional deficit with orthotic goal simplifies the process.

SPINAL FRACTURE AND POSTOPERATIVE ORTHOSES

Biomechanics

The stability of the injured spine, measured by its ability to withstand loads without causing the progression of a deformity at the injury site, is a primary biomechanical concern in the surgical and orthotic treatment of thoracolumbar injuries. The anatomic components of a spinal segment provide inherent stability to the spinal segment. The stability of a segment defined by its load-displacement behavior is affected by an injury, and the extent of such effect is a function of the type of injury (i.e., the anatomical components disrupted by the injury and the severity of the damage).

Effect of injury on the stability of the spine

The effect of progressive disruption of posterior ligamentous structure, facet joints, and a part of the annulus fibrosis on the range of motion at L1-2 interspace was studied by Nagel et al.[70] The range of motion in flexion-extension increased with statistical significance following severing of facet joints. In the fully disrupted joint that simulated a seatbelt-type injury, the range of motion in flexion and lateral bending increased to twice the value of the intact segment, whereas in axial rotation the increase was nearly ten-fold.

Jacobs et al[39] simulated three types of injuries in fresh human cadaver spines. Posterior ligamentous injury was simulated by disrupting the supraspinous, interspinous, ligamentum flavum, and facet capsular ligaments at T11-12 and a single plane osteotomy through the upper portion of T-12 vertebral body. The anterior longitudinal ligament was preserved. Anterior injury was simulated by a comminuted fracture of the entire T-12 vertebral body but preserving the anterior longitudinal ligament. The combined injury was simulated by both the posterior ligamentous injury and the anterior comminuted vertebral body fracture. The spines were tested before and after injury under a four-point bending mode, and resultant motion was measured between T-11 and L-1. The intact segments had a stiffness of 7 to 8 Nm/degree in the load range of 10 to 25 Nm, with a maximum flexion angle of 6 degrees (SD 0.8 degrees). The angular deformity at 10 Nm moment measured 17.6 degrees (SD 2.2 degrees) after the anterior injury, and 25.3 degrees (SD 3.1 degrees) after the posterior injury. Combined injury resulted in 43.4 degrees (SD 7.1 degrees) of flexion deformity at no load.

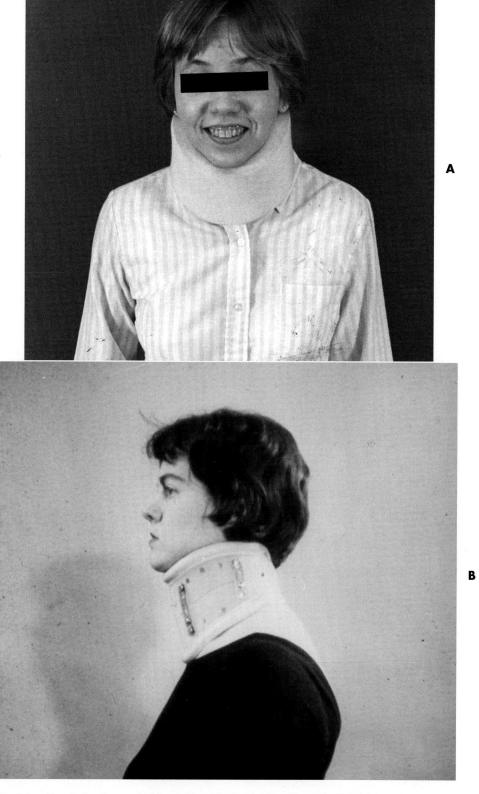

Fig. 8.9.   Cervical orthoses. **A,** Nonrigid cervical orthosis, collar style. **B,** Rigid cervical orthosis, collar style.

Table 8.2. Cervical orthoses

SEGMENTAL LEVELS	FLEXION/EXTENSION		FLEXION		EXTENSION	
	BRACE	MEAN MOTION ALLOWED (DEGREES)	BRACE	MEAN MOTION ALLOWED (DEGREES)	BRACE	MEAN MOTION ALLOWED (DEGREES)
C1–C2	(Halo)	3.4	SOMI	2.7	Cervicothoracic	2.5
C2–C3	(Halo)	2.4	SOMI	0.9	Four-poster	2.0
	Four-poster	3.7	Four-poster	1.6	Cervicothoracic	2.1
	Cervicothoracic	3.8	Cervicothoracic	1.8		
Middle (C3–C5)	Cervicothoracic	4.6	SOMI	1.7	Cervicothoracic	1.8
			Four-poster	2.0		
			Cervicothoracic	2.8		
Lower (C5–T1)	Cervicothoracic	4.0	Cervicothoracic	1.5	Cervicothoracic	2.5
			SOMI	2.9	Four-poster	2.5

From Johnson RM, et al: Cervical orthoses: A study comparing their effectiveness in restricting cervical motion in normal subjects, J Bone Joint Surg 59A:332, 1977.

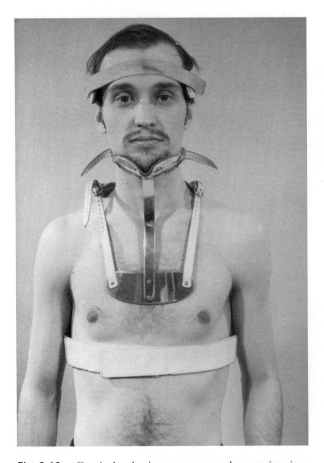

Fig. 8.10. Cervical orthosis, two-poster style, anterior view.

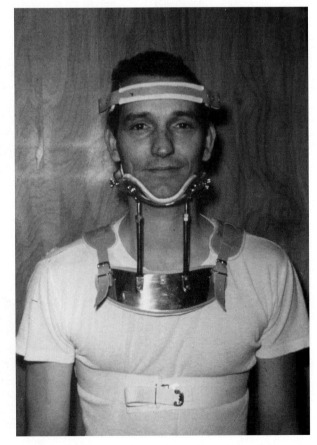

Fig. 8.11. Cervical orthosis, four-poster style, anterior view.

To classify acute thoracolumbar fractures, Denis[17] proposed that the spine has three load-bearing columns. The *anterior* column is formed by the anterior longitudinal ligament, anterior annulus fibrosis, and anterior part of the vertebral body. The *middle* column is formed by the posterior longitudinal ligament, posterior annulus fibrosis, and posterior wall of the verte-

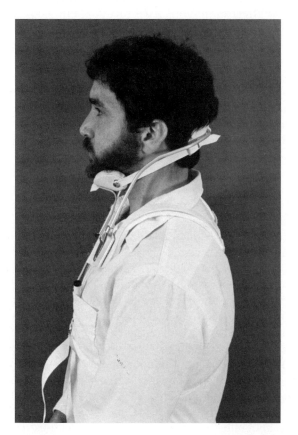

Fig. 8.12. Cervicothoracic orthosis, SOMI style.

bral body. The *posterior* column is formed by the posterior arch, supraspinous ligament, interspinous ligament, capsule, and ligamentum flavum. Compression fracture involves failure of the anterior column with the middle column being totally intact. The burst fracture involves failure of both the anterior and the middle columns. The seatbelt-type injuries represent failure of the middle and posterior columns. Finally, the fracture-dislocation injury represents failure of all three columns.

The axial load-carrying capacity (LCC) of the thoracolumbar spine as a function of injury to the three columns of the spine was studied by Haher et al.[34] Disruption of the anterior column reduced the LCC of the spine by 20%. The reduction in the LCC of the spine was 80% with disruption of both the anterior and the middle columns of the spine. Disruption of the posterior column reduced the LCC by 35%, whereas the reduction in LCC was 60% with disruption of both the posterior and the middle columns. Ferguson and colleagues[22] found that a two-column injury involving the disruption of the anterior and posterior columns caused a 78% loss in flexion stiffness of the T11-L1 segment as compared to the intact value. Thus, disruption of two of the three load-bearing columns led to substantial instability, whereas the three-column injury rendered the segment completely unstable.

Slosar and co-workers[82] investigated the three-dimensional instability patterns of L-1 burst fractures. Analysis of the burst fracture in flexion and lateral bending showed stiffness losses of 71% and 75% at low load (up to 3 Nm) applications. Subsequent loss of stiffness through higher loads (3 to 10 Nm) showed only a 5% stiffness change in flexion and 25% stiffness loss in lateral bending when comparing intact to burst. Post-injury stiffness losses for rotation were 92% and 67% for

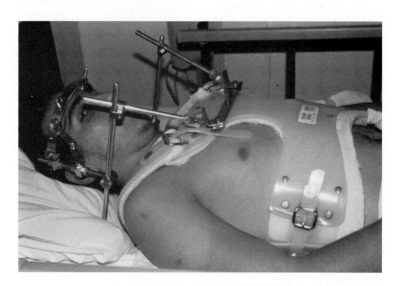

Fig. 8.13. Ambulatory Halo orthosis.

low-load and high-load applications. After the burst fracture, loss of low-load stiffness was much larger than the subsequent loss of stiffness at high loads. It may be postulated that the initial instability represents a structural collapse through the fracture itself. Once the collapse is complete, the apposition of the involved cortices limits further significant displacement. With the fracture now maximally collapsed and cortices apposed, the injured spine behaves similarly to the intact spine. The severe loss of stiffness found through both the low-load and the high-load applications in rotation may indicate that to the unprotected, injured spine, rotation is potentially the most destabilizing motion. The authors also determined that posterior column involvement in the form of an isolated lamina fracture did not alter the behavior of a two-column (anterior + middle) burst fracture. Burst fractures with extensive third-column injuries in the form of facet joint disruptions or bilateral lamina fractures were more unstable than two-column injuries.

Mechanisms of action of spinal orthoses

Orthoses for spinal injury are designed to protect the spinal column from loads and stresses that cause progression of the angular and translational deformity from the injury.[30,75,89] Orthoses for thoracolumbar injuries have two primary uses: nonoperative and postoperative. Although their mechanisms of action remain controversial, orthoses are believed to function primarily to provide biomechanical stability.

Specific orthoses

Nonoperative orthoses.   Mild injuries, such as those that affect only a single level and single column and are at low risk of progression, require minimally immobilizing orthoses, whereas the more severe two-level and two-column injuries, which have only marginal stability yet do not require surgery, need orthoses that offer maximal stabilization and resistance to further progression of the deformity.

The most basic of orthotic functions is that of a limiter of gross trunk motion. Gross trunk motion is the movement and sway of the vertebral column during activities of normal daily living. Orthoses that primarily restrict gross trunk motion provide some protection to the vertebral column by minimizing bending moments. The effectiveness of spinal orthoses in limiting gross trunk motion in flexion-extension, lateral bending, and axial rotation was studied by Dorsky and associates[18] and Lantz and Schultz.[47] The rigid TLSO resulted in the most motion restriction in all three planes, whereas the corset provided the least restriction of gross upper body motions.

The next mechanism of orthotic stabilization is the reduction of segmental motion. Orthoses that reduce segmental motion may be assumed also to reduce gross motion. The effect of orthoses in segmental immobilization has been studied by many investigators.[23,44,55,69,70] The three-point hyperextension orthosis was fair in limiting flexion-extension motion but had little effect on the motion in lateral bending or axial rotation. The TLSO (Taylor-Knight) was effective in lateral bending and fair in flexion-extension but had little effect on limiting axial rotation. The body cast performed satisfactorily in limiting motion in all three modes. The orthoses, in general, were more effective in reducing motion at the upper lumbar levels than at lower levels. The canvas corset was found to reduce the segmental motion by one third. The Raney jacket and the Baycast reduced the segmental motion by about two thirds at the midlumbar levels, and the Baycast spica was the only orthosis that was effective in limiting motion at the lower lumbar levels.

The third mechanism, limited to nonoperative treatment, is three-point sagittal plane hyperextension. Patwardhan and coworkers[75] used a finite element model to investigate the effect of the Jewett hyperextension orthosis[40] on single-level and two-level injuries and found that for single-level injuries that cause up to 50% loss of segmental stiffness, the Jewett can restore stability under normal gravitational as well as large flexion loads. In severe two-level injuries with loss of stiffness between 50% and 85% of normal, the orthosis can restore stability with restricted patient activity level in the brace. Beyond 85% loss in segmental stiffness, such as three-column injuries, the orthosis alone appears theoretically to be ineffective in preventing progression of deformity.

The effects of orthoses on trunk myoelectrical activity, abdominal cavity pressures, and intradiscal pressures have also been investigated but have shown inconsistent results.[30,46,48,66,68,88]

Postoperative orthoses.   The goal of orthotic stabilization of a thoracolumbar injury that has been surgically reduced and instrumented is to protect the surgical construct from large loads created from torso motion until solid biologic fusion occurs. The effect of the Milwaukee brace and body cast on the loads acting on spinal instrumentation was studied by Nachemson and Elfstrom[65] in patients with idiopathic scoliosis. Both the Milwaukee brace and the body cast reduced the axial force in the Harrington rod during standing and walking.

A postoperative orthosis should protect the surgical construct from the planes of motion in which the construct is vulnerable to failure. For most surgical constructs, these motions are flexion and torsion. It should be noted, however, that both the strength and the rigidity of these constructs are adversely affected by a loss of bone mineral density such as in osteoporotic bone. As a general rule, a postoperative TLSO should have enough anterior height to resist forward bending at the sternum, but it should not induce hyperextension because this additionally stresses the implant.

Profiles of the postoperative TLSO. All postoperative TLSOs should provide a stable base of support at the sacrum. This resists flexion of the lumbar spine and reduces hip flexion range to 90 degrees, thus preventing excesssive motion and bending moment at the lower levels of the spine. The cephalad trimline defines the profile of the TLSO and should extend cephalad to or slightly above the most superior point of the spinal fusion or implant. For lumbar fusions (excluding fusion for fracture or tumor), the TLSO trimline can terminate at the xyphoid process or just below the breast line, and this provides immobilization up to T-11. For procedures that exceed T11 but do not exceed T4, or for all fractures and tumors that create large bending loads on the surgical sites, the TLSO should extend to the sternal notch and the clavicles anteriorly; this is the high-profile postoperative TLSO. For procedures that include levels T3 and T2, the high-profile TLSO should come over the shoulder with shoulder straps to reduce upper thoracic motion caused from shoulder rotation, elevation, and depression. For procedures that extend to T1 or into the lower cervical to midcervical range, a SOMI or Minerva attachment must be used to reduce cervical range of motion. As the procedure that requires postoperative immobilization moves cephalad, motion reduction becomes more important than the reduction of bending moments because there is less axial load on the uppermost segments of the spine.

When spinal fusion is performed across the lumbosacral joint, a thigh extension must be applied to the TLSO to reduce lumbosacral motion in the orthosis. A TLSO without thigh extension has been shown either to have no effect or to increase lumbosacral motion.[55,69]

The role of a postoperative orthosis is to protect the implant from undue loads during the process of fusion. The segmental motion-limiting requirements of a postoperative orthosis are not as stringent as in the case of nonoperative treatment because the orthosis is being used only as an *adjunct* to protect the implant from loads and stresses.

Orthoses for thoracolumbar injury. Anterior column compression and anterior/middle column burst fractures are best treated in a hyperextension custom-molded bivalved TLSO because this reduces the segmental angle, unloads the fractured aspect of the vertebrae, and translates the injured segment in an anterior direction.[29,75,76] This usually provides enough resistance to the gibbus to stabilize the injury and allow healing. Secondarily the orthosis reduces segmental

and gross motion of the spine.[23,24,55,69] For the posterior and middle column injury through bone, known as the Chance fracture,[15] the same mechanism of action applies because this closes the fracture and allows ossification.

Figure 8.14, *A*, shows the radiograph of a Chance fracture in a 9-year-old girl. Her first bivalved hyperextension TLSO was molded in extension, and the result was only a minimal change in segmental angulation to 21 degrees (Fig. 8.14, *B*). For a period of 3 weeks, extension force was gradually increased by means of a series of different extension pads after which the orthosis was refabricated in more extension. The result, as illustrated in Figure 8.14, *C*, was a reduction of angulation to 14 degrees in the second orthosis. Four months later, the angulation reduction had maintained at 14 degrees.

Lap belt injuries such as the slice fracture of the posterior and middle column through soft tissue as well as severe burst and three-column instabilities such as the fracture-dislocation cannot be treated nonoperatively in orthoses.[76] When treating thoracolumbar injuries in an orthosis, the patient is at risk of the progression of injury if he or she does not wear the orthosis, so the clinician must thoroughly discuss the ramifications of noncompliance with the patient and family and have assurance that wearing parameters are met.

Postoperative usage

Undoubtedly, postoperative usage is presently an area of great controversy in spinal treatment. Although Nachemson and Elfstrom[65] show us that the Milwaukee brace can greatly reduce stresses on the Harrington rod, the 1980s was an era of major changes in standards of instrumentation. These newer implants such as the Cotrel-Dubousset and the Isola are much less vulnerable to failure, and the question of the need for postoperative immobilization has arisen. Pending further investigation of the role of postoperative orthoses for the newer, stiffer implants, application of postoperative spinal orthoses will continue to be subjective and variable.

SPINAL DEFORMITY

Biomechanics

The development of orthoses for scoliosis has been empiric, based on trial and error. In the 1970s and 1980s, numerous orthoses were developed, each claiming effectiveness in the treatment of scoliosis. Biomechanical models present a method of understanding about the instability patterns of spinal curvatures and the way an orthosis can function in stabilizing them. The reasons why some curves are more likely to progress than others

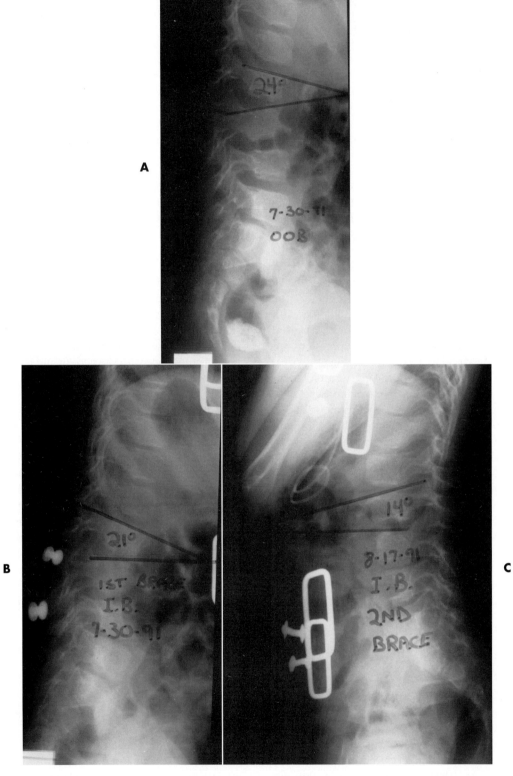

Fig. 8.14. **A,** Radiograph of 9-year-old girl with a Chance fracture. **B,** In her TLSO, the segmental angle reduced only to 21 degrees despite hyperextension fabricated into the orthosis. **C,** After gradual increase in extension and refabrication of orthosis, reduction was to 14 degrees. *(From Patwardhan AG, et al: Biomechanics of implants and orthoses for thoracolumbar injuries, Spine State Art Rev 7, 1993.)*

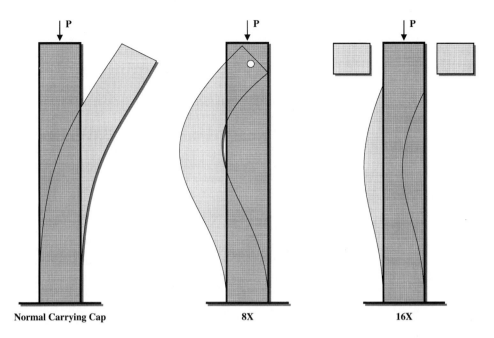

Fig. 8.15.   Elastic buckling of a straight column with different boundary conditions. **A,** Column with one end fixed and the other free. **B,** Column with one end fixed and the other pinned. **C,** Column with both ends fixed.

are important concepts in understanding treatment expectations.

Long-term studies of children with idiopathic scoliosis demonstrate that curve progression accelerates during the adolescent growth spurt. The younger the child, the higher the risk of progression because the remaining growth is greater. The relationship between the rate of growth and curve progression was studied by Duval-Beaupere[19] in 560 patients with scoliosis. There was a slow but steady increase in curvature until the accelerating portion of the growth phase. At this point, the rate of increase in curvature increased greatly and continued at this rate until the end of normal growth.

Similarly the larger the curve at any age of growth, the more likely the curve is to progress. Lonstein and Carlson[49] reviewed 727 patients with idiopathic scoliosis whose initial curves measured 5 to 29 degrees. Their data show that for curves of 20 to 29 degrees, the incidence of progression is nearly 100% for patients 10 years of age or younger. In contrast, only about half of the curves measuring 5 to 19 degrees in patients of same age group appear to progress. The incidence of progression reduces with increasing age but is still significant (37%) at the age of 14 for curves larger than 20 degrees. The relationship between the Risser sign and the incidence of progression grossly resembles that for progression as a function of age.

Biomechanics of curve progression

The long-term studies of children with idiopathic scoliosis have yielded expectations for outcomes of clinical treatment. The conceptual framework for thinking about why progression occurs is also important for treatment outcome prediction.

Curve progression in idiopathic scoliosis is sometimes explained using Euler's theory of elastic buckling of a slender column. For a straight, flexible column fixed at the base, free at the upper end and subjected to an axial compressive force (Fig. 8.15), there is an upper limit on the magnitude of this force at which point the column buckles. The buckling load of a straight slender elastic column is a function of its flexibility, length, and end support (boundary) conditions.[86] For the column shown in Fig. 8.15, this relationship is described as:

$$P_e = p^2 EI/4L^2 \tag{1}$$

where P_e is the buckling load, EI is the flexural rigidity, and L is the length.

This analogy shows the relationship between growth and progression. In a child at a given age, the weight of the upper trunk and arms may not exceed the buckling load of the spinal column, and therefore any existing curve may not progress. With height growth and weight gain, however, the buckling load of the spinal column may be exceeded and cause progression of the curvature of the column. Even if the child did not grow in height but only in weight of the upper trunk and arms, this may provide an explanation for progression of scoliosis. The formula for the buckling load indicates that an increase in the child's height greatly affects the capacity of the spinal column to carry axial load. For example, a 10% increase in height results in about 20% decrease in the buckling load. As the child grows in both height and weight, these two factors act together and explain the rapid progression seen during the growth spurt.

The phenomenon of curve progression in idiopathic scoliosis is not true elastic buckling in the engineering sense. Elastic buckling of a column implies a sudden departure from the straight configuration of the column followed by total collapse. Curve progression is a gradual deviation from the normal configuration of the spine over an extended period of time, the magnitude and shape of this deviation being of great clinical importance. Furthermore, a purely elastic buckling analysis implies that the critical load remains the same regardless of the magnitude of curvature. Clinical observations clearly document a strong relationship between the probability of progression and curve magnitude; at any age of maturity, a larger curve is much more likely to progress than a smaller curve. Progression of a spinal curvature is truly a plastic deformation. There is clearly a relationship between the magnitude of deformation and critical load. Also, as in the case of plastic deformation, the axial load may be removed without the spine returning to the original configuration. There is a residual permanent deformation in the absence of axial load.

The axial load required to cause such a permanent increase in the initial curvature of the spine because of plastic deformation is termed the *critical load* of the column. The mathematical formulation of this concept has been reported by Patwardhan and colleagues.[72]

The effect of curve magnitude or degree on the stability of a spinal curve (as measured by its critical load) is shown in Fig. 8.16, *A*. The horizontal axis is the degree of curvature. The vertical axis shows the critical load. This plot shows that with increasing curvature degree, the critical load is progressively reduced. Minor curves have only a slightly reduced critical load. Moderate curves have a more substantial reduction. Larger curves of 60 degrees or greater are severely compromised in their load-carrying ability, and the critical load is drastically reduced.

Mechanisms of action of a scoliosis orthosis

The mechanisms of action of a scoliosis orthosis to prevent the progression of a spinal curve and stabilize it may be considered as three separate but interactive events. These are end point control, transverse loading, and curve correction.

End point control.   End point control denotes the mechanical constraints provided by an orthosis on the spine. The purpose of the pelvic interface of all orthoses is to fix the orthosis rigidly to the base of the spine. The neck ring of the Milwaukee brace limits the lateral sway by keeping the head and neck centered over the pelvis.

End point control increases the critical load of a spinal curve. Stabilizing the superior end of the spine by means of a hinge (see Fig. 8.15, *B*) results in the theoretical critical load value that is eight times that for the column shown in Fig. 8.15, *A*. The mechanical analogy shown in Fig. 8.15, *B*, is an approximation of the constraints imposed by an orthosis on the end points of the scoliotic curve. For example, even though the neck ring of the Milwaukee brace limits the lateral sway of the neck, the superior end point of the scoliotic curve (usually T-5) is caudal to the neck ring and is not subjected to the same kinematic constraint as the Euler model shown in Fig. 8.15, *B*. Thus, the actual beneficial effect of the neck ring on the stability of a scoliotic curve may be much smaller than what is predicted by the aforementioned mechanical analogy. This illustration of the concept, however, does emphasize the importance of achieving end point control in orthotic stabilization of scoliosis.

Transverse load/support.   All scoliosis orthoses provide some form of a transversely directed load to the curvature of the scoliotic spine. A nontranslatory transverse load directed at the apex of the curve increases the critical load that the spine can carry. In Fig. 8.16, *B*, the solid line represents the critical load for an unsupported spine of increasing degree of curvature; the dashed line indicates the critical load of the spine with a transverse support applied at the apex of the curve. For curves of 25 to 30 degrees, the transverse support raises the critical load from about 50% of normal to about 70% of normal. This increase is shown as the vertical bar labeled *A*. This increase may be enough to prevent the curve from progressing. For curves of this magnitude, long-term maintenance of this degree of curvature is a satisfactory result because progression after skeletal maturity is rare.

With increasing curvature, however, the effect of transverse support is reduced. In contrast to the smaller curves, a curve of 45 degrees has its critical load increased from about 20% of normal to about 30%. This is shown in Fig. 8.16, *B*, as the vertical bar labeled *B*. The resultant stability may not be enough, and progression may occur in the orthosis.

Curve correction.   Curve correction in the orthosis has the greatest effect on the critical load. Reducing a curve of 30 degrees to 20 degrees in the orthosis increases the stability of the curve from 50% to about 80% of normal. This result is shown in Fig. 8.16, *C*, by the *arrow* and *vertical bar* labeled *A*.

This effect is also significant for larger curves. A curve of 45 degrees has a critical load of about 20% of normal. If the curve can be reduced to 30 degrees, the critical load increases to about 50% of normal. This is

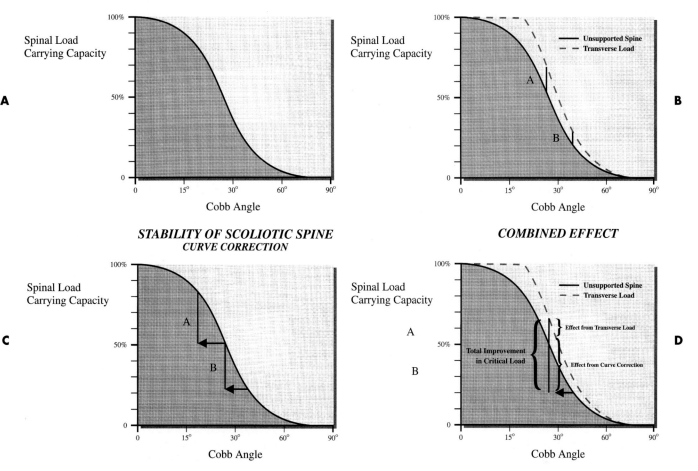

Fig. 8.16. **A,** Effect of curve magnitude on stability of the scoliotic spine. **B,** Effect of an apical transverse load on spinal stability. **C,** Effect of correcting (reducing) the scoliotic curve. **D,** This plot shows the combined effect to be optimal when using an orthosis to treat scoliosis. *(Redrawn from Bunch WH, Patwardhan AG: Scoliosis: Making clinical decisions, St. Louis, 1989, CV Mosby.)*

shown in Fig. 8.16, *C,* as the *arrow* and *vertical bar* labeled *B.*

A comparison of results shown in Fig. 8.16, *B* and *C,* illustrates that for any given curvature, reducing the curve magnitude improves the load-carrying capacity of the spine far more than does transverse support alone. This is particularly true for the larger curves. This analysis provides an explanation for the observation that satisfactory results in curves greater than 40 degrees require a reduction of curve magnitude to about 50% of the initial curve.[51]

Combined effect

The effects of curve correction and continued transverse support are additive as shown in Fig. 8.16, *D.* Once a curve of 45 degrees is reduced in the orthosis to 30 degrees, the pads can be reset to provide continued lateral support to the curve to increase further the critical load. With this cumulative orthosis adjustment,

the critical load can be increased from about 20% to approximately 70% of normal. Thus, with significant curve correction in the orthosis and continued lateral support, curves of a larger magnitude can sometimes be controlled.

Biomechanical analysis of Milwaukee and low-profile orthoses

The Milwaukee brace (CTLSO) has been the standard for orthotic management of scoliosis patients for decades.[8,14] Recent years have seen development of many low-profile scoliosis orthoses such as the Boston brace,[41] the Wilmington Jacket,[13] the Miami TLSO,[58] and the Rosenberger orthosis.[26]

Milwaukee brace. Several investigators have carried out biomechanical studies on the mechanisms of action by which the Milwaukee brace stabilizes scoliotic curves. The magnitudes of forces generated by the orthoses have been measured experimentally.[25,63] In standing, the average traction force was measured to be about 10 to 20 N, and the lateral pad forces were about 20 to 40 N. Removal of the lateral thoracic pad substantially increased the tractive forces, implying that the thoracic pad plays an important role in providing stability to the lateral curve.

Andriacchi and coworkers[3] first used a *mathematical model* of the spine to analyze curve correction achieved by the Milwaukee brace. In moderate curves of 40 to 45 degrees, lateral pad load was found to be the primary corrective component as compared with the distractive force from the superstructure of the brace. In midthoracic curves, placement of a thoracic pad at the apex of the curve produced maximum correction. Correction of the midthoracic curve decreased when the thoracic pad was placed two levels caudad to the apex and also with the addition of a lumbar pad.

The effect of the Milwaukee brace on the stability of primary thoracic and primary lumbar curves was investigated by Patwardhan and associates[73] using a *finite element model* of the spine-orthosis system. First, curve correction in the brace was obtained under the application of pad loads and axillary sling counterforce. The corrected curve was then loaded axially to simulate the weight of the body segments above the sacrum. The stability of an orthotically supported spinal curve was measured in terms of the capacity of the curve to withstand axial load without undergoing a permanent increase in curvature.[73]

Patwardhan and colleagues' predictions are derived from modelling studies of the human adolescent scoliotic spine. Although these studies have not been validated clinically, they do provide a mathematical basis for conceptualizing forces in orthoses. In addition, they correspond to a large extent with common clinical observations.

The model suggests that maximum stability of the primary thoracic curve can be achieved by applying the thoracic pad load at the apex of the thoracic curve. When the thoracic pad in the model was moved two levels caudal to the apex of the curve, the stability was reduced significantly.

In contrast, lumbar pad load at the apex of the compensatory curve decreased the theoretical correction of the primary thoracic curve. This may help to explain why orthoses reduce single thoracic curves better than they reduce the thoracic curve in double major curves. The model lumbar pad placed cephalad to the apex caused even further reduction in the potential correction of the primary thoracic curve. This may help to explain thoracic curve progression in an orthosis that is outgrown and migrating superiorly from the pelvis, thus resulting in a lumbar pad that is cephalad to the compensatory curve apex.

The model further hypothesizes that when treating primary thoracic curves with smaller, compensatory lumbar curves, a single thoracic pad without a lumbar pad provides the maximum critical load of the curve and, therefore, maximum stability. When the lumbar curve is of equal or comparable magnitude as the thoracic curve, however, maximum correction of the thoracic curve with a thoracic pad alone may result in asymmetric curve reduction and decompensation. In such instances, a lumbar pad should also be used in conjunction with a thoracic pad. Although some thoracic correction may be sacrificed (because of the addition of the lumbar pad), this is likely to yield a well-balanced and symmetrically reduced curvature in the orthosis. In reality, this is at present a clinical decision.

The model also suggested that for primary lumbar curves, the best correction and maximum stability can be achieved by application of a lumbar pad load on the apex of the primary curve with an apical thoracic counterforce of a magnitude enough to balance the upper trunk on the frontal plane. A lumbar pad alone at the apex of the primary curve without a thoracic counterforce results in nearly 25% less theoretical LCC than that achieved when a thoracic counterforce was modeled. The thoracic counterforce presumably functions to maintain a positive contact between the lumbar pad and the primary curve, thereby improving its stability. Incorrect placement of the lumbar pad too cephalad reduces its stabilizing effect in this model.

The previous theories are reviewed to underscore the importance of proper pad placement. Incorrect pad placement usually occurs for two reasons. First, it is quite possible that the lumbar pad is simply positioned too high. The apex of lumbar curves is just above the iliac crest, and it is easy to place the pad too far above it. The second mistake is much more common. The waist diameter can be easily made too small, causing the entire orthosis to move cephalad. When this occurs, the correctly placed pads are functionally one or more levels too high and the effect is lost. If the patient has grown since the last visit and the orthosis that fit previously is now too small, the curve correction is frequently diminished. Thus, a meticulous fit in the waist and pelvis is crucial for proper pad placement over time.

TLSOs (low-profile orthoses). Few biomechanical studies have analyzed the effectiveness of low-profile orthoses. Patwardhan and colleagues[73] analyzed the stabilizing effect of TLSOs such as the Boston brace and the Rosenberger orthosis with a mathematical finite element model. Such TLSOs use the trimline to provide a counterforce, which, in conjunction with the lateral pad loads, provides the forces that correct and stabilize the curve. These authors used a biomechanical finite element model to evaluate the stability of primary thoracic and primary lumbar curves

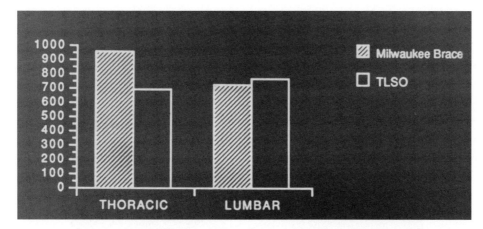

Fig. 8.17. Biomechanical comparison of optimal results clearly shows that the Milwaukee orthosis provides a more stable spine for thoracic curves; however, for lumbar primary curves, the difference between the Milwaukee and TLSO is insignificant.

under a variety of clinical situations that simulated the placement of pads and trimlines at different levels relative to the curve geometry. Their hypotheses are summarized here.

In primary thoracic curves with the cephalad end point at T5, it appears that maximum stability and curve correction are achieved with the trimline at T5-6 and a pad at the apex of the thoracic curve. As the trimline of the TLSO moves caudad relative to the cephalad end point of the curve, curve correction decreases, and there is a loss of stability of nearly 18% to 20% with *each* level.

For primary lumbar curves, the optimum result with a TLSO is theoretically achieved with the trimline counterforce at the apical level of the compensatory thoracic curve and a pad at the apex of the primary curve. Moving the trimline caudad results in progressively greater loss of stability with each lower level.

Therefore, in primary lumbar curves, a properly fitted TLSO appears to be as theoretically effective as the Milwaukee brace in stabilizing the curve. This is consistent with clinical experience. In primary thoracic curves, in contrast, the optimum stability achievable with a TLSO is approximately 25% less than that theoretically possible with the Milwaukee brace (Fig. 8.17). This may help explain why many thoracic curves are controlled with a TLSO but some apparently require the addition of a cervical control component.

Orthotic treatment

Nonoperative treatment: Cervicothoracolumbosacral orthosis (CTLSO). Present-day criteria for nonoperative orthotic treatment of spinal deformities originated with Blount and Moe in the 1950s.[8] They began using the Milwaukee brace, a device fabricated from steel and leather extending from the pelvis to the mandible and occiput, to provide longitu-

dinal distraction along with a lateral pad against the most displaced ribs on the convex side of the deformity, for the purpose of controlling scoliosis in an effort to prevent or delay surgery.

Distraction under the mandible caused orthodontic deformities.[12] The neck ring of the present-day Milwaukee brace is designed from stainless steel and no longer presses on the mandible, including instead a throat mold and two occipital pads. Some active distraction is achieved when the patient extends the neck.[8] The more recent development of low-profile neck rings (Fig. 8.18, *B* and *C*) completely abandons the concept of distraction. These rings function primarily to reduce sway of the vertebral column, keeping the upper thoracic spine constrained over the sacrum.[11,29,73,74] Euler's analogy shows a theoretical increase of eightfold when a flexible linear column is fixed at the base and constrained near the top, although the residual motion still permitted in the Milwaukee suggests much less actual increase in stability.[29]

Pad placement. Thoracic and lumbar pads are the means of achieving curve reduction by transverse loading of the deformed spine. They function as translatory variables in space, positioned directly between the constants of the neck ring and superstructure.

Thoracic pads. The thoracic pad of the Milwaukee brace is fashioned in an L shape and is often fabricated from low-density polyethylene with foam padding on the patient side. From posterior to anterior, this pad is shaped in an arc to contour to the torso. Size is specific for the patient, thus requiring a custom design. The pad is fitted on the convex side of the curve and is placed over the rib that articulates with the apical vertebra and the next rib inferior (Fig. 8.19, *A*).[27,29] The transverse span of the pad is from the medial aspect of the convex side paraspinal musculature to the midcoronal line. This covers a span of the entire posterolateral

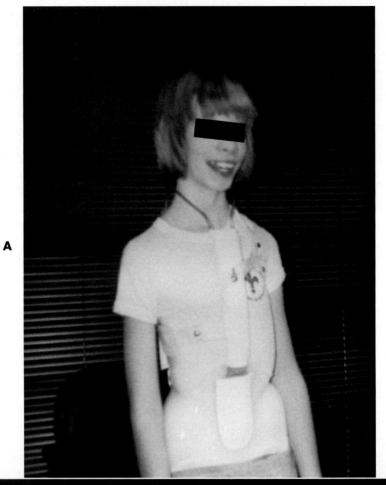

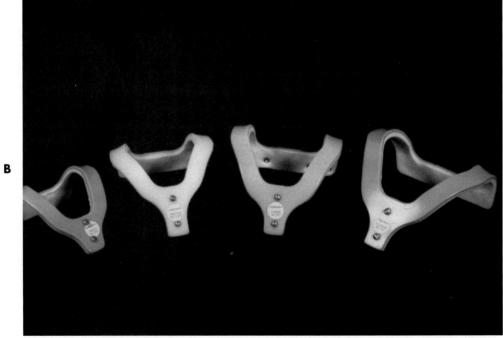

Fig. 8.18. **A,** Metal low-profile neck ring. **B,** Friddle low-profile neck rings. *(From Gavin TM, Shurr DG, Patwardhan AG: Orthotic treatment for spinal disorders. In Weinstein SL, editor: The pediatric spine, New York, 1993, Raven Press.)*

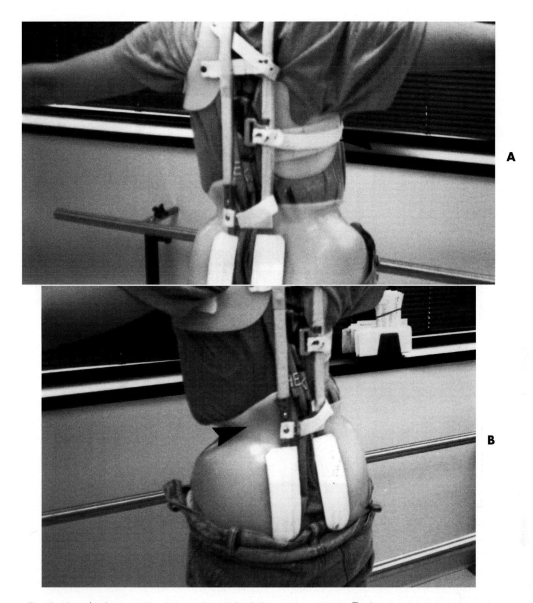

Fig. 8.19. **A,** Conventional thoracic pad for Milwaukee orthosis. **B,** Conventional lumbar pad for Milwaukee orthosis.

trunk quadrant. The posterior vertical aspect of the L pad is fitted under the convex side paraspinal bar of the superstructure so that this bar can be contoured inward to assist in the anterior, derotational force.[10,27]

Because the thoracic pad is mounted on a flexible dacron strap, a transverse outrigger made of aluminum is used on the anterior bar to bridge the strap away from the patient in the area anterior of the midcoronal line. Anterior contact is in direct opposition to the force of the thoracic pad and diminishes load.

For the patient presenting with hypokyphosis, the thoracic pad is placed directly lateral so that the anterior derotational force is eliminated.[27,29,50] This is achieved by moving the pad anteriorly on the strap to a direct lateral position and either shortening or eliminating the anterior outrigger. The neck ring on the hypokyphotic

patient should also be centered more anteriorly to midline in effort to induce a kyphotic force.

Lumbar pads.   The lumbar pad is triangular so that it can be placed inferior to the costal ribs and superior to the iliac crest. This pad is usually fashioned from a high-density foam and is contoured to the waist. Placement should be directly over the curve apex on the posterolateral convex side quadrant. The transverse span is similar to the thoracic pad, on the convex side posterolateral quadrant (see Fig. 8.19, *B*).

Pad loading.   For patients with more than one curve, it is suggested that the curve of greatest mechanical stiffness or primary curve should be loaded and shifted first. This allows the torso to shift toward the concavity of the primary curve and thus is the load of greatest trunk shift. Once that is accomplished, the

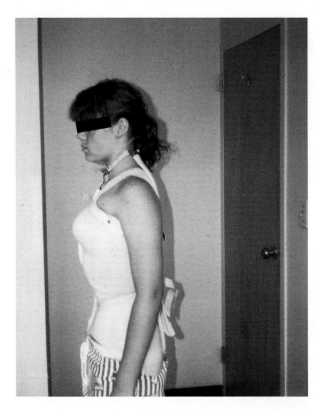

Fig. 8.20. Axillary sling. Note direct lateral placement. *(From Gavin TM, Shurr DG, Patwardhan AG: Orthotic treatment for spinal disorders. In Weinstein SL, editor: The pediatric spine, New York, 1993, Raven Press.)*

more flexible compensatory curve can then be loaded. This load on the compensatory curve is mostly transverse force and only minimally shifts the torso.[27,29]

For double primary curves, each curve should be loaded and shifted equally because the stiffness of these curves is considered equal. Thus, multiple curves with differential stiffness may be treated with differential loads, whereas those with equal stiffness should be loaded relatively equally.

Thoracic and lumbar pad force.   Pad force is the primary mechanism for reducing spinal curvature. Loading vector for thoracic and lumbar pads should be anteromedial with the exception of the thoracic pad for a hypokyphotic spine, which is medial only.[27,29,50] Pads should be kept at maximum force during treatment to optimize results. These pads are adjustable so they can be tightened periodically because viscoelastic relaxation of the spine occurs in the soft tissues and the curvature reduces.

Force is evaluated clinically by the degree of skin redness under the pads and patient comfort in the orthosis. For lighter skin, redness should be apparent in the pad areas but should disappear within 35 minutes after removing the orthosis. This ensures that force has not exceeded skin tolerance, thus avoiding skin breakdown. If redness dissipates after 15 minutes out of the

orthosis, the pads need tightening because they are not at optimal force. After the patient has worn the orthosis for 1 month, the greatest increase in pad tightening is done. Thereafter, the pads are checked every 3 months to ensure maximal force is still present and to reposition the height of the pads to compensate for growth.

Triangulation of forces.   The lumbar pad force of the Milwaukee brace is countered from both the pelvic interface and the thoracic pad. This triangulates the force into a three-point system. The thoracic pad triangulates from either the contralateral pelvic interface or the lumbar pad as a caudad counterforce but needs the addition of an axillary sling (Fig. 8.20) as the concave side cephalad counterforce. The counterforces play a primary role in not only righting and stabilizing the orthosis in the coronal plane, but also act as a mechanical constraint at the concave side cephalad end point. For double curves that require both thoracic and lumbar pads, four points of contact yield two 3-point force triangulations (Fig. 8.21).

Axillary sling load is relative to the load of the thoracic pad, and the pad is tightened to a point at which the orthosis is vertical and the patient's torso is centered or compensated.

High thoracic curves.   Orthotic treatment for scoliotic curves in the cervicothoracic spine is still controversial. The literature is devoid of orthotic treatment outcome studies, biomechanics of treatment, and natural history studies for these curves. The task of reducing these cephalad curves with an orthosis is, at best, formidable. Blount and Moe[8] reported that the shoulder ring flange (Fig. 8.22, *A*) is the component used to load these high curves as well as depress the convex side shoulder (which raises after transverse load is applied). Traditionally, these curves could only be loaded minimally because the contralateral side of the neck ring contacted the patient in reaction to the transverse axillary force, creating a neck ring reaction, a decompensated torso, and patient discomfort. Without maximal loading at the axillary (T5) level, these high curves do not reduce in magnitude, and the result is poor.

Gavin and coworkers[29] reported on a method to reorient the straps on the shoulder ring to depress the shoulder proportionate to the amount of transverse axillary load so that the patient's neck maintains a neutral position in the center of the neck ring without a neck ring reaction, thus allowing maximal transverse loading (see Fig. 8.22, *B*). Figures 8.22, *C* and *D*, show a patient with a double thoracic curve of 40 and 39 degrees that reduced in a Milwaukee brace with a well-fitted shoulder ring to 25 and 25 degrees. Because the neck ring reaction is nullified with this force system, it is theoretically possible to accomplish this method in a TLSO such as the TLSO pictured in Figure 8.23, *A*.

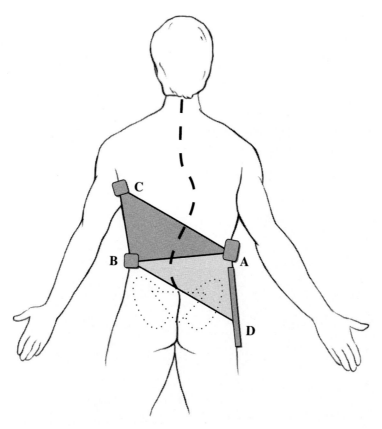

Fig. 8.21. Six-point double force triangulation provided by four points of contact. *(From Bunch WH, Patwardhan AG: Scoliosis: Making clinical decisions, St. Louis, 1989, CV Mosby.)*

Figures 8.23, *B* and *C*, show a patient with a double thoracic curve of 21 and 28 degrees who was fitted in a TLSO using proper coupling of axillary and shoulder forces, and her curves reduced to 13 and 11 degrees.

Outcome studies of results of orthotic treatment of high thoracic scoliosis are difficult because of the small demographics of high thoracic curves and the lack of data pertaining to the natural history of these curves.

Indications for treatment

The original parameters for orthotic treatment of idiopathic scoliosis with the Milwaukee brace were broad. Patients with small curves of 15 and 20 degrees as well as larger curves up to 60 degrees were prescribed Milwaukee braces despite their stage of maturity or lack of documented progression. Not until the 1970s and early 1980s were the studies of prevalence and natural history carried out that yielded current parameters for treatment.

Orthotic treatment is presently indicated for skeletally immature patients with idiopathic curves between 20 and 40 degrees. For curves from 20 to 30 degrees, previous documented progression should be shown before initiating treatment unless the patient is Risser 0–1, is premenarchal, and has much remaining growth. The younger child has the higher risk, so

orthotic treatment should begin earlier than for the older child. For the patient who is Risser 2–3 and either nearing or has exceeded menarche, the curve should be 30 degrees or greater on the first visit even if there is no documentation of progression because their risk is lower than that for the younger child. For curves greater than 40 degrees, the amount of force required to reduce the curve is usually at an intolerable level. These patients typically do not reduce enough to prevent progression after maturity and ultimately require surgery. Children who are Risser 4 or greater, more than 18 months postmenarche, and have slowed or ceased growth are too mature to initiate treatment, and the orthosis will have no long-term effect on the curve.

For the most optimal results, larger curves (35 to 45 degrees) must be reduced by at least 50% in the orthosis and maintained throughout the duration of wear. This approach yields the best chance to prevent the need for surgical intervention.[51,66] All scoliosis orthoses should achieve maximum curve reduction in the orthosis and strive to maintain the lowest possible curve magnitude in the orthosis.

Thoracolumbosacral orthoses

Current indications for the TLSO are the same as that reported for the Milwaukee except the TLSO is

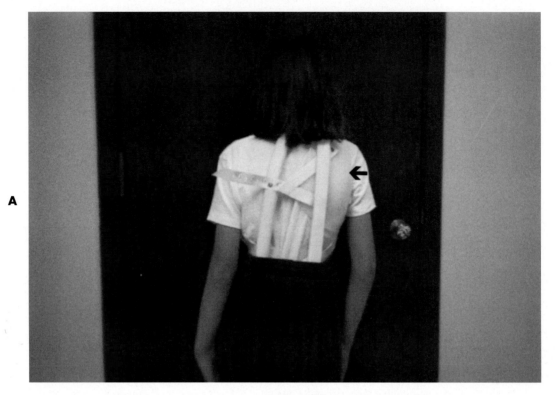

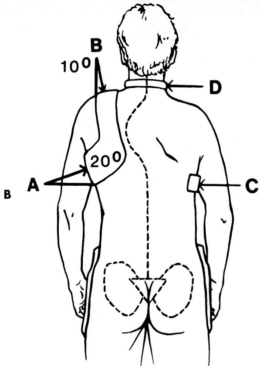

Fig. 8.22. **A,** Custom-molded shoulder ring for high thoracic curves. **B,** Clinical vectors for strap pull of shoulder ring.

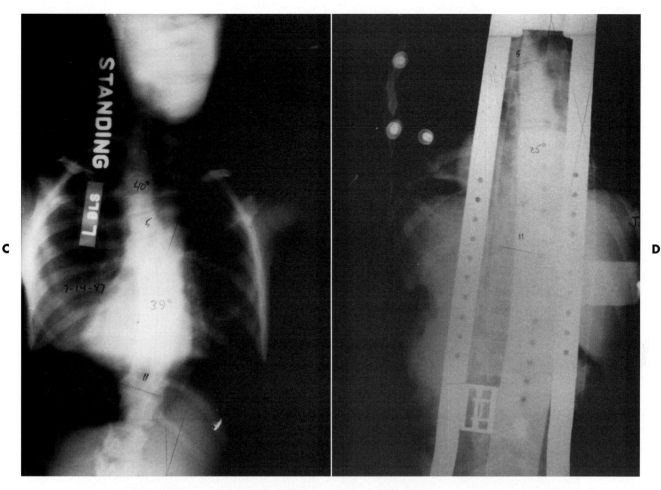

C   D

Fig. 8.22—cont'd.   **C,** Preorthosis radiograph of left high thoracic curve of 40 degrees and right midthoracic curve of 39 degrees. **D,** Milwaukee orthosis with shoulder ring and thoracic pad; both curves reduced to 25 degrees.

presently not advocated for treatment of curves with apices cephalad to T8.[26,27,29,50]

TLSO application for the nonoperative treatment of scoliosis began with the Boston brace (Fig. 8.24). The concept began as a method of treating curves with apices at and caudad to T10 with the pelvic aspect of a CTLSO, thus eliminating the superstructure.[21,41] The Boston brace has evolved into a system of prefabricated TLSO modules custom-fitted for specific patient needs and is currently used to treat all curves with apices as cephalad as T8. This is the most widely known TLSO for scoliosis treatment. In contrast to the Milwaukee brace (which is still the only CTLSO presently used for treatment of spinal deformity), a multitude of TLSOs have been developed throughout the 1970s and 1980s. The Lyonnaise orthosis was originally developed in France with modifications used in the United States (Fig. 8.25). The Lyonnaise was the first TLSO used for treatment of thoracic curves with apices as cephalad as T8 as well as treatment of the more caudad lumbar and thoracolumbar curves. The Miami orthosis[58] is a custom-molded orthosis similar to the Boston in many regards with variations in trimline. The Wilmington orthosis[13] (Fig. 8.26) is a custom-molded TLSO fabricated from a Risser frame plaster impression taken with maximal curve correction. An anteroposterior radiograph is usually obtained in the impression to predict curve correction in the orthosis. The Rosenberger orthosis[26] (Fig. 8.27) is a custom-molded TLSO fabricated from a plaster impression taken with curvature correction that uses a dacron thoracic sling to load thoracic curves.

Thoracolumbosacral orthosis profiles

The Miami orthosis is the lowest profile of the TLSOs because the anterior height is short enough to allow forward bending of the patient while in the orthosis.[58] Boston and Rosenberger orthoses are also lower-profile TLSOs. They have an anterior height to just inferior of the breasts, whereas the Lyonnaise and Wilmington are fitted up to the sternal notch, usually with breast openings for females.

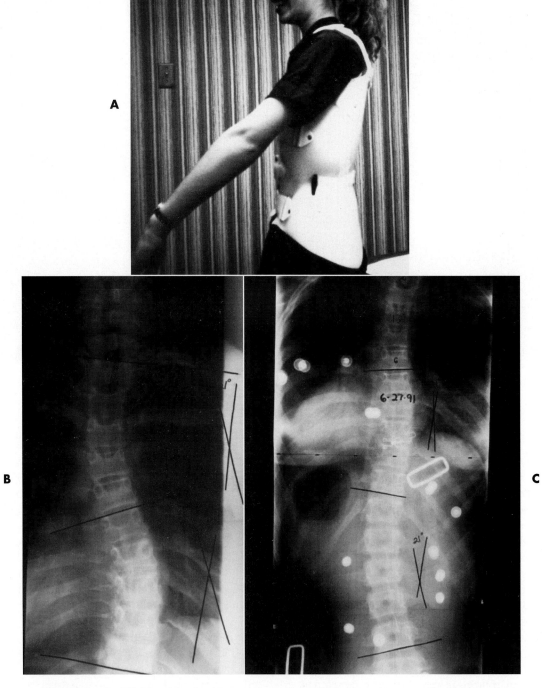

Fig. 8.23. **A,** TLSO with shoulder component for high thoracic curve. **B,** Preorthosis radiograph depicts a left high thoracic curve of 21 degrees and a midthoracic curve of 28 degrees. **C,** Orthosis radiograph shows the high thoracic curve reduced to 13 degrees and the right midthoracic reduced to 11.

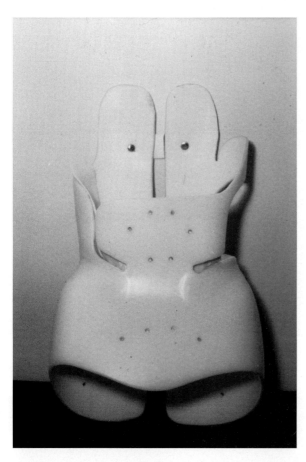

Fig. 8.24. Boston brace. *(Courtesy of Jeff Miller, C.O., National Orthotics and Prosthetics Corp. Boston, Boston Children's Hospital Medical Center. From Gavin TM, Shurr DG, Patwardhan AG: Orthotic treatment for spinal disorders. In Weinstein SL, editor: The pediatric spine, New York, 1993, Raven Press.)*

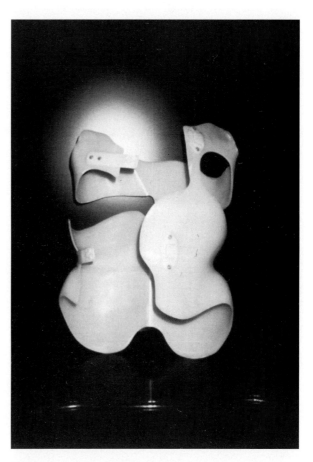

Fig. 8.25. The modified Lyonnaise orthosis. Note lack of aluminum structure and steel hinges. *(Courtesy of L. Dreher Jouett, C.P.O., Dreher-Jouett, Inc., Chicago.)*

Boston brace. The Boston brace is a modular one-piece, posterior-opening TLSO made from polypropylene. This orthosis extends anteriorly from the xyphoid process to the symphysis pubis with posterior and lateral trimlines varied for each curve pattern. This orthosis is modular and does not require a plaster impression, but it must be custom-fitted for individual size and curve pattern. On the convex side of the curve, the Boston is trimmed one level superior to the apex of the curve to provide a wall to function as a thoracic or lumbar pad mount. On the concave side of the curve, an opening is cut opposite the pad to allow an open area for the concave side trunk shift on the level of the primary curve. Above the cutout, a band of plastic is left intact to provide concave side superior end point counterforce to function in the same manner as the axillary sling of the Milwaukee (Fig. 8.28).

Rosenberger orthosis. The Rosenberger orthosis is a custom-molded, low-density, polyethylene, anterior-opening TLSO. This orthosis is fabricated from a bivalved plaster impression carried out on an examination table with corrective forces applied during

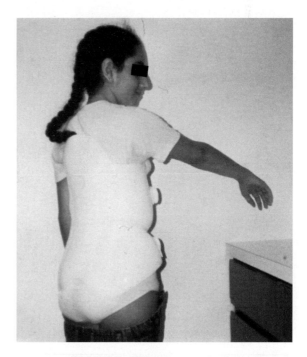

Fig. 8.26. Wilmington orthosis.

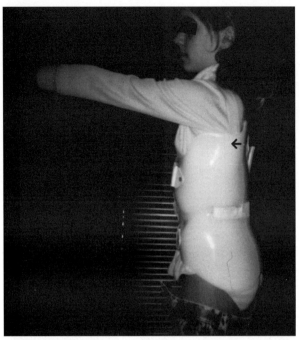

Fig. 8.27. Counterforce wall used in Rosenberger orthosis.

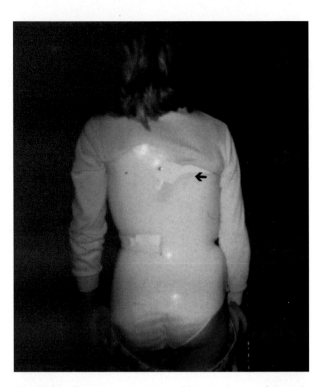

Fig. 8.29. Rosenberger orthosis. Note the usage of thoracic sling.

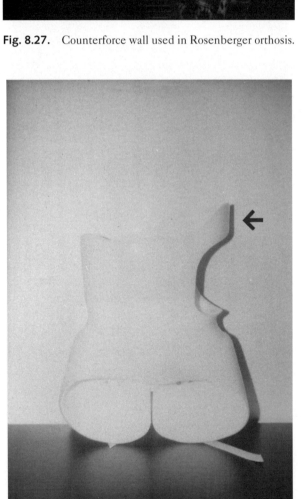

Fig. 8.28. Counterforce band used in the Boston brace. *(From Bunch WH, Patwardhan AG: Scoliosis: Making clinical decisions, St. Louis, 1989, CV Mosby.)*

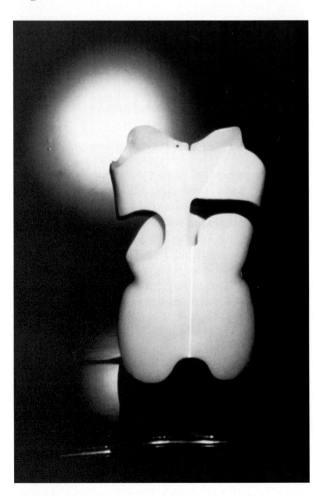

Fig. 8.30. The modified Lyonnaise lacks the superstructure of aluminum and the steel hinges used in the traditional Lyonnaise. *(Courtesy of L. Dreher Jouett, C.P.O., Dreher-Jouett, Inc., Chicago.)*

casting. Although the impression is bivalved and does not require a Risser frame, the procedure is similar to that for the Wilmington orthosis. This orthosis extends anteriorly from the pubis to the xyphoid process. Convex side trimline is one rib level superior to apical height similar to the Boston or Miami orthosis, but the concave side is similar to the Wilmington in that there is no cutout for trunk shift (because the shift is built into the orthosis). The concave side trimline terminates at the superior end point of the superior curve being treated. This orthosis is unique in that it uses adjustable floating slings for curve loading as is seen in Fig. 8.29, so that loading can exceed what is achieved by the corrected walls of the orthosis.[26,27,74]

Miami orthosis.   The Miami orthosis is a one-piece, posterior-opening polypropylene TLSO, custom-molded from a plaster impression. This orthosis offers many of the advantages of the Boston brace yet, in contrast to the Boston, is custom-molded and trimmed short enough to allow forward bending of the patient.[58] Lateral trimline heights and concave side cutout areas for trunk shift are similar to the Boston and Lyonnaise, as they are all varied according to curve pattern.

Lyonnaise orthosis.   The Lyonnaise orthosis is a one-piece, anterior-opening orthosis custom-fabricated from a plaster impression and fashioned from polypropylene. This orthosis extends anteriorly from the sternal notch to the symphysis pubis and has lateral trimlines, openings, and counterforce parameters that function similar to the Boston. The original fabrication used two lateral shells of custom-molded plastic joined posteriorly by a longitudinal aluminum bar and steel hinges allowing for function as an anterior-opening orthosis. Modifications have changed this to a one-piece molded structure, with a posterior seam used for hinge function (which eliminates the metal structure and lightens the orthosis) as seen in Fig. 8.30.

Wilmington jacket.   The Wilmington is unique in that it is casted by molding the plaster impression while the patient is on the Risser frame. This impression is designed similar to the localizer cast because the curves are reduced and analyzed by radiograph before proceeding with fabrication.[13] This orthosis was originally designed to be fashioned from low-temperature plastic (orthoplast). Many clinicians prefer the high-temperature, vacuum-formed, low-density polyethylene material as shown in Fig. 8.31 because it provides greater longevity without material degradation. This orthosis is a one-piece, anterior-opening orthosis with anterior trimline from symphysis pubis to sternal notch and bilateral heights to axilla. This orthosis does not have concave side cutouts, varied trimlines, or wall mounted pads because all loads, counterforces, and

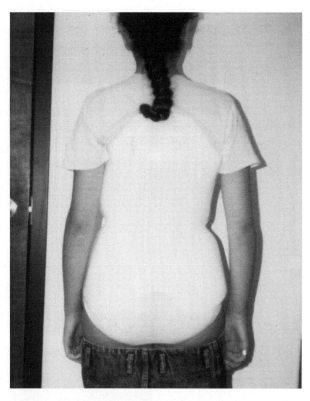

Fig. 8.31.   Wilmington orthosis. Modification includes use of polyethylene in fabrication. Note contours of orthosis walls and trimline heights. *(From Gavin TM, Shurr DG, Patwardhan AG: Orthotic treatment for spinal disorders. In Weinstein SL, editor: The pediatric spine, New York, 1993, Raven Press.)*

concave side area for trunk shift are fabricated into the orthosis.

Pad placement.   Although there are many different orthoses for nonoperative treatment of scoliosis, each with distinct characteristics, there are also some basic similarities. All scoliosis orthoses begin with the same parameters of pad placement, pad loading, pad force, and outcome expectations. All TLSOs use the same pad placement as discussed earlier for the Milwaukee brace. Because the TLSO does not have a neck ring to ensure a compensated alignment of the cervicothoracic spine, improper placement of counterforce in the TLSO can cause spinal decompensation.

Sequential pad loading.   Loading sequence for the TLSO pads is the same as that suggested for the Milwaukee brace. Primary curves must be loaded and shifted first so that compensatory curve loading is done with minimal translation of the trunk. For the Boston, Miami, and Lyonnaise orthoses (which load the curves by means of pads mounted on the wall of the orthosis), increases in loads and shifts must be done by thickening the pad. Transverse loading for the Wilmington orthosis is done in the Risser frame impression and is not adjustable in the orthosis. This requires periodic refabrication if loading needs change after the curve reduces.

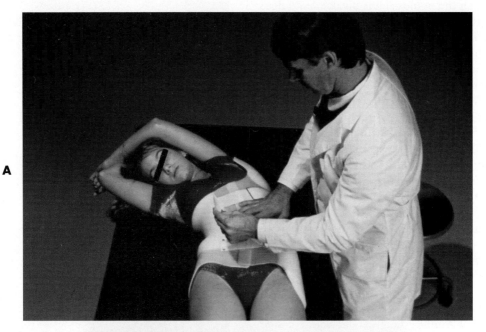

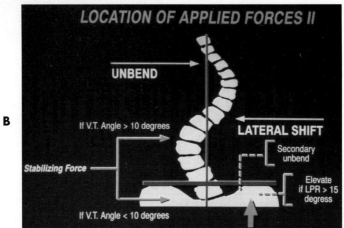

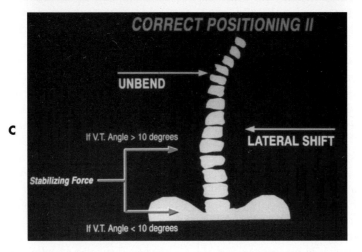

Fig. 8.32.   A, Charleston bending brace. Note side-bending contour of orthosis. **B** and **C,** The curve unbending principles of the Charleston bending brace. *(Courtesy of Ralph Hooper, C.P.O., Charleston Bending Brace Research and Education Foundation, Winter Park, Fla.)*

The Rosenberger orthosis uses an adjustable sling, so this orthosis may be adjusted with relative ease.

For the patient with idiopathic scoliosis, it is exceptionally important to monitor the fit of the orthosis periodically and to keep the pad force maximal and pads repositioned despite growth. Pad pressure is based on the criteria mentioned for the Milwaukee brace: maximum tolerable pressure.

The advantages of the TLSO are the use of a minimal orthosis for maximum result, good cosmesis, low weight, and lack of metal superstructure to tear clothes. The disadvantages of the TLSO are lack of longitudinal adjustment possible from a superstructure and lack of a neck ring to prevent sway of the cervico-thoracic spine.

Part-time orthotic treatment

Green[33] reported that part-time orthotic treatment can yield good results and the protocol of full-time treatment is not necessary. Edmonsson and Morris[20] found that patients who were not cooperative with full-time wearing did not do as well as the full-time wearers. In Edmonsson's study, the difference was 25% long-term correction for the full-time wearers and only 14% for the partially compliant. One present-day alternative for part-time orthotic treatment is the use of the Charleston bending brace (Fig. 8.32, *A*). The principle of unbending the curves for nighttime use only is demonstrated in Fig. 8.32, *B* and *C*. Acceptable results[90] have been reported using this orthosis.

Neuromuscular scoliosis

Orthotic treatment for neuromuscular scoliosis has traditionally been a method to delay spinal fusion. Because of the pelvic obliquity and decompensation from neuromuscular scoliosis common to the nonambulatory child, seating balance is frequently a major concern. A properly fitted orthosis may also assist this type of patient with seating balance to reduce fatigue and allow for longer periods of upper limb function. Custom-molded seating orthoses attached to the wheelchair are presently commonly used for this condition. These devices frequently do not incorporate continuous circumferential support, however, and therefore are not optimal for curve reduction and maintenance.

Proper orthotic selection for these patients is a difficult task. Bunch[9] reported on the use of the Milwaukee brace for paralytic scoliosis showing that the openness about the torso reduces chance of skin compromise and that the dynamic aspect of pads leads to better curve reduction. A custom-molded, total contact TLSO is also sometimes used (Fig. 8.33).

Many physicians are pessimistic about using orthoses for neuromuscular scoliosis. Orthotic treatment, however, may reduce or maintain spinal defor-

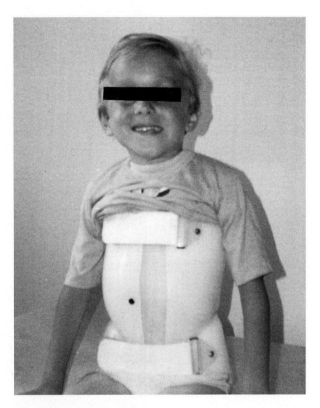

Fig. 8.33. TLSO for the neuromuscular patient. *(From Bunch WH, Patwardhan AG: Scoliosis: Making clinical decisions, St. Louis, 1989, CV Mosby.)*

mity until the patient is mature enough for spinal fusion. Although the current trend is to operate on these patients at a younger age because surgery is inevitable, many neuromuscular patients are either juvenile or infantile at the onset of progression and may benefit from the use of an orthosis.

Figure 8.34, *A*, shows the anteroposterior radiograph of a 16-month nonambulatory neuromuscular patient with a 72-degree thoracolumbar curve from pelvis to cranium. Although this patient had a high level of muscular tone, resisting the function of the orthosis, after wearing the TLSO for a month her curve reduced to 35 degrees (Fig. 8.34, *B*). The first orthosis was outgrown in approximately 10 months, when a second was prescribed. Transverse loading yielded greater trunk shift and further curve reduction to 17 degrees in the second orthosis (Fig. 8.34, *C*). The total contact TLSO is ideal for the nonambulatory patient because the patient does not have the muscle volition to shift away from the three-point pressure pads and slings of other designs. Properly constructed, the TLSO does not cause skin or pulmonary problems, reduces and maintains the curve, enhances seating stability, and is quite comfortable to the patient.

The ambulatory neuromuscular patient frequently presents with a compensatory curve and may benefit from the adjustability of the three-point orthoses as

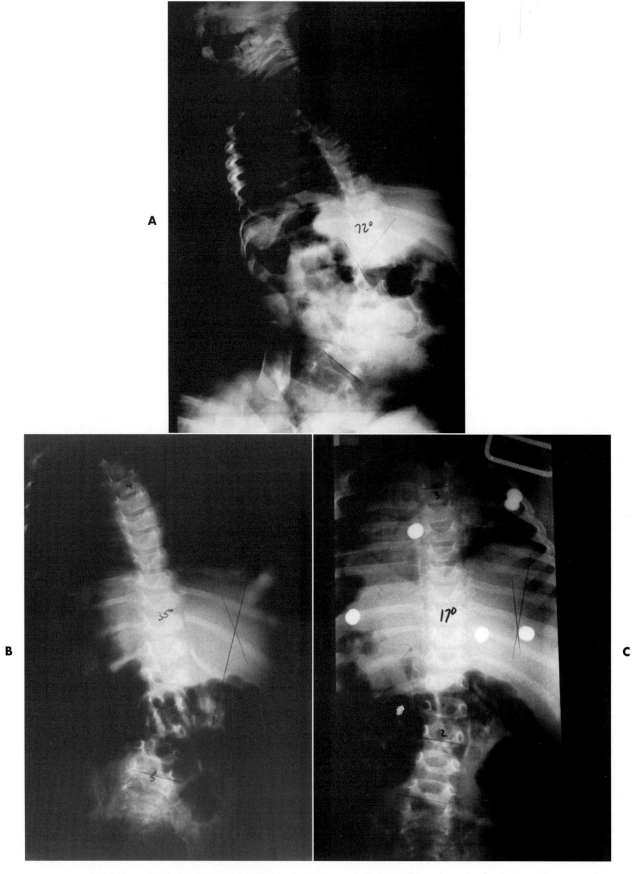

Fig. 8.34. **A,** Preorthosis radiograph of a 72-degree thoracolumbar neuromuscular curve. **B,** Radiograph in first TLSO shows an improvement to 35 degrees. **C,** Second orthosis reduced the curve to 17 degrees. *(From Gavin TM, Shurr DG, Patwardhan AG: Orthotic treatment for spinal disorders. In Weinstein SL, editor: The pediatric spine, New York, 1993, Raven Press.)*

seen in Fig. 8.35. Decision making for these patients must define primary orthotic goals. If seating stability is primary, the patient benefits from custom-molded seating. If curve reduction and delay of fusion are primary, however, the TLSO yields the optimal result.

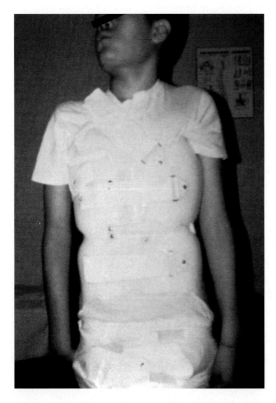

Fig. 8.35. Ambulatory neuromuscular patient in a Rosenberger TLSO.

Congenital scoliosis

The patient with congenital scoliosis challenges orthotists' creativity. Orthotic goals for congenital scoliosis are to reduce compensatory curves and to maintain a compensated alignment of the spine during growth. Changing the segmental angulation of the rigid congenital anomaly is usually not possible using any orthosis, and ill-advised attempts may lead to discomfort and skin breakdown.

Deciding which orthosis to use should include clinical needs as well as the mechanism of action. Because most of these patients begin treatment at an early age, they usually require several orthoses during the treatment course. For families with financial difficulties, the Milwaukee brace may be preferred because it is the only scoliosis orthosis that has longitudinal adjustability, allows for partial refabrication, and is easily converted for postoperative use.[27] The TLSO is otherwise often recommended because of its cosmesis. The congenital patient requires imagination in the design of the orthosis. Figure 8.36, *A,* shows a patient with several congenital anomalies in the lumbar spine causing severe decompensation to the right and the high thoracic spine causing a development torticollis. She was placed in an anterior-opening TLSO with a mandibular attachment to right the head. After 6 months of rigorous physical therapy and orthosis wear, the mandibular aspect was removed. Four years later, she maintained acceptable spinal and head alignment in the orthosis (Fig. 8.36, *B*).

Reduction of compensatory curves and correction of

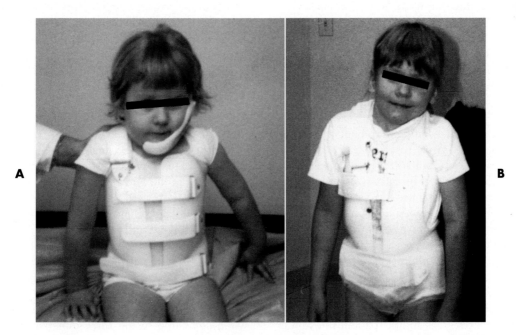

Fig. 8.36. **A,** A patient with congenital scoliosis in a TLSO with detachable mandibular support. **B,** The same patient in the TLSO 4 years later.

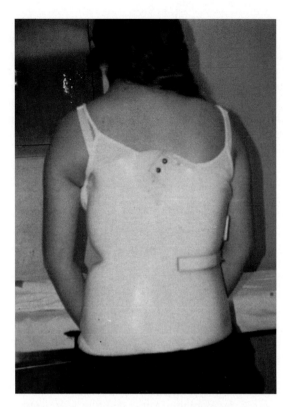

Fig. 8.37. A patient fitted with a Rosenberger orthosis for right thoracic scoliosis. Note high left shoulder.

any secondary deformity are the primary functions of orthoses for congenital scoliosis.

Spinal compensation

Orthoses may shift the torso, so it is important to assess the posture of the patient while wearing the device. Figure 8.37 shows a patient in a Rosenberger orthosis fitted for a right thoracic–left lumbar curve. Although the orthosis loads the curves adequately, is stable on the pelvis, and is comfortable to the patient, it is apparent that the left shoulder is high. On close evaluation, the patient's torso is decompensated to the left. This was due to an inadequate amount of counterforce in the left axilla with the result being the patient's tendency to raise the left shoulder to right herself. This problem was simply solved by increasing the axillary counterforce, thus centering the head and eliminating the righting reflex with the result of level shoulders.

The radiograph in Figure 8.38, A, depicts a right thoracic curve of 29 degrees with a left lumbar curve of 34 degrees. The Rosenberger orthosis was fitted with too much thoracic load and shift with a minimal lumbar pad force. The result was a reduction of the thoracic curve to 7 degrees; however, the lumbar curve reduced only to 25 degrees and the patient's head was decompensated to the left 3 cm (Fig. 8.38, B). With a minor adjustment to the pads, the thoracic force

magnitude and trunk shift were reduced to allow a greater lumbar load and shift. Curve reduction values changed to 12 and 11 degrees, and the result was a well-compensated spine (Fig. 8.38, C).

When treating patients with spinal disorders, care must be taken to ensure that secondary deformities and decompensation are not created by the orthosis.

Kyphosis

Kyphosis has several causes, including Scheuermann's disease, postural round back, neuromuscular conditions, and congenital causes. The most common type treated with an orthosis is Scheuermann's disease. This is depicted radiographically as anterior wedging of one to three consecutive vertebrae. The orthosis of choice is the Milwaukee brace because the apices of these curves are usually cephalad to T8. Figure 8.39 shows a patient with Scheuermann's disease in a Milwaukee brace for the first time. The pelvic interface and neck ring provide constraints in space, which yield the counterforce to the kyphosis pads. These pads are usually rectangular and are placed at and inferior to the apex of the curve, are mounted on the paraspinal bars, and produce anteriorly directed force to reduce the curvature, thus opening the wedges and allowing bony remodeling. The tendency is for the patient to lean on the throat mold because of the force generated by the kyphosis pads. Physical therapy plays a role in teaching these patients thoracic hyperextension exercises so that they can retract from the neck ring, thus providing an active counterforce to the kyphosis pads.

For the more caudad thoracolumbar curves, a TLSO may gain the desired result because the apex is low and the sternum is cephalad enough to be used as a counterforce without being in opposition to the kyphosis pads (Fig. 8.40).

The goal when treating Scheuermann's disease is bony remodeling of the wedges and overall reduction of the curvature. Sachs and associates[78] reviewed 75 patients who had completed an average of 34 months in the Milwaukee brace and had vertebral wedging corrected to a mean of 5 degrees. At long-term follow-up, there was an average of only 6 degrees loss of overall correction. Montgomery and Erwin[61] reported on a group that was weaned out of the orthoses 4 to 6 months after overall correction of the kyphosis and reported poor results in contrast. They showed 15 degrees average loss of correction at follow-up. Because bony remodeling is the goal of orthotic treatment, weaning from the orthosis is recommended after measurable changes have occurred in the wedges.

Because the nature of kyphosis is two-dimensional when compared to the three-dimensional aspects of scoliosis, reducing these curves is usually an easy task. Once again, proper follow-up for growth adjustment

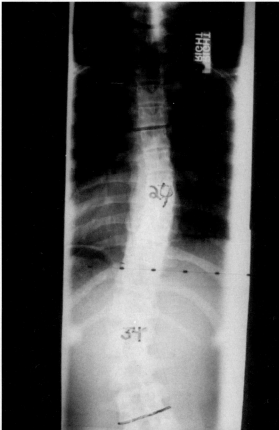

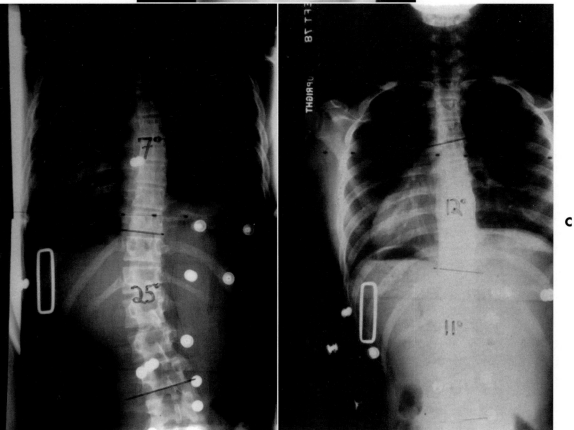

Fig. 8.38. **A,** Preorthosis radiograph of a patient with a right thoracic curve of 29 degrees and a left lumbar curve of 34 degrees. **B,** Improper pad loading reduced the thoracic curve to 7 and the lumbar curve to 25 degrees. The result was left decompensation of 3 cm. **C,** The same patient after balancing pad loads. The thoracic curve increased to 12 degrees; however, the lumbar curve reduced to 11 degrees, and the result was a compensated spine. *(From Gavin TM, Shurr DG, Patwardhan AG: Orthotic treatment for spinal disorders. In Weinstein SL, editor: The pediatric spine, New York, 1993, Raven Press.)*

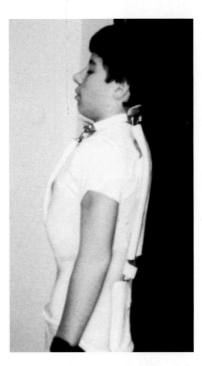

Fig. 8.39. Typical Milwaukee orthosis for Scheuermann's kyphosis.

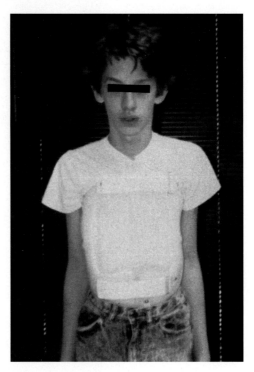

Fig. 8.40. TLSO for thoracolumbar Scheuermann's disease.

and increases in pad pressure along with sound clinical parameters for treatment yield the best possible result.

CONCLUSION

Although a body of literature exists investigating mechanisms and outcomes of orthotic treatment for spinal disorders, much work is still needed. Who will benefit from orthotic treatment and who will not are still key issues that are often unclear. Treatment compliance is an area that is also unknown.

The role of physical therapy as an adjunctive component to orthotic treatment is also unclear. Retrospective analysis of clinical data has allowed identification of the upper and lower thresholds for orthotic management of idiopathic scoliosis. This allows immediate planning for surgical correction when this result is inevitable, sparing the expense and effort of "trying a brace first" in such cases. As more research is done in the area of natural history of spinal disorders and treatment of these disorders, more data become available to quantify the effect of orthotic treatment of these disorders. This allows the clinical team to predict outcomes better and reduces the "wait and see" aspect of treatment.

Choosing the proper orthosis should be based on many factors both objective and subjective. A well-versed clinical team helps ensure that the orthosis is properly fitting the patient throughout the duration of wear. A poorly fitted orthosis or a patient that is not followed with timely visits for periodic adjustment is usually worse than no orthosis at all.

ACKNOWLEDGMENTS

The authors would like to thank Patrick Carrico from the Department of Orthopaedic Surgery at Loyola University Medical Center for his assistance with the illustrations.

REFERENCES

1. American Academy of Orthopaedic Surgeons: Atlas of orthopaedic appliances, Ann Arbor, 1952, Edwards.
2. Andersson GBJ, Ortengren R, Nachemson A: Intradiscal pressure, intra abdominal pressure, and myoelectric back muscle activity related to posture and loading, Clin Orthop Rel Res 129:156, 1977.
3. Andriacchi TP, et al: Milwaukee brace corrections of idiopathic scoliosis, J Bone Joint Surg 58A:806, 1976.
4. Andry N: Orthopaedia, Philadelphia, 1961, JB Lippincott (facsimile reproduction of the first edition in English, London, 1743).
5. Axelsson P, et al: Lumbar orthosis with unilateral hip immobilization, effect on intervertebral mobility determined by roentgen stereophotogrammetric analysis, Spine 18:876–879, 1993.
6. Axelsson P, et al: Effect of lumbar orthosis on intervertebral mobility, a roentgen stereophotogrammetric analysis, Spine 17:678–681, 1992.
7. Benzel E: A comparison of the Minerva and Halo jackets for stabilization of the cervical spine, J Neurosurg 70:411–414, 1989.
8. Blount WP, Moe JH: The Milwaukee brace, Baltimore, 1973, Williams & Wilkins.
9. Bunch WH: The Milwaukee brace in paralytic scoliosis, Clin Orthop 110:63–68, 1975.

10. Bunch WH, Keagy R: Principles of orthotic treatment, St. Louis, 1975, CV Mosby.

11. Bunch W, Patwardhan A: Clinical experience in orthotic treatment. In Scoliosis: Making clinical decisions, St. Louis, 1989, CV Mosby.

12. Bunch WH, Patwardhan AG: Scoliosis: Making clinical decisions, St. Louis, 1989, CV Mosby.

13. Bunnell WP, MacEwen GD, Jayakumar S: The use of plastic jackets in the non-operative treatment of idiopathic scoliosis, J Bone Joint Surg 62A:31–38, 1980.

14. Carr W, et al: Treatment of idiopathic scoliosis in the Milwaukee brace, J Bone Joint Surg 62A:599–612, 1980.

15. Chance GQ: Note on a type of flexion fracture of the spine, Br J Radiol 21:452, 1948.

16. Colachis SC, Jr, Strohm BR, Ganter EL: Cervical spine motion in normal woman: Radiographic study of effect of cervical collars, Arch Phys Med Rehabil 54:161, 1973.

17. Denis F: The three column spine and its significance in the classification of acute thoracolumbar spinal injuries, Spine 8:817, 1983.

18. Dorsky S, et al: A three dimensional analysis of lumbar brace immobilization utilizing a noninvasive technique, Proceedings of the 33rd Annual Meeting, Orthopaedic Research Society, San Francisco, 1987.

19. Duval-Beaupere G: Pathogenic relationship between scoliosis and growth. In Zorab PA, editor: Proceedings of the Third Symposium on Scoliosis and Growth, Edinburgh, 1971, Churchill Livingstone.

20. Edmonsson A, Morris J: Follow-up study of Milwaukee brace treatment in patients with idiopathic scoliosis, Clin Orthop 126:58–61, 1977.

21. Emans J: The Boston bracing system for idiopathic scoliosis: Follow-up results in 295 patients, Spine 11:792–801, 1986.

22. Ferguson RL, et al: Biomechanical comparisons of spinal fracture models and the stabilizing effects of posterior instrumentations, Spine 13:453–460, 1988.

23. Fidler MW, Plasmans CMT: The effect of four types of support on the segmental mobility of the lumbosacral spine. J Bone Joint Surg 65A:943–947, 1983.

24. Fishman S, et al: Spinal orthoses. In American Academy of Orthopedic Surgeons: Atlas of orthotics, biomechanical principles and applications, ed 2, St. Louis, 1985, CV Mosby.

25. Galante J, et al: Forces acting in the Milwaukee brace on patients undergoing treatment for idiopathic scoliosis, J Bone Joint Surg 52A:498, 1970.

26. Gavin T, Bunch WH, Dvonch V: The Rosenberger scoliosis orthosis, J Assoc Child Prosthet Orthot Clin 21:35–38, 1986.

27. Gavin TM: Fabrication and fitting of orthoses. In Bunch WH, Patwardhan AG, editors: Scoliosis: Making clinical decisions, St. Louis, 1989, CV Mosby.

28. Gavin TM, et al: Preliminary results of orthotic treatment for chronic low back pain, J Pros Orthos 5:5/25-9/29, 1993.

29. Gavin TM, Shurr DG, Patwardhan AG: Orthotic treatment for spinal disorders. In Weinstein SL, editor: The pediatric spine, New York, 1993, Raven Press.

30. Gilbertson LG, et al: The biomechanical function of "three point" hyperextension orthoses, Proceedings of the American Society of Mechanical Engineers 112th Winter Annual Meeting, Atlanta, 1991.

31. Goel VK, Weinstein JN, Found EM: Biomechanics of lumbar and thoracolumbar spine surgery. In Goel VK, Weinstein JN, editors: Biomechanics of the spine: Clinical and surgical perspective. Boca Raton, FL, 1990, CRC Press.

32. Goel VK, Weinstein JN, Patwardhan A: Biomechanics of the intact ligamentous spine. In Goel VK, Weinstein JN, editors: Biomechanics of the spine: Clinical and surgical perspective. Boca Raton, FL, 1990, CRC Press.

33. Green NE: Part-time bracing of idiopathic scoliosis, Orthop Trans 5:22, 1981.

34. Haher TR, et al: The contribution of the three columns of the spine to spinal stability: A biomechanical model, Proceedings of the 22nd Annual Meeting of the Scoliosis Research Society, Vancouver, Canada, 1987.

35. Hampton D et al: Healing potential of the annulus fibrosis, Spine 14:398, 1989.

36. Harris EE: A new orthotics terminology—a guide to its use for prescription and fee schedules, Orthot Prosthet 27:6–19, 1973.

37. Harris JD: Cervical orthoses. In Orthotics Etcetera, ed 3, Baltimore, 1986, Williams and Wilkins.

38. Hukins D: Disc structure and function. In Ghosh P, editor: The biology of the intervertebral disc, Boca Raton, FL, 1988, CRC Press.

39. Jacobs RR, Nordwall A, Nachemson A: Reduction, stability, and strength provided by internal fixation systems for thoracolumbar spinal injuries, Clin Orthop Rel Res, 171:300–308, 1982.

40. Jewett EL: Hyperextension back brace, J Bone Joint Surg 19:1128, 1937.

41. Jodoin A, et al: Treatment of idiopathic scoliosis by the Boston brace system: Early results, Orthop Trans 5:22, 1981.

42. Johnson RM, et al: Cervical orthoses—a study comparing their effectiveness in restricting cervical motion in normal subjects, J Bone Joint Surg 59A:332, 1977.

43. Johnson RM, et al: Cervical orthoses: A guide to their selection and use, J Bone Joint Surg, 1980.

44. Johnson RM: Influence of spinal immobilization on consolidation of posterolateral lumbosacral fusion, Spine 17:16–21, 1992.

45. Kim, et al: Factors affecting fusion rate in adult spondylolisthesis, Spine 15, 1990.

46. Krag MH, et al: The effect of back braces on the relationship between intra-abdominal pressure and spinal loads, Adv Bioeng pp 22–23, 1986.

47. Lantz SA, Schultz AB: Lumbar spine orthosis wearing: I. Restriction of gross body motions, Spine 11:834–837, 1986.

48. Lantz SA, Schultz AB: Lumbar spine orthosis wearing: II. Effect on trunk muscle myoelectric activity, Spine 11:838–842, 1986.

49. Lonstein JE, Carlson M: The prediction of curve progression in untreated idiopathic scoliosis during growth, J Bone Joint Surg 66A:1061–1071, 1984.

50. Lonstein JE: Orthotic treatment of spinal deformities. In American Academy of Orthopaedic Surgeons: Atlas of orthotics, St. Louis, 1985, CV Mosby.

51. Lonstein JE, Winter RL: Milwaukee brace treatment of adolescent idiopathic scoliosis—review of 1020 patients, J Bone Joint Surg 75A, 1993.

52. Lucas D: Spinal bracing. In Orthotics Etcetera, Baltimore, 1966, Williams & Wilkins.

53. Lucas DB: Mechanics of the spine, Bull Hosp Joint Dis 30:115, 1970.

54. Lucas D, et al: Spinal Orthotics for pain and instability. In Orthotics Etcetera, ed 3, Baltimore, 1986, Williams and Wilkins.

55. Lumsden RM, Morris JM: An in vivo study of axial rotation and immobilization at the lumbosacral joint, J Bone Joint Surg 50A:1591, 1968.

56. Lusskin R: Pain patterns in spondylolisthesis, Clin Orthop 40:125–136, 1965.

57. Maiman D, et al: The effect of the thermoplastic Minerva body jacket on cervical spine motion, Neurosurgery 25, 1989.

58. McCollough NC III, et al: Miami TLSO in the management of scoliosis: Preliminary results in 100 cases, J Pediatr Orthop 1:141–152, 1981.

59. McGill SM, et al: The effect of an abdominal belt on trunk

muscle activity and intra-abdominal pressure during squat lifts, Ergonomics 33:147–160, 1990.

60. Micheli LJ, Hall JE, Miller ME: Use of the modified Boston brace for back injuries in athletes, Am J Sports Med 8:351–356, 1980.

61. Montgomery SP, Erwin WE: Scheuermann's kyphosis—long-term results of Milwaukee brace treatment, Spine 6:5–8, 1981.

62. Morris JM, Lucas D, Bresler B: Role of the trunk in stability of the spine, J Bone Joint Surg 43-A:327–351, 1961.

63. Mulcahy T, et al: A follow-up study of forces acting in the Milwaukee brace on patients undergoing treatment for idiopathic scoliosis, Clin Orthop 93:53, 1973.

64. Nachemson A: The load on the lumbar discs in different positions of the body, Clin Orthop Rel Res 45:107, 1966.

65. Nachemson A, Elfstrom G: Intravital wireless telemetry of axial forces in Harrington distraction rods in patients with idiopathic scoliosis, J Bone Joint Surg 53A:445–465, 1971.

66. Nachemson A, Morris JM: In vivo measurements of intradiscal pressure, J Bone Joint Surg 46A:1077–1092, 1964.

67. Nachemson A, Peterson LE: Scoliosis Research Society Brace Study Report: Effectiveness of brace treatment in moderate adolescent idiopathic scoliosis—factors predicting progress in moderate adolescent idiopathic scoliosis, Proceedings of the 28th Annual Meeting of the Scoliosis Research Society, Dublin, 1993.

68. Nachemson A, Schultz AB, Andersson GBJ: Mechanical effectiveness studies of lumbar spine orthoses, Scand J Rehabil Med (Suppl. 9), 1983.

69. Norton PL, Brown T: The immobilizing efficiency of the back braces: Their effect on the posture and motion of the lumbosacral spine, J Bone Joint Surg 39A:111–139, 1957.

70. Nagel DA, et al: Stability of the upper lumbar spine following progressive disruptions and the application of individual internal and external fixation devices, J Bone Joint Surg 63A:62–70, 1981.

71. Patwardhan A, et al: Biomechanics of the spine. In Bunch WH, et al, editors: Atlas of orthotics, St. Louis, 1985, CV Mosby.

72. Patwardhan AG, et al: A biomechanical analog of curve progression and orthotic stabilization in idiopathic scoliosis, J Biomech 19:103, 1986.

73. Patwardhan AG, et al: Orthotic stabilization of idiopathic scoliotic curves: A biomechanical comparison of the Milwaukee brace and low profile orthoses. In Erdman AG, editor: Advances in bioengineering, 1987, ASME.

74. Patwardhan AG, et al: Biomechanics of adolescent idiopathic scoliosis: Natural history and treatment. In Goel VK, Weinstein JN, editors: Biomechanics of the spine: Clinical and surgical perspective, Boca Raton, FL, CRC Press, 1990.

75. Patwardhan AG, et al: Orthotic stabilization of thoracolumbar injuries: A biomechanical analysis of the Jewett hyperextension orthosis. Spine 15:654–661, 1990.

76. Patwardhan AG, et al: Stability of fractures in the thoraco-lumbar spine, Spine State Art Rev 7, 1993.

77. Perry J: The use of external support in the treatment of low back pain, J Bone Joint Surg 52A: 7.1440–1442, 1970.

78. Sachs B, et al: Scheuermann's kyphosis: Follow-up of Milwaukee brace treatment, J Bone Joint Surg 69:50–57, 1987.

79. Salter RB: Textbook of disorders and injuries of the musculoskeletal system, ed 2, Baltimore, 1983, Williams & Wilkins.

80. Schimandle JH, Weigel M, Edwards CC: Indications for thigh cuff bracing following instrumented lumbosacral fusions, Proceedings of the 8th Annual Meeting of the North American Spine Society, San Diego, 1993.

81. Schultz AB, Ashton-Miller JA: Biomechanics of the human spine. In Mow VC, Hayes WC, editors: Basic Orthopaedic Biomechanics, New York, 1991, Raven Press.

82. Slosar PJ, Patwardhan AG, Lorenz MA, et al: The three-dimensional instability patterns of the thoracolumbar burst fracture, Proceedings of the Annual Meeting of the International Society for the Study of the Lumbar Spine, Chicago, 1992.

83. Spinal Orthotics, New York University Post-Graduate Medical School, Prosthetics and Orthotics, 1973.

84. Taylor CF: On the mechanical treatment of Pott's disease of the spine—the spinal assistant, treatise, New York State Medical Society 6:67, 1863.

85. Thompson A: Appliances for the spine and trunk. In American Academy of Orthopedic Surgeons: Orthopedic appliance atlas, Vol I, Ann Arbor, 1952, Edwards Bros.

86. Timoshenko S, Gere J: Theory of elastic stability, ed 2, New York, 1961, McGraw-Hill.

87. Triggs, KJ: Length dependence of a halo orthosis on cervical immobilization, J Spinal Disord 6:34–37, 1993.

88. Waters RL, Morris JM: Effects of spinal supports on the electrical activity of muscles of the trunk, J Bone Joint Surg 52A:51–60, 1970.

89. White AA, Panjabi MM: Clinical biomechanics of the spine, ed 2, Philadelphia, JB Lippincott, 1990.

90. Wilhemy JK, Farrow B, Zeller JL: Five year study evaluating the use of the Charleston night brace for the treatment of idiopathic scoliosis, Proceedings of the 25th Annual Meeting of the Scoliosis Research Society, Honolulu, 1990.

91. Williams PC: Lesions of the lumbosacral spine—lordosis brace, J Bone Joint Surg 19:702, 1937.

92. Willner S: Effect of a rigid brace on back pain, Acta Orthop Scand 56:40–42, 1985.

93. Willner S: Test instrument for predicting the effect of rigid braces, Prosthet Orthot Intl 1990.

CHAPTER 9

Upper Limb Orthoses

Thomas R. Lunsford

Upper limb orthoses are distinct from other orthoses because of the complexity of the human hand. There are many simultaneous joint motions that have to be considered for either mobilization or immobilization (e.g., nine interphalangeal [IP], five metacarpophalangeal [MCP], wrist, forearm, elbow, three shoulder), short digital levers (which translates to high forces, high pressures, and skin intolerance), and little soft tissue padding for bands and other components. Orthotic design for the upper limb must give equal focus to mechanical efficiency and precision of fit because comfort is critical for acceptance. Therefore, the small segments, limitations in soft tissue padding, and multiplicity of joint motion create high demands, which only a skilled Certified Orthotist with both a keen problem-solving sense and finely tuned fabrication skills can meet.[4] Frequently the benefit is limited, and when the treatment goals are met, the orthosis is discontinued. The orthoses may be discarded if the patient finds another, more acceptable means to function or if the benefit of the orthosis is outweighed by the patient's lack of "gadget tolerance."

Upper limb orthoses are more likely to be accepted by clients if there is a well-defined therapeutic purpose or if the orthosis provides a desired function that cannot be accomplished by any other means, such as substitution. Because even the best upper limb orthosis lacks mechanical versatility to grasp objects that vary widely in size, shape, and weight with equal ease, upper limb orthotic design tends to be optimized for a specific purpose. Combine this mechanical shortcoming with impaired sensation, reduced skin friction, and poor subcutaneous contouring, and individuals have to produce greater prehension force than the normal hand just to accomplish routine activities. In addition, an upper limb orthosis is conspicuous and advertises the disability. Despite these limitations, upper limb

orthoses can offer appealing advantages for the limb left impaired by paralysis, deformity, or pain.

Frequently, upper limb orthoses are applied to insensate limbs, and a well-defined skin inspection regimen must be followed to avoid pressure sores. It is common to have the patient wear the orthosis initially for a relatively short period of time (5 to 30 minutes) and then remove the orthosis and inspect the skin for persistent red marks. Red marks should disappear within 20 minutes. If they do not, the orthosis should be adjusted to alleviate the excessive pressure on the skin. If the red marks disappear within the 20-minute period, wearing time can be gradually increased (e.g., by 15 minutes) until it can be tolerated for several hours.

To the novice, upper limb orthoses seem widely diversified and hopelessly unorganized. This is probably the result of the enormous versatility of the upper limb. With lower limb orthotic management, the goals are generally to reduce walking or running deviations. While the task of walking or running is defined by specific repeatable phases, no such simple definition can describe upper limb function. The upper limb is involved with so many activities that even identifying a specific goal or function can be difficult.

In fact, upper limb orthoses can be organized categorically in several ways, such as by pathology (e.g., spinal injury, arthritis, trauma, head injury), arthrosegmentally according to the joint encompassed (e.g., shoulder, elbow, wrist, hand, fingers), or treatment objective (e.g., promote healing, direct growth, prevent deformity, correct deformity, enhance function). The main categories selected for this chapter are *static* and *dynamic*. Under each of these primary categories, it is convenient to group upper limb orthoses further as either *therapeutic* or *functional*. To illustrate, one example of a static functional upper limb orthosis is a short opponens (static hand orthosis) with attachments for eating, reading, page turning, shaving, and grooming.

The temporary upper limb orthoses made from low-temperature thermoplastics are discussed separately. These devices are typically fitted immediately postsurgery or posttrauma. Designs are developed using paper patterns, the plastic is heated in hot water, and the orthoses are formed directly on the patient's limb.

STATIC ORTHOSES

Therapeutic

Orthoses in this category include the static wrist-hand orthosis (WHO), static hand-orthosis (HdO), elbow orthosis (EO), shoulder-elbow orthosis (SEO), and shoulder-elbow-wrist orthosis (SEWO). Several specific therapeutic attachments to these basic devices are described. Although there are many other static orthoses used occasionally for therapeutic purposes, space limitations preclude a listing or description of all custom-designed and custom-fabricated orthoses.

Static WHO

Clinical application.   The static WHO (Fig. 9.1) supports the wrist joint, maintains the functional architecture of the hand, and prevents wrist-hand deformities. Occasionally the static WHO is used as a platform for other therapeutic attachments (e.g., MCP extension stop, IP extension assist, thumb extension assist). The static WHO illustrated in Fig. 9.1 is of the Rancho type. Several functionally equivalent metal and plastic designs are available, including those used at the Rehabilitation Institute in Chicago, The Institute for Rehabilitation and Research in Houston, and the Institute of Rehabilitation Medicine at New York University. The reader is referred to previous editions of this text for examples of alternative designs.

Patient population.   Patients with severe weakness or paralysis of the wrist and hand musculature are appropriate candidates for the static WHO. Without support, these individuals are at risk of developing the "claw hand" deformity and/or overstretching weak muscles (Fig. 9.2). For example, quadriplegics usually exhibit the aforementioned weakness and can benefit from a static WHO to preserve the functional posture of their hand and wrist (see Figs. 9.1 and 9.2). It is important to prevent encumbering contractures or deformities in patients because they may later become a candidate for a functional WHO. The static WHO is often indicated as a positional orthosis for C1-5 quadriplegics with zero wrist extensors and an *intrinsic minus* hand.

Attachments.   Two of the most common attachments used with the static WHO are the MCP extension stop and the IP extension assist (Fig. 9.3). If there is loss of flexion range at the MCP joints and loss of extension range at the proximal PIP joints, these two attachments can help prevent a claw hand deformity by

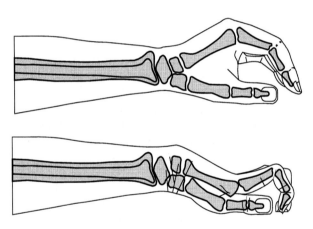

Fig. 9.2.   Claw hand deformity (wrist flexed, MCPs hyperextended, and thumb extended and abducted).

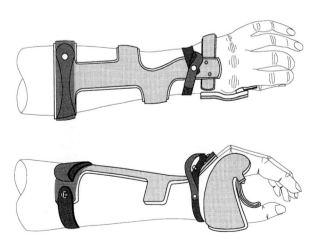

Fig. 9.1.   Static wrist-hand orthosis (WHO).

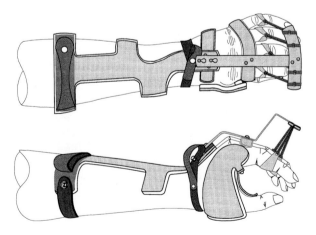

Fig. 9.3.   Static WHO with MCP extension stop and IP extension assist.

preventing hyperextension of the MCP joints while encouraging extension of the IP joints of index through little fingers. Both of these attachments can be mounted on the same outrigger bar. This outrigger bar has two keyholes that facilitate installation and removal of the assembly.

The thumb can be maintained in opposition while allowing a limited range of motion with the addition of a swivel thumb (Fig. 9.4). The swivel thumb acts as a carpometacarpal (CM) flexion assist for the thumb and consists of a custom-contoured metal band over the proximal phalanx of the thumb, which is secured to the radial extension of the palmar piece with a simple cantilevered wire spring (see Fig. 9.4).

Static hand orthosis (HdO)
Clinical application. The static HdO (Fig. 9.5) maintains the functional position of the hand and prevents deformities from developing. Occasionally the static HdO is used as a platform for other therapeutic attachments. All the attachments described for the static WHO can also be used with the static HdO. Again, the Rancho design is depicted here, and the reader is referred to previous editions of this text for

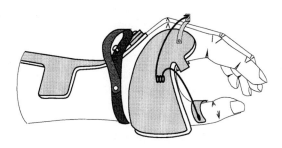

Fig. 9.4. Swivel thumb attached to static WHO.

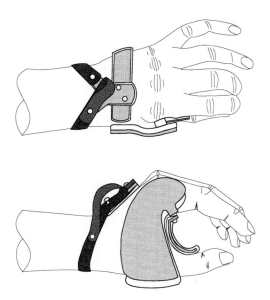

Fig. 9.5. Static hand orthosis (HdO).

examples of other functionally equivalent upper limb orthoses designs.

Patient population. Patients with weakness or paralysis of the hand intrinsic musculature and strong wrist extensors are appropriate candidates for the static HdO. Without this orthosis, these patients are at risk of developing a flat hand with the thumb carpometacarpal joint in extension. The C7 neurosegmental level quadriplegic exhibits this weakness, for example, and can benefit from a static HdO.

Elbow orthosis (EO)
Clinical application. Elbow orthoses designed for reducing soft tissue contractures must be custom-designed and custom-fabricated with structural plastic (polypropylene) bands and total contact flexible plastic (polyethylene) cuffs and straps and incorporate at least one of a variety of mechanisms for increasing the range of motion. It is preferable to apply low-magnitude, long-duration forces when attempting to reduce an elbow flexion or extension contracture (Fig. 9.6). This is necessary to avoid the antagonist response, which accompanies quick, intense stretching. With quick and/or intense orthotic forces, the outcome may be that the muscles in series and parallel with the tight collagen fibers might become tighter. Also the skin is at greater risk of breakdown with the higher forces. Particular attention must be given to mechanical/anatomical joint alignment, and the arm and forearm must be restricted to pure rotation with minimum translation to avoid joint subluxation or dislocation. The contracture reduction force must be gradually increased therapeutically (see Fig. 9.6; slowly expand or contract the turnbuckle) so that the soft tissue collagen adhesions responsible for the contracture can undergo microtears without causing trauma to the joint. The bands and cuffs should be placed near the elbow joint so that the levers of the three-point contracture reduction force system are maximized, correction forces are minimized, and skin pressure is tolerable. The edges of the bands and cuffs

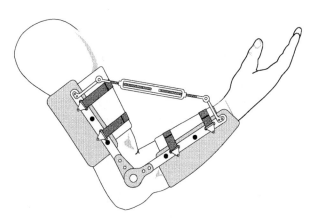

Fig. 9.6. Elbow orthosis (contracture reduction application).

should be flared to avoid excessive edge pressure and shear. The therapeutic strategy should be to tease the tissues into lengthening without provoking an antagonistic response, without causing permanent red marks on the skin, and without creating internal bruising.

Patient population.   Elbow orthoses are used for reduction of soft tissue contractures of the elbow that result in functional limitations. The need to reduce elbow flexion or extension contractures can result from trauma or disease. The largest population affected are individuals with spinal cord injury, who depend on full range of motion of their elbow for alleviating ischial sitting pressure, propelling a manual wheelchair, and bringing the hand to their face. Another common cause for restricted elbow motion may be immobilization posttrauma or postsurgery.

Shoulder-elbow orthosis (SEO)

Clinical application.   It may be necessary to support a painful shoulder or traumatized brachial plexus–injured limb with an orthosis. In many cases, a conventional arm sling suffices, provided that there is not excessive force on the base of the neck and the use is short-term. For long-term use, however, a sling offers very little function. The abduction orthosis, properly anchored on the hip, can be a successful alternative. Rancho Los Amigos Medical Center has developed a dynamic arm and shoulder support called the gunslinger (Fig. 9.7). The client's arm is strapped to a forearm trough, which is mechanically coupled to a plastic hemigirdle anchored on the patient's pelvis (iliac crest). The coupling between the forearm trough and iliac cap can be customized to permit a variety of motions, including glenohumeral joint internal/external rotation, flexion extension, and horizontal flexion/extension as well as flexion/extension of the elbow joint. The arm and hand is held in a cosmetically pleasing pose, and the hand is available for use, enabling early functional recovery. The gunslinger SEO is easy to put on and take off, and full deweighting of the arm is feasible.

Patient population.   The brachial plexus–injured patient can benefit from the application of the gunslinger SEO for both prevention of further stretch injury during the healing process and positioning of the hand in useful locations for functional activities. With a long-sleeve shirt, the iliac cap and arm trough can be concealed making the orthosis more cosmetically acceptable.

Some individuals with a brachial plexus injury have a normal hand and wrist (intrinsic plus hand and wrist, C7-8 spared) with proximal musculature weakness. The gunslinger orthosis with a simple forearm trough is sufficient in these cases to support the arm, position it in space, and allow the hand to be functional. A painful, subluxing glenohumeral joint can be deweighted and

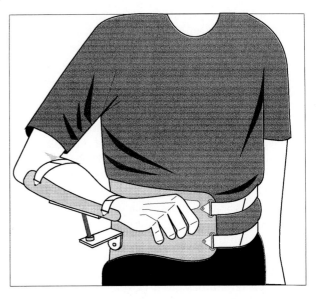

Fig. 9.7.   Gunslinger shoulder elbow orthosis (SEO).

can also benefit from the gunslinger SEO with a simple forearm trough. If the wrist or hand is also weak or painful, however, either an extension to forearm trough (cock-up palmar piece) or an attachable WHO is indicated.

Shoulder-elbow-wrist orthosis (SEWO)

Clinical application.   Shoulder-elbow-wrist orthoses are frequently used to protect soft tissues or to prevent contractures of soft tissues. Occasionally, these orthoses are used to correct an existing deformity.

The specific design depends on the therapeutic goal prescribed. Interim SEWOs, used for relief of pain or to promote healing, are frequently custom-fitted to the patient from prefabricated kits or assemblies. The hardware is usually adjustable so that a few sizes fit all. The SEWOs used for the long-term are custom-designed and custom-fabricated, with carefully selected structural and biomechanical components. The bands and joints are not adjustable, and only the straps can accommodate physical changes in the patient.

The SEWO depicted in Fig. 9.8 transmits the weight of the upper limb to the ipsilateral pelvis, and the system is stabilized with trunk straps. When this type of SEWO is used for clients with an axillary burn (3), the objective is to provide as much contact as possible while keeping the glenohumeral joint in maximum abduction. The anatomic elbow joint may be immobilized or free motion allowed. Generally the wrist is supported in extension to protect the associated soft tissues against the forces of gravity.

The disadvantage of prefabricated and custom-fitted versus custom-designed and custom-fabricated SEWOs is that the prefabricated orthoses require more follow-up to guard against excessive pressure or shear. This is especially true if the patient has sensory impair-

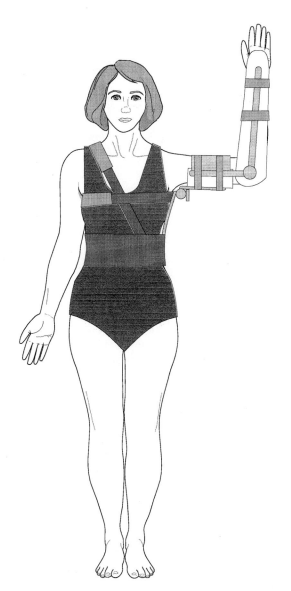

Fig. 9.8. Shoulder-elbow-wrist orthosis (SEWO).

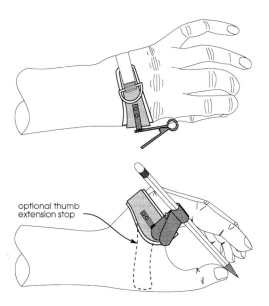

optional thumb
extension stop

Fig. 9.9. Static HdO with butterfly writing clip.

ment. Also, prefabricated orthoses have to be adjusted if the patient has episodes of edema, whereas the custom-fabricated device can be designed to reduce edema using total contact bands and cuffs.

The orthosis shown in Fig. 9.8 is also known as the airplane orthosis because of obvious appearance when it is used bilaterally. An alternate name for this orthosis is the shoulder stabilizer. By externally rotating the glenohumeral joint with the SEWO (see Fig. 9.8), the internal rotators are stretched, and the tension on the deltoid and rotator cuff is relieved, often desirable after shoulder surgery.

It is possible to design the SEWO with maximum mobility in mind for therapeutic purposes. Full range of abduction/adduction, flexion/extension, internal/external, and horizontal flexion/extension motions of the glenohumeral joint can be incorporated into the ortho-

sis by careful selection of the subaxillary mechanical joints used. This permits postoperative rehabilitation without removing the orthosis.

Patient population. The airplane SEWO is an excellent orthosis to prescribe after rotator cuff repairs, anterior-posterior capsular repairs, and postmanipulation. This orthosis is also frequently prescribed for axillary burns to prevent contracture and alternatively to help reduce soft tissue contractures owing to a variety of reasons (e.g., long-term immobility). The wearing time for the airplane SEWO can be gradually increased while avoiding skin problems by routine inspection and modification to the orthosis when indicated.

Functional

Clinical application. The static WHO and HdO can be modified to provide functional activities by attaching clips and pockets that hold utensils, writing devices, page turners, and so forth. The static HdO shown in Fig. 9.9 has butterfly type of clamp attached to the radial extension that clasps the shaft of a writing device. An alternative to the clamp is the truss stud configuration on the palmar extension of the palmar side (Fig. 9.10). Utensils and other attachments are adapted with a slotted plate that engages the truss studs on the palmar side to secure the attachments. A simple HdO can be modified with an aluminum rod to create an ulnar page turner (Fig. 9.11). The rubber end of an eye dropper is used on the end of the aluminum rod for friction to facilitate page turning. Numerous devices can be attached to an HdO or WHO, including toothbrushes, razors, combs, brushes, hygiene aids, eating utensils, arts and crafts implements, and devices unique to the injured individual's work environment.

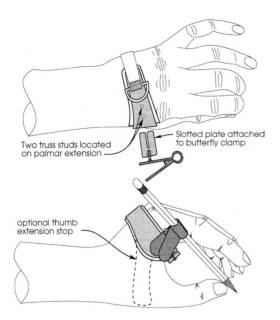

Fig. 9.10.   Static HdO with truss stud attachment.

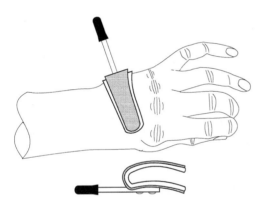

Fig. 9.11.   Static HdO with ulnar page turner.

Patient population.   Adapting the static HdO or WHO in this fashion is usually done when rigid deformities exist in the hand and finger joints and supple prehension is not feasible, precluding use of more functional dynamic WHOs. Some individuals with spinal cord injury and residual quadriplegia lose the flexibility of their fingers and hand over time and become candidates for the HdO or WHO with a variety of attachments. The HdO version is generally used when the patient's wrist extension musculature is strong enough to stabilize the hand position during use.

DYNAMIC ORTHOSES

Therapeutic
Wrist-action wrist hand orthosis (WAWHO)
Clinical application.   The WAWHO functions as a positional and therapeutic orthosis.[5] As with the static

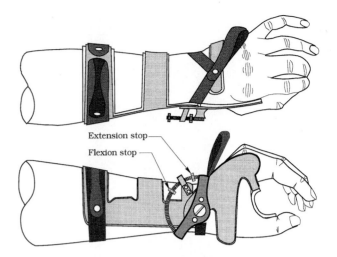

Fig. 9.12.   Wrist action wrist-hand orthosis (WAWHO).

WHO, it maintains the functional position of the hand and prevents wrist and hand deformities (Fig. 9.12). Its therapeutic function is to protect and assist weak wrist extensors with mechanical wrist motion stops. Sometimes the WAWHO is used with a rubber band and pulley arrangement to assist wrist extension (Fig. 9.13). Also, if necessary, the previously described MCP extension stop and IP extension assist are added. The protection and strengthening of weak muscles is achieved by limiting wrist motion, while the functional position of the hand is maintained by the orthosis.

Patient population.   Clients with weak (2, poor to 3, fair) wrist extensors and paralyzed hand muscles or clients who have potential for wrist extensor musculature return are appropriate candidates for a WAWHO. For those individuals with poor to fair wrist extensors or those with 3+ (fair+) wrist extensors with limited endurance, a WAWHO with extension assist is indicated (Fig. 9.13). The WAWHO has a hinge at the wrist allowing active extension and gravity-assisted flexion. A flexion stop (see Fig. 9.12 and 9.13) is used to prevent prolonged stretching to the extensors, which may cause increased weakness. A rubber band can be used to assist weak extensors (see Fig. 9.13). Patients are usually progressed by locking the wrist joint when muscles are less than fair (3) and loosening the wrist joint for periods of specific therapy. When wrist extensors are grade 3+ (fair+) or better with good endurance, static positioning is discontinued during the day allowing more advanced functional training. Positioning at night is continued until it is determined that functional hand position is maintained, and no loss of range of motion or stretching is occurring.

Elbow orthosis
Clinical application.   Elbow orthoses are frequently used immediately posttrauma or postsurgery (Fig. 9.14). Usually a three-point force system in con-

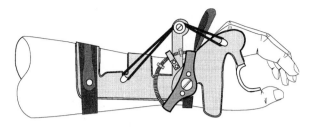

Fig. 9.13. WAWHO with wrist extension assist.

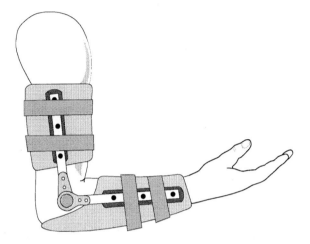

Fig. 9.14. Elbow orthosis (postsurgical application).

junction with a hydraulic lock of the semiliquid tissues surrounding the fragments is used to maintain the fracture fragments as a single unit during the healing process. In the past, this was generally done with a cast. A cast, however, does not allow normal joint motion and eventually loosens, and the bone fragments may angulate. Compared to a cast, a well-fitting custom-fabricated EO is much lighter, is more comfortable, allows self-hygiene, and provides optimum control at the fracture site. As the patient gains or loses weight, the cuffs and straps opposing the bands can be tightened to maintain control. Many mechanical elbow joints are currently available. Most permit limited and adjustable range of motion at the elbow joint, to control mobility without sacrificing vital bone fixation.

Patient population. Elbow orthoses are indicated following cast removal for stable fractures; postoperatively as an adjunct to internal fixation; for elbow dislocation management; and for strains, sprains, and muscle trauma. The design of an EO depends on the specific application. Postsurgical or posttrauma devices often are of the "off the shelf" variety because they are used for a relatively short time period. They tend to have soft cuffs with multiple straps and an adjustable mechanical elbow joint (see Fig. 9.14).

The therapeutic aim in the case of a fracture is to promote callus formation and simultaneously permit a

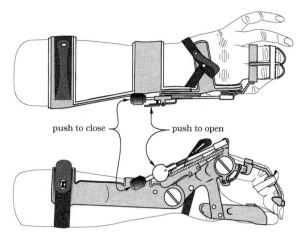

Fig. 9.15. Ratchet WHO.

safe, painless range of motion to stimulate healing and to avoid the nuisance of an iatrogenic joint contracture.

Functional
Ratchet wrist hand orthosis (ratchet WHO)
Clinical application. The ratchet WHO is a functional prehension orthosis (Fig. 9.15) that enables the patient to grasp and release objects by using external power.[1] The ratchet WHO is manually controlled and substitutes for finger flexor and extensor muscles that are less than grade 3 (fair). The wrist is stabilized for function, but the position can be changed for different activities. A thumb post is used to maintain abduction and to position the thumb in alignment with the finger pads. A finger piece assembly is provided to maintain the index and long fingers in position for pinch. A ratchet system is employed so that the hand can be closed in discrete increments. Pinch is achieved by applying force on the proximal end of the ratchet bar (black knob) or by using the patient's own chin, other arm, or any stationary object to flex the index and long fingers toward the thumb to form a three-jaw chuck. When the ratchet disk is tapped, the ratchet lock is released and spring-assisted opening of the hand occurs.

The ratchet WHO allows the individual increased independence in a variety of functional activities without needing multiple pieces of adaptive equipment (Fig. 9.16). Following a carefully organized and sequenced training program, a patient with C5 quadriplegia may attain independence in feeding, light hygiene (application of makeup, shaving, and hair grooming), desk top activities (e.g., writing and typing), and donning and doffing the orthosis. More complex desk tasks (more difficult writing, typing) are feasible using a well-organized desk arrangement. By using gross motion to close the hand, a functional three-point pinch is achievable.

There are at least two alternatives to the Rancho type of ratchet WHO that also provide dynamic prehension with a locked wrist. These are the carbon dioxide (CO_2)–powered McKibben muscle prehension WHO and the Electric-Powered Prehension Unit (EPPU) developed at The Institute for Rehabilitation and Research (TIRR) in Houston.

The McKibben device is a mechanical muscle powered by an external storage cylinder of compressed CO_2. This storage cylinder is generally attached to the back side of a wheelchair. When CO_2 is injected into the McKibben muscle, the muscle contracts and a mechanical linkage between the muscle and fingers 2 and 3 produces prehension by flexing the MCP joints of fingers onto the posted thumb. When the gas in the McKibben muscle is exhausted, the MCP joints extend with the help of a spring. The patient uses gross motion to open and close miniature pneumatic valves that allow CO_2 to enter and exit the McKibben muscle.

The EPPU is an externally powered prehension orthosis that derives energy from a rechargeable battery pack. The battery pack supplies current to a geared down DC motor that closes the hand with one polarity and opens it with the opposite polarity. Gross motion (e.g., forearm supination/pronation) operates a rocker type of electrical switch assembly that provides current from the battery pack to the motor. Typically, pronation produces prehension and supination hand opening. The EPPU and ratchet WHO have virtually replaced the McKibben muscle WHO.

Patient population. The ratchet WHO, EPPU, and McKibben WHO are appropriate for patients with paralysis or severe weakness of the hand and wrist musculature. Some functional proximal strength is required to use the ratchet WHO. For optimal use, the individual should have at least 3+ (fair+) strength in shoulder flexion, abduction, external rotation, and internal rotation. Individuals with weaker proximal muscles, however, may be able to use the ratchet WHO along with a mobile arm support (the mobile arm support [SEO] orthosis is described in a following section). Other considerations that should be evaluated are endurance, ROM limitations, spasticity, sensation, and the patient's motivation and social support. Originally, these orthoses were designed for upper limb paresis secondary to poliomyelitis. Today, these orthoses are used primarily for spinal injured patients with no hand or wrist extension strength but at least grade 2 (poor) shoulder and elbow control (e.g., patients with functional C5 quadriplegia are appropriate candidates for the ratchet WHO, EPPU, or McKibben WHO).

Wrist-driven wrist hand orthosis (WDWHO)

Clinical application. The wrist-driven WHO (WDWHO or flexor hinge WHO) is a dynamic prehension orthosis for transferring power from the wrist extensors to the fingers (Fig. 9.17). Active wrist extension provides grasp, and gravity-assisted wrist flexion enables the patient to open the hand.

The PIP and DIP joints of fingers 2 and 3 are immobilized along with the CM and MCP joints of the thumb. Active wrist extension results in the fingers approximating the posted thumb. Conversely, passive (gravity-assisted) wrist flexion causes the hand to open. An adjustable actuating lever system at the wrist joint allows the user to fine tune the wrist joint angle at which prehension occurs. This is necessary if maximum prehensile force is to be achieved. As with the ratchet WHO, the WDWHO replaces the need for multiple assistive devices.

Patient population. The WDWHO is an appropriate orthosis for the individual with paralysis or severe weakness of the hand. Wrist extensor strength must be at least grade 3+ (fair+), and proximal strength must be functional. For those individuals with wrist extensors grades of less than 3+ who are improving or are 3+ (fair+) with poor endurance, a rubber band wrist extension assist is indicated. Candidates for the wrist-driven WHO are patients with functional level of C5 with some C6 return (wrist extensors), C6, and C7 quadriplegia. By using active wrist extension, a functional three-point pinch is achieved.

If and when a patient begins to have return of function in the extrinsic muscles, the patient becomes a candidate for a wrist-driven WHO. In general, if pa-

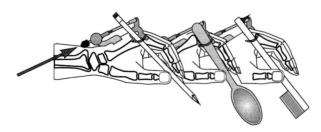

Fig. 9.16. Pen spring applications.

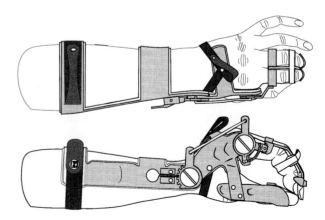

Fig. 9.17. Wrist-driven wrist-hand orthosis (WDWHO).

tients use their orthoses for function throughout the day, they gain wrist strength and consequently improved prehension.

Although rare, bilateral application of the WDWHO can be successful. Usually the patient's vocation or hobby is the determining factor. If the patient desires bilateral prehension and it cannot be achieved any other way, then bilateral application is feasible. The key is the motivation of the patient, not that of the clinician.

Mobile arm support (MAS)

Clinical application. Mobile arm support (MAS) is a shoulder-elbow orthosis (SEO) that supports the weight of the arm and provides assistance to the shoulder and elbow motions through a linkage of bearings joints (Fig. 9.18). A properly installed and adjusted MAS enables patients to perform self-care and vocational and recreational activities and can decrease the patient's dependency on family or hospital personnel.

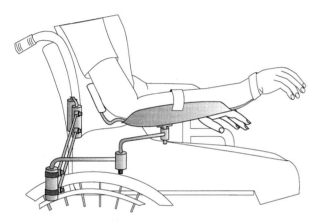

Fig. 9.18. MAS with elevating proximal arm.

An MAS is therapeutic in that it can be adjusted to complement weak muscles so they can function while being protected and strengthened. Joint range of motion can be maintained with the use of an MAS. The MAS can also provide considerable psychological value by enabling patients to do meaningful activities despite severe disability.

The MAS can provide assistance for shoulder and elbow motions by:

1. Using gravitational forces and occasionally tension from rubber bands or springs to substitute for or supplement loss of strength in shoulder and elbow musculature. For example, the inclined plane of an MAS may assist weak elbow extension, and the elastic mechanism assists shoulder elevation.

2. Supporting the weight of the arm so that weak muscles can move the arm over a useful range of motion.

The basic components of the MAS are the wheelchair mounting bracket, the proximal arm, the distal arm, and the forearm trough (Fig. 9.19). The standard proximal elevating arm is available with an optional feature to deweight the patient's arm (see Fig. 9.19). Also, the standard wheelchair mounting bracket is available with an optional pivot type of adjustment for tilting the axis of the proximal arm (see Fig. 9.19).

Patient population. The MAS can increase upper limb function for patients who have severe arm paralysis because of such disabilities as muscular dystrophy, poliomyelitis, cervical spinal cord lesion, Guillain-Barré syndrome, and amyotrophic lateral sclerosis.

Patients should have sufficient muscle weakness or endurance limitation to warrant use of the support. The

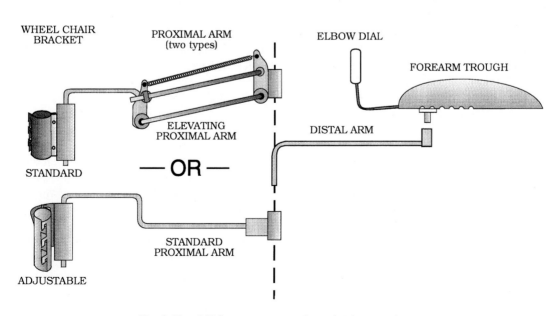

Fig. 9.19. MAS components and proximal arm options.

deltoid, elbow flexors, and external rotators are the most significant muscles to evaluate because of their importance in arm function. Criteria for MAS use are:

1. Absent or weak elbow flexion (poor to fair).
2. Absent or weak shoulder flexion and abduction (poor to fair).
3. Absent or weak external rotation (poor to fair).
4. Limited endurance for sustained upper limb activity.

The patient must have adequate muscular strength to move the MAS. Neck, trunk, shoulder girdle, shoulder, and elbow may serve alone or in combination as power sources.

An exact minimum strength requirement to power an MAS is difficult to formulate, and a clinical trial is often necessary. The patient's basic coordination may be as important as the amount of muscle strength present. To have control over the lapboard range in the planes of horizontal motion at the elbow and at the shoulder, it is essential that the patient have some controlling muscles in both elbow and shoulder to position the arm in the MAS in the horizontal plane.

The individual with at least poor muscle strength, especially in the shoulder girdle, shoulder, elbow, or trunk, can operate the MAS more effectively and do more with it, and the MAS is much easier to adjust and to stabilize for function. Some hand function widens the scope of available activities but is not always a necessity. Lack of grasp may be substituted for by the WDWHO or the ratchet WHO.

Elbow orthosis

Clinical application.   Elbow orthoses designed to assist normal motion in functional activities are definitive in nature and should be custom-designed and custom-fabricated with the highest-quality components and materials and carefully fitted to provide durable function for many years. Functional EOs usually incorporate an elastic device with a locking mechanism to assist elbow flexion with multiple angular lock points (Fig. 9.20). The user initiates elbow flexion with residual musculature or using body mechanics, and the elastic device (e.g., spiral spring) assists the flexion until one of the flexion stops is reached. A release on the stop permits the elbow either to advance to a new greater angle or to fall back into extension.

Patient population.   Individuals with selective loss of elbow flexion secondary to a brachial plexus injury or congenital deficit are appropriate candidates for the EO with elbow flexion assist. Bilateral applications may be more successful than unilateral ones. This is because the normal side becomes dominant in the unilateral case, and the additional function provided by the orthosis in the presence of a normal contralateral limb is often insufficient to offset the stigma of wearing an orthosis. In the case of bilateral involvement, however,

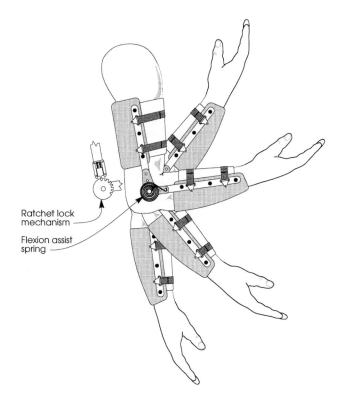

Ratchet lock mechanism ———

Flexion assist spring ———

Fig. 9.20.   Elbow orthosis.

the orthosis is more likely to be accepted because no function is available without it. Unilateral applications tend to be acceptable when the wrist and hand are functional and only the elbow needs to be stabilized to complement the other normal side. Also, if the activity desired by the individual requires use of both the normal side and the impaired side, a successful outcome is more likely.

LOW-TEMPERATURE THERMOPLASTIC ORTHOSES

Because of their ease of fabrication, this group of upper limb orthoses meet the need for quickly available devices in the clinical setting. Because of a combination of the hand-forming technique used to produce them and the poor mechanical properties of the material, however, such orthoses are not well suited for long-term use or when intimacy of fit is required for function.

Such interim upper limb orthoses are generally fabricated from low-temperature thermoplastics such as orthoplast, formsplint, or plastazote.[2,3] Orthoplast, for example, can be formed in water heated to 140°F to 170°F. Higher-temperature thermoplastics, such as nyloplex, kydex, and vinyl can be used, but a plaster mold of the patient's forearm, wrist, or hand should be made to avoid burning the patient. Also, the higher-temperature materials cannot be cut with scissors so a power must be used.

A large variety of both static and dynamic upper limb orthoses have been designed from low-temperature materials. The static orthoses may be protective, supportive, or corrective. Protective designs are intended to protect weak muscles from being stretched and therefore prevent contractures. Supportive orthoses are intended to support a joint or an arch in substitution for weak muscles. Supportive can mean *immobilize*, such as the case of a painful arthritic joint. Corrective designs may force the involved joint into a correct or near-correct alignment. The use of static orthoses must include concern for swelling and long-term immobility. Therapy should include a regimen of activities where the patient is encouraged to use his limb as often as possible.

The main advantages of the low-temperature thermoplastic orthoses are that they can be fitted early after trauma or injury and they are light in weight. For example, to prevent a deformity and position a limb in a functional position, it may be necessary to fit the patient within hours of the injury or admission. The disadvantages in using these materials is that they do not have sufficient stiffness to hold their form and prevent high-pressure spots, and hand forming results in a less precise fit.

Dynamic upper limb orthoses using low-temperature plastics must be designed to provide specific forces in the correct direction, often using outriggers that are attached to the body of the main orthosis. The use of mechanical joints in parallel with the anatomic joints can decrease joint adhesions, maintain joint function, and prevent ankylosis of the joint. A large percentage of individuals requiring low-temperature dynamic orthoses are seen in acute-care hospitals following surgery or trauma to the forearm and hand and subsequently are seen as outpatients and in rehabilitation centers.

Resting WHO

Clinical application. The resting WHO (Fig. 9.21) is designed to maintain the arches of the hand, keep the thumb abducted and flexed, and maintain the wrist in a functional position (30 degrees). This orthosis is made by placing the patient's limb on a piece of paper and drawing a pattern that encompasses the tips of the fingers, is expanded at the forearm for wraparound, and is slotted so that the thumb can be separated from the other fingers. If the affected side cannot be straightened for drawing the pattern, the unaffected side can be used and then reversed. When drawing the pattern, extra width must be allowed for padding. The pertinent joints and landmarks are noted. There are many popular patterns published that can be used as a guide in the

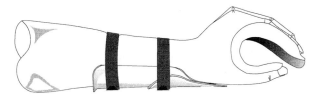

Fig. 9.21. Resting WHO.

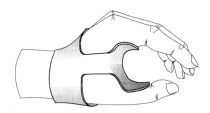

Fig. 9.22. HdO with thumb adduction stop (C-bar).

fabrication. Scissors or tin snips can be used to cut the chosen material (e.g., orthoplast). Heating the cut line with a heat gun facilitates the cutting. Orthoplast is heated until "rubbery" in a long, shallow pan of hot water, wiped dry, and then molded over the client's limb and secured with Ace wrap. After the orthosis cools, the straps can be added with rivets or contact cement or by sandwiching between pieces of orthoplast with a solvent.

Patient population. Although the resting WHO is most often used to preserve the architecture of the hand and wrist on a patient with paralyzed musculature, it can also be used to reduce hypertonicity by abducting the fingers. This modification requires angular ridges between the digits and extra straps. This resting WHO is also used to alleviate wrist or hand pain by immobilizing these tissues. Because this orthosis can be readily formed and fitted in the clinic, it is suitable for prevention of loss of motion in post–acute trauma (e.g., burns). Moreover, the large contacting area of the resting WHO can also be beneficial to the burn patient in combating scar formation. Frequent skin inspection is particularly important in these cases.

HdO with thumb adduction stop

Clinical application. This upper limb orthosis is used to position the thumb in opposition and maintain the thumb web space, leaving the hand in a functional position for use (Fig. 9.22). If the dorsal and palmar extensions are formed snugly, the orthosis may sometimes be worn without straps.

Patterns for this orthosis should be custom-designed by placing a flexible piece of paper around the appropriate portion of the patient's hand and sketching the pattern in place. The hand part is formed first before the thumb web component can be formed. The thumb web component must allow IP flexion of the thumb and flexion of the second MCP joint.

Patient population. This HdO is particularly useful for acute intervention in a painful hand or in those cases in which a thumb contracture is threatening. The burn victim with palmar hand trauma or the arthritic with tender joints may benefit from the use of this orthosis.

HdO with MCP extension stop

Clinical application. Intrinsic weakness of the hand can leave the hand in a resting posture that encourages MCP hyperextension. If the source of the weakness is expected to resolve and the potential for function is good, the HdO with an MCP extension stop is desired (Fig. 9.23). An oval-shaped piece of orthoplast is heated and wrapped around the dorsum of the patient's hand distal to the wrist and proximal to the proximal IP joints. A cutout is made in the pattern to avoid pressure on the MCP joints. A rectangular piece of orthoplast is formed into a "Tootsie Roll" shape and wrapped under the palmar aspect of the hand and secured to the ulnar and radial sides of the oval. The design requires no straps if snugly fabricated.

Patient population. This orthosis is used when a condition results in an intrinsic minus hand that, if left untreated, would flatten and the MCP joints would hyperextend. This orthosis is also used when a median and radial nerve injury causes weakening of the transverse arch. If curvature is formed into the palmar roll, the normal palmar arch is preserved.

Dynamic dorsal WHO

Clinical application. This orthosis provides a quick clinical means for positioning the hand and assisting wrist and MCP extension. This orthosis consists of three main components that accomplish these objectives (Fig. 9.24): the dorsal forearm piece, the palmar piece, and the MCP extension assist. The forearm and palmar pieces are connected with a rubber band, which assists wrist extension. For this feature to be effective, a large forearm strap is required to prevent distal migration of the forearm piece. The dorsum of the forearm piece provides a base of support for the wire outrigger to which the rubber band for MCP extension is attached. One rubber band attached to the ends of the

palmar phalangeal bar is usually sufficient to extend the MCP joint of the index through little fingers. The wire outrigger can be shaped to fine tune the extension torque.

The patterns should be custom-designed, heated to the appropriate temperature, and formed directly on the client. The small pads holding the hooks for the rubber bands are secured with a solvent (Carbona) or contact cement.

Patient population. Patients with a radial nerve injury resulting in weakness of wrist and MCP extension are typical candidates for this orthosis. For patients showing signs of muscle function return, rubber bands are used to assist clinically targeted motions. The rubber bands can be fine tuned commensurate with the therapeutic changes.

General considerations

The edges of the upper limb orthoses made from low-temperature thermoplastic, such as orthoplast, can be folded over to create a rounded, smooth finish. Reinforcing strips can be made the same way and attached to certain weak areas (such as the wrist area) of the orthosis with solvent or contact cement. Instead of rolls of plastic, it may be desirable to create small corrugations by forming a small rectangular piece of plastic around a cylindrical object and then attaching to the main body of the orthosis where reinforcement is desired.

There are hundreds of designs of low-temperature plastic upper limb orthoses. Only a few have been presented here to give the reader a general idea of their potential. The designer is limited by his imagination and to a certain degree by the poor mechanical properties and bulk of the low-temperature thermoplastic materials.

TEAM APPROACH TO ORTHOTIC MANAGEMENT

Patient acceptance of an orthosis can be high with a well-organized team approach to orthotic management.[1] Both the Certified Orthotist and the occupa-

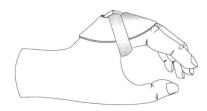

Fig. 9.23. HdO with MCP extension stop (lumbrical bar).

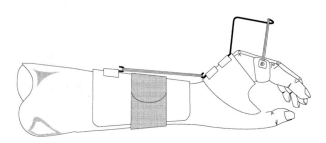

Fig. 9.24. Dorsal WHO with wrist extension assist and MCP extension assist.

tional therapist have a vital role in ensuring a successful outcome. The occupational therapist evaluates the need for orthoses, recommends them, and trains the client in their use. In some cases, the occupational therapist fabricates the less complex, low-temperature orthoses that can be readily applied during a short clinical encounter. The orthotist's role is usually to design, fabricate, and fit the more complex and definitive upper limb orthoses.

To meet best the patient's orthotic needs, a team clinic is suggested. During this clinic, the orthotists, occupational therapists, and physicians meet with the patient. The goals of the team clinic are to:

1. Ensure proper fitting and re-evaluate fit over time as the patient's hand contours and functional needs may change.
2. Facilitate the patient's compliance by incorporating their feedback to the team discussion and by teaching patients the fit and function of the orthosis.
3. Provide on-going "hands-on" training for both orthotic and occupational therapy students and staff.
4. Provide a setting for ongoing dialogue between the orthotist, the therapist, and the patient.
5. Facilitate brainstorming solutions to specific problems and consensus outcomes.

The benefits of such a clinic can best be illustrated by an example. A patient was presented after a month of using his WDWHO. The patient was able to use the WDWHO for hygiene and grooming and for tabletop activities. A problem occurred when the client was ready to begin self-catheterization. He was unable to hold the plastic tube tightly enough to insert it into the urethra. The problem was presented in the team clinic by the nurse, and after discussion the team decided to compromise finger opening for a tighter pinch by having the orthotist shorten the tenodesis bar and providing additional training by the therapist.

TRAINING

To gain maximum use of the orthosis, the patient must be thoroughly trained. The occupational therapy training process involves the following steps.[1]

Education

The patient is instructed in the purpose and function of the orthosis. This learning may be facilitated by a peer who is successfully using the same orthosis.

Exploration and experimentation

Before starting with functional tasks, the therapist puts the orthosis on the patient, and the patient gets to "feel it out," open it, move it, and examine it. Step-by-step instructions are given. At this time, the patient observes but is not expected to attempt donning the orthosis. The patient is encouraged to experiment with the orthosis and become familiar with the mechanical principles before introducing objects or activities.

Prefunctional training

This step involves practicing grasp, hold, placement, and release of objects of various sizes, shapes, textures, and weights.

Functional activities

The sequence usually begins with passive maintenance of pinch while the patient performs some activity. Typing, prewriting, and finger-food feeding (e.g., carrot sticks) are often used as initial activities. Feeding training is graded initially by providing setup for cutting meat, opening containers, and placement of utensils.

Applying and removing

One school of thought is that this task should be taught only after the patient achieves some proficiency using the orthosis because it is a more advanced skill and may be initially frustrating to the client. Training in removing the orthosis is done first because it is easier than donning the orthosis. The other school of thought, however, is that the sooner the patient can don and doff the orthosis, the sooner he or she becomes less dependent on someone else's assistance. Which philosophy to follow depends on the amount of therapy time available and the wishes of the patient.

Advanced functional training

This area includes fine motor skills such as activities using bilateral wrist-driven WHOs or ratchet WHOs. This training is done selectively only with those patients who are skilled in using one orthosis and who have a specific functional need.

Follow-up

After leaving the rehabilitation facility, the patient's orthotic needs must be reevaluated periodically for maintenance of proper fit and optimal function.

SUMMARY

The complexity of the human hand requires that orthotic design give equal emphasis to mechanical efficiency and accuracy of fit because comfort is critical for acceptance. Specific training and skill are required to meet the high design and fabrication demands that result from small segments (levers), limited soft tissue padding, and multiplicity of joints.

Upper limb orthoses are more often accepted by the patient when there is a well-defined therapeutic program, and the orthoses provide a desired function that cannot be accomplished in any other fashion.[4] Perhaps the most important factor in patient acceptance is the open recognition by the orthotic team that some level of compromise is necessary. Patients are quick to see through biased clouds of unrealistic enthusiasm.[4]

Specific orthoses are selected according to the patient's physical need. It is helpful to organize upper limb orthoses into groups that reflect need. Therefore, the orthoses reviewed for orthotic management of the patient with upper limb paresis or trauma were grouped primarily into *therapeutic* and *functional* categories. Each of these groups were further divided into *static* and *dynamic* subgroups. Examples of *static therapeutic* orthoses include the static WHO, which positions the wrist and hand for patients with absent or weak wrist and hand musculature, the static HdO, the wrist action WHO, the elbow orthosis, the shoulder-elbow orthosis, and the shoulder-elbow-wrist orthosis. The *functional static* orthoses reviewed include the HdOs and WHOs with a variety of attachments. *Therapeutic dynamic* orthoses include the wrist action wrist-hand orthosis (WAWHO) and the EO with adjustable joint range of motion for postsurgery or posttrauma. The *functional dynamic* orthoses described are the ratchet WHO, wrist-driven WHO, the mobile arm support (MAS), and elbow orthosis with flexion assist and multiple joint angle stops.

The ratchet WHO is a manually manipulated prehension orthosis for patients with C4 quadriplegia with some C5 return or C5 quadriplegia or similar loss of function and can be used in conjunction with an MAS. The wrist-driven WHO is a prehension orthosis powered by the wrist extensors and is usually prescribed for quadriplegics with 3+ (fair+) or greater wrist extensor strength and absent hand function.

The programs discussed include patient instruction in the orthotic purpose and mechanical principles, patient experimentation with the orthosis, and graded therapeutic and functional activity. With a carefully planned and implemented interdisciplinary training program, patient acceptance of an upper limb orthosis can be high. Upper limb orthoses can make major contributions to the management of dysfunction when properly selected, designed, fabricated, and fitted.

REFERENCES

1. Baumgarten JM: Upper extremity adaptations for the person with quadriplegia. In Spinal cord injury, New York, 1985, Churchill Livingstone.
2. Malick MH: Manual on dynamic hand splinting with thermoplastic materials, Pittsburgh, 1974, Harmarville Rehabilitation Center.
3. Malick MH: Manual on static hand splinting, ed 5, Pittsburgh, 1976, Harmarville Rehabilitation Center, Inc.
4. Perry J: Prescription principles. In AAOS: Atlas of orthotics, St. Louis, 1975, CV Mosby.
5. Wilson DJ, et al: Spinal cord injury: A treatment guide for occupational therapists, revised ed, Thorofare, NJ, 1984, Slack Inc.

Lower Limb Orthoses

John W. Michael

Lower limb orthoses, with their many variations, are the most commonly prescribed devices to assist individuals with neuromuscular deficits.[10] For most orthotists and most physicians, lower limb applications are therefore the most commonly encountered clinical entities.

The preponderance of lower limb orthoses reflects both the strong desire by most individuals with a disability to walk or at least stand and the fact that present orthotic technology can do a reasonably effective job of restoring gross physical functions such as walking and standing. In addition, for the extremely active competitive athlete, rather subtle interventions with foot orthoses can sometimes overcome small physiologic deficits that would otherwise limit performance. Lower limb orthoses are therefore applicable to enhance function for many deficits, large and small.

Custom footwear and modifications to commercial footwear are extremely important aspects of orthotic and pedorthic practice as well. Not only can shoe adaptations successfully treat many simpler problems, but also they can significantly enhance the effectiveness of orthotic management when more proximal devices are required.[8] Chapter 11 discusses the shoe and its functions in more detail.

FOOT ORTHOSES

Foot orthoses (FOs) are the foundation for lower limb management. Not only are they suitable for managing many of the basic problems encountered in daily practice, but also it should be noted that each and every more proximal orthosis (e.g., ankle-foot orthosis [AFO], knee-ankle-foot orthosis [KAFO], and hip-knee-ankle-foot orthosis [HKAFO]) is first and foremost an FO. In general, the FO portion should be used to manage as many deficits as possible, relying on more proximal

designs *only* when an FO alone is insufficient. This approach is the most cost-effective and enhances patient acceptance because most FOs are "invisibly" contained within the footwear.

Conceptually FOs are usually divided into three broad categories:[29]
1. Accommodative or soft devices.
2. Intermediate or semirigid devices.
3. Corrective or rigid devices.

Accommodative FOs are typically used to "cradle" and protect rigidly deformed or dysvascular feet and may be made from a variety of soft or flexible materials. Minor problems such as mild metatarsal pain may respond to over-the-counter (OTC) or prefabricated inserts of resilient materials, but most often a custom-molded FO is required.

Corrective FOs made of rigid materials can be extremely difficult to fit successfully and require meticulous attention to detail.[1] Usually a weaning period of several weeks is required for client acceptance. Most practitioners reserve the rigid materials for easily correctable, flexible deformities such as mild ankle valgus and for subtle control of a nearly normal foot with slight biomechanical deficits, such as the Olympic level sprinter with a few degrees of excess pronation.

Intermediate FOs made of semirigid materials are popular clinically because they can be fabricated from multiple layers of slightly different densities to provide graduated degrees of control, thereby enhancing client acceptance. Again, for mild problems such as metatarsalgia without ulceration, OTC, prefabricated, or modular intermediate FOs may suffice, and these may also be suitable for a clinical trial to verify the effectiveness of orthotic management in a given case. Chronic conditions as well as moderate and severe problems—including all feet with a history of ulceration or sensory limitation—typically require custom-molded devices to insure the most meticulous fit.

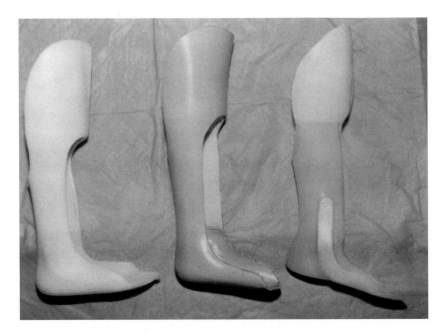

Fig. 10.1. Plastic AFO, with a rigid ankle set to accommodate various heel heights, uses floor reaction forces to reduce knee flexion indirectly.

It must always be remembered that the foot is a dynamically changing organ during the gait cycle, whereas the FO is a static device. A thorough understanding of the foot and ankle biomechanics (see Chapter 7), in addition to careful follow-up and adjustments, is essential for long-term success with this modality. Additional information on FOs may be found in Chapter 31.

ANKLE-FOOT ORTHOSES

AFOs can be designed with sufficient lever arms to fully control the ankle complex and to influence the knee joint indirectly, making them applicable for more extensive disabilities than FOs. At present, electronic AFOs based upon electrical stimulation of paraplegic muscles are research modalities in North America.[9] If they prove economical and reliable, they may become clinically available devices in the future.

For now, the clinician must choose between metal alloy–based devices, plastic-based devices, and a hybrid assembly incorporating both materials. In most cases, this choice is best left to the orthotist and patient, who can take the time to discuss the various advantages and disadvantages of each approach. In general, plastic or hybrid plastic/metal systems predominate in North America because of the greater degree of client acceptance and circumferential control they offer.[13]

The older-style metal and leather orthoses are usually reserved for selected applications, such as satisfied previous wearers; unusually large or heavy individuals;

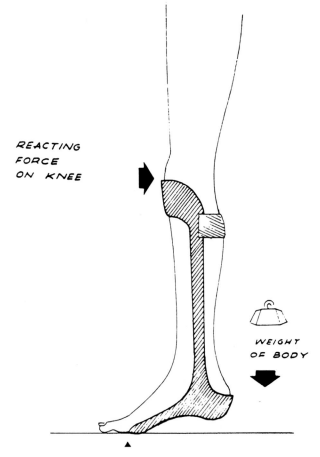

Fig. 10.2. Biomechanics of the floor reaction type of AFO. In late stance, the extended forefoot plate contacts the floor and creates a knee extension moment via the well-padded anterior contours.

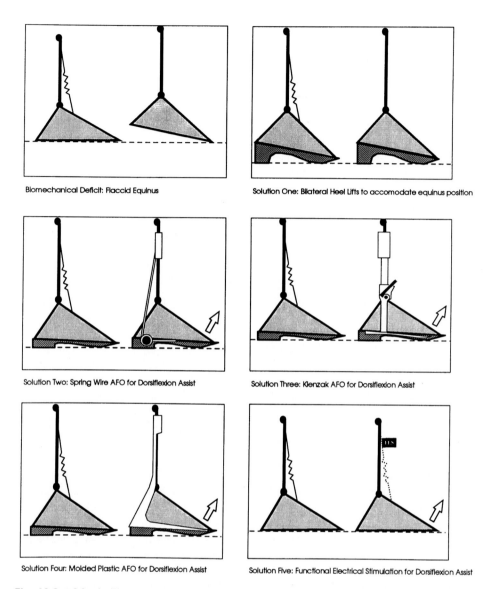

Biomechanical Deficit: Flaccid Equinus

Solution One: Bilateral Heel Lifts to accomodate equinus position

Solution Two: Spring Wire AFO for Dorsiflexion Assist

Solution Three: Klenzak AFO for Dorsiflexion Assist

Solution Four: Molded Plastic AFO for Dorsiflexion Assist

Solution Five: Functional Electrical Stimulation for Dorsiflexion Assist

Fig. 10.3. Matrix illustrates five distinct orthotic solutions for the problem of bilateral flaccid equinus.

and conditions where minimal contact with the leg is desirable, such as persons with fluctuating edema and heat-sensitive individuals who cannot tolerate the more intimately fitting plastic contours.[17] Some clinicians prefer metal systems for growing children because of their adjustability for growth, but many others believe that plastic or hybrid devices are just as versatile in this regard.[18] One of the most significant factors is client (or parent) preference, which largely determines acceptance and should predominate over all moot points in the final decision.

As has been noted in the Introduction to this Section, all orthotic devices including AFOs must fulfill one of the following fundamental goals:[3] (1) control of motion, (2) correction of deformity, and (3) compensation for weakness. Figure 10.1 illustrates one common application of *control of motion:* a rigid, plastic AFO with the

ankle locked in slight dorsiflexion and a well-padded anterior proximal segment to stabilize the tibia. This design, first reported in 1969 by an Israeli orthotist, Saltiel, is often colloquially termed a floor reaction AFO[25] because the extended, rigid forefoot section accentuates the knee *extension* moment at midstance and thereby prevents tibial collapse owing to weak or absent gastrocnemius-soleus musculature. This illustrates one of the critical treatment principles of orthotic management: The orthosis may indirectly affect remote body segments, and this characteristic can be used therapeutically. The sagittal plane biomechanics of this AFO at midstance are shown in Fig. 10.2.

As noted in Chapter 1, orthoses are rationally prescribed based on the biomechanical function desired.[14] The plastic floor reaction AFO with ankle locked in slight dorsiflexion is usually applicable when the patient has a paralyzed ankle-foot complex but good or better quadriceps and balance. Examples of pathologies that could give rise to this clinical picture include myelodysplasia, spinal cord injury, peripheral nerve injury, poliomyelitis, and gastrocnemius-soleus trauma.

One of the most common lower limb deficits is a flaccid equinus, which may result from many causes, including Charcot-Marie-Tooth disease, mild cerebrovascular accidents, muscular dystrophy, and peroneal palsies of various types. The orthotic options to *compensate for* pretibial compartment *weakness* or paralysis definitively, shown in Fig. 10.3, include:

1. Bilateral 2-inch heel lifts.
2. Piano wire AFO.
3. Klenzak style AFO.
4. Flexible plastic AFO.
5. Peroneal FES.

A functionally based prescription, as advocated in Chapter 1, such as "orthosis to compensate for weakened pretibial musculature" insures that the Certified Orthotist considers all available alternatives before selecting the optimum solution for a particular patient.[17] A more specific prescription, such as "prefabricated plastic AFO to provide dorsiflexion assist" is appropriate only if that is indeed the sole desirable solution—and all others are to be automatically ruled out.

The first alternative, which may be supplied by the 2-inch heels typical of cowboy footwear, prevents the plantar flexed forefoot from dragging in swing phase because the boot stabilizes the flaccid foot, and the heel height lengthens both legs sufficiently for clearance of a plantar flexed extremity. This is obviously the least expensive option and may be acceptable in some geographic locations.

The next two choices are essentially spring-loaded metal systems attached to the client's shoes. Use of a caliper box and removable stirrups with the Klenzak AFO allows shoe interchange (as does the spring wire AFO), but the cost and inconvenience of modifying all shoes should not be underestimated. The chief advantage of the metal systems are the limited contact with the leg, which must be balanced against the bulk, weight, and maintenance required for such mechanical solutions.

The fourth option (flexible plastic AFO) may be either prefabricated or custom-molded. In general, prefabricated solutions are applicable for short-term use with sensate extremities (such as a mild iatrogenic palsy from cast application) so long as the limb contours are within normal limits. Deformed limbs, insensate limbs, and definitive applications generally require custom-made devices to insure long-term comfort and success.

As noted previously, the fifth option (FES) is presently considered experimental. Various elastic slings available for temporary management of flaccid equinus have been omitted from the discussion because such OTC items are intended as "therapy gym equipment" to facilitate gait retraining and are usually inappropriate for long-term, outpatient use. The discussion has also excluded the compensatory steppage gait characterized by excess hip flexion, which is a common *adaptation* to untreated flaccid equinus.

The reader should note that all the devices discussed in this section offer similar function: compensation for weakness. The particular orthosis selected for an individual patient must take into consideration a variety of additional criteria, including ease of donning, weight, cost, and durability.

Correction of flexible deformities is so common in lower limb orthotic management that it has become a sine qua non for modern treatment: Reduce all flexible deformities to a neutral or balanced position.[2] Such careful alignment markedly reduces the floor reaction moments trying to collapse the limb segment further, lowers the magnitude of stabilizing force necessary, and results in a more comfortable orthosis thus enhancing long-term acceptance.[4]

Correction of more rigid deformities is feasible only in selected cases in which the cause is short-term and primarily soft tissue related. Figure 10.4 illustrates bilateral hybrid AFOs designed to allow ambulation as well as to help reduce the plantar flexion contractures caused by a hypertonic gastrocnemius following a closed head injury. Many other pathologies that result in spastic contractures can present a similar biomechanical challenge.

Initially the ankle joints were set to accommodate the full contracture, and the plastic foot and tibial shells held the limb securely, eliminating clonus. External wedges of a lightweight material were added to the plantar surface of the orthosis so the tibia-to-floor angle simulated slight dorsiflexion, which allowed ambulation without the painful hyperextension moment at the knee that occurred during barefoot walking.

Over time, neurological recovery and physical therapy mobilization decreased the spasticity, making the deformity more flexible. By incrementally readjusting the ankle joints, the orthosis was then used to maintain the limb in a less deformed attitude, 24 hours per day, to consolidate the gains made during daily treatments.

Slices of the wedge material were removed over time to restore the proper tibia-to-floor attitude as the ankle attitude approached neutral. Ultimately the patient was discharged as a community ambulator with her ankles

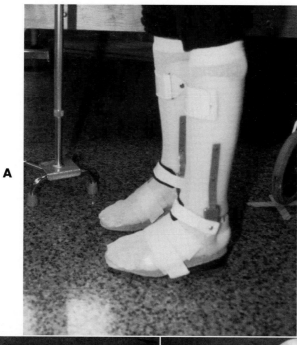

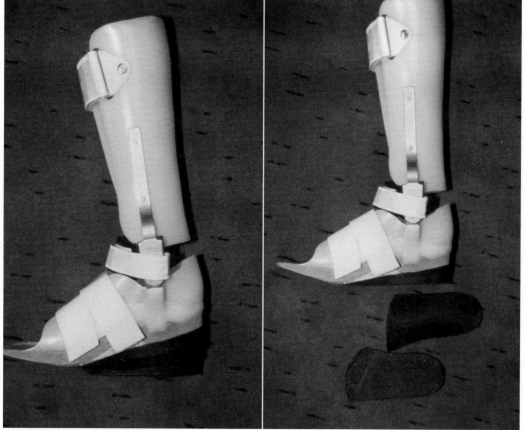

Fig. 10.4.   **A,** Bilateral hybrid AFOs combine the intimate, secure fit of molded plastic shells with the ease of adjustment of metal double action ankle joints. **B** and **C,** As the patient improves over time, the ankle joint is adjusted to maintain the improved posture, and the compensating wedge attached to the sole of the shoe can be reduced.

Orthotic Ankle Control Options

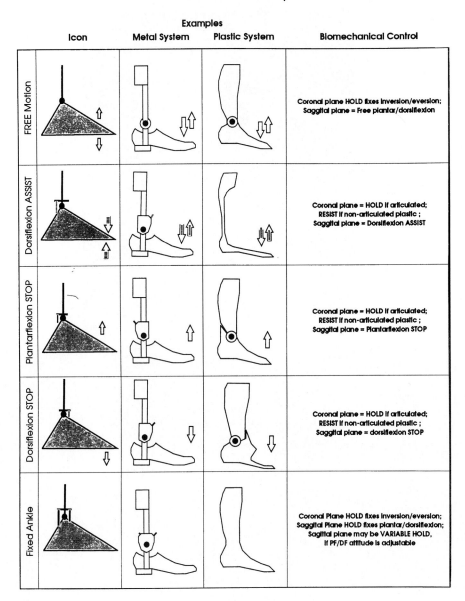

Fig. 10.5. Ankle joint componentry and plastic orthosis designs allow various modes of biomechanical control.

held in slight dorsiflexion by the orthoses, which now fit comfortably inside conventional athletic footwear.

This case example illustrates two important additional treatment principles: (1) Application of low-level, tolerable forces over an extended period may result in significant changes. (2) The tibia-to-floor angle may be varied independently of the ankle-foot attitude to facilitate gait.

The matrix in Fig. 10.5 summarizes the motion control options available at the ankle and provides

examples of both metal and plastic AFOs that offer such function. This graphic summary should help the novice visualize the available options better. Much like the ingredients in a recipe, these simple options, when properly and creatively combined, create a result that is more effective than just the sum of the individual parts. This is the clinical art of orthotic practice.

On rare occasions, orthoses may be prescribed to offer an additional function: partial axial unweighting of more distal limb segments.[24] Figure 10.6

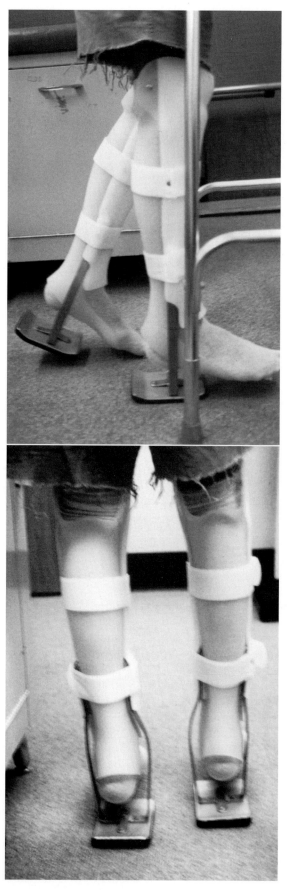

Fig. 10.6. Custom-designed AFOs were successfully used to protect calcaneal fractures until healing was complete.

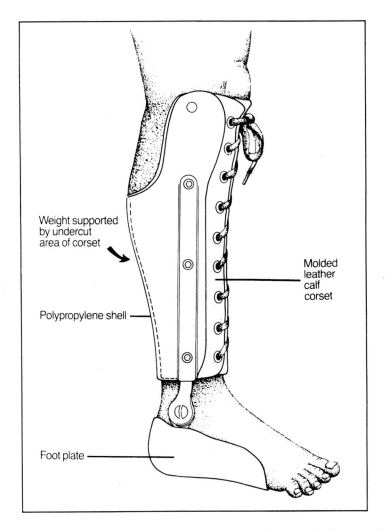

Weight supported
by undercut
area of corset

Molded
leather
calf
corset

Polypropylene shell

Foot plate

Fig. 10.7.   One type of AFO designed to unload partially the ankle/foot complex.

depicts an AFO to fully unload the calcaneus, bilaterally. Such devices may be used to protect hindfoot fractures, recalcitrant heel ulcerations, and similar pathologies. Figure 10.7 shows a hybrid system with metal uprights and ankle joints sometimes used to unload the ankle-foot complex partially during the consolidation phase of neuropathic (Charcot) arthropathy.[19] Chapter 29 discusses the insensate foot in more detail and presents additional orthoses for consideration.

KNEE-ANKLE-FOOT ORTHOSES

As noted in the Introduction to this Section, simpler orthoses enjoy a much higher long-term acceptance rate than more complex devices. Therefore, a KAFO should not be prescribed unless there is a compelling reason to

do so. The most common justification for a KAFO is the need for direct control of the knee complex, which cannot be accomplished in another fashion, *in addition to a need for ankle or foot control or suspension.*[16] Obviously, if knee control alone is the objective, the simple KO (to be discussed next) suffices.

Figure 10.8 depicts the range of controls possible at the knee joint and examples of typical applications. When combined with the plethora of ankle controls available, literally scores of orthoses can be constructed. Prescribing orthotic management on a functional basis allows the physician to direct the team's efforts, while allowing the knowledgeable Certified Orthotist to consider all available permutations before selecting the preferred approach.

Figure 10.9 presents a metal KAFO designed for a polio survivor with a flail leg from the hip distally. The offset knee joints are held in extension during stance by

Orthotic Knee Joint Options

	Examples	Biomechanical Control	Typical Application
Single Axis	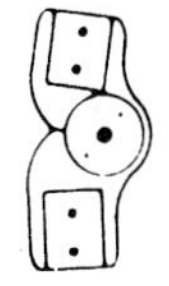	Coronal plane HOLD fixes genu varum-valgum; Saggital plane = Free flexion-extension; integral hyperextension stop	Mild to moderate genu varum or valgum
Offset	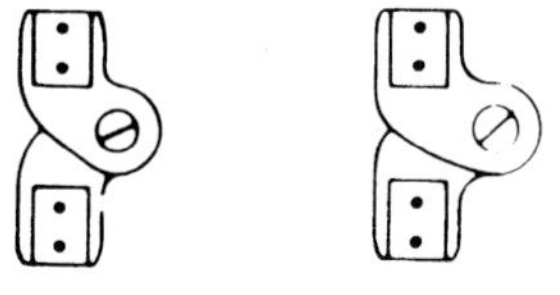	Coronal plane HOLD fixes genu varum-valgum; Saggital plane = Free flexion-extension; integral hyperextension stop	Moderate genu recurvatum
Polycentric	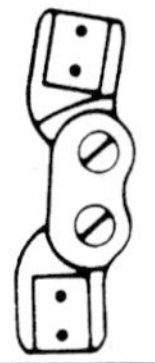	Coronal plane HOLD fixes genu varum-valgum; Saggital plane = Free flexion-extension; integral hyperextension stop	Usually, self-suspending orthoses - to track the knee axis more closely
Lock	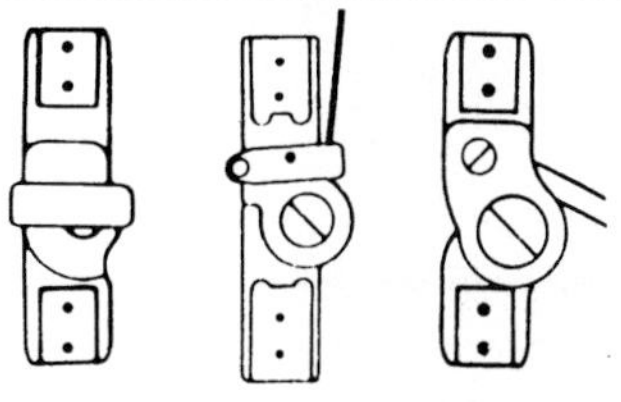 Droplock Wedge Lock Ball Lock	Coronal Plane HOLD fixes genu varum-valgum; Saggital Plane = removable LOCK in full extension	Paralysis, severe paresis, severe genu varum/valgum or recurvatum
Lock + Variable Flexion	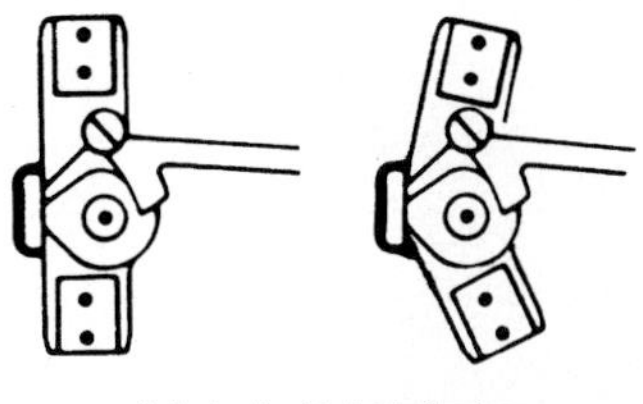 Swiss Lock + Variable Flexion	Coronal Plane HOLD fixes genu varum-valgum; Saggital Plane = removable LOCK, in variable degrees of flexion	Usually, spastic paralysis with reducible knee flexion contractures

Fig. 10.8.   Knee joint componentry allows various modes of control.

loading on the anterior proximal thigh band. The individual's knee is allowed to go into slight recurvatum, sufficient to stabilize it via floor reaction forces that occur when the dorsiflexion stop inside the orthotic ankle joint applies force to the extended steel shank placed inside the sole of the shoe. This biomechanical result is depicted in Fig. 10.10.

The biomechanics at heel strike are also crucial and are presented in Fig. 10.11. The resistance from a mild plantar flexion resist spring allows the foot to descend to the floor in a controlled manner, replacing the function of the pretibial muscles. If a rigid plantar flexion stop had been provided instead, as shown in Fig. 10.12, the resultant knee flexion moment would cause the orthotic knee joint to flex, and the individual might fall.

The Certified Orthotist must carefully analyze the resultant forces throughout the device to anticipate and deal with their effect.[28] If a rigid ankle device were prescribed in this situation, then a locked knee mechanism would also be required, for the same biomechanical reason. Particularly for individuals with good proprioception as in this case, locking the knee joint is undesirable because it disrupts the gait mechanics and may increase the effort required to ambulate.

The variety of knee lock mechanisms available suggests how often pathologic conditions require this level of security, despite the obvious gait deviation that results. Perhaps the most common application is for paraplegia, which may result from a variety of neuromuscular diseases as well as many traumatic causes, including spinal cord injury.

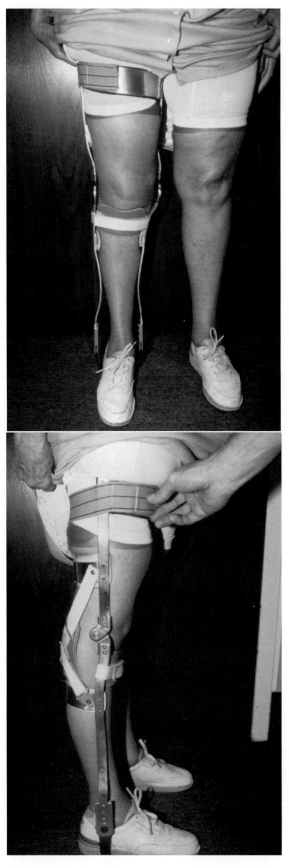

Fig. 10.9.   Metal KAFO to control genu recurvatum and toe clearance in a flail leg.

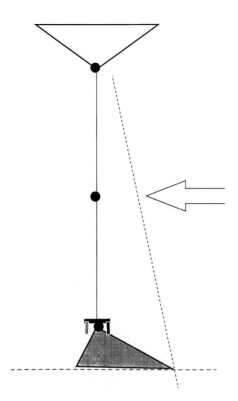

Fig. 10.10. KAFO biomechanics. In late stance, an extended steel shank inside the sole of the shoe applies an extension moment at the knee.

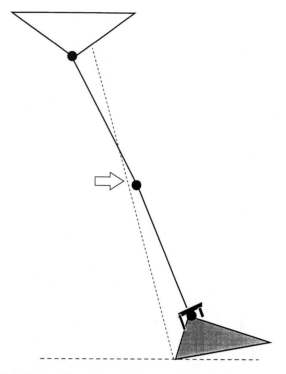

Fig. 10.12. If a rigid ankle is provided, a significant knee flexion moment is generated at heel strike. If the limb is flail, then a locked knee mechanism is required.

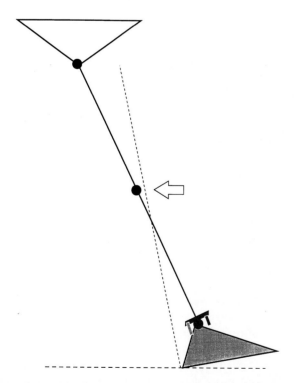

Fig. 10.11. Biomechanics at heel strike with an articulated ankle joint that resists plantar flexion and limits dorsiflexion. This results in a slight knee extension moment that helps stabilize the limb.

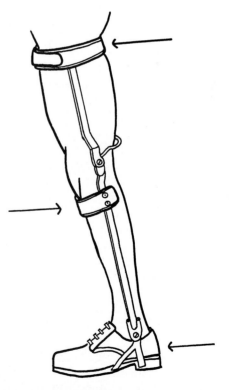

Fig. 10.13. Bilateral KAFOs with locked knees and adjustable solid ankles is one approach to paraplegic standing and walking. This design was popularized by Craig Rehabilitation Hospital in Colorado.

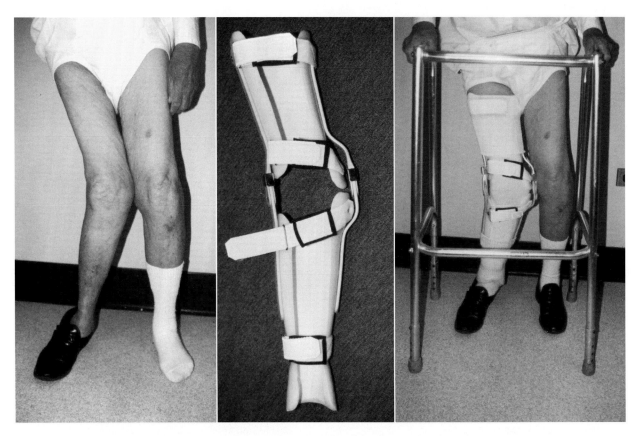

Fig. 10.14. Custom-designed KO designed to unload the lateral compartment to relieve pain and prevent further progression of osteoarthritic deformity. Note the extended lever arms on the thigh and shin, which significantly lowers the pressure per unit area, enhancing comfort despite the strong corrective forces required.

Figure 10.13 illustrates one of the simplest approaches permitting limited ambulation, using forearm crutches, despite full paralysis of the lower limbs. The fixed ankle with adjustable joints, combined with specially reinforced shoes, provides a solid base of support. Careful adjustment into a slightly dorsiflexed attitude, combined with the locked knee mechanisms and therapy training to teach the patient to extend the hips and hang on the hip ligaments, results in hands-free balance. Ambulation for limited distances is possible using crutches, at least for the young or vigorous individual. This type of KAFO bears the eponym Scott Craig after the Colorado rehabilitation hospital that popularized its application.[26]

KNEE ORTHOSES

Knee orthoses (KOs) were originally rarely prescribed, with their application limited to isolated knee pathologies—typically varus or valgus angulation secondary to advanced arthritic destruction on the condylar area (Fig. 10.14). To unload the painful condyle as well as to prevent further progression, extensive bracing with long moment arms was required. The need for

self-suspension was met by careful contouring to the deformed limb, supplemented with a supracondylar indention similar to the prosthetic suspension technique.

About two decades ago, the Lenox Hill brace was first developed, gradually becoming the first widely accepted KO for sports applications.[21] Over the ensuing years, literally hundreds of imitators have developed slight variations of a self-suspending KO with dual freely moving knee hinges. The original custom-molded designs have gradually been supplanted in many cases with prefabricated and even OTC variants. Many have only superficial differences; others are made of poor-quality materials; none has been convincingly demonstrated to be uniformly "superior" to any other variant.

Indications for sports KOs remain equivocal, other than for nonoperative applications in which surgery has been refused or is not feasible.[20] Prophylactic application to prevent injuries has never been shown definitively to be effective, and some fear transfer injuries to adjacent joints.[23] Jaded observers might comment that the advent of KOs as chic sports accessories, each with its own flamboyant sports bag, represents the nadir of rational orthotic management.

Chapter 28 reviews the literature and presents more

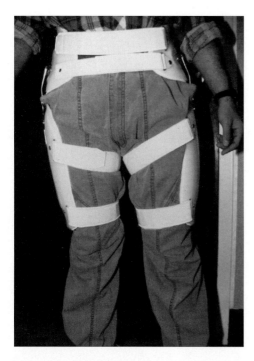

Fig. 10.15. Bilateral hinges connect the lateral thigh panels to the pelvic section on this hip orthosis [HpO], controlling the amount of abduction while permitting free motion in the sagittal plane.

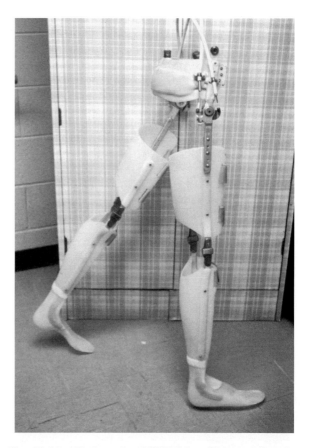

Fig. 10.16. Early style of HKAFO, which uses Bowden cables to link hip extension on one side with hip flexion on the contralateral side. This allows a reciprocating foot-over-foot gait as well as the option to swing to or swing through.

detailed commentary on the use of KOs. It is interesting to note that the majority of commercial KOs are not provided by Certified Orthotists but rather by therapists, athletic trainers, cast room technicians, and other ancillary personnel.

HIP ORTHOSES

Hip orthoses (HpOs) are indicated for isolated problems in the acetabular region, which may be the result of (1) dysplastic disorders, (2) traumatic injury, or (3) surgical procedures (total hip replacement). A variety of devices are available to treat infantile developmentally dysplastic hips, with generally good results. The prefabricated Pavlik harness is one of the most common HpOs.[22] A variety of custom-made HpOs have been used to treat Legg-Calvé-Perthes disease in adolescence, based on the containment theory, which states that if the femoral head is maintained in the acetabulum during the active phase of the disorder, a more congruent head results. The scientific evidence to support the containment theory is equivocal, and it is now being challenged in many quarters.[15]

The most common application for the HpO in adults is for postoperative protection of total hip replacement, particularly after revisions that are unstable. In general, those devices that incorporate an extensive hemishell

at the hip (and are therefore technically called lumbosacral HpOs) provide the most effective biomechanical control.[11] It should be noted that no orthosis has yet been developed that can fully protect the at-risk hip, particularly with an uncooperative or incoherent client. At best, under such circumstances, the HpO decreases the risk of dislocation.

Definitive HpO applications are rare. Figure 10.15 shows a young man with total loss of adductor power secondary to one of the muscular dystrophies. This custom-made HpO prevented the progressive abduction that would otherwise immobilize him, with his legs abducted maximally, after just a few steps—while allowing free sagittal plane motion.

HIP-KNEE-ANKLE-FOOT ORTHOSES

HKAFOs are most commonly prescribed for pediatric patients, who do remarkably well even with complex devices.[18] They are selectively recommended for adults, who tend to abandon more involved orthoses after the first year or so because of the tremendous

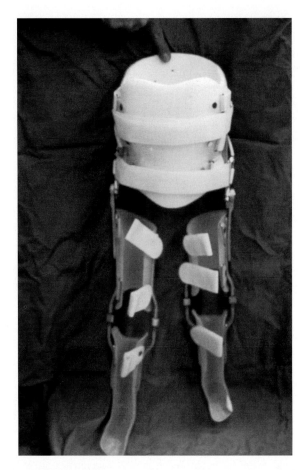

Fig. 10.17. Compound orthosis consisting of a plastic TLSO for control of paralytic scoliosis plus bilateral HKAFOs to allow paraplegic gait. Children often tolerate even such involved bracing and are usually able to ambulate reasonably well for short distances.

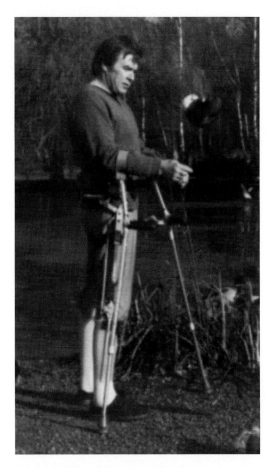

Fig. 10.18. This compound orthosis allows a reciprocal gait. The hip and knee joints are mechanically linked for coordinated locking/unlocking. Strong extension assist mechanisms at each knee help the paraplegic arise from a chair more easily.

energy required to use bilateral devices that cross the knee.[5] Unilateral applications are rare.

One of the most common HKAFOs uses a mechanical linkage to couple flexion of one hip with extension of the other. Such mechanisms allow the option of a reciprocal step-over-step gait, which has been shown to be more energy efficient albeit slower than the traditional swing-through gait. One example of such an HKAFO is illustrated in Fig. 10.16. Colloquially referred to as reciprocating gait orthoses, these HKAFOs are used for a variety of pathologies that result in paraplegia, including spinal cord injury and myelodysplasia.[7] Chapters 24 and 25 discuss paraplegic gait orthoses in more depth.

COMPOUND ORTHOSES

Devices that cross more than five body segments may be considered *compound* orthoses, composed of two or more less complex devices. The terminology reflects

this perspective as two or more individual orthoses, with the device pictured in Fig. 10.17 described as a TLSO plus HKAFO. Such extensive bracing is occasionally successful with young adults who are extremely motivated, as illustrated by the Advanced Reciprocal Gait Orthosis (ARGO) in Fig. 10.18, designed to assist the adult paraplegic in both ambulating and arising from/sitting down in a chair.[12]

Children typically do well with such complexity. Even if a TLSO is required full-time for scoliosis management and superincumbent HKAFOs are used daily for ambulation, youngsters often wear such compound orthoses without complaint and ambulate reasonably well with a reversed walker.

The TLSO + HKAFO shown in Fig. 10.19 is sometimes called a *Ferrari orthosis* after the Italian physician who advocated its use for selected children with spina bifida who have weak hip musculature and paralyzed legs.[6] The articulated plastic AFO segments allow a small degree of ankle motion, whereas the knee locks stabilize the legs bilaterally. The hip mechanisms allow

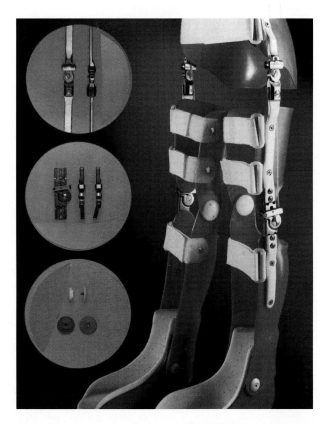

Fig. 10.19. This compound orthosis includes a simple TLSO to stabilize the paralyzed trunk linked to bilateral KAFOs with special hip joints that allow about 10 degrees of motion in any direction. The child must use available hip musculature for balance while the joint stops prevent the torso from jackknifing.

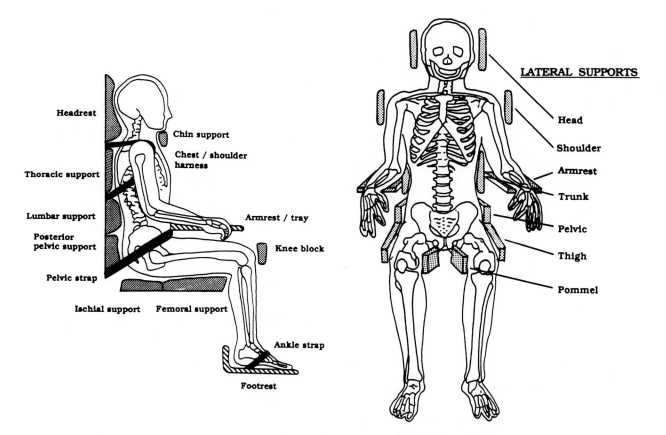

Fig. 10.20. Custom seating system to provide full body support for the severely involved individual is an example of extensive orthotic control. Conceptually, this device may be described as a static CTLSHKAFO + bilateral SEWHO.

about 10 degrees of motion in all planes (which the children can learn to control with their weakened muscles), while preventing excessive motions that would result in trunk collapse. With practice, this system allows the child to walk with a limited reciprocal gait, although the legs are not linked together as would be the case with the reciprocating gait orthoses.

The most complex orthosis involving the lower limbs could be termed a *cervicothoracolumbosacral HKAFO + bilateral SEWHOs*, and would obviously provide full body control. Although an articulated orthosis of such complexity is presently a bionic myth, the future may include electrical stimulation and other new strategies to make such complex control tolerable.

Figure 10.20 is one example of a contemporary static CTLSHKAFO plus bilateral SEWHOs. More commonly referred to as a custom-seating system, such orthoses can be effective for postural control of severely involved individuals.[27]

SUMMARY AND CONCLUSIONS

Lower limb orthoses may be fabricated from metal systems, various plastics, or a combination of both materials. They are commonly indicated to control motion, correct or prevent progression of a deformity, or to unweight partially a distal limb segment.

Orthoses are prescribed by specifying the functional outcome desired, with the individual elements selected by the Certified Orthotist to satisfy the individual patient's needs. The same orthosis may be suitable for a variety of pathologies so long as the biomechanical deficits are similar.

In general, the least orthosis is the best orthosis, so more complex devices are used selectively, and a higher rejection rate is anticipated. Children, unlike adults, generally do quite well even with more extensive orthoses. This chapter has provided an overview of the fundamentals of lower limb orthotic management including typical applications. The reader is referred to the subsequent chapters dealing with treatment of specific pathologies and populations for more information about particular applications of lower limb orthoses.

REFERENCES

1. Anthony RA: The manufacture and use of functional foot orthosis, New York, 1991, Karger.
2. Bowker P: The biomechanics of orthoses. In Bowker P, et al, editors: Biomechanical basis of orthotic management, London, 1993, Butterworth-Heinemann.
3. Bunch WH, Keagy RD: Principles of orthotic treatment, St. Louis, 1976, CV Mosby.
4. Carlson JM, Berglund G: An effective orthotic design for controlling the unstable subtalar joint, Orthot Prosthet 33:39, 1979.
5. Coughlan JK, et al: Lower extremity bracing in paraplegia: A follow-up study, Paraplegia 1:25, 1980.
6. Dittmar K: Treatment of spina bifida children from a technical orthopedic view (German), Orthop Techn 44:28, 1993.
7. Douglas R, et al: The LSU reciprocation-gait orthosis, Orthopaedics 6:834, 1983.
8. Edwards CA: Othopaedic shoe technology: II. Clinical conditions requiring orthopaedic footgear, Muncie, IN, 1985, Ball State University Press.
9. Kralf A, Acimov K, Stanic U: Enhancement of hemiplegic patient rehabilitation by means of functional electrical stimulation, Prosthet Orthot Int 17:107, 1993.
10. Lehmann JL: Lower limb orthotics. In Redford JB, editor: Orthotics etcetera, ed 3, Baltimore, 1986, Williams & Wilkins.
11. Lima D, Magnus R, Paprosky WG: Team management of hip revision patients using a post-op hip orthosis, J Prosthet Orthot 6:20, 1994.
12. Lissens MA, et al: Advanced reciprocating gait orthosis in paraplegic patients, Eur J Phys Med Rehabil 3(Suppl 4):147, 1993.
13. Lower-limb orthotics, New York, 1986, New York University Medical Center.
14. McCollough NC: Biomechanical analysis systems for orthotic prescription. In Atlas of orthotics: Biomechanical principles and application, ed 2, St. Louis, 1985, CV Mosby.
15. Meehan PL, Angel D, Nelson JM, et al: The Scottish Rite abduction orthosis for the treatment of Legg-Perthes disease: A radiographic analysis, J Bone Joint Surg 74A:2, 1992.
16. Merritt JL: Knee-ankle-foot orthotics: Long leg braces and their practical applications, Phys Med Rehabil State Art Rev 1:67, 1987.
17. Michael JW: Orthotic treatment of neurological deficits. In Good DC, Couch JR, editors: Handbook of neurorehabilitation, New York, 1994, Marcel Dekker.
18. Michael JW: Pediatric prosthetics and orthotics, Phys Occup Ther Pediatr 10:123,1990.
19. Michael JW, Isbell MA, Harrelson JM: Orthotic management of diabetic neuropathic arthropathy, J Prosthet Orthot 4:55, 1991.
20. Montgomery DL, Koziris PL: The knee brace controversy, Sports Med 8:260, 1989.
21. Nicholas JA: The five-one reconstruction for anteromedial instability of the knee—indications, technique, and the results in fifty-two patients, J Bone Joint Surg 55A:899, 1973.
22. Pavlik A: The functional method of treatment using a harness with stirrups as the primary method of conservative therapy for infants with congenital dislocation of the hip, Clin Orthop 281:4, 1992.
23. Requa RK, Garrick JC: Clinical significance and level of prophylactic knee brace studies in football, Am Sports Med 9:853, 1990.
24. Rose GK: Orthotics principles and practice, London, 1986, Heinemann Medical Books.
25. Saltiel J: A one-piece laminated knee locking short leg brace, Orthot Prosthet 23:68, 1969.
26. Scott BA: Engineering principles and fabrication techniques for the Scott-Craig long-leg brace for paraplegia, Orthot Prosthet 25:14, 1971.
27. Silverman M: Commercial options for positioning the client with muscular dystrophy, Clin Prosthet Orthot 10:159, 186.
28. Wiest DR, et al: The influence of heel design on a rigid ankle-foot-orthosis, Orthot Prosthet 33:3, 1979.
29. Wu KK: Foot orthoses, Baltimore, 1990, Williams & Wilkins.

Shoes

Carol Frey

The manufacturers of shoewear depend on scientific research and prior experience in the development of their products. Much of the progress made in the shoe industry over the past few years has been made in the athletic shoe industry and carried over to other types of shoewear. This chapter covers important aspects of technology, design, specific functional needs, medical considerations, and orthopedic considerations in the development of athletic, conventional, and therapeutic shoewear.

CONSTRUCTION

Although the product marketing and development methods are different, similar construction techniques are used in the manufacturing of sports, conventional, and therapeutic shoes (Fig. 11.1).

Last

The last is a three-dimensional model (Fig. 11.2) on which the shoe is made and is the foundation for shoe production and development. The shape of shoe instep, girth, toe box, and foot curvature are determined by the last. Because foot shape may vary with activities, this must be considered in the development of the last. The biggest last variations occur in girth (or widest part of the forefoot) and in heel width.

Straight and curved lasts

The majority of feet have a mild inward curve. Most athletic shoe manufacturers use a last with an inward curve of about 7 degrees. More foot mobility is allowed as the inward curve increases, a desirable feature for the hypopronator. A straighter shoe with less inward curve provides more medial support, a desirable feature for the hyperpronator.

Combination lasts

A combination last is any last that varies from a standard proportional last. This type of last can accommodate a combination of fitting or movement requirements.

MATERIALS

Upper materials

Rubber, leather, plastic injection molding, nylon, PVC-coated fabrics, polyurethane-coated fabrics, and canvas have been used in the production of uppers. Most uppers used in sports shoes are made of soft or mesh nylon, leather, canvas, suede, and synthetic materials such as Kangoran.

Sole materials

Because of its versatility, performance, and durability, the most widely used sole material is rubber. A highly compressed molded rubber or a blown microcellular rubber are the most commonly used forms. Styrene-butadiene and carbon rubber are the two most common rubber compounds used in athletic shoes. Black carbon rubber is the hardest-wearing form of rubber and is often used in running shoe soles. Also hard, styrene-butadiene rubber is commonly used in tennis and basketball shoes.

Microcellular rubber (MCR). MCR is composed of natural rubber plus additives. MCR contains a powder blowing agent that decomposes during vulcanization, forming a cellular structure. MCR is mainly used for wedges and midsoles but has also been used as an outsole material.

Polyurethane (PU). Polyurethane is a liquid polymer that can be made into a blown cellular structure. Alone or in combination with ethyl vinyl acetate,

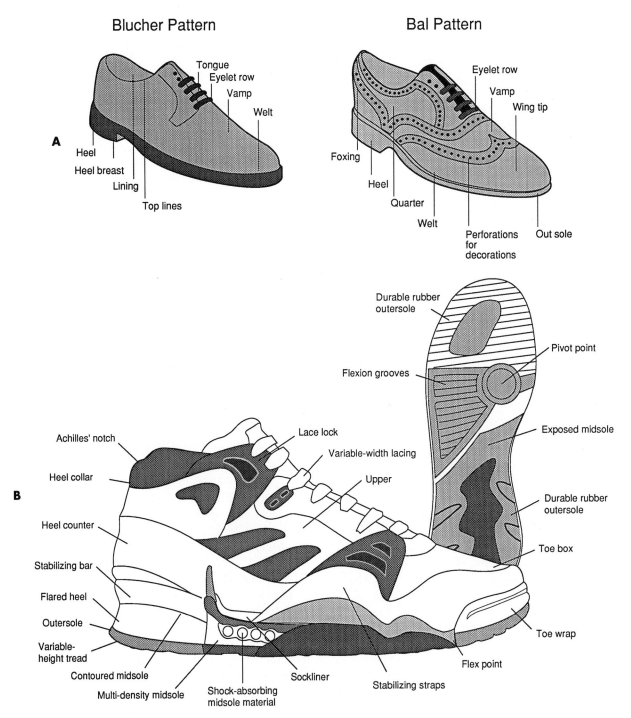

Fig. 11.1.   A, Anatomy of a shoe. **B,** Anatomy of a sports shoe. *(From Pfeffer GB, Frey C, editors: Current practice in foot and ankle surgery, Vol II, New York, 1994, McGraw-Hill.)*

PU is commonly used as a midsole and heel wedge material. PU is also light and durable enough to make a satisfactory outsole material. PU can be used in hardened elastomer form or in the blown cellular state.

Ethyl vinyl acetate (EVA).   EVA is composed of ethylene and vinyl acetate, in addition to a blowing agent in powder form that decomposes during vulcanization to form a cellular structure. EVA is flexible, light,

and resistant to impact, making it a common material used in the manufacture of good-quality athletic shoes. EVA is available in compression molded forms and prefabricated sheets.

Nylon.   Nylon is a polymer resin with a high melting point that can be used to form a hard outsole. Nylon is used as a base for screw-in studs and for spike plates.

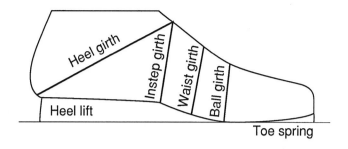

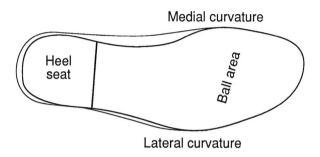

Fig. 11.2. Three-dimensional model on which the shoe is made. It is thought by many to be the foundation for shoe production, development, and fit. *(From Pfeffer GB, Frey C, editors: Current practice in foot and ankle surgery, Vol II, New York, 1994, McGraw-Hill.)*

The hardness grade of nylon refers to the number of carbon atoms in the nylon molecule and is graded as nylon 6, 11, and 12 (the lowest number is the hardest).

Leather

Split leather and coarse full hides are commonly used in the construction of conventional shoewear.

LASTING TECHNIQUES

In the manufacturing of shoes, the most common methods of lasting are slip lasting, board (flat) lasting, and combination lasting (Fig. 11.3).

1. *Slip lasting:* A slip-lasted shoe is made by sewing together the upper like a moccasin and then gluing it to the sole. The last is usually forced into the upper, which then takes on the shape of the last. With this technique, the insole is usually replaced with a sock liner. This lasting method results in a flexible, lightweight shoe without much resistance to torsion.

2. *Flat or board lasting:* With this technique, the upper is formed over the last and then attached to the insole with staples, cement, or tacks. This construction technique decreases flexibility but promotes stability and torsional rigidity in the resultant shoe.

3. *Combination lasting:* More than one lasting technique can be used in the production of a shoe. Commonly the shoe is board lasted in the rear foot

for stability and slip lasted in the forefoot for flexibility.

UPPER DESIGNS AND CUTS

1. *U-throat:* The U-throat provides a U-shaped lacing pattern that extends down to the toes.

2. *Blucher pattern:* This upper has a design with no seams across the dorsum of the midfoot, and the tongue piece is continuous with the vamp (the part of the shoe upper behind the toe box). This upper pattern gives more room allowance at the throat and instep and is adjustable for throat fit.

3. *Balmoral or brogue pattern:* This design is a front-laced shoe, in which the quarters meet, and the vamp is stitched over the quarters at the front of the throat. The tongue, throat, and lace stays are seamed as one unit. This type of upper construction allows less space for the dorsal aspect of the midfoot and is not recommended for the growing foot.

4. *Lace-to-toe pattern:* This pattern provides a lacing system similar in design to the U-throat pattern, but, in addition, both quarters are pulled together across the foot for maximum support.

BOTTOMING PROCESS

Bottoming is the process in which the upper is attached to the sole components of the shoe. Although

BOARD-LASTED

SLIP-LASTED

COMBINATION-LASTED

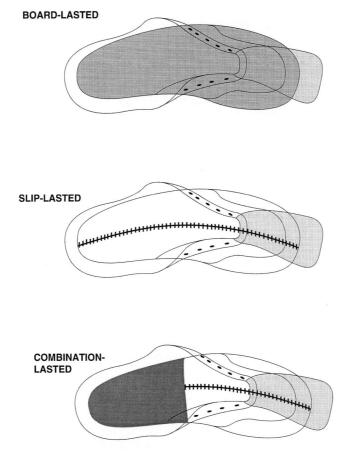

Fig. 11.3.   The most common methods of lasting are slip lasting, board lasting, and combination lasting. *(From Pfeffer GB, Frey C, editors: Current practice in foot and ankle surgery, Vol II, New York, 1994, McGraw-Hill.)*

the upper determines the shoe fit and provides support, it is the sole that provides traction and cushioning.

OUTER SOLE

The outsole is the surface of the shoe that makes contact with the ground and is usually attached to a midsole to form a complete sole. Most sports shoes have outer soles of hard carbon rubber or blown rubber compounds. Not as durable as carbon rubber, blown rubber is the lightest outsole material. Many outsoles are composed of both blown and carbon rubber, with blown rubber in the forefoot and midfoot and carbon rubber used in the high-impact heel area. Gum rubbers grip well on most surfaces and are hard-wearing. PU is less versatile than rubber but can provide a durable satisfactory outsole material. Nylon, leather, and PVC have specific outsole applications for certain sports.

Outer sole designs

Outsole design patterns can enhance traction and stability. Certain patterns can decrease the weight of a shoe by exposing the middle part of the midsole, thereby eliminating part of the outsole and the associated weight. The design of the outsole can provide cushioning, traction, flexpaths, pivot points, and wear plugs. Outsoles can be made for specific surfaces, weather conditions, and sports. Outsole options include (Fig. 11.4):

- Wear area reinforcement (running shoes)
- Cantilevered designs for shock absorption (running shoes)
- Herringbone (court shoes)
- Pivot points (court shoes)
- Radial edges (court shoes)
- Suction cup designs (court shoes)
- Multiclaw or stud designs (field shoes)
- Asymmetric studs (field shoes)
- Traction and wear lugs (hiking and climbing boots)

The traction provided by the outsole is an important design feature of a shoe and is directly related to the ability of the shoe to develop frictional forces with the ground. Traction requirements depend on the specific occupational, sports, and environmental needs. Too

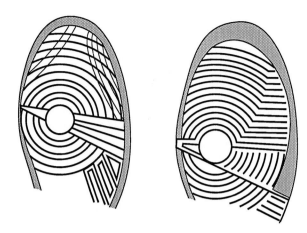

Fig. 11.4. Typical outsole patterns for a court shoe including a pivot point and flexion grooves. These outsole patterns are typically seen in court shoes. *(From Pfeffer GB, Frey C, editors: Current practice in foot and ankle surgery, Vol II, New York, 1994, McGraw-Hill.)*

little traction may have a negative effect on performance, and too much traction may increase the risk of injury.

A running shoe must create a firm enough grip with the ground so that propulsion forces created by the runner are not lost with push-off. Push-off has the highest traction needs, and therefore the forepart of the outsole should provide the most traction. The material used in the outsole of a running shoe is usually blown rubber (air injected to lighten it) or hard carbon rubber.

The design of cleated shoes must make a compromise between performance and protection of the athlete. Rotational traction, expressed by the torque about a normal axis that is developed to resist rotation of a shoe on a playing surface, must be reduced to decrease the incidence of injury while still providing adequate traction. Both cleat length and outsole material influence friction. Torg and Quendenfeld[13] concluded that the increased rotational traction properties of some football shoes are related to an increased number of significant knee injuries.

The necessity for lateral movement with court sports makes the traction characteristics of court shoes important. A flat outsole pattern produces the greatest frictional forces, whereas a herringbone pattern produces less.[14]

With sprinting, ground contact is initially made with the front part of the shoe. At foot strike, a large horizontal velocity is created resulting in a high braking force, which can cause a backward slide. Anterior spikes help to prevent backward slippage.

With jumping events, an athlete converts the large horizontal momentum of the run-up to a vertical momentum as the foot is planted. Spikes prevent the foot from slipping and allow the development of the large propulsive forces needed for the long and triple jump.

Motion is primarily stationary with little horizontal velocity in golf. Golf shoes provide a base of support that allows the coordinated body movements necessary to hit the ball. A nonvertical alignment of the spikes prevents slipping.

MIDSOLES AND WEDGES

Most of the recent advances in the shoe industry have been made in midsole materials and design. The midsole and heel wedge are sandwiched between the upper and the outsole, attaching to both. Midsole components provide shock absorption, cushioning, heel lift, and control.

Unit soles

Unit soles usually contain the outsole, midsole, and heel wedge as one unit. This design is used in ice skates, roller skates, and in the shoes of other sports where the sole does not make contact with the ground. This design is usually heavy and provides little flexibility but excellent torsional rigidity.

Combination or prefabricated soles

Midsoles are usually made from a combination of two basic materials: EVA and PU. EVA is light and has excellent cushioning properties and can be manufactured in a variety of densities. PU is a denser, heavier, and more durable material than EVA. The firmest densities in a multidensity midsole are usually designated by a darker color. The firmer materials may be placed at critical points in the midsole to aid in motion control. Both EVA and PU are used to encapsulate other cushioning materials such as air bags and silicone gel.

OTHER COMPONENT PARTS

Heel counters

The heel counter is a firm cup incorporated into the rear of the shoe upper that helps hold the heel in position and control excessive motion. Most heel counters today are made of a durable plastic, thermoplastic, or polyvinyl. The medial side of the heel counter may be extended or reinforced to control pronation. Contoured or notched heel counters can reduce irritation of the Achilles tendon, especially in plantar flexion.

Toe box

The toe box is constructed of a stiff material inserted between the shoe lining and upper to prevent collapse and protect the toes.

Foxing

Foxing is a stripping material that provides medial and lateral support to the outside of the shoe and is usually made of suede or rubber. In running shoes, the most important foxing is at the toe, where it is referred to as the toe cap. In court shoes, the foxing runs completely around the sole for added lateral support.

Shank

The shank is a reinforcing material that bridges between the ball area and the heel of the shoe. It is arched and somewhat narrowed to conform roughly to the arch area of the midfoot. Shanks are not commonly used in wedge-soled shoes but provide important torsional rigidity in shoes with heels.

Tongues

The tongue of the shoe is primarily designed to protect the dorsum of the foot from lace pressure and the environment. Lacing loops and tongue slits may be added to prevent the tongue from slipping.

Sock linings, arch supports, and inserts

The sock liner lines the inside of the shoe and primarily functions as a buffer between the shoe and the foot. Sock linings are molded, soft support systems that can function in moisture absorption, aeration, hygiene, shock absorption, and motion control.

Arch supports, heel cups, and other types of pads can also be placed in the shoe to provide support, cushioning, and motion control.

Custom-molded "foothotics" have been popularized by the ski industry. These semirigid insole devices are custom-molded to the foot and may help increase comfort, performance, and shock absorption.

Custom insoles can be added to any shoe, provided that there is enough room to accommodate the insert.

NEW COMPONENTS AND DESIGNS

Air soles

NIKE first introduced the idea of air cushioning in 1979, using encapsulated air units in the midsole to enhance cushioning. Depending on the shoe model, the air units may be placed in the heel, forefoot, or both. Initial reports indicated that although air systems had excellent shock absorption, stability was poor. Stability in the context of sports shoes refers to the ability of the shoe to resist unwanted or excessive motions of the foot and ankle. Shoes with soft cushioned midsoles allow more motion than firmer shoes and, in some cases, encourage instability. Newer shoe designs incorporating air systems have addressed the stability problem with success. Air systems are thought to be more durable and not as susceptible to compaction as PU, EVA, and other midsole materials.

Energy return

Compression of a viscoelastic midsole material allows a small amount of strain energy to be stored in the compressed elastic components. Theoretically, when weight is released, the elastic components spring back, and stored energy is returned to the athlete. Theoretically, by increasing the energy return of a shoe, the oxygen cost of an activity is reduced and athletic performance enhanced. There is little scientific evidence, however, to support these claims. Of interest, the arch of the human foot is also a viscoelastic system and therefore can return energy.[1,9]

Pumps

Shoes with "pump" devices are constructed with inflatable linings in the tongue and other parts of the shoe that are pumped up by a device built into the top of the shoe. This feature is reported to provide a tight secure fit. Both NIKE and REEBOK use this fit feature.

Pronation control devices

Shoe designs that control overpronation are a major concern of the sport shoe industry. Most motion control features of a shoe fall into two categories: (1) a harder density material built into the medial aspect of the midsole and/or heel to resist pronation, and (2) an added medial heel component to the inside or outside of the shoe that limits pronation.

SHOE FIT

Ill-fitting shoes have been implicated as being responsible for a variety of forefoot deformities.[2,3,4,7,8,10,12] The deforming effects of a poorly fit shoe on a normal foot can cause hallux valgus, hammertoes, bunionette, calluses, corns, neuromas, and metatarsalgia. In one study,[4] more than 80% of women were found to wear shoes that were at least one width size smaller than their feet (Fig. 11.5).

Shoes should feel comfortable and fit well the first time they are put on. It is recommended that shoes should be fit at the end of the day, when feet are at their largest. While standing, the shoe should be fit to the largest foot. There should be a ½ inch from the end of the longest toe to the end of the toe box, and all the toes should be able to extend fully.

The most common fashion shoe width is C for men and B for women, and the average athletic shoe width is D for men and C for women. This reflects additional allowances for movement and foot expansion during sport.

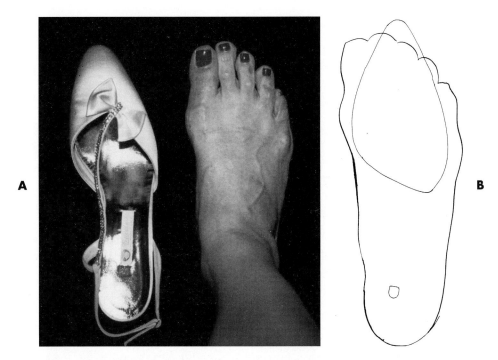

Fig. 11.5. **A,** Poor-fitting shoes have been implicated as the primary cause of forefoot problems seen in women. The majority of women that Frey et al studied wore shoes that were smaller than their feet. **B,** Tracings and measurements of the weight-bearing foot and shoe showed that the shoe was often smaller than the foot. *(From Frey C, et al: AOFAS women's shoewear survey, Foot Ankle 14:78–81, 1993.)*

When fitting new shoes, one should wear the socks one normally would use. If orthoses are needed, the sock liner of the shoe should be removed and the orthosis inserted before fitting the shoe.

SPORTS-SPECIFIC SHOES

Athletic shoes are grouped by the manufacturers into the following categories:
1. *Running, training, and walking shoes.*
2. *Court sport shoes:* This category includes all shoes used for major and minor court sports.
3. *Field sport shoes:* This category includes cleated, studded, and spiked shoes.
4. *Winter sport shoes:* All winter sport activities are included in this category.
5. *Outdoor sport shoes:* Large recreational sports such as hunting, fishing, and boating are included.
6. *Track and field shoes.*
7. *Specialty sport shoes:* All specialized minor sports and some major ones not included in other groups, such as golf and aerobic dancing, are included in this category.

Running, training, and walking

This category includes hiking, race walking, exercise walking, and running.

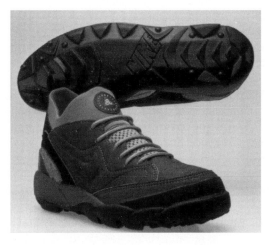

Fig. 11.6. Hiking boots have soles with heavy lugs for traction and durability.

Hiking boots. The upper of a hiking boot (Fig. 11.6) should be water resistant and possess few seams for both comfort and water resistance. Heavily lugged soles, which provide traction and durability, are usually made of rubber, PU, or PVC compounds. Some flexibility is needed in the forepart of the shoe at the metatarsophalangeal joints. Other features of a good hiking boot include a firm heel counter, a padded ankle area, a smooth or seam-free lining, and a high wide toe box. A wedge or a heel with a shank is required.

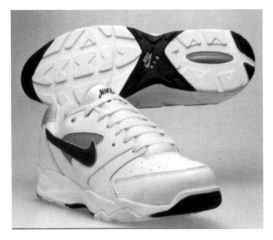

Fig. 11.7. Walking shoes should have a flexible forefoot, good shock absorption, and a rocker sole design.

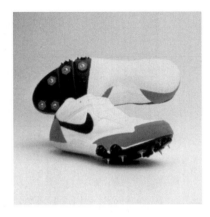

Fig. 11.8. Sprinting shoes have just enough padding in the heel to prevent a contusion. The toe box is semipointed, and the shoe contains a maximum of six sole and two heel spikes.

Climbing boots differ from hiking boots in that they have inflexible soles and a thicker upper.

Race walking shoes. The construction of a race walking shoe is similar to that of a track shoe. A firm light midsole is important. Outsoles are made from carbon or gum rubber. A firm heel counter is desirable.

Exercise walking shoes. The features needed in a good walking shoe (Fig. 11.7) include lightness, a flexible forefoot, a comfortable soft upper, and good shock absorption. Because weight is not as important a consideration for the urban walker, leather is often used for the upper material. An ample toe box and soft sock liner are added for comfort. The sole is also different, with a wedge incorporated into the design. The tread has a smooth, low profile with a herring-bone pattern. Many outsoles have a rocker profile to encourage the natural roll of the foot during the walking motion and to reduce excessive flexion at the metatarsophalangeal joints.

A walking shoe should have a firmer landing area on the heel than most running shoes. The bias-out or up-swept heel of many running shoes does not offer the landing platform needed by walkers. A heel height of 10 to 15 mm is recommended for exercise walking to promote the correct walking motion and reduce over-stretching of the Achilles tendon.

Running

Spikes. Little body weight is placed on the heel in sprinting. For most track runners, even those who run long distances, landing and propulsion are carried out on the ball and middle part of the foot. For faster and shorter races, track shoes generally have just enough padding at the heel to prevent a contusion (Fig. 11.8).

Track shoe lasts are designed to hug the foot at the heel, waist, and girth. The toe box is semipointed to prevent the toes from splaying under the pressure of landing and take-off. Torsional rigidity is often omitted in lightweight track shoes, but a slight wedge is often added to shoes used in longer races to provide more torsional rigidity and support.

Certain specifications for track spikes may vary depending on the event. A maximum of six sole and two heel spikes is allowed; spikes must not project more than 25 mm or exceed 4 mm in diameter. Additional spike receptacles may be present for optimal adjustment and may be filled with flat screws when not in use.

With the use of synthetic and rubber tracks, track spikes have been shortened to around 9 mm, and six spikes are used for better traction. With the use of shorter spikes, shoe manufacturers invented removable plastic "claws." When used in conjunction with replaceable variable-length spikes, track shoes have more versatility for different track surfaces. A spikeless track shoe, usually made with a thin rubber outsole covering a midsole with a maximum heel height of 13 mm, may be preferred if the track surface is hard.

Following the same pattern as sprint shoes, middle distance shoes vary only in the midsole area. A thin wedge or shank may help control overpronation and torque during bend running.

Participants in short and long hurdles require sprint shoes with lasts wider in the toe and shorter front spikes to avoid clipping the hurdle with the lead foot. A more heavily padded heel is desirable to cushion the landing.

Flats. More research and design has been done in the development of running flats than in all other areas of athletic footwear (Fig. 11.9). The features most required in a running shoe used for training on hard road surfaces are shock absorption, control, flexibility and stability in the heel counter area, torsional rigidity in the waist or shank, lightness, traction, comfort, motion control, and good fit.

Because of the specific needs of individual runners, athletic shoewear companies now produce models for

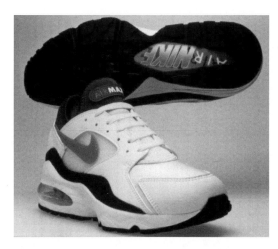

Fig. 11.9. A good running shoe should include cushioning, flexibility, lightness, traction, motion control, and good fit.

specific foot types, gait patterns, and training styles. There are designs for light runners, heavy runners, heel strikers, motion control, stability, lightweight trainers, and rugged terrain. This segmentation of the market is crossing over into other sports specialty shoes such as tennis and basketball.

Uppers are usually made of lightweight soft or mesh nylon. A rigid heel counter is a requirement because like walkers, most runners land heel first. The midsoles of training shoes should be lightweight and offer good shock absorption. PU and EVA are the most commonly used materials, but ambient air, freon, and silicone gel can also be used. All these materials have good-to-excellent shock absorbency and are built into heel wedge and midsole combinations. The shape of the sole is wedged from heel to toe. A flared heel increases stability in the heel area.

Traction is obtained by rubber outsole materials and a good tread design. To obtain the best traction on loose or open terrain surfaces, a deeper sole tread is recommended. On smoother, harder surfaces such as pavement, a lower-profile sole offers better stability.

Throwing events. Shoes for throwing events, where athletes tend to be larger, are primarily made of leather or suede for maximum durability and support. Because of tremendous stresses applied to the medial and lateral portion of the shoe, the uppers are made with extra support around the girth. A shot put shoe should provide reinforced leather uppers, a sturdy heel counter, firm toe box, and reinforcement in the quarter for lateral support. Good grip provided by a rubber sole and an adequate shank gives some control for anterior and lateral movements across the circle. Discus shoes are similar to shot put shoes but with more flexibility in the forefoot and a wrap-up sole for improved turning motion in the circle. Javelin boots are the only throwing shoes provided with spikes for run-up and foot plant.

Soles have a heavy-duty forefoot and heel spike plates containing six front and two back spikes that may be as long as 25 mm for competition on grass runways. A buckle or strap may be used across the girth to provide additional support.

Jumping events. For jumping events, spike placement changes from the asymmetric pattern, with two spikes in front for stability (the IAAF rules that there may be a maximum of six forepart spikes and two heel spikes). Most long jumpers do not use heel spikes. The forepart spike plate is sturdy for extra support. Heel cushioning is provided for shock absorption.

Similar to long jump shoes, triple jump shoes vary only in the midsole, where a sturdy wedge gives better support for landing during the midstance and toe-off stress during this event. Most triple jumpers use heel spikes.

Regardless of their style, high jumpers use a one-foot take-off. Because foot plant and take-off are critical for a successful jump, the jump foot shoe is emphasized by designers. The take-off shoe is made in right and left foot versions. Forward and backward ascent styles ("Fosbury Flop") have different spike placements and gradient on the sole for take-off. The jump shoe can be built with a maximum elevation of 10 mm in the forepart to assist in lift-off. Six forepart and two heel spikes may be used. Most shoe companies now produce counterpart trailing shoes that are lighter, with fewer spikes and more flexibility to assist the run-up.

Court sport shoes

Racquet sports. These sports require forward, backward, and side-to-side movements. Movements are multidirectional and controlled. From the wear patterns produced in even a short time, it is apparent that court shoes used in racquet sports are subjected to heavy abuse.

Tennis. Tennis requires body control with quick side-to-side movement, sprinting, jumping, and stretching. The sport is played on lawn, asphalt, clay, synthetic, and rubberized courts. The selection of an appropriate sole must be made for each surface. On clay courts, soles with an overly deep tread pattern may be prohibited because of excessive court maintenance even though most players would prefer the traction. On artificial or synthetic surfaces, harder soles with high rubber content or dual-density PU are recommended for durability.

A tennis shoe (Fig. 11.10) should provide good lateral support, light-to-medium weight, a flat sole with a good heel wedge, a firm heel counter, a well-cushioned insole and midsole, ample toe box, good ventilation, nonslip traction, a pivot-point, and reinforcement for toe drag. The upper should provide a

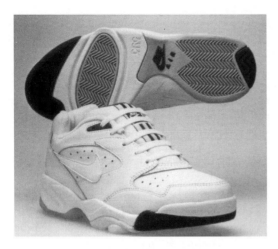

Fig. 11.10. A tennis shoe should provide good lateral support, a firm heel counter, cushioning, ample toe box, traction, a pivot point, and reinforcement of the toe box.

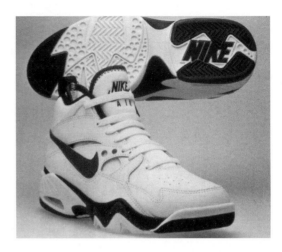

Fig. 11.11. A basketball shoe should provide good lateral and medial support, a flat sole, cushioning, a large firm heel counter, reinforcement of the toe box, ventilation, a pivot point, and good traction.

sufficiently high quarter pattern to give good ankle and lateral foot support. Over the ankle line, midcut models are available for those players who prefer more ankle support.

Manufacturers of tennis shoes recommend more cushioning in the ball of the foot for the serve-and-volley player. For the baseline player, a solid heel counter, strong reinforcement in the heel and midfoot area, and good rear foot stability are recommended.

Basketball. Basketball requires backward, forward, and vertical accelerations; quick stops; and side-to-side movements. The playing surface is usually wood but may be synthetic or rubberized material. The shoe (Fig. 11.11) should provide good lateral and medial support, light-to-medium weight, a flat sole, a slight heel wedge, good cushioning, a large firm heel counter, toe drag reinforcement, a pivot-point, and good traction. A high rubber content in the sole is recommended. Soles with multiple-edge patterns, such as circles, squares, or diamonds, offer better traction than herringbone patterns (which is excellent for forward stop but not good for lateral stops). High-cut designs are available for added ankle support. While offering added ankle support, high-cut uppers must not restrict ankle flexion. Proprioceptor straps are popular. Low-cut uppers are preferred by some players for increased ankle flexibility, but the incidence of ankle injuries may increase with use of these shoes.[5]

The emphasis of design research in basketball shoes has been the reduction of ankle inversion injuries. Studies have shown that shoes with increasing restriction of the ankle by the upper significantly reduce ankle joint inversion.[11] It was also shown, however, that with increasing amounts of ankle restriction, movements were not only restricted in the sagittal plane, but also the frontal plane, which led to reduced agility. There-

fore, a design compromise must be met between performance and protection of the athlete from injury.

Field sport shoes

Field sports combine many types of movement and a variable degree of body contact. Running is basic to all these sports.

Spike and stud formations vary from sport to sport but are almost all replaceable or detachable cleats, studs, or spikes affixed into nylon soles. Generally, smaller studs in a denser pattern help prevent ankle and knee injuries secondary to less penetration of the cleat into the playing field. In addition, weight distribution is better in multistudded designs.

Soccer. Soccer involves mainly running, kicking, jumping, sliding, stretching, and multidirectional movements. The playing surfaces are natural grass and artificial turf. Soccer is played almost entirely by the feet with the ball being kicked off the medial, lateral, and dorsal aspects of the foot. Soccer shoe lasts tend to be snug fitting, often using European lasts, which are somewhat more narrow than American. Thinner soft leathers are preferred for the upper because players like to feel the ball, but the tongue should be well padded to reduce lace pressure and cushion the dorsal kicking area of the foot (Fig. 11.12). Some players use the tongue and lace area to produce spin and control the ball. Soles should be flexible at the metatarsophalangeal joints for running and have torsional stability.

Football. Running is the primary motion in football along with quick lateral movements and the production of great forces secondary to blocking and hitting. Studies have shown that injuries may be caused from wearing fewer, longer cleats, which produce excessive pressure beneath the cleats from increased foot fixation.[13] More specifically, the excessive resistance to

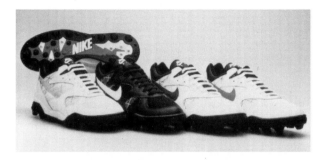

Fig. 11.12. The upper of a soccer shoe often is made of soft leather because players like to feel the ball. The tongue should be well padded to reduce lace pressure and protect the kicking area of the foot.

rotation causes knee injuries during the twisting motions of football. As a result of these studies, it has been determined that the maximum diameter of a cleat tip should be $\frac{7}{16}$ inch and a maximum overall length $\frac{1}{2}$ inch. A seven-stud pattern is preferred on natural grass. Nylon soles are preferred because they shed dirt easily and prevent caking of mud between the studs. Commonly, multistudded rubber soles are used on natural grass (Fig. 11.13).

Special shoewear requirements exist for linemen, backs, and kickers. Uppers for linemen must provide support and protection. High-cut or semi–high-cut boot designs are preferred. A sturdy toe box and firm heel counter are recommended. Astroturf linesmen's shoes are multistudded for grass with shorter, more numerous studs for traction and stability.

The uppers used for backs are similar as for linemen. For added mobility, a low-cut design is usually preferred. Lightweight Astroturf shoes with nylon or cotton mesh uppers reinforced with suede are preferred by many players. These shoes usually have a rubber outsole with a waffle design that wraps up at the toe and front quarter for better lateral support.

For place-kickers, a shoe with a square toe box is usually handmade for the kicking foot. A conventional shoe is worn on the nonkicking foot. The shoe is usually custom-made for the individual kicker at the professional level. A soccer shoe is usually preferred for kickers who kick from the side of the foot. For punting, either a soccer or a back's shoe is used. Some players kick in a traditional football back's shoe.

Baseball. Baseball requires sprinting, throwing, and complex batting movements. The playing surface is usually natural but may be artificial turf with dirt or clay on infield basepaths. A traditional baseball shoe has a U-throat and conventional lacing system. Lasts are similar to a football shoe. On natural turf, steel cleats with a design of three in the front and two in the heel are used extensively. Removable cleats are available in steel, PU, and nylon. For pitchers, a pitching toe is often added for toe drag reinforcement.

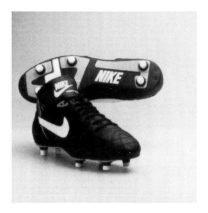

Fig. 11.13. American football shoe.

Winter sports

Skating. Skating maneuvers are similar for all skating events, although footwear and blades are specialized. Ankle movement and support are essential to skating performance. The subtalar joint, however, must be free to allow positioning of the blade on the ice.

The traditional leather boot and the injection-molded model are the two main types of boots on the market. A leather boot should have good ankle support and a firm heel counter with elongation of the medial side. Uppers are made from thick-grade leather or split leather with a leather or textile lining, which gives the foot and ankle stability but allows some flexibility. Metal eyelets are used in the lower portion of the throat and metal hooks above the ankle.

Ice hockey skates were the first to use injection molded models. A viscous plastic is injected under pressure into molds to form the lower and upper parts of the boot. The two parts are placed together, completing a hinged outer shell. A soft foam liner is then added.

The hinged two-piece design gives the boot some lateral flexibility needed in ice skating. Leather boots tend to become more flexible with age.

Figure skating. Figure skating requires the athlete to jump, skate, balance, spin, dance, and lift. The performing surface is ice on artificial or natural rinks.

The upper is either full or top grain cowhides. Good-quality boots are lined with lightweight top grain leather or suede. A firm heel counter, usually elongated on the medial side for added arch support, is important. Soles are PVC or PU molded units with a shank for added support. Screw-in blades are often used so that the position of the blades may be changed. The lasts used in figure skating are semipointed with a narrow shank and heel to contain the foot and maintain position.

The quality of the blades helps determine the quality of the skate. Blades are commonly made of tubular steel or plastic frame with high tempered steel, which is hollow ground to give two skating edges to the

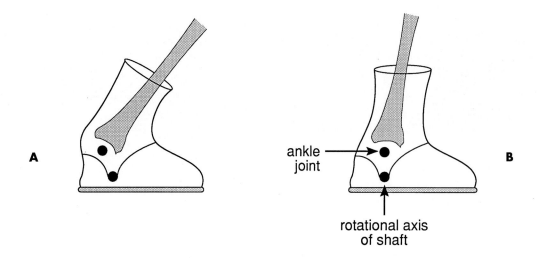

A   Unfavorable lever relationships

ankle joint

rotational axis of shaft

B   Favorable lever relationships

Fig. 11.14.   During dorsiflexion and plantar flexion, the motion of the shaft of the ski boot should correspond to the motion of the ankle and the tibia. **A,** Unfavorable lever relationships. **B,** Favorable lever relationships.

blade. The blades can be nickel or chrome plated. Figure skating and freestyle blades have a front-to-back curvature called a radius or rocker. The placement of the blades is usually slightly medial to the midline of the sole. For jumps or spins, a toe rake or pick is used. With forward motion, the picks can also help prevent the blade sliding sideways. For figures, a pair of skates without a pick and less sharply ground blades is often preferred.

Ice hockey.   Ice hockey requires skating, quick stops, quick turns, and balance on the ice of artificial and natural rinks. A high-cut model of leather or ballistic nylon with leather reinforcement is available. A good skating boot requires a firm protective leather toe box of polyethylene or firm fiber and a comfortable ankle padding with a high cut over the Achilles tendon for protection. A molded boot with a hinged upper can provide additional protection and durability. High-grade boots have a leather lining.

The goalie wears a special design of either a molded or leather boot with a protective casing. The boots have a low-cut design at the ankle, which allows increased flexibility and accommodates goalie pads. The blades are thick and reinforced with increased surface area in contact with the ice to block shots at the goal.

Speed skating.   Speed skating requires balanced skating with a low center of gravity in the lunge position. Skaters often compete with bare feet in skates. The skating surface is ice on artificial or natural ice tracks. The uppers have a deep-cut U-throat with a full lacing pattern to the toes. A ¾ ankle boot is the preferred design with a firm heel counter elongated on the medial side.

Thin (¹⁄₁₆ inch) straight blades are used of either tubular steel or plastic frames. The blade is long (30 to 45 cm) and is placed distal to the skating boot via a high-profile frame to allow a lean of low angle between the skate and the track. Higher-quality blades are chrome plated.

Alpine skiing.   Alpine skiing requires ankle and knee flexion, forward lean, and balance on snow-covered surfaces. Ski boots (Fig. 11.14) provide a high-cut upper of a hinged or one-piece injection molded plastic outer shell to support the lower leg. The boot should provide rigid support for the foot and ankle and allow forward ankle flexion. Adjustable buckles, dial closure devices, or straps are used for instep support and a comfortable snug fit. Rearentry and midentry boots have eliminated buckles and overlaps on the vamp, instep, and ankle regions to reduce pressure. Inner liners can contain a footbed, a variety of wedges, or adjustable canting devices. To relieve pressure, conforming foam or pressure flow bags can be used.

Ski boots are one of the last categories of athletic footwear to accommodate the female athlete. Important design differences include an elevated heel for a shorter female Achilles tendon, easier forward flexion, and a more flared ankle cuff.

Cross country skiing.   Cross country skiing requires fast walking movements, running, jogging, downhill skiing, and balance on snow-covered terrain. Boot and bindings act together as a hinge between the foot and the ski and must be compatible. Boots are made of leather, Gore-tex, nylon, or poromeric materials that allow the air to circulate and transpire. Boots should be waterproof and as seam free as possible with

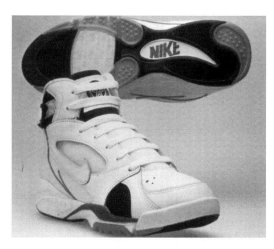

Fig. 11.15. The aerobic shoe requirements combine those of a well-cushioned running shoe and a modified indoor court shoe.

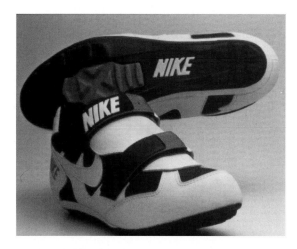

Fig. 11.16. The bicycle shoe has a last similar to the sprinting shoe with a semipointed toe, narrow waist, and narrow heel.

rigid heel counters. Good forefoot flexion is essential. For use on the snow and ice, rubber soles are preferred.

Other sports

Aerobic dancing. Aerobic dancing requires stationary running, skipping, jumping, stretching, dancing, and stair climbing. The dance surface is on carpet or covered surfaces. The shoe requirements are a combination of a lightweight shock-absorbent running shoe and a modified indoor court shoe (Fig. 11.15). Medial and lateral support is needed as well as a wrap-up toe and heel protection. The forefoot requires stabilization and good shock absorption. EVA and PU combinations, air systems, and gel are used in shock-absorbing forefoot pads. Flexibility in the forepart is important.

Bicycle. Bicycling involves use of the gluteus, quadriceps, hamstrings, and calf muscles to generate the power necessary to perform upward and downward thrusts through the forefoot. The foot is often placed into a valgus or varus position on the pedal causing pressure to develop on the lateral or medial sides of the foot. Cleat and pedal placement can be changed to prevent this canting.

A cycle racing shoe has a last similar to a sprinting shoe with a wide girth, semipointed toe, narrow waist, and narrow heel (Fig. 11.16). A high toe box is required for toe movement. Uppers are usually made of smooth calf or kid leather with perforations for ventilation. Racing shoes are usually unlined and tend to stretch. Rigid soles are made of reinforced steel, nylon, or PU and can protect the foot from pedal pressure. Depending on the system, shoes are affixed to pedals by cleats, which improve cycling efficiency by locking the foot to the pedal for upward and downward thrust. Adjustable cleats are available on most shoes that allow angular and fore/aft adjustments.

CORRECTIVE SHOES

The term *corrective shoes* has been used to describe shoewear that use lasts of a particular shape to accommodate a specific condition. Although shoewear can accommodate for deformity, disease, and pathology, it cannot correct. A corrective shoe, however, can be used for maintenance of a correction that has been made by manipulation, casting, or surgery.

Children's corrective shoes

Children's corrective shoes are pictured in Fig. 11.17.

1. *Outflare lasts* are used for maintenance of correction after treatment for metatarsus adductus. The prewalker laces to the toe and has an instep strap for foot control.
2. *Straight lasts* are neutral from toe to heel. The right and left shoes have little difference. The prewalker style has open toes, and the lacing pattern extends to the toes.
3. *Conventional lasts* are a standard shape from heel to toe. Shoe modifications can be made for minor corrections.
4. *Inflare lasts* can be used to maintain correction after the treatment of overpronation.

Adult corrective shoes

1. *Postoperative shoes* are similar to a cast boot but usually possess a wooden sole, canvas upper, open toe, and velcro or lace closures. This shoe limits foot motion.
2. *Extra-depth* shoes are one size longer (⅓ inch) and two sizes wider (½ inch greater in girth) than the patient's normal size and can accommodate a custom-molded insert. These shoes are often recommended for neuropathic or hypersensitive

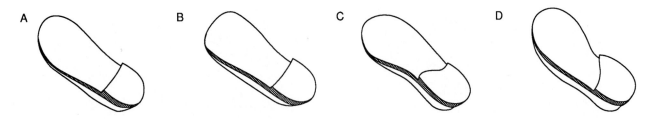

Fig. 11.17.   Children's corrective shoes. **A,** Conventional last. **B,** Straight last. **C,** Outflare last. **D,** Inflare last.

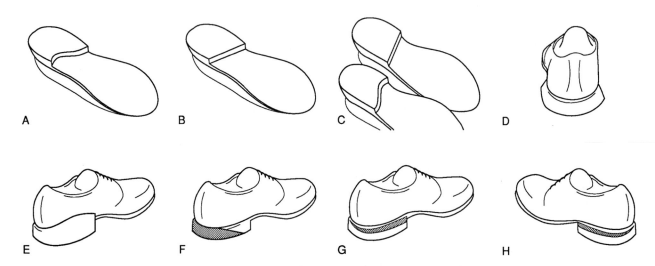

Fig. 11.18.   Heel corrections. **A,** Thomas's heel. **B,** Stone's heel. **C,** Reverse Thomas's and Stone's heel. **D,** Flare heel. **E,** Offset heel. **F,** Plantar flexion heel. **G,** Medial heel wedge. **H,** Lateral heel wedge.

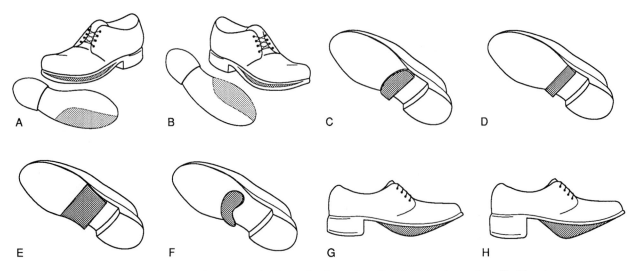

Fig. 11.19.   Outsole corrections. **A,** Lateral sole wedge. **B,** Medial sole wedge. **C,** Mayo's metatarsal bar. **D,** Flush's metatarsal bar. **E,** Denver's heel or bar. **F,** Hauser's bar. **G,** Rocker sole. **H,** Rocker sole (extended and steeper).

feet such as seen in diabetes and rheumatoid arthritis.

3. *Bunion-last shoes* provide a soft leather upper and a high wide toe box to provide adequate room for toe deformities.

4. *Custom-molded shoes* are also referred to as space shoes. These shoes are made from a cast mold of the foot and accommodate all foot deformities.

Heel corrections

Figure 11.18 shows several heel corrections:

1. A *Thomas heel* extends medially for about ½ inch to provide added support under the sustentaculum tali.

2. A *reverse Thomas heel* extends laterally.

3. A *flared heel* provides a broad base of support for the hindfoot.

4. An *offset heel* is broader than the flare heel and provides reinforcement for the sides of the heel counter.

5. A *SACH heel* incorporates a soft posterior wedge in the heel to cushion heel strike. This heel modification is useful for patients who have limited ankle motion, arthritis, or anterior impingement.

6. A *medial heel wedge* may be used to control hyperpronation and decrease excursion of tendons on the medial side of the ankle.

7. A *lateral heel wedge* may be used to control supination and decrease excursion of tendons on the lateral side of the ankle.

Outsole corrections

Outsole corrections are shown in Fig. 11.19.

1. A *lateral sole wedge* can be used to control forefoot inversion.

2. A *medial sole wedge* can be used to control forefoot eversion.

3. A *Denver heel* or *bar* is usually ¾ inch wide and is placed ¼ inch proximal to the widest part of the shoe. The heel tapers to a straight distal edge and is recommended for metatarsalgia.

4. A *metatarsal bar* should be positioned proximal to the metatarsal heads to decrease pressure across the metatarsal heads. This modification is recommended for metatarsalgia from a variety of causes.

5. A *Hauser bar* is a comma-shaped metatarsal bar that may be combined with a Thomas heel. It has been reported to prevent supination of the forefoot.[6]

6. A *rocker sole* provides a rocker pattern from heel to toe to allow for rigid protection of forefoot fractures, hallux rigidus, arthritis, and insensitive feet. This sole pattern limits weight bearing on the forefoot.

REFERENCES

1. Alexander RM: How elastic is a running shoe? New Scientist 123:45–46, 1989.

2. Didia BC, Omu ET, Obuoforibio AA: The use of footprint contact index II for classification of flat feet in a Nigerian population, Foot Ankle 7:285–289, 1987.

3. Engle ET, Morton DJ: Notes on foot disorders among natives of the Belgian Congo, J Bone Joint Surg 13:311–318, 1931.

4. Frey C, et al: AOFAS women's shoewear study, Foot Ankle 14:78–81, 1993.

5. Garrick JG, Requ RK: Role of external support in the prevention of ankle sprain, Med Sci Sports Exerc 5:200–203, 1973.

6. Gould N: Shoes and shoe modifications. In Jahss, editor: Disorders of the foot and ankle, Philadelphia, WB Saunders.

7. Hoffman P: Conclusions drawn from a comparative study of the feet of barefooted and shoe-wearing peoples, Am J Orthop Surg 3:105–136, 1905.

8. Holmes G Jr: Arthrodesis of the first metatarsophalangeal joint using interfragmentary screw and plate, Foot Ankle, 13:333–335, 1992.

9. Kerr RF, et al: The spring in the arch of the human foot, Nature 325:147–149, 1987.

10. Janisse D: The art and science of fitting shoes, Foot Ankle 13:257–262, 1993.

11. Robinson JR, Frederick EC, Cooper LB: Systematic ankle stabilization and the effect on performance, Med Sci Sports Exerc 18:625–628, 1986.

12. Sim-Fook L, Hodgson A: A comparison of foot forms among the non-shoe and shoe-wearing Chinese population, J Bone Joint Surg 40A:1058–1062, 1958.

13. Torg JS, Quendenfeld T: Effect of shoe type and cleat length on incidence of severity of knee injuries among high school football players, Res Quart 42:203–211, 1971.

14. Valiant GA: The effect of outsole pattern on basketball shoe traction. In Terauds J, Gowitzke BA, Hole LE, editors: Biomechanics in sports III & IV, Del Mar, CA, 1986, Academic Publishers.

SPINAL ORTHOSES

INTRODUCTION
John E. Lonstein

This section on Spinal Orthoses builds upon the principles laid out in the preceding sections. This section continues the process with chapters on the clinical application of spinal orthoses covering different areas.

Spinal pain is an important topic, and the role of the different orthoses in the treatment and relief of the painful condition is presented in Chapter 12. The pros and cons of the devices used in different areas of the spine give basis for the orthotic treatment of these problems. The treatment of spinal trauma involves the use of both surgical and orthotic modalities, either separately or in conjunction with each other. Chapter 13 covers these areas, discussing the different regions of the spine and the role of the different orthoses. This understanding is essential for effective treatment of spinal trauma. Both Chapters 12 and 13 use standard orthoses, with cross references to Chapter 8, which is

on the different spinal orthoses and their principles. For those who have an interest in understanding the rationale used in the treatment of spinal orthoses these two chapters should be read together.

The first historical use of orthoses for the spine was for the treatment of spinal deformities, and this remains the major use of spinal orthoses. These principles and application gained from the experience with spinal curve control serve as a basis for the effective treatment of spinal deformities orthotically as covered in Chapter 14.

With this section, it is hoped that the reader will gain an appreciation of the use of spinal orthoses in numerous different areas and for a variety of problems. Only with this background can a logical and effective treatment plan be formulated for a patient with a spinal problem.

Orthoses for Spinal Pain

Joan E. Edelstein

Pain in the neck, thorax, or low back is sometimes reduced by the use of an appropriate orthosis. Although the mechanism of pain relief with orthoses remains controversial, most clinicians recognize that orthoses remind the wearer to avoid extreme, abrupt, stressful movements and promote rest for the affected anatomic structures.[86] Orthoses may also limit the range through which the wearer can move[13,41] and foster more satisfactory vertebral alignment. These functions can lessen pain by minimizing faulty muscle action.

Because an external device does not contact or act solely on the spine, force that an orthosis transmits is influenced by the surrounding tissues. Skin and subcutaneous tissue do not tolerate high pressure. Force must therefore be applied not only to relatively rigid bone, but also to fat, muscle, superficial vessels, and viscera, which are viscoelastic tissues having low stiffness.[95] Prolonged use of a spinal orthosis is to be avoided because muscles begin to weaken and become fibrotic, and the individual is likely to develop psychological dependence on the device.[55] An orthosis, however, should be part of a comprehensive plan of management, which may include therapeutic exercise and other conservative treatment, with or without medication.

CERVICAL ORTHOSES

Neck pain, whether caused by muscle spasm related to maintaining one position for a continuous period, arthritic impingement or subluxation, or acceleration or deceleration trauma to the connective tissues or muscles, may respond to use of a flexible or rigid collar. Orthotic prescription is common empiric practice without scientific evidence to substantiate its efficacy.[86] Individuals with more severe pain may wear a post orthosis, which includes vertical posts joining plates on the head and chest. Cervical orthoses are usually mass produced but often can be adjusted to suit the needs of a particular individual. They differ in the extent to which they restrict motion and realign the vertebrae.

Unlike thoracolumbosacral (TLSOs) or lumbosacral orthoses (LSOs), which are usually worn under clothing, cervical orthoses are conspicuous. Therefore, the individual may be reluctant to display the device and fail to comply with treatment guidelines or may persist in wearing it when it is no longer medically required to garner sympathy or be persuasive in litigation pertaining to a claim of negligence.[31]

Therapeutic rationale

Cervical orthoses may reduce pain primarily by restricting motion[3,14] and, in the case of collars, by also reducing body heat loss.[22,31,33,79] Keeping the neck warm aids resolution of temporary strain[63]; heat retention with a collar, however, is about the same when a wool scarf is worn.[6] Although the therapeutic benefits of heat application are well-known,[63] it remains unclear whether heat retention by a collar is useful.

Motion restriction contributes to bony stabilization, muscle relaxation, prevention of deformity, and tissue healing. Although collars minimally restrict voluntary neck motion, they do remind the wearer not to move abruptly or through the extreme limits of available excursion, thereby resting painful tissues.

To restrict movement, orthoses must be worn moderately snugly. Nevertheless, cervical orthoses fitted tighter than 25 mm Hg do not provide substantially greater immobilization and may cause discomfort that the wearer is apt to relieve by loosening the orthosis excessively.[23] Cervical orthoses overlie superficial blood vessels and the throat; consequently an overly tight orthosis can cause the wearer to choke or faint. The orthosis is adjusted to place the head and neck in the best tolerated position during the phase of acute pain. Subsequently the orthosis should maintain the head directly over the center of gravity to flatten the cervical lordosis and thus maintain sufficient opening of the intervertebral foramina to decrease nerve root pressure. This posture also decreases the need for neck muscles to support the head.[11] Slight flexion opens the intervertebral foramina and separates the articular facets.[56,79] Depending on its trim lines, a broad rigid collar may also alter vertebral alignment. Similarly a post orthosis can be set to increase or decrease cervical lordosis.

The design and rigidity of the orthosis influence the extent of motion limitation. Most published reports involve adults who have no neck pain and thus are able to move freely in all directions.[13,24,34,41,42,44,54] When these people wore orthoses of various designs, radiographic studies indicated that no orthosis eliminated vertebral motion, although wearing rigid appliances was associated with reduction in cervical motion. The picture is quite different with individuals who have pain and are thus reluctant or unable to move easily. For such patients, orthoses help to remind the wearer to moderate motion, avoiding extreme or irritating actions. Collars, whether manufactured or custom-made, block neck flexion slightly and limit rotation much less than do orthoses that encompass the mandible and occiput[13,43]; rigid orthoses are more restrictive than flexible ones.[34,41] Sternal and dorsal plates reduce flexion and rotation of lower cervical vertebrae, without much effect on upper cervical motion. Lateral posts decrease lateral flexion, rotation, and sagittal motion of the upper segments. Consequently the Philadelphia collar restricts extension at all cervical levels substantially more than does the sternal-occipital-mandibular immobilizer (SOMI) orthosis.[42] Motion limitation in all planes is greater with the cervicothoracic version of the four-post orthosis; orthoses in decreasing order of motion limitation are the basic four-post, SOMI, Philadelphia collar, and flexible collar.[24,41]

With regard to the SOMI and four-post orthosis, the SOMI is somewhat more effective at limiting flexion, whereas the four-post orthosis restrains extension better.[24] Control of atlantoaxial subluxation is difficult to achieve orthotically; the occipital plate tends to force the atlas forward when the patient extends the head.[3] Some investigators report that orthoses with chin pieces control motion of the upper portion of the cervical spine,[13] whereas others dispute orthotic effectiveness at the first two intervertebral joints.[41]

Although it is claimed that collars which do not contact the skull or chest reduce load through the vertebral column,[32,79] thereby reducing compressive stress, such effect probably is minimal. If the patient holds the neck in moderate flexion while a basic collar is fitted, the anterosuperior portion of the orthosis does

offer some chin support.[6] Orthoses having mandibular, occipital, and thoracic plates support more vertical load.

Collars are indicated for clients with cervical sprain without bony injury,[60] intervertebral disc injury, or disease without herniation or significant root compression. For more severe or persistent pain, either an orthosis with mandibular and occipital supports or a post orthosis should be prescribed. Pain resulting from cervical spondylosis and spondylitis may respond to a combination of a soft collar worn at night and a firm collar used during the day.[55]

Although cervical orthoses may provide temporary pain relief, they do not prevent progression of arthritic changes.[65,74,85] Early mobilization is desirable for most cervical sprains[60]; in fact, wearing a collar for more than 6 weeks is likely to cause neck stiffness.[55]

Types of cervical orthoses

Collars.   The simplest cervical orthosis is a flexible collar made of polyethylene foam, sponge rubber, felt, or quilted cotton.[51] Such a device serves primarily as a reminder to the wearer to avoid twisting or bending the neck. Flexible, soft collars are generally well tolerated.

Slightly more restrictive is a hard plastic collar, either manufactured or custom-made. Collars made in the clinic of moderately rigid polyethylene foam (Plastazote) can be quite comfortable.[6,18]

Both the soft and the hard collars cover approximately the same area, with the superior border usually at the base of the mandible and slightly below the superior nuchal line and the inferior border at the manubrium and the lower posterior border in the vicinity of the seventh cervical vertebra. Some manufacturers offer a hard collar with one portion slightly broader; with this design, the clinician can position the client's head in moderate flexion or extension, depending on the client's tolerance. The superior border should not impinge onto the mental protuberance, which would interfere with swallowing. In addition, the orthosis should not irritate the cervical or brachial plexin or the temporomandibular joints.

The Philadelphia collar features anterior and posterior struts of semirigid plastic. The soft portion encompasses the lower mandible and occiput. This orthosis limits cervical motion, particularly flexion, more than narrow collars.[41] High interface pressures have been recorded at the chin, particularly when the subject flexed the neck, whereas occipital pressures increased substantially during extension.[6] A modification of the Philadelphia collar is the Yale cervical orthosis, which has anterior and posterior plates extending from the collar to a belt around the lower ribs.[42] The Nec-Lock collar, which resembles a Philadelphia collar but stores flat, restricts motion more than the Philadelphia collar.[44] Collars are generally easier than post orthoses for clients to don.

Post orthoses. A typical post orthosis has rigid plates at the mandible, occiput, midsternum, and upper back. The plates, usually padded, are joined by straps and vertical metal posts. The two-post orthosis has an anterior and a posterior post. The four-post version has a pair of anterior and posterior posts. The posts are threaded to facilitate adjustment of head position. Post orthoses are more restrictive than collars. The four-post design limits lateral flexion and rotation more effectively than does the two-post orthosis. Post orthoses are cooler than collars but do not offer the therapeutic benefit of heat retention. Patients may object to the mandibular plate because it interferes with eating, and accumulated saliva can irritate the skin.

The SOMI is a three-post orthosis, consisting of a central bar joining the sternal to the mandibular plate and two anterior lateral bars from the sides of the sternal plate to the occipital plate. The sternal plate is secured with a waist belt and shoulder straps. The SOMI can be applied to the supine client without having to rotate the individual.

THORACOLUMBOSACRAL ORTHOSES (TLSO)

Some clients find pain relief from thoracolumbosacral corsets that extend superiorly to the upper chest and usually include axillary straps. Inferiorly the corset terminates at the lower border of the buttocks and at the inguinal ligaments. Corsets remind wearers to avoid jerky, extreme movements. A rigid, custom-molded plastic TLSO may be required for the client with pain caused by osteoporotic compression fractures.

Therapeutic rationale

TLSOs are rigid orthoses that encompass the thorax as well as the abdomen. They are prescribed primarily to restrict motion in the presence of vertebral fracture, paralytic instability, or scoliosis or following spinal surgery. The primary reason for considering a TLSO is to restrict lower thoracic, midthoracic and lumbosacral movement. TLSOs are not as frequently prescribed as are cervical or lumbosacral appliances, probably because of the cumbersome quality, cost, and lack of scientific evidence of efficacy of most TLSOs.

Fitting a rigid orthosis is relatively difficult, particularly to make the orthosis tolerable when the client is sitting. The plastic retains body heat; consequently a cotton undershirt worn under the orthosis is necessary to protect the skin and absorb perspiration.

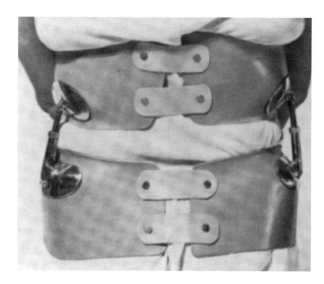

Fig. 12.1. Experimental LSO (body jacket), investigated by the Veterans Administration in the early 1970s, using adjustable distraction as a stimulus to withdrawal encouraging postural unloading of the lumbar spine. *(Bul Prosthet Res 10-18:79, 1972.)*

Types of thoracolumbosacral orthoses

TLSO: triplanar control (plastic jacket). The TLSO: triplanar control is a semirigid plastic jacket extending from the lower ribs to the groin, with a marked indentation over each iliac crest. Anterior horizontal straps provide closure. The posterior portion is molded to reduce lumbar lordosis; models range from 0 to 30 degrees lumbar lordosis.[61] The Veterans Administration Prosthetic Center (VAPC) LSO encircles the lower torso with semirigid plastic molded into an upper and a lower portion, joined by threaded metal posts. The orthosis is intended to unweight lumbar disks by supporting the lower thorax.[80] An independent clinical trial confirmed that it provided pain relief to most patients who had chronic lumbosacral pain (Fig. 12.1).[77]

Other rigid TLSOs. Framelike devices include TLSO flexion control (Jewett), flexion-extension control (Taylor), and flexion-extension-lateral control (Knight Taylor).[48,88,91] As compared with the plastic jacket, these orthoses are less restrictive, lighter in weight, allow more air circulation, and are less expensive.

LUMBOSACRAL ORTHOSES (LSO)

Low back pain may resolve with the use of a corset. Corsets for relief of low back pain are popular among orthopedists,[75] physiatrists,[20] and patients.[1,2,59] Some individuals, however, respond better to the greater restriction provided by a rigid LSO. At present, despite abundant anecdotal evidence, few scientific studies support the use of orthoses for relief of low back pain.[86]

For maximum restriction of lumbosacral motion, the orthosis requires a thigh cuff. Most LSOs are mass produced and then custom adjusted to suit the physique of a given client.

Therapeutic rationale

Refinement of diagnostic procedures to establish the organic basis of low back pain[92] should aid clinicians in selecting appropriate therapeutic interventions, including orthoses. Definition of the desired outcome of treatment for low back pain is essential for rational management, especially in view of the rarity of complete cure.[17] For example, an orthosis may contribute to the patient's willingness to return to work; although one can record the number of work days lost as the outcome measure, it remains exceedingly difficult to ascribe resumption of usual activity specifically to the use of a particular orthosis. Nevertheless, one can analyze orthotic design to suggest probable advantages.

Lumbosacral corsets and rigid orthoses may provide the following therapeutic benefits:

- Motion restriction
- Abdominal compression
- Muscle relaxation
- Postural realignment

As with orthotic management of the neck and thorax, lumbosacral corsets and rigid orthoses help the client avoid motion that might be irritative. They may foster more normal vertebral alignment.[15,52,95] Motion control is achieved through three-point systems, in which a force in one direction is balanced by two opposite forces that the orthosis applies above and below the first force. Fluid compression contributes to resting and unloading the spine.[97]

In laboratory testing of isolated trunk motions, the corset reduced lumbar intervertebral movement by approximately a quarter[71] to a third,[21] particularly flexion and lateral flexion.[49] A posterior plate in the orthosis increased pain relief, without altering trunk motion.[64] Subjects with and without back pain could move through approximately the same range whether wearing an elastic or fabric corset or a lumbosacral corset.[26,73] When performing functional tasks, individuals wearing a corset exhibited more trunk flexion whether or not they had back pain.[29] Perhaps the corset gave the subjects confidence that activity would not be injurious. One would assume that restriction of lumbar movement would compel the individual to improve body mechanics when lifting, using the hips and knees rather than flexing the trunk. Trunk flexion increases the demand on the erector spinae to maintain postural equilibrium and imposes relatively high intervertebral pressure. Reducing flexion is desirable to lessen the load on the lumbar spine. A corset, being less restrictive, allows the client to regain mobility faster; it should be discontinued as soon as possible in favor of an active exercise program[8,27,81] or used in conjunction with therapeutic exercise.[9,10,66] Orthotic support, however, tends to increase movement at the lumbosacral level.[53,73]

Corsets and most rigid LSOs increase intra-abdominal pressure, which may lessen the demand on the erector spinae to maintain upright posture.[4,66–69] Muscle relaxation reduces painful spasm. Effectiveness of trunk orthoses is limited by physical and psychological dependence.[26] Intra-abdominal pressure is raised by corsets and rigid frame and jacket-type orthoses.[26,46] The precise role of intra-abdominal pressure has been questioned.[57] Without an orthosis, the abdominal muscles convert the abdomen into a nearly rigid-walled cylinder that contributes substantially to trunk support, especially when one lifts heavy weights. Intra-abdominal pressure increases when one lifts heavy loads and is assumed to reduce load on the vertebral column.[69] Abdominal muscle contraction increases intra-abdominal pressure but also creates a flexion moment that must be counteracted by the back extensors, magnifying disk compression. Abdominal action may therefore serve primarily to stiffen the trunk, enabling one to withstand high compressive loads and resist shearing at the facet joints.[44] Orthoses have been shown to reduce intradiscal pressures when healthy subjects wearing corsets or rigid orthoses bent forward.[71,72]

LSOs, whether rigid or flexible, reduce erector spinae, transversospinalis, and abdominal muscle activity with normal subjects at rest and when walking at moderate pace; rapid walking, however, is associated with increased rotatores activity among those wearing the rigid LSO, probably because the wearer has to overcome orthotic restriction of transverse trunk rotation, necessary in normal gait.[94] The corset may decrease muscle spasm, which splints the inflamed low back. Healthy subjects exhibited similar myoelectric activity in the erector spinae whether wearing a corset or a rigid appliance while performing standardized tasks; in some activities, muscular contraction increased, whereas in other activities, muscle contraction decreased regardless of type of orthosis.[50,72] Abdominal muscle activity reduces when one wears a corset.[68] Results from these brief laboratory studies should not be extrapolated to long-term orthotic wear, particularly among individuals who have healthy musculature. Clients with pain may relax into the orthosis, reducing antagonistic muscle activity.

Orthoses may foster postural changes that alleviate pain. Lumbar flexion shifts the weight of the trunk, head, and arms forward, away from irritated posterior vertebral and neural structures. Flexion also reduces intervertebral shear forces.[12]

Obese clients with weak abdominal muscles and elderly individuals with vertebral compression fractures may feel more comfortable with a corset.[8] Other indications for corsets include acute and chronic osteochondrosis, muscle strain, degenerative disk disease, osteoporotic fracture, and low back pain owing to pregnancy.[83] The corset must be designed and fitted so that the wearer does not experience local pressure at the groin or breasts from vertical metal stays.

Although clients complaining of low back pain but having no evidence of radiculopathy had greater pain relief with spinal manipulation as compared with those who wore corsets,[15,28,38,40] one must recognize that, regardless of treatment, with time most low back disorders are likely to heal. Audiofeedback[29] and back schools[36] are other alternatives that may be more efficacious than corsets.

Increasing popularity of elastic abdominal belts as prophylaxis for industrial workers and health care personnel who lift patients is based on wearers' perceptions of improved trunk stability (Fig. 12.2). Objective measurements of intra-abdominal pressure and muscular activity are not consistent. The belt or a lumbosacral corset had minimal effect on abdominal pressure and muscular activity,[58] was associated with higher pressure,[30] or was associated with an increase in abdominal strength and fewer days lost from work.[93] The belt reminds the worker to restrict trunk flexion and rotation and offers a sense of security. Belts are prescribed for postpartum, posttraumatic, and arthritic pain in the sacroiliac region. The sacroiliac belt causes slight posterior pelvic tilt, keeping the lumbosacral joint from excessive movement in the end range of extension, and approximates the posterior lumbopelvic tissues, adding to stabilization.[76]

A rigid LSO, or low-profile TLSO, provides intermediate restriction, as compared with corset and thoracolumbosacral jacket, and may be more effective.[64] The orthosis encompasses the lower ribs and thus is more accurately designated as a TLSO; however, it is considerably shorter than the usual TLSO. Extension is controlled more than flexion.[49] A rigid orthosis is recommended for severe osteochondrosis, arthrosis of facet joints, and spondylolisthesis.[83] An orthosis may be prescribed to relieve pain aggravated by exaggerated lordosis and relieved when the client sits or bends forward[37] or for control of excessive lordosis.[91] The orthosis creates a flexion attitude in the lumbar area that induces extensor activity at the hips and dorsal spine, thereby reducing lordosis.[9]

Favorable results have been achieved with a plastic jacket worn by clients with pain resulting from athletic back injuries, spondylosis, spondylolysis, spondylolisthesis, apophyseal fractures, and disk disease.[61,87,95] Reducing lordosis with the jacket set in flexion pro-

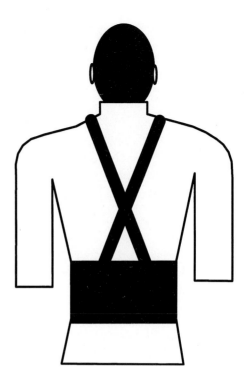

Fig. 12.2. Commonly applied LSO (elastic abdominal binder with suspenders) offers a kinesthetic reminder to workers but does not restrict undesired motion. Prophylactic value and the effect on intra-abdominal pressure are equivocal.

motes healing of pars defects via immobilization and decreased sagittal plane shear stresses. The antilordotic posture decreases vertical inclination of lower lumbar interspaces, thereby decreasing shear stress.[12,87] Plastic lumbosacral jackets promote substantial reduction of segmental sagittal motility of the lumbosacral spine.[21]

Types of lumbosacral orthoses

Corsets. Corsets, fabric garments encircling the torso, have been worn for centuries by men and women as part of everyday dress to create a fashionably narrow waist and slim silhouette.[84] The contemporary therapeutic corset is made of lightweight canvas or similar sturdy fabric or of elastic.[45] It has rather straight vertical contours. Vertical reinforcing stays are often used to prevent the upper margin from curling away from the trunk. In the front, the lumbosacral corset extends from a point just below the xiphoid process to a point just above the pubic symphysis. The corset covers the back from a point immediately below the scapulae to the gluteal fold.[25] As is the case with the rigid LSO, because the lumbosacral corset covers the lower thorax, it may be more accurately designated as a low-profile thoracolumbosacral corset. It may include a posterior reinforcement in the form of a rigid thermoplastic plate that is custom-molded to the client.[64] Perineal straps are included in men's corsets to prevent the garment from

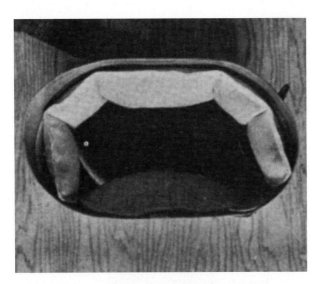

Fig. 12.3. Top view of custom-molded TLSO (body jacket) with inflatable pads allowing patient to control the amount of pressure applied. First reported in 1973, such devices are now available commercially in prefabricated sizes. *(From Morris JM, Markolf KL, Hittenberger H: Semiflexible body jacket with inflatable pads, Bull Prosthet Res 10-20:227, 1973.)*

sliding upward when the wearer bends forward; many individuals, however, find the straps uncomfortable and remove them. Women's corsets usually are manufactured with garters to be clipped to stockings; garters also prevent the corset from displacing upward.

The sacroiliac corset, also known as the abdominal belt, covers the pelvis extending from the iliac crests to the pubic symphysis and gluteal fold.[47] The sacroiliac belt, also known as a lumbopelvic support or trochanteric belt, encircles the torso at the level of the sacroiliac joints, between the iliac crests and the greater trochanters. It often includes a pad over the sacrum.[76]

Rigid orthoses. In contrast to a corset, which has no horizontal reinforcement, rigid trunk orthoses include rigid plastic or upholstered metal horizontal and vertical bands. Orthoses prescribed for pain relief typically include at least a pelvic and thoracic band. The bands should lie flat on the torso and should terminate at the lateral midline. Many variants have been described in the literature.

The framelike construction of such trunk orthoses makes them cooler alternatives to corsets. Because the pelvis tilts when one moves from standing to sitting, it is important that the orthosis be fitted in the seated position when the pelvis is posteriorly tilted to avoid undue pressure by the posterior uprights. Rigid orthoses, however, are more expensive than corsets.

A variant may include inflatable pads in the back (Air-Back Spinal System, Orthomerica Products, Inc.) or front, or both aspects, enabling the client or the clinician to adjust the snugness of the orthosis (Fig. 12.3).[70,77] LSOs may also be custom-molded.[7,90] Commercial versions, such as the Boston Overlap Brace,[61,62] Raney flexion jacket,[78] and Flexaform,[95] are also available.

CONCLUSIONS

Although various designs of orthoses are used to ameliorate pain in the neck, thorax, and low back, it is evident that prescription is based largely on empiric data or anecdotal comment, with little scientific evidence to support or refute indications for a specific version. Regardless of design, however, prolonged use of spinal orthoses is associated with psychological dependence and physical changes, including muscle weakness and joint stiffness. Clearly, although much remains to be done to establish valid prescription criteria,[5,16,19,86,89] based on scientifically rigorous research[39,82] and analysis,[35] the current state-of-the-art indicates that some patients do achieve a measure of pain relief from the use of spinal orthoses.

REFERENCES

1. Ahlgren SA, Hansen T: The use of lumbosacral corsets prescribed for low back pain, Prosthet Orthot Int 2:101–104, 1978.
2. Alaranta H, Hurri H: Compliance and subjective relief by corset treatment in chronic low back pain, Scand J Rehabil Med 20:133–136, 1980.
3. Althoff B, Goldie IF: Cervical collars in rheumatoid atlanto-axial subluxation: A radiographic comparison. Ann Rheum Dis 39:485–489, 1980.
4. Bartelink DL: The role of abdominal pressure in relieving the pressure on the lumbar intervertebral discs. J Bone Joint Surg 39B:718–725, 1957.
5. Battie MC, Cherkin DC, Dunn R, et al: Managing low back pain: Attitudes and treatment preferences of physical therapists, Phys Ther 74:219–226, 1994.
6. Beavis A: Cervical orthoses, Prosthet Orthot Int 13:6–13, 1989.
7. Bertrand ST, Walters DC: A new orthosis for selective use in low back pain, Arch Phys Med Rehabil 74:1269, 1993 (Abstract).
8. Borenstein DG, Wiesel SW: Low back pain: Medical diagnosis and comprehensive management, Philadelphia, 1989, WB Saunders.
9. Bunch WH, Keagy RD: Principles of orthotic treatment, St. Louis, 1976, CV Mosby.
10. Cailliet R: Biomechanics of the spine, Phys Med Rehabil Clin North Am 3:1–28, 1992.
11. Cailliet R, Neck and arm pain, ed 3, Philadelphia, 1991, FA Davis.
12. Chase A, Pearcy M, Bader D: Spinal orthoses. In Bowker P, et al, editors: Biomechanical basis of orthotic management, Oxford, 1993, Butterworth Heinemann.
13. Colachis SC, Strohm BR, Ganter EL: Cervical spine motion in normal women: Radiographic study of effect of cervical collars, Arch Phys Med Rehabil 54:161–169, 1973.
14. Covery P: Orthoses for head and neck. In Bowker P, et al, editors: Biomechanical basis of orthotic management, Oxford, 1993, Butterworth Heinemann.
15. Coxhead CE, et al: Multicentre trial of physiotherapy in the management of sciatic symptoms, Lancet 1:1065–1068, 1981.

16. Delitto A: Are measures of function and disability important in low back care? Phys Ther 74:452–462, 1994.

17. Deyo RA, et al: Outcome measures for studying patients with low back pain, Spine 19:2032S–2036S, 1994.

18. Dudgeon P: The effectiveness of cervical orthoses: The patients' viewpoint, Br J Occup Ther 47:242–250, 1984.

19. Edelman B: Federal agency to draft low back pain guidelines, Orthop Today 12:1, 1992.

20. Fast A: Low back disorders: Conservative management, Arch Phys Med Rehabil 69:880–891, 1988.

21. Fidler MW, Plasmans CMT: The effect of four types of support on the segmental mobility of the lumbosacral spine, J Bone Joint Surg 65A:943–947, 1983.

22. Fisher SV: Cervical orthotics, Phys Med Rehabil Clin North Am 3:29–44, 1992.

23. Fisher SV: Proper fitting of the cervical orthosis, Arch Phys Med Rehabil 59:505–507, 1978.

24. Fisher SV, et al: Cervical orthoses effect on cervical spine motion: Roentgenographic and goniometric method of study, Arch Phys Med Rehabil 58:109–115, 1977.

25. Fishman S, et al: Spinal orthoses. In American Academy of Orthopaedic Surgeons: Atlas of orthotics, ed 2, St. Louis, 1985; CV Mosby.

26. Grew ND, Deane G: The physical effect of lumbar spinal supports, Prosthet Orthot Int 6:79–87, 1982.

27. Hadler NM: Diagnosis and treatment of backache. In Hadler NM, editor: Medical management of the regional musculoskeletal diseases, New York, 1984, Grune & Stratton.

28. Hadler NW, et al: A benefit of spinal manipulation as adjunctive therapy for acute low-back pain: A stratified controlled trial, Spine 12:703–706, 1987.

29. Haig AJ, et al: The relative effectiveness of lumbosacral corset and trunk inclination audio biofeedback on trunk flexion, PMR 2:29–37, 1991.

30. Harman EA, et al: Effects of a belt on intra-abdominal pressure during weight lifting, Med Sci Sports Exerc 21:186–190, 1989.

31. Harris JD: Cervical orthoses. In Redford JB, editor: Orthotics etcetera, ed 3, Baltimore, 1983, Williams & Wilkins.

32. Hart DL: Spinal immobility: Braces and corsets. In Gould JA, editor: Orthopaedic and sports physical therapy, ed 2, St. Louis, 1990, CV Mosby.

33. Hart DL, et al: Review of cervical orthoses, Phys Ther 58:857–861, 1978.

34. Hartman JT, Palumbo F, Hill BJ: Cineradiography of the braced normal spine: A comparative study of five commonly used cervical orthoses, Clin Orthop 107:97–102, 1975.

35. Haselkorn JK, et al: Meta-analysis: A useful tool for the spine researcher, Spine 19:2076S–2082S, 1994.

36. Hayne CR: The use of spinal supports and education in back pain, Practitioner 227:1069–1073, 1983.

37. Hipps HE: Back braces: Types, functions and how to order and use them, Med Clin North Am 51:1315–1343, 1967.

38. Hoehler FK, Tobis JS: Appropriate statistical methods for clinical trials of spinal manipulation, Spine 12:409–411, 1987.

39. Hoffman RM, et al: Therapeutic trials for low back pain, Spine 19:2068S–2075S, 1994.

40. Hsieh CJ, et al: Functional outcomes of low back pain: Comparison of four treatment groups in a randomized controlled trial, J Manipu Physiol Ther 15:4–9, 1992.

41. Johnson RM, et al: Cervical orthoses: A study comparing their effectiveness in restricting cervical motion in normal subjects, J Bone Joint Surg 59A:332–339, 1977.

42. Johnson RM, et al: The Yale cervical orthosis: An evaluation of its effectiveness in restricting cervical motion in normal subjects and a comparison with other cervical orthoses, Phys Ther 58:865–871, 1978.

43. Jones MD: Cineroentgenographic studies of the collar-immobilized cervical spine, J Neurosurg 17:633–637, 1960.

44. Kaufman WA, et al: Comparison of three prefabricated cervical collars, Orthot Prosthet 39:27–28, 1986.

45. Kirkaldy-Willis WH, Read SE: An elastic support for the lumbar and lumbosacral spine, Clin Orthop 59:131–135, 1968.

46. Krag MH, et al: The effect of back braces on the relationship between intra-abdominal pressure and spinal loads, Adv Bioeng 2:22–23, 1986.

47. Kumar VN: Corsets and soft supports. In Redford JB, editor: Orthotics etcetera, ed 3, Baltimore, 1986, Williams & Wilkins.

48. Lambert GH, Nattress LW: A survey of spinal bracing, J Bone Joint Surg 46A:1146–1150, 1964.

49. Lantz SA, Schultz AB: Lumbar spine orthosis wearing: I. Restriction of gross body motions, Spine 11:834–837, 1986.

50. Lantz SA, Schultz AB: Lumbar spine orthosis wearing: II. Effect on trunk muscle myoelectric activity, Spine 11:838–842, 1986.

51. Lewin P: Cotton collar: A physical therapeutic agent, JAMA 155:1155–1156, 1954.

52. Lucas DB, Jacobs RR, Trautman P: Spinal orthotics for pain and instability. In Redford JB, editor: Orthotics etcetera, ed 3, Baltimore, 1986, Williams & Wilkins.

53. Lumsden RM, Morris JM: An in vivo study of axial rotation and immobilization at the lumbosacral joint, J Bone Joint Surg 50A:1591–1602, 1968.

54. Lunsford TR, Davidson M, Lunsford BR: The effectiveness of four contemporary cervical orthoses in restricting cervical motion, J Prosthet Orthot 6:93–99, 1994.

55. Lusskin R, Berger N: Prescription principles. In American Academy of Orthopaedic Surgeons: Atlas of orthotics, St. Louis, 1975, CV Mosby.

56. Marsolais EB: Spinal pain. In American Academy of Orthopaedic Surgeons: Atlas of orthotics, ed 2, St. Louis, 1985, CV Mosby.

57. McGill SM, Norman RW: Reassessment of the role of intra-abdominal pressure in spinal compression, Ergonomics 30:1565–1588, 1987.

58. McGill SM, Norman RW, Sharratt MT: The effect of an abdominal belt on trunk muscle activity and intra-abdominal pressure during squat lifts, Ergonomics 33:147–160, 1990.

59. McKenzie AR, Lipscomb PR: Corsets on and off, J Bone Joint Surg 61B:384, 1979 (abstract).

60. Mealy K, Brennan H, Fenelon GCC: Early mobilisation of acute whiplash injuries. BMJ 292:656–657, 1986.

61. Micheli LJ: The use of modified Boston brace system (B.O.B.) for back pain: Clinical indications, Orthot Prosthet 39:41–46, 1985.

62. Micheli LJ, Hall JE, Miller ME: Use of modified Boston brace for back injuries in athletes, Am J Sports Med 8:351–359, 1980.

63. Michlovitz SL: Thermal agents in rehabilitation, ed 2, Philadelphia, 1986, FA Davis.

64. Million R, et al: Evaluation of low back pain and assessment of lumbar corsets with and without back supports, Ann Rheum Dis 40:449–454, 1981.

65. Moncur C, Williams HJ: Cervical spine management in patients with rheumatoid arthritis: Review of the literature, Phys Ther 68:509–515, 1988.

66. Morris JM: Biomechanics of the spine, Arch Surg 107:418–423, 1973.

67. Morris JM: Low back bracing, Clin Orthop 102:126–132, 1974.

68. Morris JM, Lucas DB: Biomechanics of spinal bracing, Ariz Med 21:170–176, 1964.

69. Morris JM, Lucas DB, Bresler B: Role of the trunk in stability of the spine, J Bone Joint Surg 43A:327–351, 1961.

70. Morris JM, Markolf KL, Hittenberger H: Semiflexible body jacket with inflatable pads, Bull Prosthet Res 10-20:222–227, 1973.

71. Nachemson A, Morris JM: In vivo measurement of intradiscal pressure: Discometry, a method for the determination of pressure in the lower lumbar discs, J Bone Joint Surg A:1077–1092, 1964.

72. Nachemson A, Schultz A, Andersson G: Mechanical effectiveness studies of lumbar spine orthoses, Scand J Rehabil Med suppl 9:139–149, 1983.

73. Norton PL, Brown T: The immobilizing efficiency of back braces: Their effect on the posture and motion of the lumbosacral spine, J Bone Joint Surg 39A:111–138, 1957.

74. Pellicci PM, et al: A prospective study of the progression of rheumatoid arthritis of the cervical spine, J Bone Joint Surg 63A:342–350, 1981.

75. Perry J: The use of external support in the treatment of low back pain, J Bone Joint Surg 52A:1440–1442, 1970.

76. Porterfield JA: Dynamic stabilization of the trunk, J Orthop Sports Phys Ther 6:271–276, 1985.

77. Quigley MJ: Evaluation of two experimental spinal orthoses. Orthot Prosthet 28:23–41, 1974.

78. Raney F: Royalite flexion jacket, Report on the Spinal Orthotics Workshop sponsored by the Committee on Prosthetics Research and Development of the Division of Engineering of the National Research Council, Washington, 1969, National Research Council.

79. Rose GK: Orthotics: Principles and practice, London, 1986, Heinemann.

80. Rubin G, Greenbaum W, Molack D: The VAPC lumbosacral orthosis, Orthot Prosthet 28:9–22, 1974.

81. Russek AS: Biomechanical and physiological basis for ambulatory treatment of low back pain, Orthop Rev 4:21–26, 1976.

82. Ruta DA, et al: Developing a valid and reliable measure of health outcome for patients with low back pain, Spine 19:1887–1896, 1994.

83. Schroeder S, et al: Bracing and supporting of the lumbar spine, Prosthet Orthot Int 6:139–146, 1982.

84. Schwartz GS: Society, physicians and the corset, Bull NY Acad Med 55:551–590, 1979.

85. Smith PH, Benn RT, Sharp J: Natural history of rheumatoid cervical luxations, Ann Rheum Dis 31:431–439, 1972.

86. Spitzer WO, et al: Scientific approach to the assessment and management of activity-related spinal disorders, Spine 12(suppl 7):S1–S59, 1987.

87. Steiner ME, Micheli LJ: Treatment of symptomatic spondylolysis and spondylolisthesis with the modified Boston brace, Spine 10:937–943, 1985.

88. Stillo JV, Stein AB, Ragnarsson KT: Low-back orthoses, Phys Med Rehabil Clin North Am 3:57–94, 1992.

89. Stratford PW, et al: Assessing change over time in patients with low back pain, Phys Ther 74:528–533, 1994.

90. Turner MS, Carus DA, Troup IM: Custom moulded plastic spinal orthoses, Prosthet Orthot Int 10:83–88, 1986.

91. von Werssowetz OF: Back braces and supports, Clin Orthop 5:169–183, 1955.

92. Waddell G, et al: Objective clinical evaluation of physical impairment in chronic low back pain, Spine 17:617–628, 1993.

93. Walsh NE, Schwartz RK: The influence of prophylactic orthoses on abdominal strength and low back injury in the workplace, Am J Phys Med Rehabil 69:245–250, 1990.

94. Waters RL, Morris JM: Effect of spinal supports on the electrical activity of muscles of the trunk, J Bone Joint Surg 52A:51–60, 1970.

95. White AA, Panjabi MM: Clinical biomechanics of the spine, Philadelphia, 1978, JB Lippincott.

96. Willner S: Effect of a rigid brace on back pain, Acta Orthop Scand 56:40–42, 1985.

97. Williams PC: The lumbosacral spine, New York, 1965, McGraw-Hill.

C H A P T E R
13

Orthoses for Spinal Trauma and Postoperative Care

Courtney W. Brown
Gregory H. Chow

The use of orthoses following surgery or spinal trauma varies considerably depending on the type of surgery or injury that has occurred and whether or not surgical stabilization has been performed. As new and better methods of internal fixation of the spine have been developed, the need for rigid external immobilization has decreased. This chapter discusses the orthoses that are used for nonsurgical treatment of spinal injuries as well as those that are used for external immobilization following surgery.

SPINAL TRAUMA

Orthoses serve several purposes in the treatment of spinal trauma. The external support of the orthoses can help to reduce pain as well as provide some added stability while fractures and soft tissue injuries heal. In addition, orthoses can help to prevent deformity during the healing phase of the injury. The duration of time that an orthosis is used depends largely on the function it is serving. Bracing for symptomatic reasons in patients with stable fractures or only minor soft tissue trauma can be discontinued when the patient can tolerate the discomfort without the brace. In cases of unstable fractures and significant ligamentous disruptions, the orthosis is used for a minimum of 6 weeks to allow time for bone healing and may sometimes be continued up to 3 months.

Patients who suffer suspected cervical spine trauma are usually first treated by emergency medical technicians. Paramedics and rescue workers generally use prefabricated cervical collars such as those shown in Fig. 13.1. These devices are satisfactory for temporary immobilization; however, supplemental immobilization with sandbags on both sides of the head and taping the head to a backboard while in these collars is generally necessary to restrict rotation. This method of immobilization using the collar and sandbags is usually continued throughout the emergency evaluation. Depending on the severity of the injury, a variety of orthoses are available to the treating physician. The different types of orthoses differ widely in the amount of immobilization provided as well as in the amount of discomfort and inconvenience the patient experiences.

The standard soft cervical collar (Fig. 13.2), which is made of foam rubber and covered with a cotton stockinette, is generally considered to be the most comfortable of all the cervical orthoses. The soft collar, however, has been shown to provide almost no immobilization, allowing up to 75% to 80% of normal motion of the cervical spine.[2] Therefore, a soft cervical collar should not be used for any injury that involves significant damage to the ligamentous or bony structures of the cervical spine. The use of these collars is controversial in patients who suffer hyperextension injuries or muscular or ligamentous strain injuries to the cervical spine. Although the soft cervical collar may provide some symptomatic relief, there is also some concern that the use of such a device may lead to disuse atrophy of the cervical muscles and thus to prolonged impairment from these injuries.

Hard cervical collars, such as the Miami, Malibu, Philadelphia, and Turtle collars (Fig. 13.3) are designed to provide more rigid stabilization of the cervical spine. These collars have a molded chin support as well as an occipital support. The lower portion of the collar extends down across the upper thorax to about the level of the sternal notch anteriorly and down to about the T3 spinous process posteriorly. Experimental studies on normal subjects have shown that the Philadelphia collar allows for approximately 30% of normal flexion and extension, approximately 44% of normal rotation, and as much as 66% of normal lateral bending.[2] These different types of hard cervical collars differ in the amount of rigid or semirigid plastic or metal supports

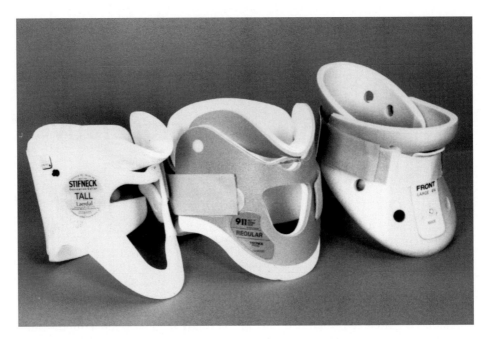

Fig. 13.1.   Hard cervical collars commonly used in emergency situations. *Left to right:* Stifneck (Laederl), 911 Collar (Technol), and Philadelphia Collar (Depuy).

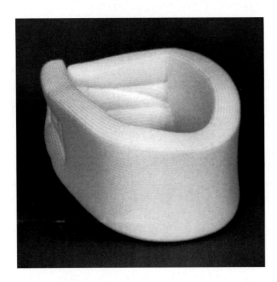

Fig. 13.2.   Soft cervical collar.

that they contain. The collars that contain more rigid plastic support, such as the Turtle collar, probably provide better protection against rotation.

A variety of cervicothoracic orthoses (CTOs) (Fig. 13.4) are available. These devices are designed to hold the head immobile by controlling the chin and the occiput and then provide fixation to the trunk with a combination of a chest and back plate, which are then connected to the head support. The CTOs come in a variety of different designs. The SOMI brace consists of a rigid metal frame with padded shoulder straps and a strap that goes around the trunk. The chin and occipital supports are connected to the chest piece

using metal bars and straps. Some of the CTOs use four metal posts to connect the chin and occipital supports to the chest piece; some also use rigid or semirigid pieces of plastic. The size of the chest piece of the various CTO designs is also quite variable. Depending on the size of the chest piece, the various CTOs can eliminate flexion and extension by as much as 70% to 85%. Rotation can be eliminated by as much as 65% to 80%, and lateral bending can be eliminated by as much as 45% to 55%.[2] The hard cervical collars and the CTOs provide better immobilization between the occiput and C4 than they do in the lower cervical spine from C4 to T1. The CTOs tend to provide better immobilization while patients are standing rather than lying down because of the fit of the chest piece.

The best immobilization of the cervical spine is provided by the halo-vest apparatus (Fig. 13.5). The halo-vest apparatus consists of a cranial ring that is attached to the skull using pins (Fig. 13.5, *A*). This ring is then attached by rigid bars to a vest, which goes around the patient's thorax. The halo eliminates as much as 90% to 95% of the normal motion of the cervical spine.[2] Most of the motion that does take place with halo immobilization comes from the lower cervical spine segments from C4 to T1.

The original halo devices were made of a steel cranial ring, steel pins, and metal bars. The vests were fabricated out of plaster and rigidly fixed to the rings. Although the well-molded plaster vest probably provides better immobilization than the modern prefabricated plastic vest, client acceptance of the plaster vest has been poor. In addition, skin problems because of

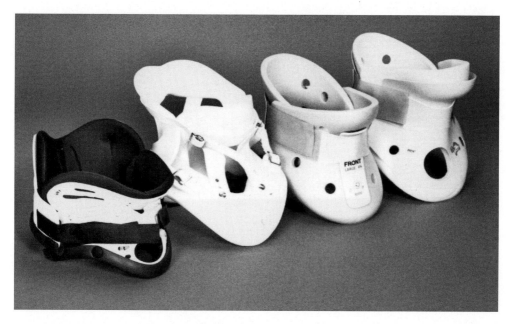

Fig. 13.3.   Hard cervical collars for traumatic cervical instability and postoperative management. *Left to right:* Miami collar, Malibu collar, Philadelphia collar, and Turtle collar.

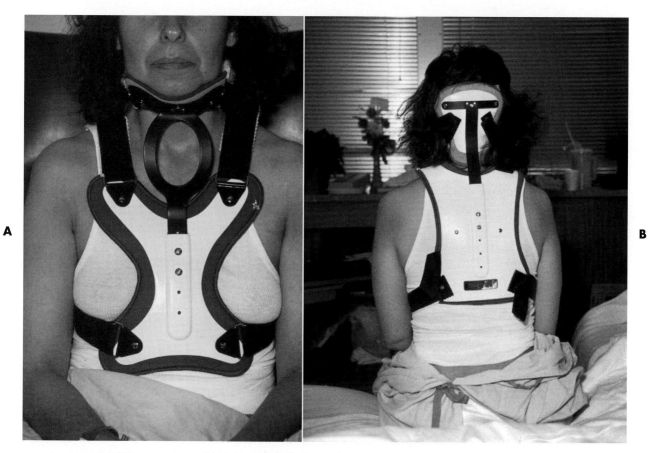

A   B

Fig. 13.4.   **A** and **B,** CTO as seen from the front and back, respectively. The chest and back pieces are strapped to the client and then connected to the head support by way of rigid plastic pieces.

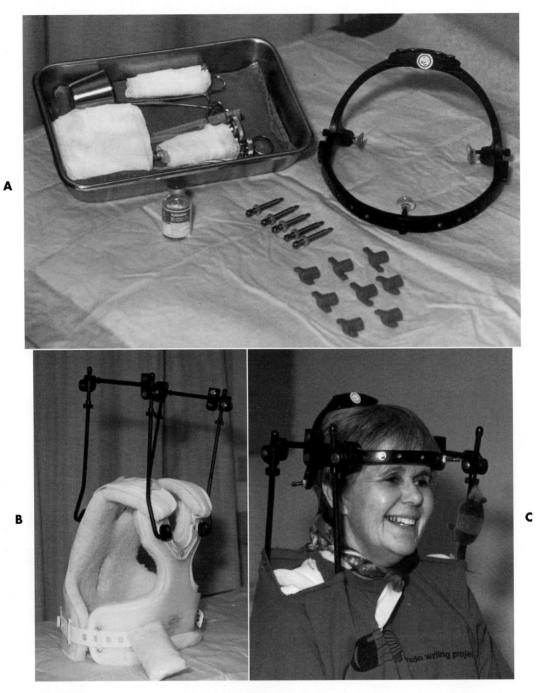

Fig. 13.5.   Halo-vest apparatus. **A,** Halo ring and pins and equipment needed for pin insertion. **B,** Halo-vest. **C,** Halo-vest apparatus in use.

pressure sores are not uncommon, particularly in patients with impaired sensation such as those with spinal cord injury. For these reasons, it is common to use the modern prefabricated plastic vest along with rings, pins, and bars (Fig. 13.5, *B,* and *C*), which are made of carbon fiber or titanium, thus enabling magnetic resonance imaging of the cervical spine with the halo apparatus in place. Occasionally a custom-made plastic thoracolumbosacral orthosis (TLSO) (body jacket) may be used for

more intimate control of the thorax, with the halo superstructure added for cervical immobilization.

Although the halo device does provide the best immobilization, it is also the least accepted by patients and also has been associated with a fairly high rate of complications. Garfin et al[1] in a review of 179 patients found that pin loosening occurred in 36%; pin infections in 20%; skin problems in 11%; and more urgent complications, such as dysphasia, nerve injury, and dural penetration, 1% to 2% of patients. In light of these complications, the treating physician must determine whether the risk of such complications warrants the benefit of the additional immobilization provided by the halo. Certain injuries, such as the facet fractures with dislocation or subluxation, may not be effectively realigned and immobilized even with the halo device because the halo vest cannot produce traction.[5]

Surgical stabilization of the spine can be accomplished with an anterior fusion, a posterior fusion, or both. A variety of internal fixation devices exist for improving the stability of the cervical spine. These devices include anterior cervical plates, posterior lateral mass plates, and wires and cables. If these internal fixation devices can be used effectively, the use of a less restrictive orthosis is possible. Occasionally, with unstable injuries, patients may require both surgical stabilization and external halo vest immobilization. In most surgical cases, however, immobilization with a hard collar is adequate. The duration of immobilization depends on the amount of time needed for healing and the adequacy of internal fixation. Often, in the immediate postoperative period, a more rigid form or immobilization is used, and then as healing progresses, it may be possible to change to either a Philadelphia collar or a soft collar.

THORACIC AND THORACOLUMBAR FRACTURES

Thoracic fractures from T2 to T9 have the benefit of internal immobilization from the rib cage. In the absence of rib and sternal fractures, fractures of the thoracic spine in this region are inherently stable. Below T10, however, the rib cage becomes less effective in immobilizing the thoracic spine. Fractures from T10 to L2 require internal or external immobilization to prevent collapse and deformity and possible neurologic injury.

There are two basic types of orthoses available for the thoracic and thoracolumbar spine. The first is the simple three-point pressure TLSOs such as the Jewett (Fig. 13.6) or cruciform anterior spinal hyperextension (CASH) braces (Fig. 13.7).[4] These consist of a front chest piece that has pads that contact the patient at the sternum and at the symphysis pubis; a third pad goes across the back and attaches to the rigid chest piece with a strap. The Jewett brace shown in Fig. 13.6 has a gibbus pad posteriorly, which is relieved in the midline to avoid direct pressure over the posterior elements of the spine or the incision. The pad across the back provides an anterior force, whereas the pads at the sternum and symphysis pubis provide a posterior force. This three-point contact is most effective at preventing

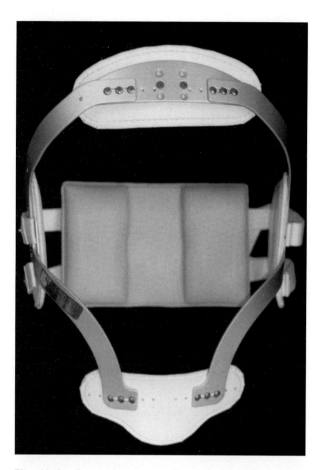

Fig. 13.6. Jewett hyperextension orthosis with posterior gibbus pad to relieve pressure directly over the incision or posterior elements.

forward flexion of the thoracic spine. The Jewett brace is most effective in preventing flexion and extension between T6 and L1. Above T6, the sternal pad may act as a fulcrum and actually increase the amount of motion in the upper thoracic spine. Clinically the Jewett appears to be more effective than the CASH.

The second type of orthosis is the more encompassing TLSO (Fig. 13.8), which can be either prefabricated or custom-molded.[4] The prefabricated TLSO provides a significant cost advantage over custom-molded devices. In addition, there is no significant time delay required for fitting the prefabricated brace. However, the prefabricated braces tend to be less comfortable and also less effective at providing support and control. The treating physician must determine how much support is necessary for the given injury and weigh this need against the difference in cost when determining whether to use a prefabricated or custom-molded TLSO.

The circumferential TLSO provides somewhat better immobilization of the thoracic and thoracolumbar spine than the three-point braces. The modern TLSO is usually made from a rigid plastic material and is

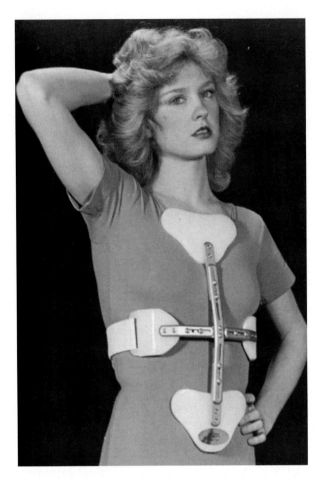

Fig. 13.7. CASH brace.

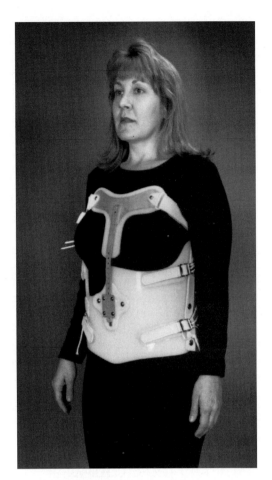

Fig. 13.8. A prefabricated TLSO.

usually designed to be a full contact brace. Because of the full contact design, it provides better immobilization of flexion and extension as well as rotation and lateral bending. If immobilization of the upper thoracic spine is necessary (above T7), it is possible to attach anterior shoulder outriggers to extend the TLSO to provide better immobilization in this region. If compliance is a significant concern, it should be noted that these braces are quite easily removed by patients. In such cases, a hyperextension plaster or fiberglass body cast for thoracic and thoracolumbar injuries may be used.

The Milwaukee brace is also an effective orthosis for immobilizing the upper thoracic as well as the midthoracic and thoracolumbar spines, particularly for managing idiopathic scoliosis.[4] Unfortunately, for patients with fractures, it tends to be uncomfortable, and acceptance is poor. For these reasons, it is rarely used in fracture cases. Following surgical stabilization of thoracic and thoracolumbar spine fractures, immobilization with a Jewett brace is usually sufficient. On some occasions, particularly with osteoporosis and compromised fixation, a circumferential TLSO may be needed.

LUMBAR FRACTURES

Fractures of the lumbar spine (L3-L5) may be stable or unstable. Stable fractures can be treated with a corset type of a brace for comfort. Lumbosacral corsets (Fig. 13.9) tend to be minimally restricting.[3] They are usually made of canvas or an elastic fabric. If more immobilization is necessary, some corsets can be supplemented with a rigid plastic insert, which can be custom-molded for the patient. The chair-back brace is probably most effective in controlling flexion and extension from L1 to L4. Lateral bending is also restricted with the chair-back brace; however, rotation is probably minimally limited.[3] The original rigid spinal orthoses such as the Knight-Taylor brace had rigid metal supports along the back and a canvas corset across the front. They have been supplanted in many cases by thermomolded variants. The modern chair-back Orthomold brace has a rigid plastic back piece that can be custom-molded for the patient (Fig. 13.10). The plastic back piece is then inserted into the canvas and elastic corset, which is then strapped around the patient.

A custom-molded TLSO or a Jewett brace may also

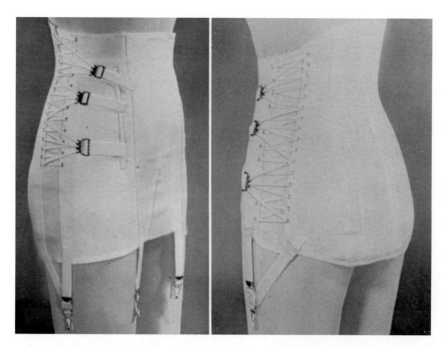

Fig. 13.9. Lumbosacral corset.

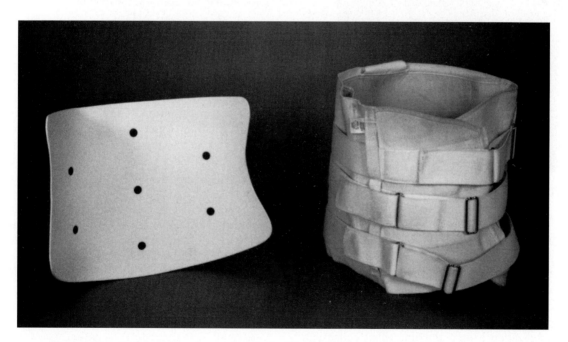

Fig. 13.10. Orthomold lumbosacral orthosis. The moldable rigid plastic insert *(left)* and the canvas corset with velcro strap closures *(right).*

be useful, particularly for injuries in the upper lumbar spine. The benefits and limitations of these orthoses in the lumbar spine are similar to those previously discussed in the thoracic and thoracolumbar spine.

There is some evidence that motion at the L5-S1 level may actually be increased by the use of a rigid lumbosacral orthosis.[3] If it is necessary to immobilize this level, the most effective external immobilization must incorporate one leg in the brace as well. This can be done either with a single leg spica cast that extends up to the lumbar region or with a leg extension added to a custom-molded TLSO (Fig. 13.11) or lumbosacral orthosis (LSO). Following surgical stabilization of lumbar fractures, a rigid LSO is usually sufficient for external immobilization. If added stability is needed, a TLSO may be used.

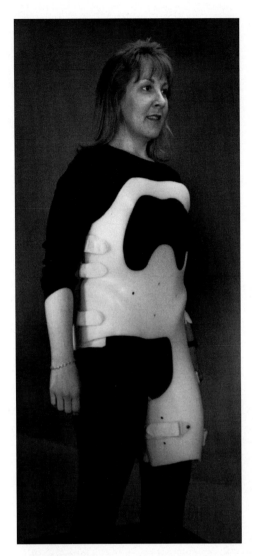

Fig. 13.11.   Custom-molded TLSO with single leg extension.

POSTOPERATIVE ORTHOSIS CARE

Cervical

The amount of bracing required after surgery varies and depends on the type of surgery performed. A single-level anterior interbody fusion needs only minimal immobilization. Most of the time, a hard collar such as a Philadelphia, Miami, or Turtle collar is used, but in certain cases when internal fixation is used, a soft collar may be sufficient. Usually, immobilization is continued until solid fusion is evident; typically in 6 to 8 weeks. If multiple levels of anterior diskectomy and fusion are performed, at least a rigid collar such as a Philadelphia or Turtle is suggested; if internal fixation is not used, the use of a CTO or halo may be indicated. If internal fixation with an anterior cervical plate is used and stable fixation is obtained, a soft cervical collar alone may be

adequate in the postoperative period. A halo is rarely needed following surgery for degenerative cervical spine disease. Use of a halo is usually reserved for special circumstances, such as correction of deformity, multilevel corpectomy and strut grafting, cases in which there is posterior instability, and in cases with compromised fixation.

Thoracic and thoracolumbar surgery

Bracing following surgery for thoracic and thoracolumbar deformity is highly controversial. With modern techniques in segmental instrumentation, many authors believe that supplemental bracing is not necessary. Traditionally, following surgery for scoliosis using the Harrington rod system, external immobilization consisted of a body cast. As instrumentation methods have improved and techniques of segmental instrumentation have become more popular, the use of body casts has waned. Some surgeons state that no immobilization is necessary, whereas others continue to use either a three-point brace or a custom-molded TLSO for added stability, especially in patients with neurogenic spinal deformity or those who are unreliable.

Lumbar

Posterior lumbar and lumbosacral fusions performed without instrumentation may require significant external immobilization. If a multiple-level fusion extends to the sacrum, external immobilization using a TLSO with a leg extension may be necessary. If segmental instrumentation is used, however, a lesser amount of external immobilization is needed. Often, with an instrumented one-level or two-level lumbar or lumbosacral fusion, a rigid LSO is sufficient. If the fusion is done both anteriorly and posteriorly, the duration of postoperative bracing can be shortened to 6 to 10 weeks rather than waiting until solid fusion is seen radiographically. Rarely, with noncompliant patients or with multiple-level fusions that extend into the upper lumbar and lower thoracic spine, a TLSO with or without a leg extension may be necessary.

REFERENCES

1. Garfin SR, et al: Complications in the use of the Halo fixation device, J Bone Joint Surg 68:320–325, 1986.
2. Johnson RM, et al: Cervical orthoses: A study comparing their effectiveness in restricting cervical motion in normal subjects, J Bone Joint Surg 59A:332–339, 1977.
3. Norton PL, Brown T: The immobilizing efficiency of back braces, J Bone Joint Surg 39A:111–139, 1957.
4. White AA III, Panjabi MM: Spinal braces: Functional analysis and clinical applications clinical biomechanics of the spine, Philadelphia, 1978, JB Lippincott.
5. Whitehill R, Richman JA, Glaser JA: Failure of immobilization of the cervical spine by the Halo vest: A report of five cases, J Bone Joint Surg 68A:326–332, 1986.

Orthoses for Spinal Deformities

John E. Lonstein

The use of orthoses for the treatment of spinal deformities is controversial; some are strong advocates of their use, whereas others are negative about this application. This chapter reviews the orthoses used for the treatment of spinal deformities: idiopathic, congenital, and neuromuscular scoliosis and Scheuermann's disease. The choices are reviewed, with the biomechanics and advantages and disadvantages of each orthosis, and the results of orthotic treatment of that disorder. Some repetition is necessary because the same orthoses are used for a number of conditions, but this will be kept to a minimum. Because idiopathic scoliosis is the most common spinal deformity treated, this is discussed first, with referral back to it in discussing the treatment of congenital and neuromuscular spinal deformities.

IDIOPATHIC SCOLIOSIS

With the widespread use of school screening for early detection of spinal deformities, a larger number of patients are presenting for care, and the role of orthotic treatment is becoming increasingly important. Spinal deformities seen are scoliosis and kyphosis. The most common type of scoliosis detected is idiopathic. With the lateral curvature, there are resultant torso changes that may need to be treated: decompensation, change in thoracic shape, and rotational prominence. In addition, hypokyphosis is a part of the deformity in thoracic curves.[18]

The aim of orthotic treatment of scoliosis is to control the curvature, preventing the curve from increasing and perhaps requiring surgical stabilization, while the balance and cosmetic appearance are improved. In the juvenile years, the aim of orthotic management is curve control until maturity or until the onset of the adolescent growth spurt. With the growth spurt, control of the scoliosis may not be possible, and curve increase sometimes occurs. In these cases, the orthosis helps in delaying surgery until optimal spinal height has been achieved. Ideally a fusion should not be performed in the juvenile years because it results in a stunting of truncal growth.

The first effective orthosis for the treatment of spinal deformities was the cervicothoracolumbosacral orthosis (CTLSO), known as the Milwaukee brace, which was developed by Blount and Schmidt in 1948 for the postoperative control of postpolio spinal deformities. It was subsequently found to be an effective means of nonoperative treatment of spinal deformities. Because of its 35 years of experience, the CTLSO is the orthosis against which all others are measured.[3,34]

In the 1960s, a large number of low-profile thoracolumbosacral orthoses (TLSO) appeared in Europe and from the 1970s onward in North America. These are usually named for the town or area where they were developed and play an important role in the orthotic treatment of spinal deformities.

A team approach, with the Certified Orthotist and orthopedist working together, is essential to the orthotic treatment of spinal deformities. Only with this cooperation in prescribing, fitting, and subsequent monitoring of the orthosis is a successful orthotic program possible.

The two main groups of orthoses are described for the treatment of scoliosis and kyphosis. The biomechanical principles of the orthoses are discussed, with the results of treatment and the problems encountered enumerated. Following this, the questions "Whom to brace?" and "What brace to use?" are addressed.

Cervicothoracolumbosacral orthosis (Milwaukee brace)

Description. The CTLSO (Milwaukee brace) (Fig. 14.1) consists of a molded pelvic section with three

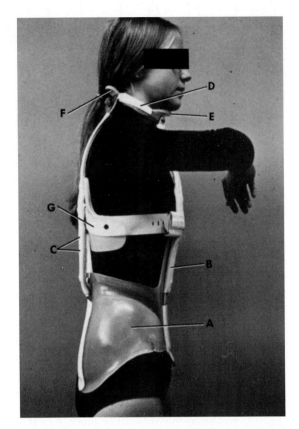

Fig. 14.1. The CTLSO (Milwaukee brace). Molded pelvic section *(A)* with one anterior *(B)* and two posterior *(C)* uprights connected to the neck ring *(D)*. There is a throat mold *(E)*, and occipital pads *(F)* are fastened to the neck ring. A thoracic pad *(G)* is attached to the uprights.

uprights—one anterior and two posterior—connected to a neck ring, the pelvic section and neck ring opening posteriorly. The neck ring helps stabilize the uprights (and attached pads) and does not exert a distractive force. For comfort, a molded throat piece and occipital rests are fitted to the neck ring. The pelvic section was originally fabricated of leather, but with the widespread use of thermoplastics, these materials have replaced leather in most centers, the most popular being polypropylene.[39]

The pelvic section may be custom-molded (from a positive mold of the patient's torso), or a prefabricated girdle may be used. Custom molding has the advantage of a better pelvic fit, allowing for variations in size of the individual and the different amounts of lumbar lordosis. Its obvious disadvantage is the longer time of fabrication. Prefabricated girdles are quicker to use and, with many sizes available, generally fit 90% of patients.[57] Individual size variations are compensated by the foam lining, but a standard control of lumbar lordosis is present. This does not, however, take into account individual variations in lordosis or the variable control of lordosis that may be necessary.

The pelvic section is extended laterally over the greater trochanter as a trochanteric extension to help stabilize the pelvic section and orthosis. This is done in cases of decompensation to help balance the torso, correcting the imbalance. The extension is placed on the side of the decompensation (i.e., with decompensation to the right, the trochanteric extension is placed on the right side).

The uprights are added to the pelvic section, with pads as necessary for the curve pattern present. Based on standing and supine bending radiographs, the curve pattern is identified; a pad is necessary for every major curve present.

Major curve	*Pad*
High thoracic	Trapezius
Thoracic	Thoracic
Thoracolumbar	Oval and lumbar
Lumbar	Lumbar

Compensatory curves do not need to be treated unless decompensation exists, and then a lumbar pad is added to improve the balance but not to treat the curve.

Biomechanics.   Biomechanically, spinal orthoses work on the three-point or four-point corrective system, which is generally a passive system. An active element is present because of the discomfort of the pads, with the individual actively moving away from the pads.

When the CTLSO (Milwaukee brace) is first fitted, a different set of forces act compared to those that act later. In a thoracic curve (Fig. 14.2, *A*) the thoracic pad *(C)* acts against the convexity of the curve and is counteracted by the axillary sling *(B)* and the lateral aspect of the pelvic section *(D)* below. After a few months, the force exerted by the axillary sling is less important, and the righting reflex induced by the neck ring *(A)* acts to counteract the force of the thoracic pad. The presence of this righting reflex can be tested by removing the axillary sling after the patient has been in the brace for 6 months. If the neck remains centralized in the neck ring, the sling is discontinued. If not, the sling is still necessary, and this reflex can be again tested 4 to 6 months later. After removal of the sling, three forces are necessary to stabilize the orthosis: the thoracic pad (*C* in Fig. 14.2, *B*), the lateral aspect of pelvic section on the opposite side *(D)*, and the inferior aspect of pelvic section on the same side *(E)*.

The pads exert their force through the ribs in the thoracic or thoracolumbar area, with the lumbar pad acting more directly on the spine via the paravertebral muscles. Because of their position, the pads exert both medially directed and anteriorly directed vectors. This force couple is important in the thoracic area because often there is hypokyphosis associated with the scoliosis. The configuration and position of the thoracic pad

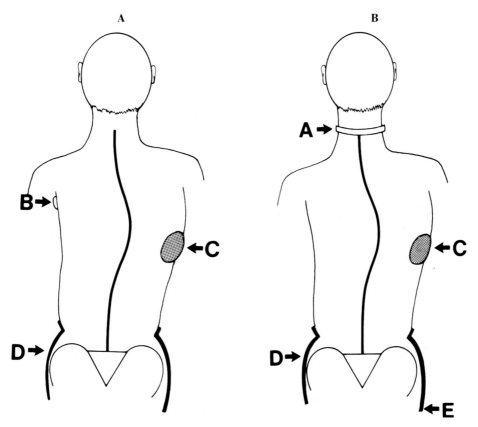

Fig. 14.2.   Biomechanics of the CTLSO (Milwaukee brace) for a right thoracic curve. **A,** The force against the thoracic pad *(C)* is counteracted by the axillary sling *(B)* and the lateral aspect of the pelvic section *(D)*, both on the opposite side. The axillary sling becomes less important, and after its removal **(B)** the righting reflex induced by the side of the neck ring *(A)* counteracts the force exerted by the thoracic pad *(C)*. To stabilize the orthosis, the inferior edge of the pelvic section, on the same side as the thoracic pad *(E)*, acts as the third point.

are thus important, the two variables being the amount of the thoracic kyphosis and the magnitude of the rib hump or rotational prominence (Fig. 14.3). The thoracic pad is centered on the rib of the vertebra just below the apex of the scoliosis so its force is at and slightly below the apex of the curve. With hypokyphosis, the posterior uprights are set more posteriorly, the anterior outrigger is eliminated, and the thoracic pad is placed lateral to the posterior upright. This placement of the thoracic pad tends to shift the vector of its corrective force more laterally, minimizing the anterior force. In extreme cases of hypokyphosis, kyphosis can be encouraged by setting the neck ring more anteriorly and adding a lower rib gusset anteriorly over the lower ribs. This tends to push the spine posteriorly (Fig. 14.4). When the thoracic hypokyphosis approaches a straight spine or is true lordosis (thoracic sagittal profile of +15 to −5 degrees), these modifications can be attempted. Careful monitoring of x-ray views is necessary in these cases because orthotic failure is common. With true thoracic lordosis (less than −5 to 10 degrees), orthotic treatment is probably contraindicated. The orthotic

modifications with increased kyphosis or a larger rib rotational prominence are shown in Fig. 14.3.[59]

The importance of control of the lumbar lordosis in the correction of scoliosis has been shown by Lindh.[27] With reduction of the lumbar lordosis in a prefabricated Boston system pelvic girdle, there can be a concomitant decrease in the lumbar scoliosis, sometimes without the addition of a corrective pad. Two possible reasons for this are as follows: (1) Spine motion is coupled, insofar as lateral deviation and rotation change together. Thus, if the sagittal curve (rotation) is altered, there can be a concomitant change in the lumbar scoliosis. (2) The orthosis, by its circumferential fit, exerts a closed cylinder effect on the abdomen and thorax with an increase in the intracavitary pressure with a resultant lengthening of the spine and thus correction of the scoliosis.

Advantages.   The CTLSO (Milwaukee brace) has many advantages. Because of its open design with uprights and attached pads, it restricts respiration minimally—an ideal situation in treating a condition in which one of the complications if untreated is respira-

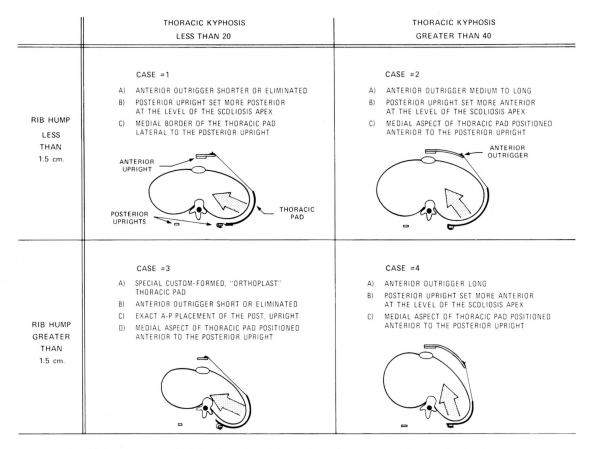

Fig. 14.3. Attachment of the thoracic pad depends on the amount of thoracic kyphosis present and on the magnitude of the rotational prominence. Four possible combinations are present, with specific modifications necessary in each case. *(From Winter RB, Carlson MJ: Modern orthotics for spinal deformities, Clin Orthop Rel Res 126:74, 1977.)*

tory. With poor fabrication and too close contouring of the uprights, however, restriction can occur. Overall restriction in activities is minimal, dictated by the child's activity level rather than by the orthosis.[2] The open design allows good air circulation so that use in hot climates is not a problem. It can be lengthened as the child grows. Pad placement is altered with growth or when curve correction dictates such a change. Control of curves with an apex above T8 is possible, and high left thoracic curves in the double thoracic curve pattern can be treated.

Disadvantages. The main problem with the CTLSO (Milwaukee brace) today is psychological, with poor acceptance by some patients and some physicians. The neck ring is visible and thus tends to make the teenager different at a time in his or her life when acceptance by peers is important. This problem varies greatly among patients. In a 1986 study by Emans and colleagues[21] of the Boston prefabricated system with and without a superstructure (i.e., CTLSO and TLSO), brace compliance was analyzed. There was no difference in compliance in the two designs, suggesting that

patient acceptance of an orthosis does not depend on the design but rather on patient factors. Treating spinal deformity patients together in a clinic situation may help minimize the self-consciousness many children and teenagers feel and thus improve their attitude toward the CTLSO. An early problem existed with the original chin piece, which exerted a distractive force and pressure against the mandible, leading to bite deformities. With the realization that distraction was not important plus a change to a molded submandibular throat piece, this difficulty has been eliminated.[22,40,42]

In the treatment of thoracic scoliosis, if care is not taken with positioning the thoracic pad and contouring the uprights, too much of an anterior vector may be present, and this can reduce a thoracic kyphosis and even produce a hypokyphosis. Thus, the fitting of the thoracic pad is important and should follow the guidelines just laid out. Because of its position, the neck ring is potentially hazardous if the child participates in gymnastics or tumbling. If the child is interested in participating in these activities, this participation has to be out of the orthosis.

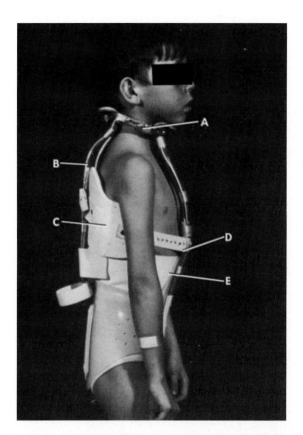

Fig. 14.4. Milwaukee brace modifications in a case of true thoracic lordosis or extreme hypokyphosis. The neck ring is set more posteriorly *(A);* the posterior uprights are contoured so they do not touch the back *(B);* and the thoracic pad is large *(C)* and lies lateral to the posterior upright, being attached anteriorly directly to the anterior upright *(D).* An elastic gusset *(E)* is added to force the ribs posteriorly and to try to induce a kyphotic vector on the spine.

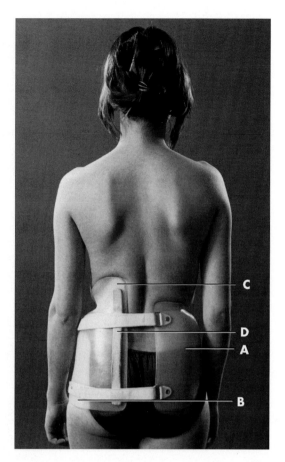

Fig. 14.5. Low-profile TLSO for a single left lumbar curve. The pelvic section *(A)* has a left trochanteric extension *(B)* with the left lumbar pad under the left lumbar extension of the orthosis *(C)*. Note the reinforcing metal bar *(D)* supporting the lumbar pad.

Thoracolumbosacral orthoses (low profile)

Low-profile TLSOs extend from the thorax to the sacrum. The numerous models available can be divided into prefabricated and custom-fabricated designs. In addition, they can be divided into designs for lumbar and thoracolumbar curves (Fig. 14.5) and for thoracic and double thoracic and lumbar curves (Fig. 14.6).

Prefabricated. The prefabricated Boston system is a series of 16 sizes of orthoses that are fitted and then trimmed according to the curve pattern. A foam lining helps form the orthosis to the variations in body contour. Pads are added to the prefabricated module according to the curve being treated. This is a useful system when a good fit is obtained, but it can present fitting problems. In addition, a drawback is the uniform reduction of the lumbar lordosis. It is impossible to take into account all the variations in size, shape, and contour of individual patients.

Custom-fitted. Numerous custom-fitted TLSOs exist, named usually for the town or area where they were designed.[10,24,31,32,41,43,44,50,57] They differ in the material used and in the way the forces are applied. Generally, they work on the three-point or four-point force system (see later) and have either an open design with specific pads added or a pad correction that is built in when the positive mold is modified. Examples are the Newington (Orthoplast),[12] Pasadena (Lexan),[24] Miami (polypropylene),[32] Charleston (polypropylene),[44] and Riviera (aluminum plus polypropylene) orthoses.[31]

Biomechanics. All TLSOs work on the three-point or four-point corrective system, the three-point system being operative in single curves and the four-point system in double curves. A TLSO cannot be used for all thoracic curves but is restricted to curves with an apex generally below T7-8, the exact level depending on the specific orthosis being used and the philosophy of the treating physician.

For a single lumbar or thoracolumbar curve, the three-point corrective system is operative, the low-profile design generally being used. The pad is applied just below the lumbar or thoracolumbar curve *(B* in Fig.

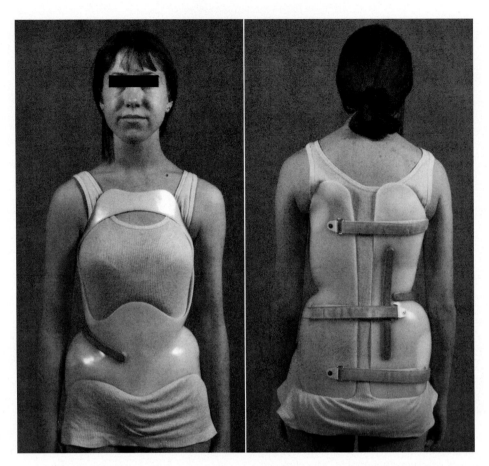

Fig. 14.6.   Low-profile TLSO for thoracic curves with an apex at T8 or below.

14.7) opposed by the thoracic extension above *(A)* and the lower end of the pelvic section below *(C)*. The latter two points are on the side opposite the corrective pad. In some TLSOs, the cranial point is not added, the counterforce being the body's righting reflex. (*A₁* in Fig. 14.8) Three forces, however, are still present to stabilize the orthosis: that against the curve (*B* in Fig. 14.8), that of the pelvic section on the opposite side *(C)*, and that of the inferior edge of the pelvic section on the same side *(D)*. Generally, because of the forces exerted, there is a tendency for the orthosis to rotate. This can be counteracted by extending the pelvic section *(D)* over the trochanter (trochanteric extension) on the same side as the corrective pad *(B)*. In addition, the Boston module with pads in place exerts a derotating force.[1] In a single thoracic curve treated with a TLSO (low profile), the force couple acting on the thoracic curve are the force on the apex of the curve (*B* in Fig. 14.9) counteracted by the axillary extension on the opposite side *(A)* and the orthosis in the lumbar area or over the pelvis also on the opposite side *(C)*.

With a double thoracic plus lumbar curve, the four-point corrective system is operative, the TLSO (low profile) design being used. Two forces act against the convexity of the thoracic (*B* in Fig. 14.9) and lumbar *(C)*

curves and are counteracted by an extension into the axilla on the side opposite the thoracic curve *(A)*. The pelvic section on the same side as the thoracic curve is the fourth point *(D)*. Depending on the design of the TLSO, the whole orthosis may be a solid shell with no cutouts or completely open with only the force areas and pelvic section remaining (Fig. 14.10). A trochanteric extension is added to this orthosis to stabilize the orthosis if there is decompensation, being added on the side of the decompensation.

Advantages.   The chief advantage of the TLSO over the CTLSO (Milwaukee brace) is its acceptance by teenagers. Because the TLSO is low profile (i.e., an underarm orthosis without a neck ring), it is well hidden by clothes and thus is well tolerated by patients. Children feel less restricted, which may lead to better acceptance, although Emans and colleagues[21] showed no difference in the compliance with orthotic use between the Boston module with and without a superstructure (i.e., TLSO versus CTLSO). In addition, fabrication is easier and quicker than for the CTLSO (Milwaukee brace).

Disadvantages.   The solid design of the TLSO limits adjustment for growth. Although both the TLSO and the CTLSO (Milwaukee brace) need refabrication

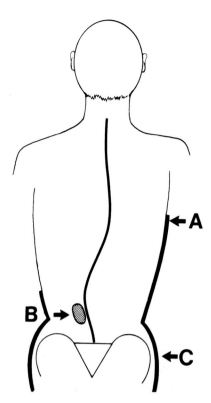

Fig. 14.7. Biomechanics of a TLSO with thoracic extension for a lumbar curve. The force applied to the lumbar (or thoracolumbar) curve *(B)* is counteracted by the thoracic extension *(A)* and by the lower end of the pelvic section on the side of the thoracic extension *(C)*.

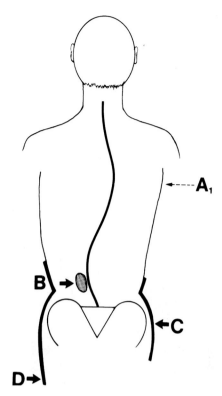

Fig. 14.8. Biomechanics of a TLSO without thoracic extension for a lumbar curve. The force applied to the lumbar (or thoracolumbar) curve *(B)* is counteracted by the righting reflex *(A₁)* and the side of the pelvic section on the opposite side *(C)*. The third point to stabilize the orthosis is the trochanteric extension *(D)*, on the same side as the lumbar curve.

with an increase in pelvic size, when there is an increase in height the CTLSO is adjustable, but the TLSO is not. When the patient outgrows the TLSO in the vertical direction, a new one must be made.

The more "closed" design of the TLSO may sometimes result in skin problems from retained heat and restricted air circulation next to the skin.

Furthermore, orthoses that are designed to treat thoracic curves and that extend from the upper thorax to the pelvis have inherent problems because of thoracic compression.[10] Normal respiration is restricted, and this leads to a reduction in pulmonary function. Also, in younger adolescents and juveniles, thoracic compression can, over time, alter the thoracic shape—producing the so-called tubular thorax. The long-term effect of this on pulmonary function is unknown. Because of the design of low-profile TLSOs, thoracic curves with an apex above T8 cannot be treated. The exact upper limits of a TLSO's use depend on its design and on the orthopedic surgeon prescribing it. This excludes, however, the single thoracic curve whose apex is above T8 and also the double thoracic curve.

When a decision is made to treat with low-profile TLSO, the foregoing advantages and disadvantages should be considered. In general, a physician and

orthotist use one design for all clients, basing their choice on these facts.

Orthotic choice in idiopathic scoliosis

With the foregoing description of the CTLSO and TLSO (low profile), the questions "What brace to use" and "Whom to brace" in idiopathic scoliosis can now be answered. Because the decisions are different for juvenile and adolescent idiopathic scoliosis, these two types of idiopathic scoliosis are discussed separately.

Juvenile idiopathic scoliosis. The orthosis of choice in the juvenile is the CTLSO (Milwaukee brace). This is because of its adjustability with growth as well as to minimize thoracic compression with resultant rib deformity and pulmonary restriction. In the rare case of a single lumbar or thoracolumbar curve in the juvenile years, a TLSO can be used.

The indications for bracing in juvenile idiopathic scoliosis are a curve that on presentation is greater than 25 degrees or that has shown documented progression. Of importance in the juvenile is the exclusion of other causes of scoliosis, as Mehta has described many causes of curves at this age (benign progressive infantile

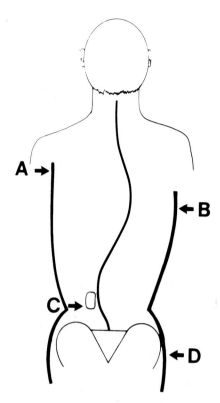

Fig. 14.9. Biomechanics of a TLSO for a thoracic plus lumbar curve. The forces against the curves *(B and C)* are counteracted by the extension into the axilla *(A)* and by the side of the pelvic section *(D)*.

idiopathic scoliosis, syndromic scoliosis, syringomyelic scoliosis, juvenile idiopathic scoliosis, and early-onset adolescent idiopathic scoliosis). A detailed neurologic examination is mandatory (including abdominal reflexes), and every juvenile should have the neural axis evaluated with a magnetic resonance imaging scan because of the high incidence of abnormalities on routine scans, as high as 17% to 20%.[60]

Adolescent idiopathic scoliosis. For single lumbar or thoracolumbar curves, a low-profile TLSO is better for patient acceptance. In thoracic curves, especially with an apex above T8, the CTLSO (Milwaukee brace) is better because it is more effective in exerting the corrective force system. In addition, pulmonary function is less restricted, and there are fewer rib cage deformities and skin problems. For single thoracic curves with an apex at T8 or below, the choice is between a CTLSO and low-profile TLSO. The same choice holds with regard to double curve patterns (thoracic and lumbar curves). The choice between a CTLSO (Milwaukee brace) and a TLSO depends on the philosophy and biases of the treating orthopedic surgeon.

Whom to brace is difficult at times to decide. Numerous factors must be taken into consideration—age, skeletal and physiologic maturity, cosmesis, amount of rotational prominence, size of the thoracic sagittal curve, and geographic and social factors.

The size of the curve is the most important of these: (1) Curves over 40 to 45 degrees in adolescents do not respond to bracing. (2) Curves under 20 degrees should not be treated but observed. (3) Approximately one third of the curves between 20 and 29 degrees in growing children do not progress.[9,28] Thus, in this range, treatment may be withheld until progression is documented. (4) In curves of less than 29 degrees, bracing may be indicated for cosmetic reasons alone (usually decompensation) and not for curve magnitude or progression. (5) Many curves greater than 30 degrees increase, and thus treatment is immediately instituted.

In the growing adolescent (Tanner maturity grade of 1 to 3[54], Risser iliac apophysis sign of 0 or 1[47]), the treatment thus depends on the curve magnitude: Curves under 29 degrees are treated when progression has been documented; curves of 30 to 40 (or 45) degrees are treated on presentation; curves greater than 40 (or 45) degrees are usually treated surgically. In the immature adolescent (Tanner 1, Risser 0) with a curve of 25 to 29 degrees, it is best to treat the child on presentation rather than waiting for progression because the results of bracing in this case are much better if the curve is under 30 degrees.[29]

Brace wearing

Juvenile idiopathic scoliosis. In the juvenile years, the brace is worn full-time initially, usually for 12 to 18 months. At this time, if the curve is controlled, and in fact corrected, weaning to part-time use may be attempted (see later). If the curve control continues with part-time wearing, the weaning can continue to only nighttime wearing and in some cases to brace discontinuation before the growth spurt. In many cases, there is curve increase at the onset of the adolescent growth spurt, necessitating a change from part-time to full-time brace wear. The effectiveness of part-time wear in juvenile idiopathic scoliosis has been reported by Kahanovitz and by Lonstein and Winter.[30]

When weaning occurs in the juvenile, the curve control may not be maintained, and part-time wear is not possible. The child remains in the brace full-time until the adolescent growth spurt. At this time, curve control may not continue, with the curve increasing and surgery being indicated. If curve control is maintained, bracing continues till the end of growth, when the child is then weaned from the orthosis. Thus, in juvenile idiopathic scoliosis, there are three main brace scenarios: (1) weaned before the growth spurt, (2) increase at the onset of the growth spurt with surgery performed, and (3) bracing to maturity.[30]

In both the juvenile and the adolescent, full-time bracing is brace wear of 20 to 23 hours per day. The child

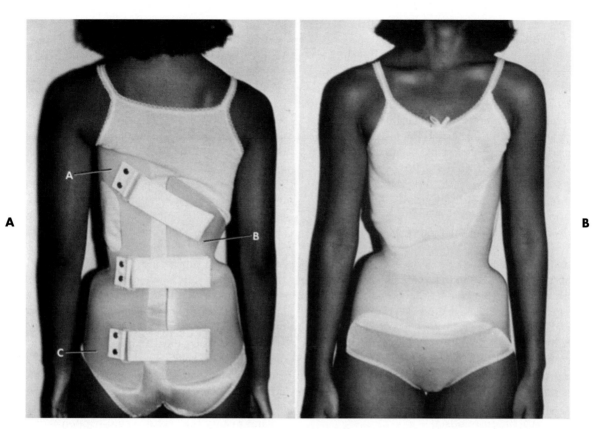

Fig. 14.10. Miami TLSO for a right thoracolumbar curve. **A,** Back opening orthosis with axillary extension. Note the cutout *(A),* force over the thoracolumbar curve *(B),* and counterforce at the lower end of the pelvic section on the opposite side *(C).* **B,** Large area free anteriorly. (Courtesy Newton McCollough, III.)

is allowed out of the brace for bathing, swimming, and physical education class at school. If the child is involved in other sports or physical activities (gymnastics, soccer, football, basketball), extra time is allowed out for these activities, the extra time out being an average of 1 to 2 hours per day. The brace is removed because either the activity is not possible in the brace (gymnastics, football) or participation with the brace on may injure the other players (soccer, basketball). This regimen allows the child to remain active and aids compliance.

Adolescent idiopathic scoliosis. The role of part-time orthotic use in the adolescent is controversial. There is only one study on part-time use of the CTLSO (Milwaukee brace).[23] It is a small series and states that the curves were controlled, but the results were not as good as with full-time wear. The Charleston night bending brace is a new bending brace that is used only during sleep.[44] Preliminary results show curve control, but the series is small and includes patients still under treatment. It must be remembered that the treatment of double curves is not possible and that two things are being evaluated—part-time wear and a new bending orthosis.[44]

During full-time brace wear in both the juvenile and the adolescent, the best way to assess the effect of the orthosis is to take all radiographs in the orthosis, rather than to take an out-of-brace film. Thus, on return visits every 3 to 4 months, the brace fit is checked, and a posteroanterior radiograph is taken in the orthosis and is compared with the original prebrace film and the film of the previous visit. In this way, the effect of the orthosis on the scoliosis and control of the curve can be assessed. A lateral radiograph is taken when there is concern about the sagittal profile (i.e., in the presence of thoracic hypokyphosis or thoracic lordosis).

Weaning

Until growth is complete, orthoses are worn full-time (as above) for idiopathic scoliosis treatment. Cessation of growth is evidenced by no increase in height on serial measurements and a Risser sign of 4 or 5. Removal of the orthosis can be either gradual (over 1 or 2 years) or rapid (over 6 months or less). Because some curve increase commonly occurs with discontinuance of the orthosis as stabilization of the curve occurs, a gradual weaning process is usually recommended.

At the end of growth, the stability of the curve is

tested with a radiograph out of the orthosis 4 hours (i.e., the child removes the orthosis 4 hours before the visit). With less than 5 degrees of curve increase, the child is allowed to be out of the orthosis 4 hours daily. Three or four months later, another radiograph is taken with the child out of the orthosis for 8 hours. With curve control, 8 hours is allowed out of the orthosis. This is repeated with 12 hours out of the orthosis, then only sleeping in the orthosis. If minimal increase has occurred, the child is progressively weaned from the orthosis. Then for another 6 to 12 months the orthosis is worn just during sleeping hours. Finally, orthosis wear is discontinued entirely, with follow-ups remaining only to evaluate the long-term effectiveness of the treatment.

Exercises

A special exercise program was originally an integral part of the orthotic management of scoliosis.[3,35] These are either corrective shifting exercises in the orthosis or exercises to maintain muscle tone.[3] No studies are available to show that the curves are improved by an exercise program or that the results are better with an exercise program. For these reasons, the use of exercises has disappeared. It is far better to get the child involved in sports on a regular basis to establish a lifetime physical fitness mindset.

Results

The literature on CTLSO (Milwaukee brace) treatment of idiopathic scoliosis, with follow-ups at the time of brace discontinuance and as much as 1 year later, shows an average curve correction of 18% to 20%, with slightly less for high left thoracic curves and slightly more for lumbar curves.[4,19,25,35,48] Long-term results with Milwaukee brace treatment of idiopathic scoliosis fall into two groups. Mellencamp and co-workers[33] and Carr and associates,[14] with follow-ups of more than 5 years after brace discontinuance, showed that on average the final correction was close to the initial prebrace curve. This suggested that generally orthotic treatment of scoliosis results in curve control not curve correction. These two studies included a large number of curves that were initially over 40 degrees and documented the results of two strong proponents of the Milwaukee brace, Blount and Moe.[3] Two other studies,[20,48] with an average 10-year follow-up of adolescent and juvenile idiopathic scoliosis, showed a final correction of 14% to 16%, some modest curve correction. The larger curves in these series were also controlled rather than corrected. The average curve, however, was smaller than those of Mellencamp and co-workers and Carr and associates.

The results in juvenile idiopathic scoliosis are different. Either these curves are well controlled or at the onset of the adolescent growth spurt, control is lost and surgical intervention is necessary. This has been well shown by Tolo and Gillespie,[55] Shuffelbarger and Keiser,[51] and Lonstein and Winter,[30] where the surgical rate for the juvenile treated with a CTLSO is 50%.

Interpretation of the studies on adolescent idiopathic scoliosis is difficult because the curve magnitudes and patterns vary greatly, most studies including juveniles and adolescents and evaluating curves rather than curve patterns (i.e., the right thoracic curve is evaluated as a curve regardless whether it is a single right thoracic curve or part of a double thoracic or double thoracic and lumbar pattern). Studies on the natural history of untreated idiopathic scoliosis by Bunnell[9] and Lonstein and Carlson[28] have shown that a high percentage of these curves do not progress, even in an immature, rapidly growing child. Many patients in the series may thus show good results because a nonprogressive curve is treated. In addition, with a larger curve or one that shows documented progression, the results of orthotic treatment may vary greatly, even with an ideal orthosis, ideal curve selection, and ideally cooperative patient.

To evaluate the effectiveness of the orthotic treatment of adolescent idiopathic scoliosis is thus difficult and can be judged only by comparing brace results to natural history (i.e., what would happen without any treatment). There are only two studies that do this, the larger one of Lonstein and Winter[29] evaluating 1020 adolescents treated with the CTLSO (Milwaukee brace). Failure of bracing was taken as those that underwent surgery, plus those treated in a brace who at the end of bracing had curves that were 5 or more degrees larger than their prebrace curve. The four main curve patterns (single right thoracic, double thoracic, double thoracic and lumbar, and double thoracic and thoracolumbar patterns) with curves between 20 and 39 degrees were evaluated. For curves of 20 to 29 degrees and immature children with a Risser sign of 0 or 1, the failure rate with the CTLSO (Milwaukee brace) was 40% compared to the natural history prediction of 68%,[28] a statistically significant difference ($P = 0.0001$ Chi-square). With more mature children with a Risser of 2 or more, the failure rate for the brace was 10% compared to natural history progression of 23%, again a statistically significant difference ($P = 0.0022$ Chi-square). For curves of 30 to 39 degrees, the figures for Risser 0 and 1 were 43% versus 57% and 22% versus 43% for a Risser of 2 or more. It would appear that these differences are significant, but this could not be shown because of the small number of cases in the natural history series.[9]

The use of TLSOs in the treatment of scoliosis has not been studied for as long as CTLSOs. Excellent curve correction has been reported, however,[11,24,32,41,50,57] ranging from 32% to 70%. Some retention of correction was also reported when the brace was discontinued and ranged from 30% to 35%.[10,24,32] The average curve treated with a TLSO is smaller than the average curve treated with the CTLSO (Milwaukee brace), which makes interpretation difficult because of the knowledge that the incidence of nonprogressive curves under 29 degrees, and especially under 19 degrees, is high.[9,15,28] In addition, the natural history studies indicate that the prevalence of progression of lumbar and thoracolumbar curves is low.

A Scoliosis Research Society sponsored project has evaluated the effectiveness of treatment of adolescent idiopathic scoliosis.[38] This was a multicenter, multinational prospective study evaluating observation, electrical stimulation, and bracing with a TLSO. The subjects were all girls of 10 to 15 years of age with single curve of 25 to 35 degrees with an apex from T8 to L1. Each center treated the patients with one treatment method (observation, electrical stimulation, or bracing), a failure of any method being a curve increase of 6 or more degrees. The first finding was that electrical stimulation was no different than observation, these two groups of patients thus making up the natural history group. Using survival analysis, and taking all the cases lost to follow-up as failures (the worst case scenario), it was found that the failure rate of orthotic treatment was 40% versus 70% failures with observation—a statistically significant difference ($p < 0.0002$).[38] From this study and the one of Lonstein and Winter, it is seen that orthoses are effective statistically in altering the natural history of adolescent idiopathic scoliosis. Thus, the orthosis should be thought of not as turning large curves into small curves but as preventing progression and keeping small curves small.

SCHEUERMANN'S KYPHOSIS

Adolescent kyphosis or Scheuermann's disease is of unknown origin. It affects the growth areas of the vertebral body, altering the normal growth and causing vertebral wedging, kyphosis, and often back pain.[6,36] Orthotic treatment is indicated for pain alone or for pain combined with hyperkyphosis measuring greater than 60 to 65 degrees. Two orthoses are used for the treatment of Scheuermann's disease: the CTLSO (Milwaukee brace) and a TLSO.

Bracing principles

There are age differences in starting brace wear for idiopathic scoliosis and Scheuermann's disease. A successful result in idiopathic scoliosis requires an actively growing child. Bracing in Scheuermann's disease can be instituted as long as there are active vertebral ring

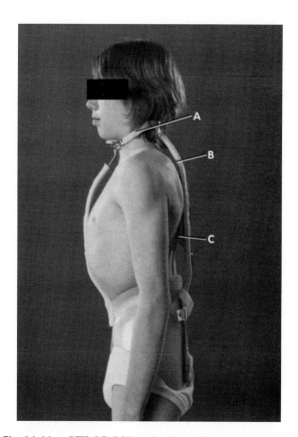

Fig. 14.11.   CTLSO (Milwaukee brace) for the treatment of thoracic kyphosis. The neck ring *(A)* is set posteriorly. The posterior uprights *(B)* are contoured close to the back. Kyphosis pads *(C)* are positioned behind and just below the apex of the curve.

apophyses, a later stage of growth than with scoliosis. The CTLSO (Milwaukee brace) is used, with some modifications in its fabrication. To encourage extension, the neck ring is set somewhat posteriorly. The posterior uprights are contoured to lie close to the back, with kyphosis pads positioned behind and just below the apex of the curve (Fig. 14.11). In thoracic kyphosis, the corrective force system consists of the kyphosis pads (*B* in Fig. 14.12) counteracted by the righting reflex induced by the throat mold *(A)* and the abdominal apron of the pelvic section *(C)*. Force A (in Fig. 14.12) is active; therefore, the posteroinferior edge of the pelvic section *(D)* acts as the third force to stabilize the orthosis. If the apex of the kyphosis is in the lower thoracic or thoracolumbar area, a TLSO (Fig. 14.13) can be used. It consists of a pelvic section with posterior extensions of either plastic or metal and kyphosis pads. The corrective system consists of a force over the kyphosis (*B* in Fig. 14.14) counteracted by forces from the sternal pad *(A)* and the anterior portion of the pelvic girdle *(C)*. The TLSO is well accepted, and thus it is tempting to use it for Scheuermann's kyphosis with apex in the midthoracic area. In this case, it is ineffective biomechanically because the apical force *(B)* and

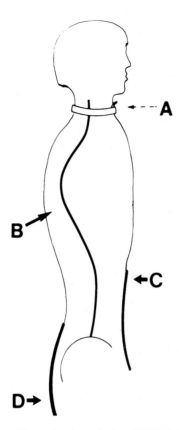

Fig. 14.12. Biomechanics of the CTLSO (Milwaukee brace) for a thoracic kyphosis. The kyphosis pads exert pressure just below the apex of the deformity *(B)*, with the righting reflex induced by the throat mold *(A)* and the abdominal apron *(C)* being the two opposing forces. The lower end of the pelvic section posteriorly *(D)* helps to stabilize the orthosis.

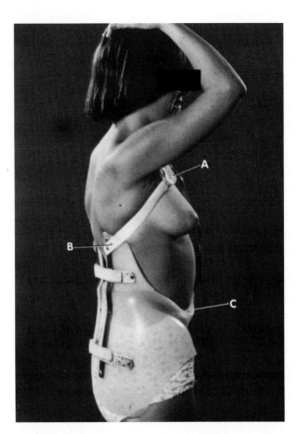

Fig. 14.13. TLSO for a thoracolumbar kyphosis with low kyphosis pads built into the pelvic section *(B)* counteracted by the sternal pad *(A)* and abdominal apron *(C)*.

the sternal force *(A)* (in Fig. 14.15) are too close together, making the corrective moment poor. Thus, the TLSO should not be used for thoracic hyperkyphosis but should be reserved for cases in the thoracolumbar area. An alternative TLSO is similar to the low-profile TLSO used for scoliosis with metal reinforcement strips posteriorly supporting the kyphosis pads.

Orthotic treatment of Scheuermann's kyphosis is quite effective because the force is applied directly to the spine over the paravertebral muscles and not through the ribs, as in scoliosis. With the extension force of the orthosis, pressure on the anterior vertebral growth cells is relieved, and these cells recover enough to reconstitute the vertebral shape. The correction obtained in the orthosis tends to be permanent, with little loss after brace wear is discontinued.

Brace wearing and weaning

Patients with Scheuermann's kyphosis can be divided into two groups—those with minimal vertebral wedging and those with significant wedging of the apical vertebrae.

With minimal wedging, and usually a more flexible curve, the correction of the kyphosis is usually rapid, taking 9 to 18 months. When the correction has been obtained, the child can be weaned from the brace by being allowed progressively longer times out of it every month (e.g., 4, 6, 8, 10, 12 hours). With maintenance of correction, the total weaning phase is approximately 9 months.

With marked apical vertebral wedging and usually a more rigid kyphosis, a longer period of orthotic wear is required. Although the kyphosis may be corrected fairly rapidly, reconstitution of anterior vertebral height with reduction of the wedging is necessary for a successful result. Bracing is continued until the wedging is corrected, usually until the end of growth and fusion of the vertebral ring apophyses. The weaning program in these cases is gradual, following that described for the treatment of scoliosis (see earlier).

Exercises

An exercise program plays a more important role in the treatment of Scheuermann's disease than in the treatment of scoliosis. Back extensor strengthening and pelvic tilt exercise programs are useful because they aid in both obtaining and maintaining the correction with strengthening of the spine extensors.

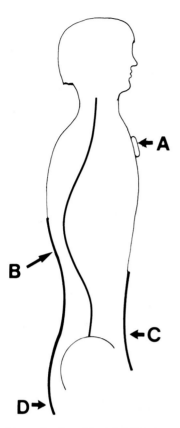

Fig. 14.14. Biomechanics of the TLSO for a thoracolumbar kyphosis. The pressure just below the apex of the kyphosis *(B)* is counteracted by the forces of the sternal pad *(A)* and the abdominal apron *(C)*, with the lower end of the pelvic girdle posteriorly *(D)* helping to stabilize.

Results

The short-term results of orthotic treatment of Scheuermann's disease are excellent. After a time in the orthosis, the curve is corrected to the normal range, and the vertebral wedging is reduced.[5,17,26,45,53,56] The best results of improvement of vertebral wedging have been shown by Bradford and associates,[5] who found that an average wedging of 8.5 degrees was corrected using a brace regimen of 34 months to 2.8 degrees. No long-term results have been published, but the general experience is that the correction is maintained with little if any loss into early adulthood.

CONGENITAL SCOLIOSIS

Congenital scoliosis is due to abnormal development of the vertebrae with the vertebral anomaly being present at birth. The deformity is thus noted at an early age. The vertebral anomaly is failure of a part of the vertebra to form (failure of formation, hemivertebra); or it is due to failure of the vertebral anlage to segment into individual segments, either completely (block vertebra) or partially (unsegmented bar); or it may be a

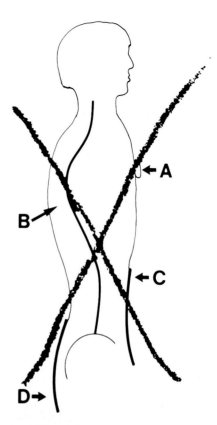

Fig. 14.15. Biomechanics of the TLSO for a thoracic kyphosis. The force over the apex of the curve *(B)* is too close to the sternal pad *(A)*, making the forces ineffective for correction of the kyphosis.

combination of formation and segmentation defects. In addition, the anomaly can occur in any part of the vertebral ring (anterior, anterolateral, lateral, posterolateral, or posterior). The anomaly gives rise to a deformity because of absent growth potential in a part of the vertebral ring, the resultant growth in the remainder of the ring giving rise to the deformity. Depending on where the anomaly is in the vertebral ring, the resultant deformity can pure scoliosis, kyphosis, or lordosis, or a combination of scoliosis plus kyphosis or lordosis.

Because congenital spine deformities are due to abnormal development in the embryo, it is fairly common to have associated anomalies elsewhere. The most common of these are kidney and urinary tract anomalies, which occur in 25% to 30% of patients with congenital spine deformities. Congenital heart defects also occur, and there can be additional congenital spine anomalies, the most common being a failure of segmentation in the cervical spine, which is classified as Klippel-Feil syndrome.

Indications for bracing in congenital deformities

Because the primary deformity is in the bones rather than the soft tissues, the curves tend to be rigid and thus are not as amenable to orthotic treatment as are idiopathic or neuromuscular curves. The role for orthoses in congenital deformities is limited. They have little effect in the treatment of congenital kyphosis, congenital lordosis, and rigid scoliosis. In patients with flexible scoliosis in which the anomaly is a part of the curve, and the remainder of the curve is made up of normal segments, orthotic treatment is effective. Thus, the curve is longer than the anomalous area with the anomalies being in the cranial, center, or caudal part of the curve. In addition, orthotic treatment is used for secondary curves to control them during growth, often after surgical treatment of the congenital curve. In many of these cases, surgical treatment of the secondary curve becomes necessary with curve increase at the onset of the growth spurt.

Another role for orthoses in congenital scoliosis is for the effect of the curve on the coronal balance. When there is coronal imbalance associated with the congenital anomaly, bracing may be indicated. This may be coronal decompensation or head tilt. With single or multiple anomalies and decompensation, the orthosis can restore the spinal balance with the flexibility in the normal uninvolved segments, allowing the spine to be balanced with growth. In cervicothoracic or upper thoracic anomalies, the often accompanying head tilt can correct this head tilt.

This limited role for orthotic treatment of congenital scoliosis must be appreciated. In addition, as with any orthotic treatment, when curve progression occurs, it must be promptly diagnosed and surgically treated.

Orthoses available

Kalibus splint. This is a three-point splint used in children too young and small to fit with a CTSLO (Milwaukee brace)—usually under 9 to 12 months (Fig. 14.16). It consists of a custom-molded pelvic section with straps attaching a thoracic pad over the apex of the curve and straps attaching to a shoulder ring on the other side. For stability, the shoulder ring is attached with a bar to the pelvic section.

CTLSO (Milwaukee brace). The CTLSO is the orthosis of choice in congenital scoliosis. The TLSO rarely plays a role in these children because it is a circumferential orthosis with marked restriction of thoracic expansion. In addition, it is not possible to treat high thoracic curves with the TLSO or affect head

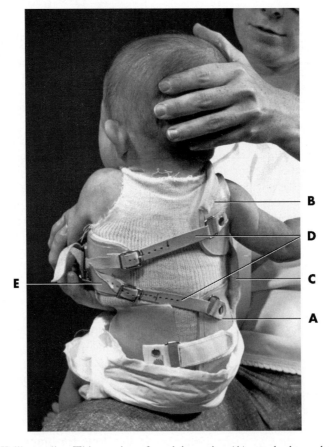

Fig. 14.16. Kalibus splint. This consists of a pelvic section *(A)*, attached to a shoulder ring *(B)* with a metal bar *(C)*. Straps from the pelvic section and shoulder ring *(D)* connect to a thoracic pad *(E)* on the other side. This orthosis works on the three-point principle—between the shoulder ring *(B)*, thoracic pad *(E)*, and pelvic section on the opposite side *(A)*.

tilt—both being common in congenital scoliosis. Children with congenital scoliosis are diagnosed at a young age, and thus bracing is started early, sometimes with a Kalibus splint in the very young, followed by a CTLSO in children as young as 9 to 12 months. Pads are added to the brace to treat the curves as described previously for idiopathic scoliosis. Two additional pads are used in congenital scoliosis. For the high thoracic curve, a shoulder ring is added to control this area (Fig. 14.17). In patients with head tilt, a head support is added—a support either posterior to the ear or on the skull from the occipital area over the ear (Fig. 14.18). All these pads are custom-fabricated, and they are trimmed and fitted so that there is equal pressure exerted without any area of concentrated pressure.

Advantages. The CTLSO (Milwaukee brace) used in congenital scoliosis has the same advantages as in idiopathic scoliosis. Its open design minimally restricts respiration, allows good air circulation, is adjustable for growth, and allows control of the upper thoracic spine and head.

Disadvantages. In congenital scoliosis, the CTLSO (Milwaukee brace) is usually well accepted by young children and their parents. In fact, it is easy for a young child to accept this orthosis because they adjust to it and it does not restrict their activities. The chin piece in the small child is different than in later years because there is little space between the mandible and thorax owing to the short neck in these small children, especially with cervical spine anomalies. The neck ring is padded, this being the support at this age (Fig. 14.19).

Results. There is only one study on the treatment of congenital scoliosis with the CTLSO (Milwaukee brace). A study by Winter and colleagues[59] showed that certain patients did well in the CTLSO for many years, a few even not needing surgery. The best results were in those patients with flexible mixed anomalies or those with progressive secondary curves. The brace was found to be effective for flexible deformities and plays no role in those with rigid deformities.

NEUROMUSCULAR DEFORMITIES

Neuromuscular spine deformities form a diverse group of conditions that share principles of natural

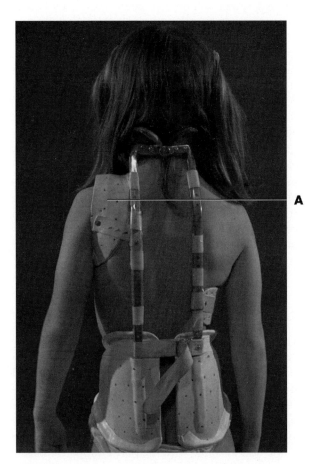

Fig. 14.17. CTLSO (Milwaukee brace) with shoulder ring *(A)* to control a high thoracic congenital curve.

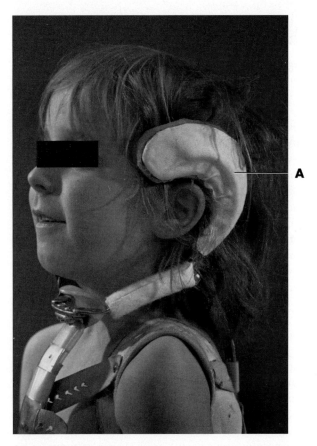

Fig. 14.18. Head support *(A)* attached to the neck ring of a CTLSO (Milwaukee brace) to control head tilt in a congenital cervicothoracic curve.

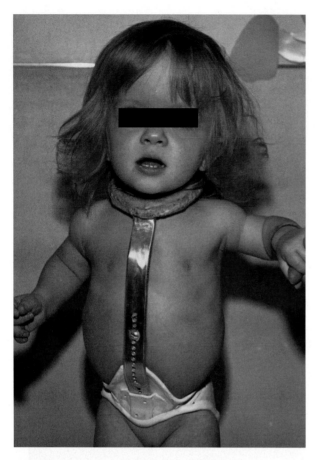

Fig. 14.19.   CTLSO (Milwaukee brace) with a padded neck ring for a young child placed in this orthosis.

history, evaluation, and treatment. The neuromuscular involvement has been classified into neuropathic and myopathic conditions. The neuropathic conditions involve the nervous system and have been subdivided into upper and lower motor neuron lesions. The upper motor neuron group include diseases such as cerebral palsy, syringomyelia, and spinal cord injuries; the lower motor neuron group include poliomyelitis and spinal muscle atrophy. Certain conditions such as myelodysplasia and spinal trauma have both upper and lower motor neuron involvement. The myopathic conditions include the diseases involving the muscle—arthrogryposis, Duchenne muscular dystrophy, and the other myopathies.

The prevalence of spinal deformities in these conditions is much higher than in idiopathic scoliosis, varying from 25% in cerebral palsy to nearly 100% in spinal trauma in a child under age 10 years. In general, the greater the neurologic involvement, the greater the likelihood and severity of the scoliosis. In addition, these deformities have a great chance of progressing, the progression continuing into adulthood.

Although these conditions vary in their cause, they share many features and can be considered together. Many are genetic in origin, and they all tend to involve multiple systems with multiple attendant problems—contractures, dislocated hips, seizures, mental retardation, insensate skin, and pressure sores. Thus, the evaluation of these children is not confined to the spine alone but must cover all these areas, best accomplished with the multidisciplinary team approach.

The aforementioned conditions are associated with either spasticity or flaccidity. There is no consistent curve pattern associated with a particular pattern of weakness, a combination of the weakness and muscle imbalance giving rise to the spinal deformity in each individual case. The most common deformity seen is scoliosis, followed by kyphosis, with lordosis being uncommon. The curve patterns in scoliosis can resemble those seen in idiopathic scoliosis, whereas others are long C curves. The most common curve pattern is a long C thoracolumbar curve extending to the pelvis, with the sacrum being part of the curve and associated with pelvic obliquity.

A collapsing kyphosis is also common, but often with severe scoliosis the apparent kyphosis is not due to posterior angulation of the vertebrae but is due to vertebral rotation. This has been termed *kyphosising scoliosis* by Stagnara.[52]

Nonoperative treatment of neuromuscular deformities is directed to two areas—seating and curve control. Seating systems are used for patients unable to sit without support, whereas orthoses—CTLSO (Milwaukee brace) or TLSO—are used for curve control.

Seating devices

In clinics with a large number of patients with neuromuscular diseases, seating plays a large role in treatment. These patients with absent or reduced sitting ability need help to maintain a balanced upright sitting posture. Where hand support is used to maintain this posture, the patient becomes a functional quadriplegic as the hands are used for support not for upper extremity functional activities.

The main principle of any sitting support is progressive trunk and spine control. The support of the base (i.e., pelvis) is primary, typically involving lateral pelvic support and a lap belt that holds the pelvis firmly back in any seat. The spine and trunk are controlled by lateral thoracic supports and a thoracic vest. When necessary, the head is supported with appropriate head supports. The amount of control and the seating support needed depend on the sitting balance of the patient. If control of the pelvis allows a good sitting posture, this minimal support is all that is needed. If the trunk is still unstable with the pelvic support, thoracic support is added. If at this stage the head is not controlled, a head support is added. To better control

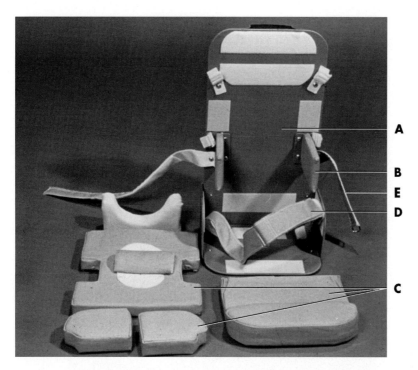

Fig. 14.20. Unholstered SSO consisting of a one piece plastic base *(A)* with lateral supports *(B)* and pads added *(C)*. There is a pelvic/lap *(D)* strap with an additional strap *(E)* to secure the support in the wheelchair.

the head it is often useful to tilt the whole sitting support backward.

The tendency of the spine, an unstable column, to collapse is shown biomechanically by Euler's laws, which state the critical load able to be supported by an unstable column. In a column with the lower end stabilized and the upper end free, the formula is as follows: $cEI/4L^2$, where c = constant, E = elasticity of the column, I = area moment of inertia, and L = length of column. If the length increases, or the size or weight increases (smaller area moment of inertia), the critical load able to be supported by the column decreases, and the column (spine) is more unstable. This explains why the child becomes more difficult to support with growth as the height and weight increase.

Types of seating devices. Many devices are available for sitting support, either commercially made or custom-fabricated. The commercial supports have the advantage of being easily available with some adjustment for growth. The disadvantage is that spine control is not optimal, and difficult seating problems cannot be treated. The custom-fabricated supports give better spine support but are labor intensive taking time to fabricate, and they are less adjustable for growth.

Tumbleform seat. This is one example of a commercial foam-molded seat that comes in three sizes and is used for infants and small children. It is effective in supporting these small flexible spines and becomes less effective as the child grows older.

Commercial chairs. A large number of commercial chairs are available in different parts of the United States (e.g., Orthokinetic chair, McClarren buggy, Mullholland chair, Transporter chair). They generally have some sort of pelvic and thoracic support, with abduction pads, and some type of head support. They are useful for flexible, easily controlled spines and are less effective for larger individuals or when more spine control is necessary.

Firm seat and back. In cases where minimal support is necessary, a firm seat and back are all that is necessary to stabilize the pelvis. These are usually padded plastic or wood added to the wheelchair.

Upholstered sitting support orthosis (SSO). This consists of a padded base (consisting of the seat and back) made of wood or plastic. A lap belt or pelvic strap is added to contort the pelvis, and a thoracic vest is added as needed (Fig. 14.20). The SSO is secured in a wheelchair or on a base. They are easily adjustable for growth by lengthening the seat and back, and altering the padding.

Molded SSO. In cases where more control is needed, a custom-fabricated total contact SSO is used.[13] This is made from a mold of the patient and extends from the distal thighs to the upper back with extensions around the pelvis and thorax (Fig. 14.21). A lap belt is added to maintain the position of the pelvis in the SSO, and a thoracic vest is used to hold the trunk back in the orthosis. Some adjustments for growth are

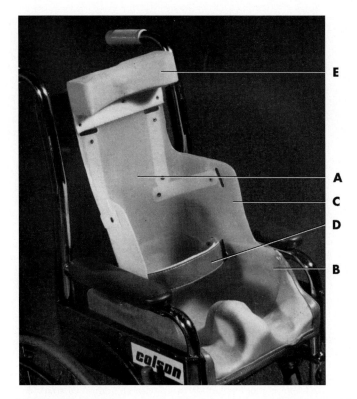

Fig. 14.21.   Molded SSO consisting of a molded sitting support with a seat and back *(A)* with lateral pelvic *(B)* and thoracic *(C)* supports. There is a pelvic/lap *(D)* strap with a head support *(E)*. This support is in a wheelchair.

possible with the addition of plastic to the seat or back portion and with widening of the orthosis. Like the upholstered SSO, it is secured in a wheelchair or to a base.

Results.   Sitting supports control flexible postural curves and have no effect on structural curves. They allow functional hand use and aid in the mobility of the patient. The greatest effect is in facilitating nursing care. Less time is necessary for constant repositioning, and mobility and transportation are easier. In addition, feeding is easier, with less time being necessary because the thorax and head are supported.

Curve control

In idiopathic scoliosis, the aim of nonoperative treatment is curve control and to prevent the need for surgery. In neuromuscular deformities, the aim of bracing is to control the curve during growth, allowing spinal growth to occur and delaying the time of surgical stabilization.

Orthotic treatment of neuromuscular deformities is more demanding than in idiopathic scoliosis. The duration of treatment is longer, and there are more skin problems because of the high incidence of insensate skin. In addition, full-time bracing is not always necessary. In flexible curves that are well controlled by the orthosis, bracing is necessary only when the patient is upright under the effect of gravity. During sleep, brac-

ing is unnecessary because gravity is not loading the spine causing the curve to collapse.

Orthoses available

CTLSO (Milwaukee brace).   A CTLSO is rarely used for curve control in neuromuscular deformities unless patients are ambulatory.

Advantages.   Great adjustability for growth is present, and there is minimal thoracic compression because of its open design.

Disadvantages.   The neck ring poses a problem in a large number of these patients—in whom there is less than optimal head control and in patients in whom the neck ring restricts head movement necessary for the functioning of the child. In addition, the force of the thoracic pad is localized and can result in localized rib deformity because of this pressure as the ribs are malleable in the growing child, especially when there is intercostal muscle paralysis or weakness.

TLSO.   A custom-fabricated low-profile TLSO is the most common orthosis used for curve control in neuromuscular deformities. This is usually the two-piece design, commonly called the two-piece body jacket or TLSO (Fig. 14.22). The orthosis is removed for skin care, especially with insensate skin. Care must be taken in fabrication of this orthosis to have a good total contact fit. In addition, the anterior thoracic win-

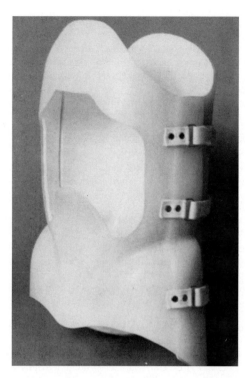

Fig. 14.22. Two-piece TLSO or body jacket consisting of anterior and posterior shells secured with lateral straps. There is a large thoracic window anteriorly.

dow must be as large as possible to minimize the respiratory restriction in the orthosis.

Advantages. The total contact fit minimizes the skin problems. Head and neck function are not affected with this design. The two-piece design allows easy donning and doffing by the parents for their child, as the child is placed in the orthosis in the supine position, which is much easier with the children.

Disadvantages. Because of the total contact design with the large surface area covered by the orthosis, use in hot climates without air conditioning is difficult. In addition, in some paralyzed patients, restricted heat loss is possible. Because the orthosis is not adjustable, modifications for growth are limited to relief over pressure areas and flaring. The need for replacement with growth depends on the growth rate of the child and averages every 2 years. In patients with intercostal paralysis (spinal muscle atrophy, high paraplegia, or high thoracic level myelodysplasia), there can be thoracic cage growth restriction or deformity or flaring of the lower ribs because the diaphragm is accentuated. These latter two effects of the orthosis are difficult to prevent, and when they occur, bracing may have to be discontinued and the curve treated surgically.

Results

The use of orthoses to control the curve in neuromuscular scoliosis is possible, being restricted to the juvenile years. With the onset of the pubertal growth spurt, this control is lost, and surgical stabilization is necessary. It must be remembered that these children's growth is in many cases unpredictable, and thus the age of the pubertal growth spurt varies tremendously. It is important to monitor the child's sitting and supine heights and to check the development of secondary sexual characteristics (Tanner grading). It is foolhardy to delay fusion to the end of growth, as at the onset of puberty 85% to 90% of spinal growth has already occurred. If surgery is delayed, the curve increases during puberty, with loss of flexibility. Thus, the additional spinal growth does not result in a longer spine, but rather in one that is more curved, shorter, and stiffer.

This control of the curve during the juvenile years slows down the rate of curve increase rather than giving dramatic curve correction. With flexible curves, some dramatic correction is possible, but this is only temporary. This control during the juvenile years has been documented for Duchenne muscular dystrophy,[12,37] spinal muscle atrophy,[46,49] myelodysplasia,[8] and paralytic scoliosis.[16] Nonoperative treatment is not effective for the rigid deformities in spastic cerebral palsy and arthrogryposis, although it has some effect in the smaller, less rigid deformities in these conditions.

SUMMARY

Orthotic nonoperative care plays an important role in the treatment of spinal deformities in idiopathic, congenital, and neuromuscular scoliosis. It must be recognized that these conditions are different, and the use of orthoses and their results differ with the condition and the orthosis used. The care must be individualized to the patient and carefully monitored for orthotic fit and curve response. Curve increase must be promptly diagnosed and surgically treated.

REFERENCES

1. Aaro S, Burstrom R, Dahlborn M: Derotating effect of the Boston brace, Spine 6:477, 1981.
2. Benson DR, Wolf AW, Shoji H: Can the Milwaukee brace patient participate in competitive athletics? Am J Sports Med 5:7, 1977.
3. Blount WP, Moe JH: The Milwaukee brace, Baltimore, 1973, Williams & Wilkins.
4. Bonnett CA, Tosoonian R: Results of Milwaukee brace treatment in seventy patients, Orthop Rev 7:79, 1978.
5. Bradford DS, et al: Scheuermann's kyphosis and roundback deformity, J Bone Joint Surg 56A:740, 1974.
6. Bradford DS, Moe JH, Winter RB: Kyphosis and postural roundback, Minn Med 56:114, 1978.
7. Breed A, et al: A PFT in adolescents with spine deformities being treated in a brace, Nashville, Pediatric Orthopaedic Study Group, 1981.
8. Bunch WH: Treatment of the myelomeningocoele spine, Instructional Course Lect 25:93, 1975.

9. Bunnell WP: A study of the natural history of idiopathic scoliosis, Orthop Trans 7:6, 1983.

10. Bunnell WP, MacEwen GD: Use of Orthoplast jacket in the nonoperative treatment of scoliosis, J Bone Joint Surg 58A:156, 1976.

11. Bunnell WP, MacEwen D, Jayakumar S: Use of plastic jackets in nonoperative treatment of idiopathic scoliosis, J Bone Joint Surg 62A:31, 1980.

12. Cambridge WR, Drennan JC: Scoliosis associated with Duchenne muscular dystrophy, J Pediatr Orthop 7:436–440, 1987.

13. Carlson JM, Winter RB: The "Gillette" sitting support orthosis, Orthot Prosthet 32:35, 1978.

14. Carr WA, et al: Treatment of idiopathic scoliosis in the Milwaukee brace, J Bone Joint Surg 62A:599, 1980.

15. Clarisse P: Prognosis of the evaluation of minor idiopathic scoliosis—from 10 to 29 degrees during growth of patients, Thesis, Claude Bernard University, 1974.

16. Dearolf WW III, et al: Scoliosis in pediatric spinal cord injuries, J Pediatr Orthop 10:214–218, 1990.

17. de Smedt A, Fabry G, Mulier JC: Milwaukee brace treatment of Scheuermann's kyphosis, Acta Orthop Belg 41:597, 1975.

18. Dickson RA, et al: The pathogenesis of idiopathic scoliosis: Biplanar spinal asymmetry, J Bone Joint Surg 66B:8, 1984.

19. Edmonson AS, Morris JT: Followup study of Milwaukee brace treatment in patients with idiopathic scoliosis, Clin Orthop Rel Res 126:58, 1977.

20. Edmonson AS, Smith GR: Long term followup study of Milwaukee brace treatment in patients with idiopathic scoliosis, Orthop Trans 7:10, 1983.

21. Emans JB, et al: The Boston bracing system for idiopathic scoliosis: Follow-up results in 295 patients, Spine 11:792, 1986.

22. Galante J, et al: Forces acting in the Milwaukee brace on patients undergoing treatment for idiopathic scoliosis, J Bone Joint Surg 52A:498, 1970.

23. Green NE: Part-time bracing of adolescent idiopathic scoliosis, J Bone Joint Surg 68A:738, 1986.

24. Gustafson B: Pasadena brace (Lexan), AAOS course on spine deformities, San Diego, 1976.

25. Keiser RP, Shuffelbarger HL: The Milwaukee brace in idiopathic scoliosis: Evaluation of 123 complete cases, Clin Orthop 118:19, 1976.

26. Keller B: Vitrathene hyperextension underarm jacket for Scheuermann's disease, Presented at the Pediatric Orthopaedic Study Group, Rochester, MN, 1978.

27. Lindh M: Effect of sagittal curve changes on brace correction of idiopathic scoliosis, Spine 5:26, 1980.

28. Lonstein JE, Carlson MJ: The prediction of curve progression in untreated idiopathic scoliosis, J Bone Joint Surg 66A:1061, 1984.

29. Lonstein JE, Winter RB: Milwaukee brace treatment of adolescent idiopathic scoliosis—review of 1020 patients, J Bone Joint Surg 76A:1207, 1994.

30. Lonstein JE, Winter RB: Milwaukee brace treatment of juvenile idiopathic scoliosis, Orthop Trans 13:91, 1989.

31. Mariani G, DeGiorgi D: The treatment of lumbar scoliosis with a three-piece brace, Ital J Orthop Traumatol 6:207, 1980.

32. McCollough NC, et al: Miami TLSO in management of scoliosis—preliminary results in one hundred cases, J Pediatr Orthop 1:141, 1981.

33. Mellencamp DD, Blount WP, Anderson AJ: Milwaukee brace treatment of idiopathic scoliosis: Late results, Clin Orthop Rel Res 126:47, 1977.

34. Moe JH: The Milwaukee brace in the treatment of scoliosis, Clin Orthop Rel Res 77:18, 1971.

35. Moe JH, Kettelson DN: Idiopathic scoliosis: Analysis of curve patterns and the preliminary results of Milwaukee brace treatment in one hundred and sixty-nine patients, J Bone Joint Surg 52A:1509, 1970.

36. Moe JH, et al: Scoliosis and other spinal deformities, ed 3, Philadelphia, 1994, WB Saunders.

37. Moseley CF, Koreska J, Miller F: Treatment of spinal deformity in Duchenne muscular dystrophy, Paper read at the 52nd Annual Meeting of the American Academy of Orthopaedic Surgeons, Las Vegas, 1985.

38. Nachemson AL, Peterson LE: Effectiveness of brace treatment of moderate adolescent idiopathic scoliosis, J Bone Joint Surg 77A:815, 1995.

39. Nash CL Jr: Current concepts review: Scoliosis bracing, J Bone Joint Surg 62A:848, 1980.

40. Northway RO, Alexander RG, Riolo MI: A cephalometric evaluation of the old Milwaukee brace and the modified Milwaukee brace in relation to the normal growing child, Am J Orthod 65:341, 1974.

41. Park J, et al: A modified brace (Prenyl) for scoliosis, Clin Orthop Rel Res 126:67, 1977.

42. Persky SL, Johnston LE: An evaluation of dentofacial changes accompanying scoliosis therapy with a modified Milwaukee brace, Am J Orthod 65:364, 1974.

43. Ponte A: An orthopaedic brace for the nonoperative treatment of lumbar and thoracolumbar scoliosis, J Bone Joint Surg 56A:1764, 1974.

44. Price CT, et al: Nightime bracing for adolescent idiopathic scoliosis with the Charleston bending brace, preliminary report, Spine 15:1294, 1990.

45. Ravaglia L, Caruso G: Treatment of dorsal kyphosis with the Milwaukee brace, Ital J Orthop Traumatol 7:61, 1981.

46. Riddick MF, Winter RB, Lutter LD: Spinal deformities in patients with spinal muscle atrophy: A review of 36 patients, Spine 7:476–483, 1982.

47. Risser J: The iliac apophysis: An invaluable sign in the management of scoliosis, Clin Orthop 11:111, 1958.

48. Salanova C: Le corset de Milwaukee dans le traitement des scolioses idiopathiques: Resultats et indications, Rev Chir Orthop 61:585, 1975.

49. Savin R, et al: La scoliosi nelle atrofie muscolari prossimali infantili. In Grupo Italiano di Studio della Scoliosi: Progressi in pathologia vertebrale, Bologna, Editore Aulo Gaggi.

50. Schmitt EW, Whitesides TE: Ponte orthosis in idiopathic scoliosis, Orthop Trans 5:23, 1981.

51. Shuffelbarger HL, Keiser RP: Nonoperative treatment of idiopathic scoliosis—a ten year study, Orthop Trans 7:11, 1983.

52. Stagnara P: Examen du scoliolique. In Deviations laterales du rachis: scolioses. Encyclopedie mediocochirurgicale, Paris, Apareil Locomoteur, 1974.

53. Stagnara P, Du Peloux J, Fauchet R: Traitement orthopedique ambulatoire de la maladie de Scheuermann en periode d'evolution, Rev Chir Orthop 52:38, 1966.

54. Tanner J: Growth at adolescence, ed 2, London, Blackwell, 1962.

55. Tolo VT, Gillespie R: The characteristics of juvenile idiopathic scoliosis and results of its treatment, J Bone Joint Surg 60B:181, 1978.

56. Von Riere D: Die konservative Behundlung fixierter juvenile thorakal Kypbosen, Beitr, Orthop Traumatol 22:175, 1975.

57. Watts HG, Hall JE, Stanish W: The Boston brace system for the treatment of low thoracic and lumbar scoliosis by the use of a girdle without superstructure, Clin Orthop Rel Res 126:87, 1977.

58. Winter RB, Carlson MJ: Modern orthotics for spinal deformities, Clin Orthop Rel Res 126:74, 1977.

59. Winter RB, et al: The Milwaukee brace in the nonoperative treatment of congenital scoliosis, Spine 1:85, 1976.

60. Winter RB, et al: Presence of spinal canal or cord abnormalities in idiopathic, congenital and neuromuscular scoliosis, Orthop Trans 16:135, 1992.

UPPER LIMB ORTHOSES

INTRODUCTION
William W. Eversmann, Jr.

As the surgeon and orthotist develop orthotic systems for the upper extremity, the kinesiology of the upper extremity that Johns outlined in Chapter 6 is essential to design an orthotic system that fills its intended purpose to protect the extremity, harness remaining motion of the extremity, and augment that motion in the face of disease or injury. Section Four gives the reader the available orthotic solutions for a constellation of upper extremity problems that require the attention of the surgeon and orthotist on a day-to-day basis. Some of these problems, as Keenan illustrates in Chapter 15, are client specific and need orthoses to be custom-designed. Other orthotic systems can be modified to groups of clients, such as clients with spinal cord injury, clients with burned hands, and clients with peripheral nerve and brachial plexus injuries in the upper extremity. Chapter 22 by Griffin and Chandler on protective devices that have been designed specifically for the sports-injured upper extremity emphasizes the protection of the extremity as the athlete continues to participate insofar as is possible.

The devices in Section Four emphasize the function of the upper extremity and the augmentation of that function and support of the extremity in the face of disease. Hand prehension patterns such as cylindric grasp, tip pinch, spherical grasp, hook or snap grasp, and lateral pinch require orthoses of different designs depending on which function is to be preserved for the client. The frequency of the use of the prehension patterns often dictates the most useful orthoses and orthotic systems for clients.

The importance of sensibility of the extremity that is fitted with an orthosis cannot be overemphasized. All of the authors of this section would agree that when neurologic injury prevails, whether it be central or peripheral, a portion of the client's skin may be anesthetic and the fitting of the orthosis and the monitoring of the anesthetic skin by physician and orthotist is necessary to avoid the occurrence of blisters and pressure sores from an ill-fitting orthosis. These chapters emphasize the necessity of proper fit of either thermoplastics or metal that is padded as desirable to prevent the adverse reactions to skin. The authors in this section have outlined the prevailing techniques in each of their chosen subjects. Adherence to their principles should provide the physician, orthotist, and client with a satisfactory outcome and final result.

Upper Extremity Orthoses for the Brain-Injured Patient

Mary Ann Keenan

GENERAL PRINCIPLES

Serious brain injury is frequently complicated by spasticity.[9,10,18] Often, this spasticity is severe and prevents adequate range-of-motion therapy of joints or maintenance of acceptable limb position. Contractures can occur despite the most conscientious and aggressive treatment attempts by family members, nursing staff, and therapists.[3]

Even when joint motion can be maintained by knowledgeable therapists, it commonly requires much force that is painful for the patient, potentially harmful to limbs, and time-consuming for the caregivers. Lesser degrees of spasticity also can impede a patient's function or require the use of positioning devices that interfere with the use of an extremity.

Prevention of deformity or fixed myostatic contracture in the face of severe spasticity is challenging. Splints applied to only one side of an extremity are not sufficient to control excessive spasticity and may result in skin breakdown from motion of the extremity against the splint (Fig. 15.1).[1,9,17,19] If used inappropriately, the orthosis may serve to conceal the severity of a deformity or may even cause additional deformity. It is therefore important to treat the underlying spasticity to use orthotic or positioning devices effectively.[2,7,8,9,14,22]

TIMING OF TREATMENT

Spontaneous neurologic recovery occurs for a prolonged time after a traumatic brain injury. Definitive surgical procedures to reduce spasticity, such as neurectomies, tendon releases, and transfers, are delayed until the patient shows minimal further improvement in motor control.[4,5,10,11,12,16] The prolonged period of spontaneous neurologic recovery (6 to 18 months)

combined with the intense level of spasticity, the common additional problem of rigidity (resistance to slow stretch), and strong muscles found in the young patient with brain injury make the temporary control of spasticity difficult but essential in these patients. Nerve blocks and casting techniques are used commonly and aggressively.

Nerve blocks done with local anesthetic agents are useful in assessing joint motion in a spastic limb. Repeated local anesthetic blocks provide some relief when severe spasticity prevents adequate range of motion. Repeating nerve blocks on a daily basis, however, is generally not practical. In this situation, a longer-acting agent, such as phenol, is used to block nerve function.[2,7–9,14] Phenol denatures the protein in a peripheral nerve causing axonal degeneration. The axons then regenerate, because the continuity of the nerve sheath has not been disrupted. The average duration of a phenol block is 6 months when performed as a surgical procedure, because the phenol is mixed with glycerine to prolong its action. When phenol nerve blocks are done percutaneously, the phenol is mixed with normal saline to allow greater dispersion of the solution. The average duration of a percutaneous block is 2 months. The action of phenol is nonspecific, contrary to original theories, and affects all nerve fibers alike.

The brain-injured patient is likely to have quadriplegic involvement, concomitant peripheral nerve injuries, residual deformities from fractures, and limitation of joint motion from heterotopic ossification.

CAUSES OF LIMITED JOINT MOTION

In a head-injured patient, it is often difficult to distinguish between several possible causes of de-

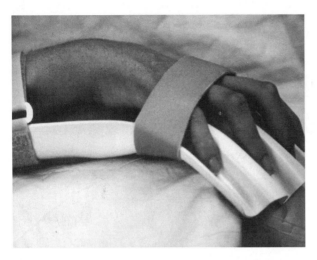

Fig. 15.1. A volar wrist hand orthosis applied to a hand with excessive spasticity does not adequately control position and may cause skin breakdown or boutonnière deformities of the fingers.

creased range of motion, such as increased muscle tone, myostatic contracture, heterotopic ossification, an undetected fracture or dislocation, pain, or lack of patient cooperation secondary to decreased cognition. A fracture or dislocation may or may not exhibit a clinical deformity but can easily be ruled out by radiographs. Early heterotopic ossification is accompanied by an inflammatory reaction with redness, warmth, severe pain, and steadily decreasing range of motion. Generally a radiograph shows evidence of the heterotopic bone as a hazy area of calcification forming in a periarticular location when it is suspected clinically. On occasion, a technetium bone scan is necessary to make the diagnosis.

Differentiating between the relative contributions of pain, increased muscle tone, and contracture can be more difficult. Diagnostic blocks using short-acting local anesthetic agents are extremely useful in assessing a spastic limb. The blocks can be performed at bedside or in the clinic setting without the use of special devices. By temporarily eliminating pain and muscle tone, patient cooperation is gained, and the amount of fixed contracture can be measured. The strength and control of antagonistic muscle groups can also be determined.

USES OF ORTHOTIC DEVICES

Contracture prevention

A combination of peripheral nerve blocks and casting or splinting techniques is commonly used to give temporary relief of spasticity. Positioning a limb in the desired position for later function is important. Because the clinical situation may change quickly after a trau-

matic brain injury, a short-term orthosis such as a cast is often a practical choice.[1,9,17] Casting maintains muscle fiber length and diminishes muscle tone by decreasing sensory input. Lidocaine blocks are helpful when done before cast application, because relieving the spasticity allows for easier limb positioning. Casts are used prophylactically to prevent contracture formation in nonfunctional position. A well-applied circular cast also protects the skin in an unconscious patient. Casts are commonly used to treat pressure sores in these patients. Close neurovascular observation is necessary in patients with head injury after circular plaster application because many cannot complain of pain secondary to a tight cast.

Contracture correction

Correction of contracture deformities can be obtained by serial cast application done at weekly intervals or by the use of dropout casts.[1] Serial casting is most successful when a contracture has been present for less than 6 months' duration. The patient is sedated, and an anesthetic nerve block is given if necessary to decrease the spasticity. The limb is manipulated for 10 minutes before cast application to gain the increased joint motion. A well-padded cast is then applied holding the arm in the improved position. Care must be taken not to exert excessive force while applying the cast. The major correction in joint position should have been obtained by the manipulation.

Drop out casts use the force of gravity to assist passively in correction of an early contracture. These are casts that have been modified to allow motion in one direction while preventing motion in the opposite direction. Because gravity is needed for correction, these casts are used in a patient who can be seated in an upright position or who is ambulatory.

Maintaining limb position

When the desired limb position has been achieved by serial or drop out casts, bivalved casts are frequently used. Bivalved casts or splints maintain the limb in the desired position but can be removed several times daily to perform joint range of motion and skin care. Bivalved casts or splints should not be used if severe spasticity persists. They do not adequately immobilize the arm to prevent shearing of the skin against the cast, which quickly leads to decubitus formation.

Functional aids

Orthoses can also be used to improve or assist function by positioning the limb adequately for use. Lapboards, arm slings, and other positioning devices should be considered as well as more conventional orthoses.

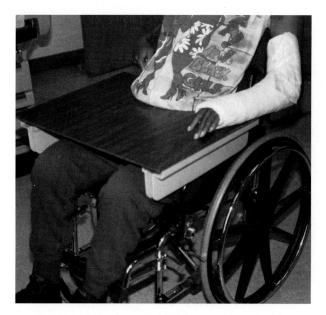

Fig. 15.2. A lapboard applied to a wheelchair can be used to support the shoulder and prevent inferior subluxation in the presence of proximal muscle weakness. The thickness of the board is adjusted to aid in upright sitting posture.

SHOULDER ORTHOSES

Spasticity can develop slowly after the onset of a brain injury. The extremity often begins in a flaccid state. Even as spasticity develops, the muscles supporting the shoulder are weak. The weight of the arm hanging can cause the shoulder to sublux inferiorly.

A prospective study revealed that 34% of brain-injured patients admitted for rehabilitation had peripheral neuropathies that had not been previously diagnosed.[21] The most common were ulnar nerve compression at the elbow, median nerve impingement, and brachial plexus injuries.[13,20] Many neuropathies are potentially preventable by careful positioning, padding, and treatment of spasticity.

Lapboard

A lapboard placed over the arms of a wheelchair can serve as a support for the upper extremity (Fig. 15.2). The thickness of the board is adjusted to support the arm. This device also assists the patient in maintaining an upright posture while seated.

Arm supports

A weak upper extremity can be supported using a sling suspended with springs from an overhead bar attached to a wheelchair. This simple device is comfortable, inexpensive, and easy for the patient and caretakers to use. It provides support to prevent inferior subluxation of the glenohumeral joint and can be positioned to hold the arm in slight abduction and

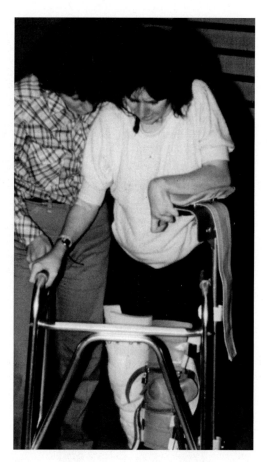

Fig. 15.3. A forearm trough support is used to support a nonfunctional arm or an arm with an elbow flexion contracture. The trough can be attached to the arm of a wheelchair or an ambulation device.

neutral rotation. This position is desirable to prevent adduction and internal rotation contractures of the shoulder from forming. Such contractures are painful and interfere with hygiene and upper body dressing.

A forearm trough device can be used to support and position the arm (Fig. 15.3). This can be attached directly to the arm of a wheelchair or on an ambulation device. The trough is used to position statically a nonfunctional arm. The patient's forearm can be secured in position with padded straps. This is useful when there is a mild-to-moderate degree of spasticity in the adductor and internal rotator muscles of the shoulder.

A forearm trough can be attached to a hinged mobile support on the arm of the chair (Fig. 15.4). This allows the arm to be placed in a variety of positions for functional use or training of the hand. By decreasing the amount of friction in the hinges, a relatively weak motion of the shoulder can be enhanced to place the hand and arm in a desired position. Alternatively the friction can be increased to provide greater stability.

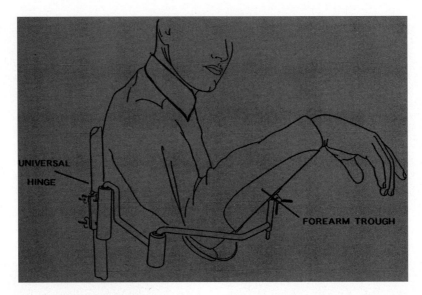

Fig. 15.4. A mobile arm support attached to a wheelchair can be used to provide support to a weak shoulder and enhance function of the upper extremity.

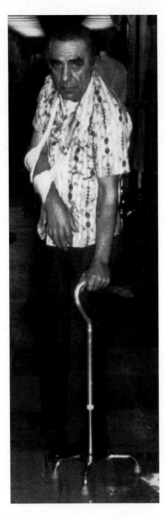

Fig. 15.5. A hemisling is useful to support a flail arm and prevent inferior subluxation of the shoulder in an ambulatory patient.

Sling

A sling is the simplest and most common orthotic device used to position the arm (Fig. 15.5). Its advantages are low cost, ease of use, light weight, and portability. This is the apparatus of choice in an ambulatory patient with hemiplegic involvement. The sling should be removed periodically to do range-of-motion exercises of the shoulder and elbow.

Abduction pillow

A bed-bound patient with paralysis or spasticity of the shoulder musculature is prone to develop an adduction and internal rotation contracture of the shoulder from prolonged immobility.[2] A foam pillow is a useful device to position the shoulder in slight abduction and neutral rotation. This position facilitates care and prevents contractures and hygiene difficulties in the axilla.

ELBOW ORTHOSES

Flexor spasticity is common and frequently severe in the brain-injured patient. Flexion contractures are therefore common. These are painful and lead to maceration of the antecubital skin. The flexed posture of the elbow places traction on the ulnar nerve in the cubital tunnel and positions the relatively immobile patient to place excess pressure directly on the nerve. Compression neuropathy of the ulnar nerve is seen in 10% of patients with brain injury.[13,21]

The elbow flexor spasticity must be diminished to allow correction of a contracture or permit static positioning of the elbow. During the initial 6 to 9 months after injury, the spasticity is customarily treated by

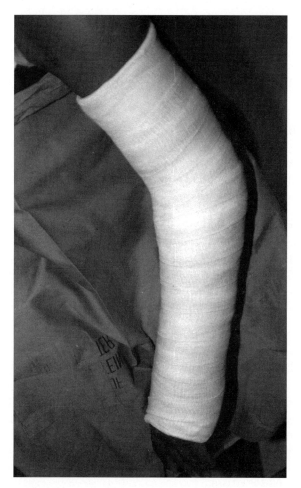

Fig. 15.6. A long arm cast is an effective device to control elbow position or to correct a flexion deformity.

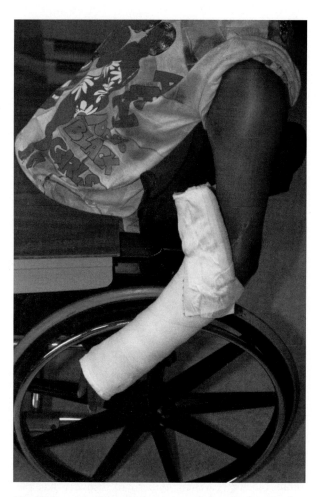

Fig. 15.7. An elbow drop out cast allows elbow extension while preventing flexion. The weight of the cast stretches the tight anterior joint capsule. The upper arm can then "drop out" of the posterior window in the cast.

performing a percutaneous phenol block of the musculocutaneous nerve in the upper arm.[9,14] This block decreases spasticity in the biceps and brachialis muscles. Because the brachioradialis muscle is usually the most spastic of the elbow flexors, it must be addressed also.[15] This is done by performing a phenol motor point block of the brachioradialis muscle.

When neurologic recovery has stabilized, residual elbow flexor spasticity is treated surgically. In an extremity that exhibits some volitional movement, the elbow flexor tendons are lengthened.[10,15,16] When a contracture is present in an elbow that lacks volitional movement, the flexor tendons are transected. It is common to be faced with a residual flexion deformity even after surgical release.

Long arm cast

A long arm cast is an excellent orthotic device for positioning the elbow (Fig. 15.6) and is the most frequently used device for correcting a flexion contracture. After the spasticity has been diminished by blocks or surgery, the elbow is casted in maximum extension.

The cast is then changed every 5 to 7 days and, with each change, the elbow is gently manipulated into further extension. When full extension has been obtained, the cast is bivalved and a clamshell splint is fabricated. The elbow is immobilized in full extension for an additional 3 to 4 weeks to prevent recurrent deformity, with the splints being removed several times daily for range-of-motion exercises.

Drop out cast

A drop out cast is a modification of a long arm cast in which the posterior portion of the cast above the elbow joint is removed (Fig. 15.7). This cast allows the elbow to extend further but prevents flexion. The cast is purposefully made heavy or weights are added to the wrist to provide an extension force on the elbow. A dropout cast is effective only in a patient who is in an upright position for much of the day, because the arm must be hanging freely for the device to work. As the elbow extends further, the arm "drops out" of the cast.

The cast is changed periodically as further elbow extension is gained.

Bivalved long arm cast

A bivalved cast or clamshell cast is another modification of the long arm cast. The cast is lined with stockinette to provide a smooth inner surface. Straps are added to secure the anterior and posterior halves of the cast together. The cast can be removed several times daily to allow active or passive joint motion of the elbow to prevent stiffness. A bivalved cast cannot be used in the presence of severe spasticity, because it does not sufficiently immobilize the arm to protect the skin from friction and breakdown. A bivalved cast must be reapplied carefully to assure proper alignment and prevent pressure on bony prominences. It requires a cooperative patient and a knowledgeable caretaker.

WRIST AND HAND ORTHOSES

Spastic forearm flexor muscles causing wrist and finger flexion deformities are commonplace. Again, it is important to diminish the muscle spasticity. Casts and orthotic devices are used in an adjunctive manner to correct residual contractures or position the wrist and hand.

During the first 6 to 9 months after onset of injury, extrinsic flexor spasticity is treated by phenol motor point blocks.[7-9] When neurologic recovery has plateaued, the spastic extrinsic flexors are surgically lengthened.[10,12,16]

Short arm cast

When only the wrist is contracted, a short arm cast is an excellent device for positioning the wrist (Fig. 15.8). Most commonly, there is also a flexion contracture of the elbow, and the entire arm is treated using a long arm cast.

Bivalved short arm cast

A bivalved cast or clamshell cast is another modification of the short arm cast. The cast is lined with stockinette to provide a smooth inner surface. Straps are added to secure the anterior and posterior halves of the cast together. The cast can be removed several times daily to allow active or passive joint motion of the wrist to prevent stiffness. A bivalved cast cannot be used in the presence of severe spasticity, because it does not sufficiently immobilize the arm to protect the skin from friction and breakdown. A bivalved cast must be reapplied carefully to ensure proper alignment and prevent pressure on bony prominences. It requires a cooperative patient and a knowledgeable caretaker.

Thumb spica cast

The thumb-in-palm deformity is a frequent deformity in the spastic hand.[4] This deformity is generally secondary to spasticity in the flexor pollicis longus muscle as well as the median and ulnar innervated thenar muscles. If a flexion deformity of the interphalangeal joint of the thumb is present, the flexor pollicis longus is spastic.

A thumb spica cast is an excellent orthotic device for positioning the thumb (Fig. 15.9) and is a commonly

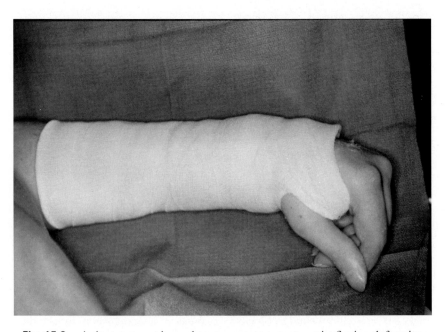

Fig. 15.8.   A short arm cast is used to prevent or correct a wrist flexion deformity.

used device for correcting a thumb-in-palm contracture. As with all deformities in the spastic upper extremity, a thumb spica cast is used in conjunction with phenol blocks or surgery.[4,7–9,16] The cast is applied as a circular device initially. It can later be modified to a bivalved splint if needed.

Finger casts

Individual finger casts can be applied to correct flexion deformities of the interphalangeal joints (Fig. 15.10). The underlying noxious spasticity must be resolved or diminished before casting. The casts must be applied with extreme caution to prevent excessive pressure and skin breakdown. A minimum of padding must be used or the small cylinder casts may fall off. The casts should be changed every 1 to 2 days to allow inspection of the skin.

Dynamic finger splints

Dynamic spring splints can be applied for short periods several times each day to correct flexion contractures of the interphalangeal joints. Dynamic splints should not be used if flexor spasticity is present. The splints must be carefully positioned and checked frequently because the brain-injured patient cannot be expected to be compliant with treatment.

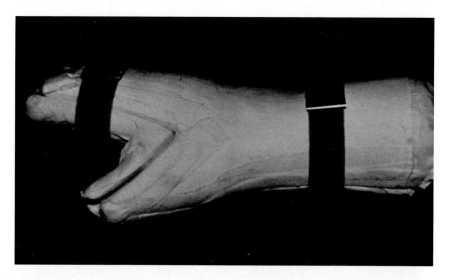

Fig. 15.9. A thumb spica cast that has been bivalved to allow removal for skin care and range-of-motion exercises.

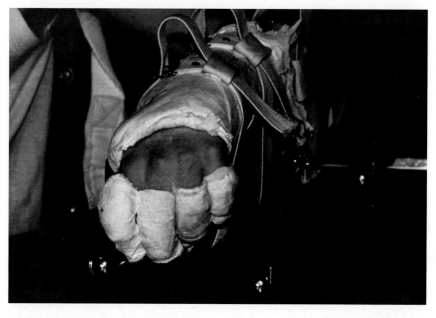

Fig. 15.10. Individual finger casts can be applied to correct flexion deformities of the interphalangeal joints of the fingers.

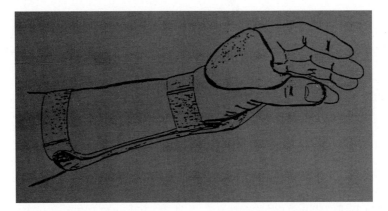

Fig. 15.11.   A volar wrist splint can be used to maintain the wrist in neutral position after the spasticity has been reduced using phenol nerve blocks or surgical lengthening of the involved muscles.

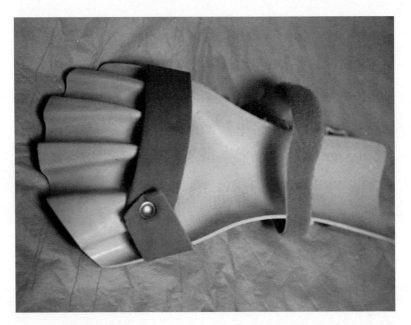

Fig. 15.12.   A wrist hand orthosis is useful for passive positioning of the wrist and fingers after the spasticity has been eliminated by surgical lengthening of the flexors.

Volar wrist splint

A lightweight volar splint can be useful to maintain the wrist in an extended position for hand function (Fig. 15.11). This splint most commonly is indicated after surgical lengthening of spastic extrinsic finger flexor muscles in a hand with modest volitional movement. By holding the wrist in slight extension, the patient can proceed with occupational therapy and functional training of finger motion.

Wrist hand orthosis

A volar splint that holds the wrist, thumb, and fingers in an extended position is useful as a positioning device after surgical lengthening of the extrinsic flexors (Fig. 15.12). The orthosis is worn at night for sleeping to maintain the hand in a corrected position and is removed for functional activities during waking hours.

A nonfunctional hand with severe flexion deformities is best treated surgically by performing a superficialis-to-profundus tendon transfer combined with wrist arthrodesis.[5,11] These patients tolerate orthotic devices poorly and tend to develop skin maceration. Because these patients commonly reside in skilled nursing facilities, the orthotic devices are easily lost or are improperly applied.

Thumb abduction splint

A lightweight splint that holds the thumb metacarpal in an abducted and slightly opposed position can be used to improve thumb function and pinch (Fig. 15.13).[6] This type of orthosis is gener-

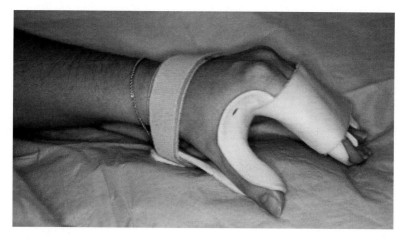

Fig. 15.13. A thumb abduction orthosis can be used to passively position the thumb. An orthosis can also be devised to hold the thumb abducted while allowing for use of the hand.

ally used after surgical correction of a thumb-in-palm deformity.

SUMMARY

Orthoses have a limited but important role in preventing or correcting upper extremity deformities in brain-injured patients. Spasticity must be diminished or eliminated using phenol nerve blocks or surgical tendon lengthening. Most often, the orthoses must completely encase the extremity to adequately control position without the danger of skin breakdown.

REFERENCES

1. Booth BJ, Doyle M, Montgomery J: Serial casting for the management of spasticity in the head-injured adult, Phys Ther 63:1960, 1983.
2. Botte MJ, Keenan MAE: Percutaneous phenol blocks of the pectoralis major muscle to treat spastic deformities, J Hand Surg 13A:147–149, 1988.
3. Botte MJ, Nickel VL, Akeson WH: Spasticity and contracture: Physiologic aspects of formation, Clin Orthop 233:7–18, 1988.
4. Botte MJ, et al: Surgical management of spastic thumb-in-palm deformity in adults with brain injury, J Hand Surg 14A:174–181, 1989.
5. Braun RM, Vise GT, Roper B: Preliminary experience with superficialis to profundus tendon transfer in the hemiparetic upper extremity, J Bone Joint Surg 56A:466–472, 1974.
6. Currie DM, Mendiola A: Cortical thumb orthosis for children with spastic cerebral palsy, Arch Phys Med Rehabil 68:214–216, 1987.
7. Garland DE, Lilling M, Keenan MA: Phenol blocks to motor points of spastic forearm muscles in head-injured adults, Arch Phys Med Rehabil 65:243–245, 1984.
8. Katz J, Knott LW, Feldman DJ: Peripheral nerve injections with phenol in management of spastic patients, Arch Phys Med Rehabil 48:97–99, 1967.
9. Keenan MAE: The orthopaedic management of spasticity, J Head Trauma Rehabil 2:62–71, 1987.
10. Keenan MAE: Management of the spastic upper extremity in the neurologically impaired adult, Clin Orthop 233:116–125, 1988.
11. Keenan MAE, et al: Results of transfer of the flexor digitorum superficialis tendons to flexor digitorum profundus tendons in adults with acquired spasticity of the hand, J Bone Joint Surg 69A:1127–1132, 1987.
12. Keenan MAE, et al: Results of fractional lengthening of the finger flexors in adults with upper extremity spasticity, J Hand Surg 12A:575–581, 1987.
13. Keenan MAE, et al: Late ulnar neuropathy in the brain-injured adult, J Hand Surg 13A:120–124, 1988.
14. Keenan MAE, et al: Percutaneous phenol block of the musculo-cutaneous nerve to control elbow flexor spasticity, J Hand Surg 15A:340–346, 1990.
15. Keenan MAE, Haider T, Stone LR: Dynamic electromyography to assess elbow spasticity, J Hand Surg. 15A:607–614, 1990.
16. Keenan MA, Waters RL: Surgical treatment of the upper extremity after stroke or brain injury. In Chapman E, editor: Operative Orthopaedics, Philadelphia, 1993, JB Lippincott.
17. King TI: Plaster splinting as a means of reducing elbow flexor spasticity: A case study, Am J Occup Ther 36:671–673, 1982.
18. Kraus JF, et al: The incidence of acute brain injury in a defined population, Am J Epidemiol 119:186, 1984.
19. Mills VM: Electromyographic results of inhibitory splinting, Phys Ther 64:190–193, 1984.
20. Orcutt SA, et al: Carpal tunnel syndrome in patients with spastic wrist flexion deformity, J Hand Surg 15A:940–944, 1990.
21. Stone L, Keenan MAE: Peripheral nerve injuries in the adult with traumatic brain injury, Clin Orthop 233:136–144, 1988.
22. Wainapel SF, Haigney D, Labib K: Spastic hemiplegia in a quadriplegic patient: Treatment with phenol nerve block, Arch Phys Med Rehabil 65:786–787, 1984.

Upper Limb Orthoses for the Spinal Cord Injured Patient

Darrell R. Clark
Robert L. Waters
Jane M. Baumgarten

The individual with tetraplegia resulting from spinal cord injury experiences varying degrees of functional loss in the upper limb, depending on the neurologic level of the lesion. Goals in the treatment of the upper limb include preventing deformity, maintaining range of motion, restoring function, and maximizing functional capability.[3,11] An organized interdisciplinary team approach is essential to meet these goals. Orthotic management can play an important part and can allow the individual to gain independence in various activities of daily living. This can help restore self-esteem and provide a sense of accomplishment that would not otherwise be attainable.

HISTORICAL BACKGROUND

Historically, upper limb orthoses were designed for patients with paralysis that resulted from conditions other than spinal cord injury. One of the earliest of these was the flexor-hinge hand splint (Fig. 16.1). Originally designed for the patient with polio, this orthosis transmitted force generated by active wrist extension via a mechanical linkage to paralyzed index and long fingers, enabling finger closure against the thumb. The design of this orthosis evolved into what is today known as the wrist-driven, wrist-hand orthosis (WDWHO). The prehension offered by this orthosis had obvious application for the spinal cord–injured patient with strong wrist extensor musculature and paralyzed finger flexors. The WDWHO harnesses wrist extensor power and uses the power of wrist extension to flex the fingers at the metacarpophalangeal joints.

Many patients lacked sufficient wrist extensor strength to use the flexor-hinge splint. Interest in providing external power to the basic mechanical design of the splint led to a system that used a CO_2-powered "artificial muscle" to provide proportionally controlled prehension. This system was designed in 1957 at Rancho Los Amigos Hospital in collaboration with McKibben, a physicist whose daughter was a patient.[2] It featured a helically-woven fabric surrounding a rubber bladder (Fig. 16.2). When pressurized with CO_2, the bladder expanded against the woven fabric and shortened in length. This, in turn, operated the linkage, which propelled the fingers into flexion. A two-way valve, operated by shoulder shrugging, released the pressure to allow finger extension.

By 1964, the advent of smaller, more powerful electric motors caused a shift away from CO_2 as a source of external power for upper limb orthoses. Electrical external power was coupled to the WDWHO through the use of cables and battery-powered motors (Fig. 16.3). Again the potential benefits to the patient with partial upper limb paralysis were obvious.

Encouraged by results of the work with the WD-WHO, Certified Orthotists and biomedical engineers at Rancho Los Amigos undertook a much more ambitious project—a battery-powered, multidimensional upper extremity orthosis that would attempt to duplicate all major motions of the arm and hand. Designed using anthropometric measurements, this tongue-switch–controlled device offered the opportunity for high-level tetraplegic patients to achieve greater independence in activities of daily living (Fig. 16.4).

In actual practice, however, externally powered systems often proved difficult to maintain. Unless there was ready access to technical support personnel who could repair delicate electronic parts, the orthoses fell into disrepair and became unusable. Equally crucial for useful function was patient training. The complexity of these systems required a well-planned, well-implemented training program. These two factors often proved a deterrent to continued use by all but the most committed patients.

Designs that used simple mechanical components proved easier to operate and maintain. One example was the adoption of prosthetic harnessing systems to

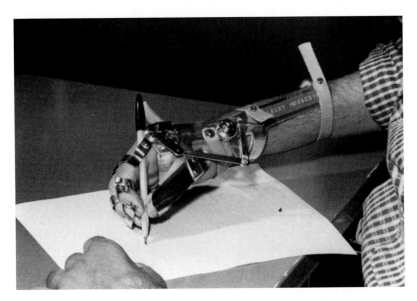

Fig. 16.1. Flexor hinge hand splint.

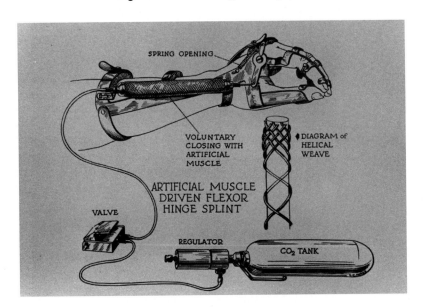

Fig. 16.2. Artificial muscle.

the WDWHO. Upper limb prostheses have long been powered by the use of strapping systems that use contralateral shoulder protraction to operate a cable that opens the terminal device. This principle was applied to the WDWHO with limited success. Current designs, although less elaborate, continue to use simple mechanical components, which are more easily maintained.

Today, orthoses for the spinal cord–injured patient population can be divided into two broad categories: static orthoses for positioning and dynamic orthoses for function. To help prevent deformity, static hand orthoses and WHOs are designed to maintain thumb opposition, thumb web space, and palmar arch as well as proper angulation between the hand and forearm. Dy-

namic orthoses, such as the wrist-driven WHO and the ratchet WHO, provide prehension to increase independence in activities of daily living.

DEFINITIONS

The American Spinal Injury Association (ASIA) and the International Medical Society of Paraplegia (IM-SOP) have developed the *International Standards for Neurological and Functional Classifications of Spinal Cord Injury.*[5] These standards identify and define appropriate terms and concepts for this patient population.

Injuries are classified as either complete or incomplete with respect to sensory and motor function.

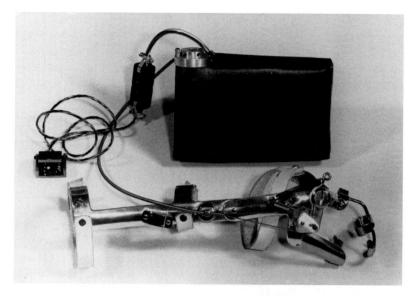

Fig. 16.3. Electric-powered WHO.

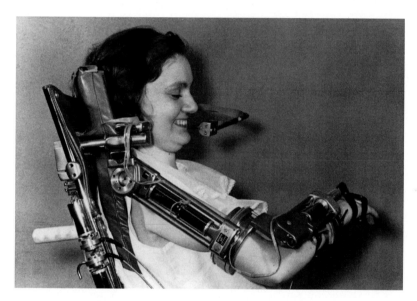

Fig. 16.4. "Golden arm."

Complete is defined as an absence of sensation at S4-5 segments and inability to contract the external anal sphincter. *Incomplete* is defined as at least partial preservation of S4-5 sensation or external sphincter motor function.

Injuries are further classified as to neurologic, sensory, and motor level. ASIA/IMSOP defines these terms as follows:

Neurological level: The most caudal segment of the spinal cord with normal sensory and motor function on both sides of the body. Because segments at which normal function is found often differ by side of body, up to four different segments may be identified in determining neurologic level (i.e., right or left sensory, right or left motor).

Sensory level: The most caudal segment of the spinal cord with normal sensory function on both sides of the body. The level is determined by neurologic examination of key sensory test points (Table 16.1) within each of 28 dermatomes on each side of the body (Fig. 16.5).

Motor level: The most caudal segment of the spinal cord with normal motor function on both sides of the body. The level is determined by neurologic examination of key muscle test points (Table 16.2) within each of 10 myotomes on each side of the body.

With respect to function and orthotic management, the motor level is more significant than the neurologic level. It is often useful to think in terms of *functional level* rather than *neurologic level*. Functional level is defined as the lowest segmental level at which the key muscles are grade 3 or stronger and sensation is intact at that dermatome level and above.

The importance of sensation is that it provides tactile feedback. Lack of sensation results in diminished functional capability. In spinal cord injury, sensation is generally intact at, and slightly above, the motor level. This means, for example, that a C6 quad typically has sensation on the side of the thumb and index finger, which greatly facilitates hand function. Although a C5 quad may or may not have this specific sensory distribution, it is important to examine for this possibility.

Muscle grades are an important factor as well. Assigning an accurate grade is often difficult, especially with regard to interrater testing. Although it is generally agreed that a grade 3 is required for function, it can be argued that functionally to pick up an object with the fingers, strength higher than grade 3 is necessary. *Plus* or *minus* subdivision of the grades, however, creates difficulty in maintaining interrater accuracy. The ASIA/IMSOP five-point motor scale (Table 16.3) is based on international standards and should be adhered to as closely as possible in classifying patients.

Waters and colleagues[10] found that reasonable predictions about muscle return can be made using 1 month postinjury baseline examinations. Overall, key upper extremity muscle groups with grade 1 or 2 strength at 1 month postinjury have a 97% chance of recovering to grade 3 or greater 1 year postinjury (Table 16.4). Concomitantly a grade 0 muscle one level below the most caudal voluntary muscle has a 27% chance of functional recovery ≥ grade 3; a grade 0 muscle two levels below the most caudal voluntary muscle has only 1% chance of functional recovery. With this information, it is possible to predict reasonably the orthotic needs early in the rehabilitation period and prescribe accordingly. For example, if a patient is grade 2 at 1 month, it may be more cost-effective to use a prefabricated splint rather than a custom static WHO because it can be anticipated that further motor recovery will occur.

Table 16.1.   Key sensory test points

C2	Occipital protuberance
C3	Supraclavicular fossa
C4	Top of the acromioclavicular joint
C5	Lateral side of the antecubital fossa
C6	Thumb
C7	Middle finger
C8	Little finger
T1	Medial side of the antecubital fossa
T2	Apex of the axilla

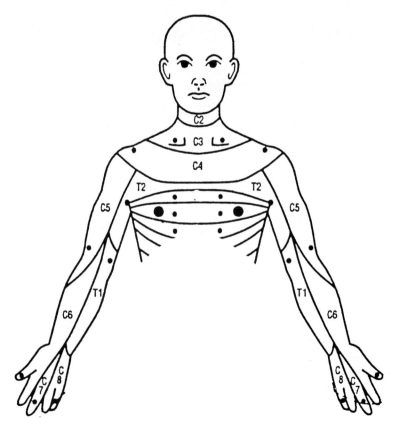

Fig. 16.5.   Upper limb dermatomes.

ORTHOTIC DESIGN PRINCIPLES BY FUNCTIONAL LEVEL

C4 motor level

The patient with a complete C4 motor level has neck and upper trapezius muscle function. Although C4 represents the first level with potential for arm function, without wrist extensor strength an individual cannot use tenodesis provided by active wrist extension to accomplish prehension. Even though there is no expectation of hand function, it is important to prevent hygiene problems and skin breakdown.

The static WHO (Fig. 16.6) is used for individuals with injuries from C1 through C4 who lack wrist extension.[3] The purpose of the orthosis is to maintain the functional position of the hand and wrist, thereby reducing the risk of contracture and deformity. This is accomplished by supporting the wrist in approximately 20 degrees of extension and holding the thumb in a position of abduction. The orthosis also preserves the palmar arch of the hand. This position approximates that required for many functional activities. It is also important to maintain correct position and range of motion in the event of neurologic return distal to the injury.

Although the static WHO is designed for positioning only, it may be worn during certain functional activities requiring wrist stability. For example, control of an electric wheelchair is more easily accomplished when the paralyzed wrist is immobilized.

Mouthsticks. The C4 or higher motor level tetraplegic may use mouthsticks for certain functional activities.[3] Mouthsticks are typically either a wooden or a metal rod with attachments designed to accomplish specific functions, such as page turning, typing, or writing (Fig. 16.7). Similar to WHOs, mouthsticks may be thought of as either static or dynamic. Static designs are passive in nature with a simple rubber tip for pushing or a clamp to hold a utensil. Dynamic designs allow the individual to pick up and move small objects. Typical dynamic designs provide a tongue-operated plunger, which allows opening and closing of a pincer mechanism on the distal end. Forceful thrusting of the tongue opens the pincer, and a rubber band or spring closes it when the tongue is relaxed.

Table 16.2.	Key muscle test points
C5	Elbow flexors
C6	Wrist extensors
C7	Elbow extensor
C8	Finger flexors to the middle finger
T1	Small finger abductors

Table 16.3. ASIA-IMSOP five-point motor scale	
0	Total paralysis
1	Palpable or visible contraction
2	Active movement, full range, gravity eliminated
3	Active movement, full range, against gravity
4	Active movement, full range, against moderate resistance
5	Normal active movement, full range, full resistance

ASIA-IMSOP, American Spinal Injury Association-International Medical Society of Paraplegia.

Table 16.4. Motor grade at 1 month versus motor grade at 1 year*		1 YEAR FOLLOW-UP (MANUAL MOTOR GRADE)					
		0	1	2	3	4	5
One month follow-up (manual motor grade)	0	213	14	12	22	5	0
	1			5	25	15	6
	2				10	9	24
	3				7	5	16
	4					2	4
	5						56

*Summary key muscles from C5 to T1.
From Waters RL, et al: Recovery following complete quadriplegia, Arch Phys Med Rehabil 74:242, 1993.

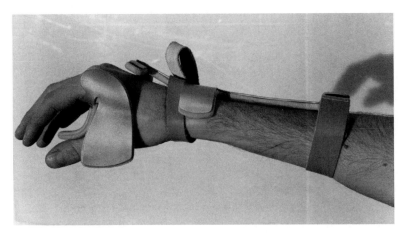

Fig. 16.6.   Static WHO.

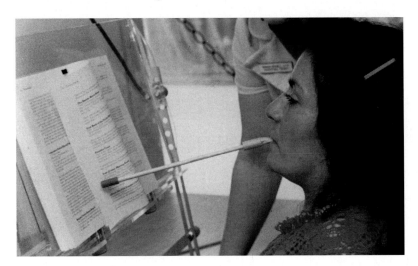

Fig. 16.7.   Mouthstick.

Mouthsticks vary in length but are generally 12 to 18 inches long. This distance is measured from the patient's lips to the work surface. Weight can also vary: Lighter weight is useful for desktop activities, and heavier mouthsticks are useful for activities requiring more force. Endurance is compromised as weight increases.

The patient must have a means of "docking," or holding, the mouthstick when it is not being used. Docking designs vary considerably, and careful evaluation of the patient's abilities and needs is important.

Patients need to meet certain minimum criteria to use a mouthstick. Full range of motion in the neck and grade 3 or greater strength in neck muscles allow optimal use. Motivation is also a critical factor, and, frequently, patients are not psychologically ready to use mouthsticks early in their program.

Training must begin slowly and with positive expectations. Initial activities should be simple and easily accomplished. The first few sessions should be only a few minutes in length with frequent rest periods.

C4 motor level (with some C5 return −1/5 or 2/5)

The complete C4 patient may develop some return at the C5 level. Recovery of at least grade 3/5 of elbow flexion is necessary to attain the C5 motor level category. Recovery of less than grade 3 in the deltoids or biceps may be sufficient for arm function, although it must be assisted to be functional. Mobile arm supports (MAS) may provide sufficient antigravity support to grade 2/5 or 3/5 muscles to enable functional upper extremity use.[3]

Mobile arm supports.   Patients with shoulder and elbow strength grade 3 or below, or who lack adequate endurance, may still be able to place their hand for functional activities through the use of a MAS. This device, which attaches to the patient's wheelchair, supports the arm and allows horizontal motion at the shoulder and elbow, thereby allowing the hand to be positioned for function (Fig. 16.8).

The system consists of a mounting bracket, proximal arm, distal arm, and forearm support trough. Simple

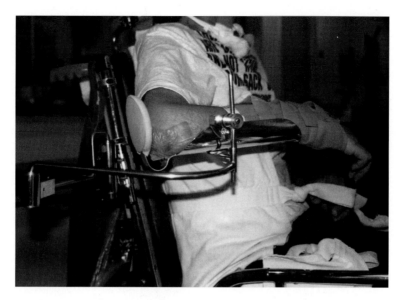

Fig. 16.8. MAS.

pivot joints are analogous to the shoulder, elbow, and wrist. The component parts are individually fitted and adjusted to assist the patient in gaining maximum functional and therapeutic benefits from the support.

Once deltoids are grade 2 or better, the patient may benefit by the addition of an elevating proximal arm to the MAS. This component replaces the standard wheelchair mounting bracket and allows vertical motion of the arm via a spring-assisted piston. This greatly increases the area of arm motion and enhances function. It is also beneficial in helping to strengthen the deltoids.

The standard MAS system significantly increases the overall width of the wheelchair and may cause problems going through doorways. An alternate design, the linear MAS (Fig. 16.9) solves this problem. This system uses linear bearings and straight rods without joints to accomplish the desired motions. For long-term users, the linear MAS is the system of choice.

Muscle function in the shoulder, elbow, neck, or trunk is used to operate the system. Varying combinations of muscle strength and coordination permit operation of the system. Even patients with strength less than grade 2 may be able to accomplish electric wheelchair control, feeding, light hygiene, and simple tabletop activities with the device, once set up. The ability to contract and relax muscles smoothly is important in obtaining full benefit from the support. Excessive spasticity interferes.

Patients must have adequate passive range of motion at the shoulder, elbow, and forearm to use the MAS effectively. At least 90 degrees of hip flexion is also required for proper sitting position. Although the MAS may be adjusted for use in a semireclined position, an upright position is preferable for functional activities. Wheelchair trunk supports may be used to obtain adequate upright position and stability.

The same indications and guidelines for use of the static WHO apply as with C4. In some cases, attachments can be added to the static WHO that allow the patient to hold utensils for such activities as feeding or typing. Another device, called the universal cuff, attaches directly to the patient's hand and provides a pouch for inserting the various specially modified utensils such as a fork or toothbrush. Many other prefabricated items are available for specific tasks.

Ratchet wrist-hand orthosis.   For patients with wrist extensor strength below grade 3 to accomplish prehension, the ratchet WHO (Fig. 16.10) may be used.[37] Designed primarily for the C5 patient, some C4 patients with weak return in the C5 musculature find it useful when used in conjunction with MAS.

The ratchet WHO holds the wrist joint in a static position. The thumb post holds the thumb abducted and aligned in opposition to the index and middle fingers to allow prehension. Finger pieces hold the index and middle fingers in enough flexion to allow pad-to-pad contact with the thumb. A ratchet bar (Fig. 16.11) connects the finger pieces to the main body of the orthosis. Closing is typically accomplished by motion of the contralateral hand against the finger pieces to flex the fingers against the thumb. Alternate methods may be used, however, such as the chin or the side of a chair or table. Release is accomplished through a return spring, which is activated by pressing a release button. Individual muscle strength and experimentation determine the easiest way for the patient to manage operation of the orthosis. This simple mechanical design is

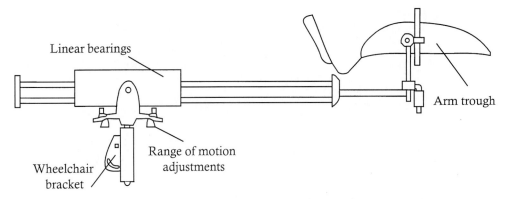

Linear bearings

Arm trough

Range of motion
adjustments

Wheelchair
bracket

Fig. 16.9. Linear MAS.

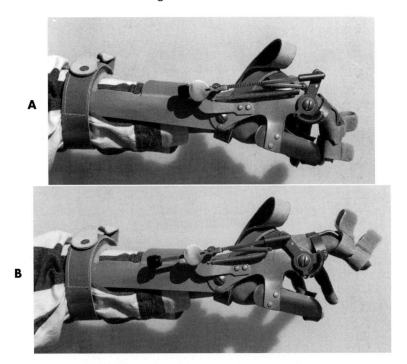

Fig. 16.10. Ratchet WHO. **A,** Closed. **B,** Open.

more easily maintained than more complex electrical systems. With a properly managed training program, a motivated individual can become proficient in a variety of functional activities using the ratchet WHO, including independent feeding, hygiene, and writing.

When the person requires the use of MAS with a ratchet WHO, functional capabilities are more limited. The person needs assistance donning the orthosis, and the work area must be set up carefully. Once the optimal setup is achieved, however, the individual is able to perform a variety of activities of daily living and leisure activities.

C5 motor level

At the C5 level, there is grade 3 or greater motor strength in the elbow flexors. The wrist extensors are less than grade 3/5, requiring orthotic prescription at the wrist. Deltoid motor function generally parallels elbow flexion, and, therefore, the patient is able to flex and abduct the shoulder against gravity. Muscles that are only grade 3/5, however, may fatigue early, and the patient may benefit from MAS temporarily until muscles reach grade 4/5.

Proper positioning of the hand in a static orthosis helps to protect against excessive stretch of the weak or absent wrist extensors. This is crucial to maximum function in later phases of treatment or recovery. In addition, a position of natural finger flexion facilitates the development of flexor tendon tightness, on which tenodesis function relies.

Patients with potential for neurologic return at the C6 level need a period of therapeutic training to strengthen wrist extensors, while still maintaining proper wrist-hand position. A wrist-action, wrist-hand

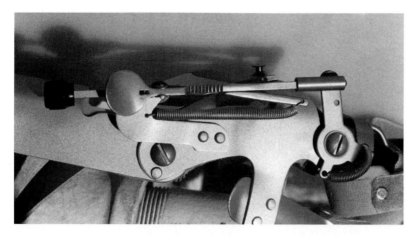

Fig. 16.11. Ratchet bar.

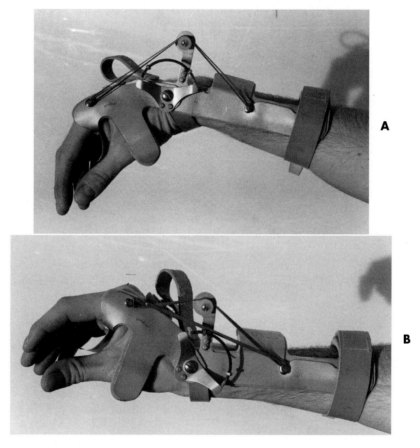

Fig. 16.12. WAWHO. **A**, Flexed. **B**, Extended.

orthosis[2] (WAWHO) (Fig. 16.12) may be used as a transition system for the patient at less than 6 months postinjury. The orthosis allows free wrist motion with adjustable stops to limit motion to a prescribed range. The stops may be adjusted to accommodate existing and changing strength in wrist extensors. If extensors are absent, the stops may be adjusted to eliminate motion and provide static support in the desired position. As strength increases, increased range of motion may be allowed. Elastic bands may also be attached to provide extension assist and augment weak muscles. Using Waters' data,[10] it is possible to predict the likely muscle strength at 1 year postinjury. Once this has been established, a definitive orthosis (either a ratchet or WDWHO) may be prescribed.

The WAWHO offers the patient with returning control of wrist extensors the combination of free assisted motion into extension with protection of weak

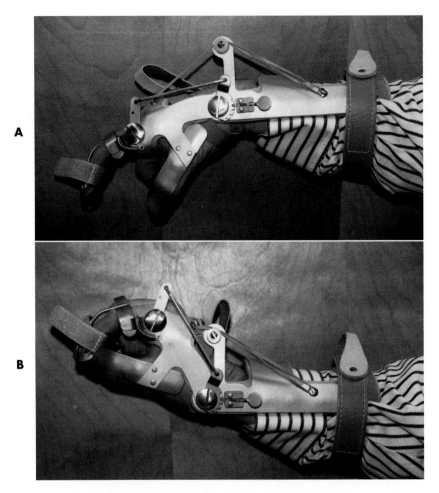

Fig. 16.13.   WDWHO. **A,** Flexed. **B,** Extended.

muscles from overstretch. This allows the patient to continue wrist exercises during nontherapy hours within a prescribed range of motion.

C6 motor level

At the C6 level, the patient has intact radial wrist extensors, along with some strength in the serratus anterior and clavicular pectoral muscles. The significance of pectoral strength is the ability to bring the arm across the chest to midline, which allows activities requiring bilateral arm use. Intact wrist extensors means the individual has the potential to harness the tenodesis action at the wrist to accomplish dynamic prehension for feeding and hygiene.

The (WDWHO)[3,8] (Fig. 16.13) is a dynamic orthosis that provides a transfer of power from the wrist extensors to the fingers for the purpose of prehension. It requires an experienced orthotist to design and fabricate and a knowledgeable therapist to train the patient in proper usage. Consequently, unless there is ongoing demand, patients in many rehabilitation settings do not receive this orthosis. Given adequate resources, how-

ever, the wrist-driven WHO can replace a variety of alternative devices and simplify the equipment needs of the patient.

Prehension with the WDWHO is produced by active wrist extension, which operates a mechanical linkage transferring power from the wrist extensors to flex the index and middle fingers against the thumb. Gravity-assisted wrist flexion creates hand opening. An adjustable component at the wrist joint allows varying degrees of hand opening associated with maximum prehension force. Experimentation and practice are required to determine optimal settings for specific tasks. Wrist extension can be assisted with elastic bands across the wrist joint, then discontinued when there is sufficient muscle strength.

C7 motor level

The key muscle for the C7 level is the triceps. There may also be some strength in finger extensors or flexors (or both). Triceps strength helps in many activities of daily living, such as transfers, dressing, pressure relief, and driving. Hand function remains a problem, how-

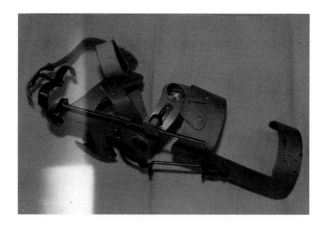

Fig. 16.14. Radial-deviation WHO.

ever. Natural tenodesis may be sufficient for some activities but insufficient for activities requiring a power grip or endurance.

Active finger extension may be present in the C7 patient. This presents a special challenge, however, because active finger extension may prevent development of natural tenodesis of the finger flexors. This level represents a significant increase in independence from the C6 level. With muscle strength that is adequate for a limited number of daily activities, the patient finds it difficult to appreciate the value of an orthosis and, therefore, is reluctant to use a WDWHO. Unless muscle strength exceeds grade 3, however, the patient cannot perform as many tasks without the orthosis as he or she can with it. In addition, daily use of the orthosis helps strengthen weak hand muscles. With adequate strength and training with the orthosis, the patient can then decide for which activities he or she needs to use the system and which he or she can accomplish without it.

Many patients exhibit a tendency to drift into radial deviation during wrist extension with the WDWHO.[1] This results in decreased prehension force and loss of stability in the wrist. A design modification addresses this problem with some success. A radial deviation WDWHO (Fig. 16.14) allows the orthosis to track with the hand as it goes into deviation while maintaining maximum prehension force. This orthosis has been used only experimentally but shows promise.

C8 motor level

The C8 patient typically has intact finger flexion. Static WHOs, which hold the thumb in position for function, are indicated. These are designed to maintain the thumb in opposition to the index and middle fingers for prehension and to maintain the thumb web space. An MP extension stop (lumbrical bar) on the orthoses help substitute for the intrinsic-minus hand to prevent clawing and improve hand opening.

Other considerations

Two other factors must be considered in the use of WHOs. One is the degree of spasticity. The patient with moderate-to-severe spasticity in the finger flexors may not be able to achieve optimal function with a dynamic orthosis because the increased tone does not allow for adequate hand opening. In addition, the resting position may be in more flexion than is optimal for pad-to-pad prehension. The other is the question of whether to use bilateral orthoses. Although it may be tempting to fit some patients with bilateral orthoses, it is uncommon that patients achieve a higher level of function with two.[3] Typically the patient is as functional using an orthosis on one hand and using the other hand as an assist. Inadequate strength in the pectoral muscles make it difficult to bring the arms to, or across, midline for bilateral activity. In addition, if sensation in the radial fingers or thumb is impaired or absent, the patient must compensate visually, and this makes bilateral use of the orthoses less effective. A higher level of function may be achieved with the use of bilateral orthoses on patients who have intact sensation and well-defined goals for bilateral use.

ORTHOTIC FITTING AND PATIENT EDUCATION

Along with good orthotic design, proper fit and training are essential. Successful fit is accomplished through collaboration between the certified orthotist, who understands the principles of orthotic fit, and the therapist, who, by monitoring the patient, is aware of problems that occur with prolonged usage. Initially the orthosis is placed on the hand for 30 minutes, after which it is removed and any red areas noted and evaluated again 1 hour later. If the redness has not disappeared, adjustments may be necessary. The patient must be instructed in the importance of skin inspection to prevent excessive pressure and skin breakdown. Wearing tolerance is gradually increased until all-day tolerance is achieved.

The patient must be educated about not only the use, but also the purpose of the orthosis, whether it is positional or functional. This understanding is important in obtaining the patient's cooperation and willingness to use the orthosis consistently. This is especially true of the positional orthosis, when functional gains are not obvious to the patient. It is important that the patient be knowledgeable about wearing tolerance and schedule. It is helpful for new patients to interact with experienced and successful users of similar equipment, and this may be initiated even before the patient receives his or her own orthosis.

On delivery, the orthosis must be carefully evaluated for fit and function. Optimum fit of the orthosis is mandatory for maximum function. An ill-fitting orthosis is of no benefit to the patient. Close communication between the therapist, orthotist, and patient is essential.

PATIENT TRAINING

When the patient understands the basic operation of the orthosis, an activity training program may be started. At first, the patient may practice simply opening and closing the fingers. The patient should be oriented to the components of the orthosis, particularly the actuating lever at the wrist, which controls the size of the opening and the resultant prehension. With the lever in the lowest notch, the opening is smaller, and firm prehension is accomplished with the wrist slightly flexed. This is useful for fine activities. With the lever in the highest notch, the opening is wide, and firm prehension is accomplished with the wrist in extension. This setting is useful for grasping large objects such as a cup. Other settings are fine-tuned through experimentation. For example, writing is often best accomplished in a position near the middle of the range. If sensation is impaired or absent on the hand and forearm, the patient must be instructed in the importance of skin inspection to avoid excessive pressure from the orthosis or from the forceful prehension achieved.

The patient should practice grasping, placing, and releasing objects. Soft, medium-sized objects are best to start with. Training should involve activities at various heights and that require pronation and supination to accomplish. Specific items may include pegs, blocks, disks, and the use of a key.

Once basic manipulation is mastered, functional training may follow. Patients can help identify specific tasks they wish to accomplish. Writing and self-care are activities most patients are interested in relearning as soon as possible. The patient using the WDWHO can be expected to become independent in these tasks, whereas the patient using the ratchet orthosis may continue to need assistance in setting up for the activity.

The ability to don and doff the orthosis is crucial to achieving independence. Initially the patient cannot be expected to accomplish this alone. Removal is easier than application, and training is often started here first. Loops may be added to the ends of the retaining straps to allow the patient to use the thumb of the other hand to unfasten the straps. Then the patient simply pushes, or shakes, the orthosis off. With training, donning may be accomplished within 2 or 3 minutes for the ratchet and less than 1 minute for the WDWHO. Obviously, success in this

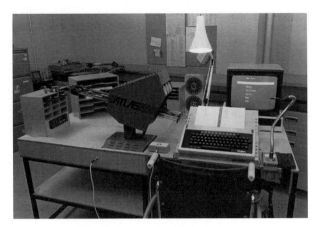

Fig. 16.15.   Robotic manipulator.

area influences ultimate acceptance and use of the orthosis.

FUTURE TRENDS

The increased use of robotics in industry to perform complex tasks suggests potential application for the disabled population. Experimental work has been done on robotic arms, which can manipulate items such as a computer or feeding utensils. Hillman and coworkers[4] designed a workstation using a commercially available robot manipulator controlled by a microcomputer (Fig. 16.15). The arm chosen was of relatively low cost and offered five degrees of freedom, plus an open/close gripper.

The module sits on a table and may be controlled in real-time, under direct control of the user. Initial tasks included loading music into a cassette, loading disks into a computer, and manipulating books. Preprogrammed routines were also provided for some tasks. Eight patients were tested, and reactions were generally favorable, although more success was achieved through the use of preprogrammed routines than through real-time direct control.

Another design uses shape memory alloys as the actuator to convert electrical energy into mechanical work.[6] The alloy deforms at low temperatures and recovers its original shape on heating. The design uses a shape memory alloy wire and electrical current to accomplish finger flexion against the thumb, thereby providing prehension.

These and other devices are available to assist the tetraplegic patient with activities of daily living. Careful evaluation, creative problem solving, appropriate orthotic design, and specific training are necessary to provide sufficient encouragement and support to allow people to achieve maximum independence and function.

REFERENCES

1. Allen VR: Follow-up study of wrist-driven flexor-hinge splint use, Am J Occup Ther 25:420, 1971.
2. Barber LM, Nickel VL: Carbon dioxide-powered arm and hand devices, Am J Occup Ther 23:215, 1969.
3. Baumgarten JM: Upper extremity adaptations for the person with quadriplegia, Spinal Cord Injury, 19
4. Hillman MR, et al: Development of a robot arm and workstation for the disabled, J Biome Eng 12:199, 1990.
5. International standards for neurological and functional classification of spinal cord injury, American Spinal Injury Association/International Medical Society of Paraplegia, 1992.
6. Markarm JE, et al: The SMART wrist-hand orthosis (WHO) for quadriplegic patients, J Prosthet Orthot 5:73/27.
7. McKenzie MW: The Ratchet handsplint, Am J Occup Ther 27:477, 1973.
8. Shepherd CC, Ruzika SH: Tenodesis brace use by persons with spinal cord injuries, Am J Occup Ther 45:82, 1991.
9. Symington DC, Mackay DE: A study of functional independence in the quadriplegic patient, Arch Phys Med Rehabil 47:378, 1966.
10. Waters RL, et al: Motor and sensory recovery following complete tetraplegia, Arch Phys Med Rehabil 74:242, 1993.
11. Werssowitz OF: Biophysical principles in selection of hand splints, Am J Occup Ther 9:59, 1955.

Orthoses for the Burned Hand

John A. I. Grossman
Lorna E. Ramos
Enricho B. Robotti

This chapter summarizes the basic principles and techniques for the use of splints and other orthoses and associated devices for management of the burned hand during the various stages of treatment. Each phase in the management of upper extremity burns requires integration of medical, surgical, and rehabilitation techniques. Correct application of splints and associated devices is critical to maximize ultimate form and function of the extremity (Fig. 17.1).

HISTORICAL PERSPECTIVES

Although Galen (131–201 A.D.) paid only minimal attention to the treatment of burns, in the sixth volume of the 1609 Venetian edition of his works, the chapter *De Fasciis* (Fig. 17.2) illustrates what may be considered

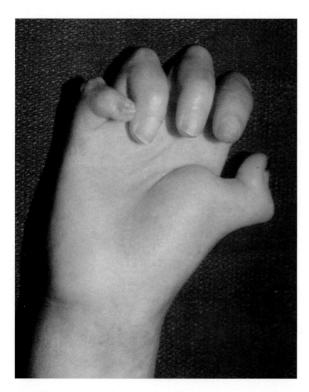

Fig. 17.1. Severe hand deformity (intrinsic minus) following second-degree burn with 1 month splinting in *resting* or *functional* position. These severe deformities could have been limited by proper splinting.

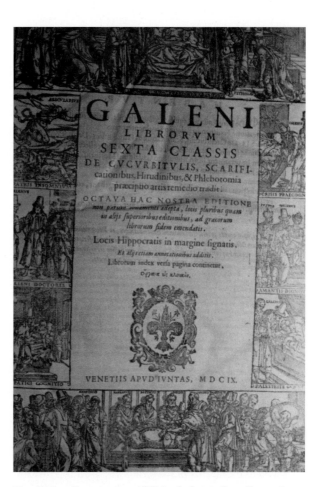

Fig. 17.2. Frontis piece of Galen's *Omnia Quae Extant Opera in Latinum Conversa*, Sixth Volume, Venice, Giunta, 1609. *(Courtesy Dr. Riccardo Mazzola.)*

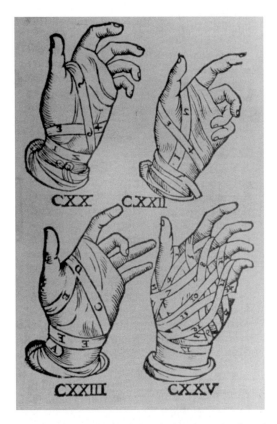

Fig. 17.3. Illustrations of hand dressings in functional position from Galen's *Omnia Quae Extant Opera in Latinum Conversa*, Sixth Volume, Venice, Giunta, 1609. *(Courtesy Dr. Riccardo Mazzola.)*

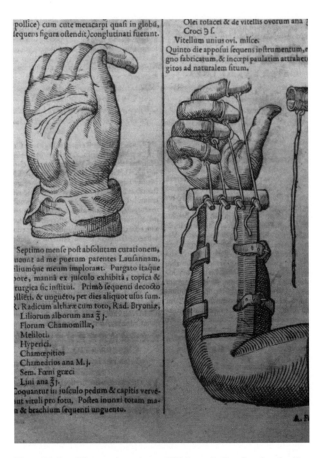

Fig. 17.4. Illustration from Hildanus' *De Combustionibus* showing a splint for correction of a burn contracture. *(Courtesy of Dr. Riccardo Mazzola.)*

the first reference on management of the burned hand by splinting (Fig. 17.3). With the advent of gunpowder, pioneer war surgeons such as Ambrose Pare, William Clowes, Fabricius Hildanus (Fig. 17.4), and Richard Wiseman took special interest in burn management and paid careful attention to the use of splints for the management of contractures.

Contemporary approaches to the splinting of the burned hand evolved during the late 19th and early 20th centuries. Bunnell, Koch, Mason, and others, the founders of the specialty of hand surgery, emphasize the correct positioning of the burned hand and the role of dynamic and static splints in the acute management and successful rehabilitation of these injuries.

SPLINTING MATERIALS

Two general kinds of materials are used to fabricate splints for burned upper extremities. Low-temperature thermoplastic materials are most commonly used be-

cause they allow a high degree of conformability, while sacrificing control. This makes them particularly applicable for custom-designed finger-based and hand-based orthoses. Rubber materials are much less commonly used to treat upper extremity burn injuries because the high degree of control provided sacrifices the ability to conform the material precisely to the digits, hand, and wrist. Table 17.1 summarizes the characteristics of the recommended and most commonly used splint materials for the burned hand. Selection of a particular material is often dictated by the experience of the treating therapist.

BIOMECHANICS

Adherence to certain basic principles of splint biomechanics assists in the fabrication of a well-fitting orthosis for the burned hand that provides maximum benefit to the patient. It is necessary to appreciate the considerable internal (joint, tendon, ligament) and ex-

Table 17.1. Commonly used splinting materials

	TEMPERATURE (°F)	STRETCH	STRENGTH	SPECIAL FEATURES	ABILITY TO REHEAT	BONDING
Polyfoam/K-Splint	160	Malleable Controlled stretch	Excellent No reinforcement necessary	Good for intricate shapes Conforms easily	Yes, but it loses its shape if done often	Coating must be removed
Ezeform	170	Nonstretch Rubberlike	Excellent No reinforcement necessary	Easy to handle Resists finger prints Slight tackiness when soft	Yes	Self-adhesive No solvent or scraping necessary
Polyflex II/Isoprene	160	Moderate stretch	Excellent	Easy to handle Good for large circumferential splints	Yes	Self-adhesive
Orthoplast	160	Minimal stretch	Very good	Increased working time Hardens in 8–10 min Not pliable for contouring	Yes	Coating must be removed
Aquaplast/Aqua-T	140	Moderate stretch Shrinks back Memory	Excellent	Clings to person's skin for precise impression Hardens slowly Material is clear when hot Sticky surface, use hand lotion on skin or scissors	Yes	Self-adhesive No solvent or scraping necessary

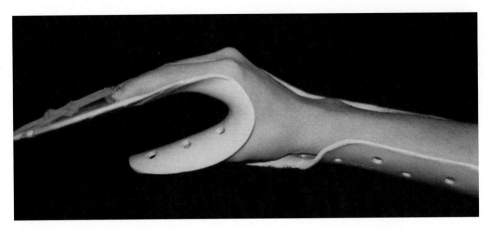

Fig. 17.5.   Orthoplast splint for positioning acutely burned hand in protective position. Note use of traction bands. This splint is also used for management of dorsal or volar skin grafts.

ternal (skin) stresses created by a splint to avoid skin ulceration or damage to underlying structures. During the acute phase of treatment, the splints must be adjusted daily to insure both a proper fit and maintenance of correct position.

SPLINTING FOR ACUTE HAND BURNS

The correct splint for management of the acutely burned hand has three purposes: (1) protection against deforming forces from the cutaneous injury as well as secondary soft tissue edema, (2) facilitation of wound care and topical therapy, and (3) facilitation of the management of the hand after tangential incision and split-thickness skin grafting. The initial splint is fabricated with the commencement of treatment. In general, the splint is volar, maintaining the wrist in approximately 10 degrees of extension with the digits in an intrinsic plus position and the thumb in maximum abduction for protection of the first web space (Fig. 17.5). Aside from simplifying elevation of the hand and protecting against deforming forces secondary to the acute edema of the soft tissues, a proper splint significantly aids in the application of topical antimicrobials and avoids the need for cumbersome, bulky dressings. During the first 3 to 4 days after a burn injury, the splint is easily modified at the bedside as edema is reduced. For patients not requiring surgical excision of the burn, this initial splint design is adequate until complete epithelialization is achieved. These splints are easily removed for active range-of-motion exercises. If tangential excision and split-thickness skin grafting are performed, this splint design is useful for immobilizing

the hand postoperatively with close monitoring of the graft (Fig. 17.6).

SPLINTING DURING THE HEALING PHASE

Once wound closure has been obtained either by epithelialization or split-thickness skin grafting, the burned hand is subject to tremendous, deforming contractile forces. Splints must be carefully designed to address the problems of the individual patient. Static splints are particularly useful in managing the first web space and dorsal contractures. Dynamic splints play a major role in dealing with metacarpophalangeal and interphalangeal joint contractures. The technique of serial casting is often useful in managing flexion contractures of the proximal interphalangeal joint. Hand splints employed during the subacute healing phase can serve as the carrier vehicle for scar management modalities, including silicone gel sheeting and elastomer products (Fig. 17.7). Also the orthoses used during the subacute healing phase are often incorporated into the use of compressive garments (Fig. 17.8).

ORTHOSES DURING THE RECONSTRUCTIVE PHASE

During reconstructive surgery of the burned hand, the basic principles of splint fabrication relevant to other aspects of reconstructive hand surgery are applied. Again, individualization is the key to successful orthotic fabrication. In some cases, the fabricated orthoses assumes a prosthetic role (Figs. 17.9 and 17.10).

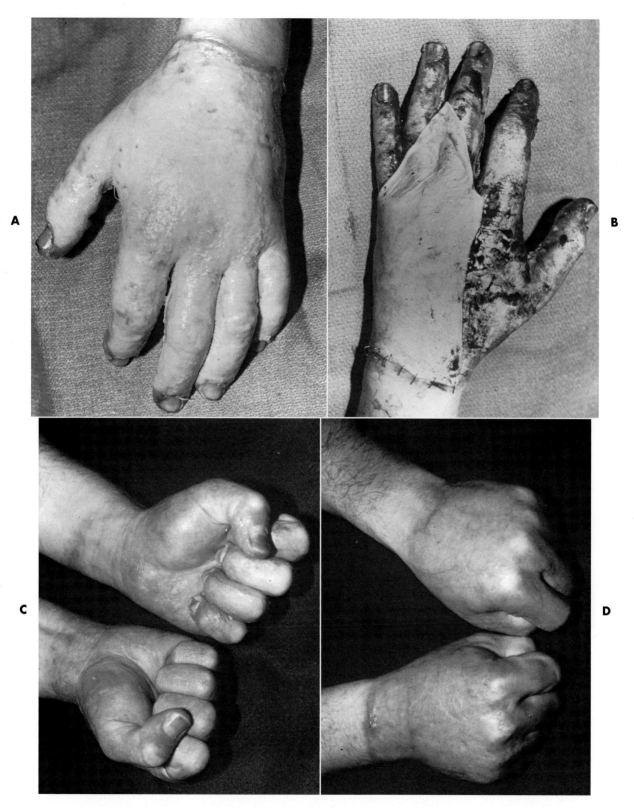

Fig. 17.6.   **A,** Example of a deep burn on dorsum of hand (bilateral symmetric injury) with eschar. **B,** Intraoperative view after tangential excision and placement of sheet split-thickness skin graft. **C,** Postoperative result. **D,** Postoperative result.   *Continued.*

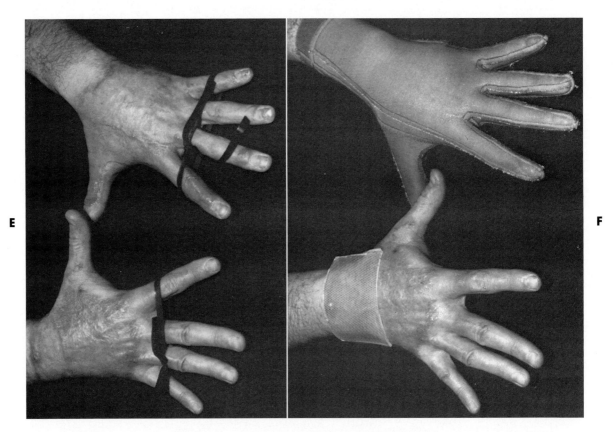

Fig. 17.6, cont'd.   E, Elastic devices for stretching web space and strengthening intrinsic muscles. F, Left hand uses a custom compression (JOBST) glove. Right hand has silastic gel, which can be incorporated into glove.

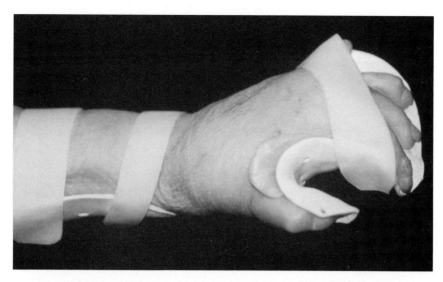

Fig. 17.7. Splint for postoperative management in functional position with a first web component for elastomere.

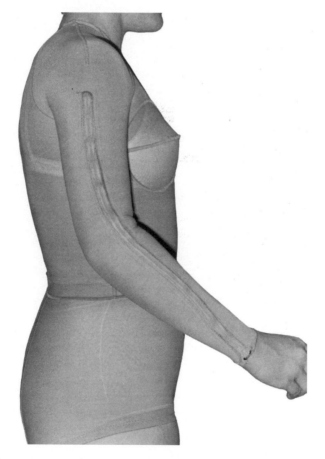

Fig. 17.8. Custom compression garment for more extensive upper extremity burn. *(Courtesy of JOBST Co.)*

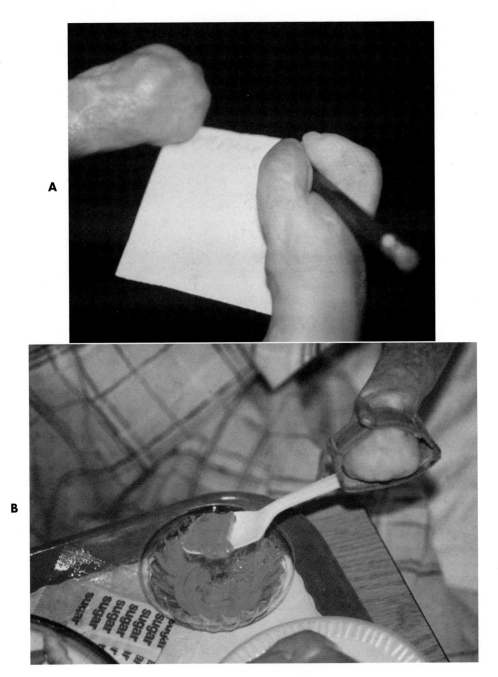

Fig. 17.9. **A,** Severe bilateral hand burns in a child. The right hand has been reconstructed with pollicization and a groin flap for reconstruction of the first web space. **B,** The left hand has lost all digits and uses an orthosis/prosthesis.

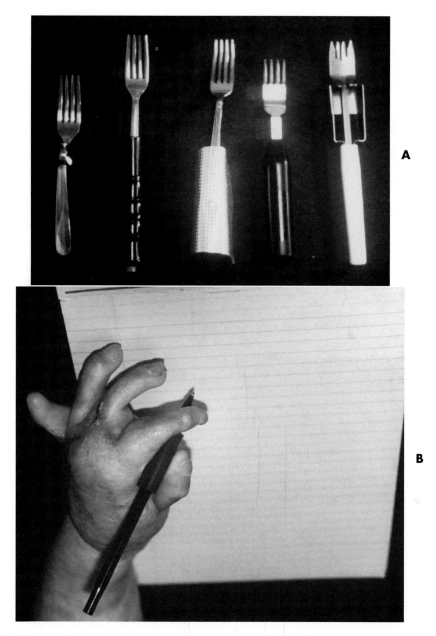

Fig. 17.10. **A,** Adapted equipment useful for severe hand burns. **B,** Standard adaptive pencil used after severe burn during reconstruction phase.

BIBLIOGRAPHY

Deitch EA, et al: Hypertrophic burn scars: Analysis of variables, J Trauma 23:895–898, 1987.

Gibbone M, et al: Experience with silastic gel sheeting in pediatric scarring, J Burn Care Rehabil 1:69–73, 1994.

Grossman JAI: Burns of the upper extremity, Hand Clin 6:2, 1990.

Hammond JS, War CG: Complications of the burn patient, Crit Care Clin 3:175, 1985.

Larson DL, et al: Contracture and scar formation in the burn patient, Clin Plast Surg 1:653–666, 1974.

Linares HA, et al: Historical notes on the use of pressure in the treatment of hypertrophic scars or keloids, Burns 19:17–21, 1993.

Parry SW: Reconstruction of the burned hand, Clin Plast Surg 7:577–586, 1989.

Quinn KJ, et al: Non-pressure treatment of hypertrophic scars, Burns 12:102–108, 1985.

Salisbury RE, Pruitt, BA: Burns of the upper extremity, Philadelphia, 1976, WB Saunders.

Ward RS: Pressure therapy for the control of hypertrophic scar formation after burn injury: A history and review, J Burn Care Rehabil 12:247–262, 1991.

Orthoses for the Arthritic Hand and Wrist

Alfred B. Swanson
Troy D. Pierce
Judy Leonard
Geneviève de Groot Swanson

Certified orthotists, hand therapists and surgeons commonly see patients with some form of arthritis, usually rheumatoid arthritis and osteoarthritis. The greatest crippler from the standpoint of severity and prolonged disability is rheumatoid arthritis.[15] Rheumatoid arthritis is a progressive, chronic systemic disease marked by inflammatory changes of the joints, tendons, and their sheaths resulting in pain, weakness, and dysfunction. Inflammation caused by proliferative synovium results in erosions of articular cartilage, articular bone, and soft tissue. This can cause rupture of tendons and the weakening of ligaments around the involved joints. In the hand, this eventually leads to muscle and tendon imbalance, ligamentous laxity, instability, and subluxation or complete dislocation of the joints.[15] Orthoses for the arthritic hand increase function and decrease pain by helping correct deformities, stabilize joints, and support segments of the hand.

The application of an orthosis (splint or brace) for a patient with an arthritic hand condition requires a thorough knowledge of the disease process to expect a good result from treatment. To apply the proper orthosis, the orthotist and/or therapist and physician must possess knowledge of normal hand anatomy and be familiar with the pathomechanics of the arthritic hand. Communication between the physician, orthotist, and patient and a thorough evaluation of the patient by both the physician and the orthotist are required for adequate orthotic management of an arthritic hand condition. The evaluation should include activities of daily living function, range of motion, dexterity, grasp and pinch, and understanding of the patient's expectations.[12]

Initially, it must be determined if orthotic treatment is appropriate. The main reasons chosen to splint the arthritic hand include to decrease inflammation, to properly position joints, to rest and support weakened structures, to improve function through better stability and position, to prevent joint contractures, and to aid in postoperative rehabilitation.[6] After establishing a need for orthotic treatment, the correct type of splint must then be chosen. Orthoses used in the rheumatoid hand are classified according to their function.[6] Resting orthoses provide passive immobilization during the acute stage of inflammation alleviating pain by resting involved joints, allowing the use of uninvolved joints.[5,6,10,12] Static orthoses provide stability and help correct joint deformity as it develops. Dynamic orthoses counteract the deforming forces of rheumatoid arthritis by providing a constant gentle traction, which is used to stretch scar tissue without excessive reaction.[6] Controversy exists between physicians and therapists as to whether an orthosis can prevent or retard the deforming process of rheumatoid arthritis.[5,10]

Dynamic orthoses are essential for postoperative rehabilitation of the rheumatic hand after implant resection arthroplasty and reconstruction.[18] Orthoses used after hand reconstruction help maintain surgically achieved mobility and alignment, assist postoperative strengthening, and decrease postsurgical adhesions.[10] The greatest challenge in postoperative rehabilitation of finger joint arthroplasty is maintaining a proper balance between good healing of the surrounding scar tissue while applying proper amounts of tension across the scar to obtain a desired range of motion.[19]

Orthoses are also used in the treatment of osteoarthritis. Osteoarthritis of the hand most commonly affects the finger distal interphalangeal (DIP) and proximal interphalangeal (PIP) joints and the thumb carpometacarpal (CMC) joint. Preoperatively, static splints can be used particularly in resting the thumb CMC joint to decrease pain.[10] Postoperatively, dynamic splints may be used in the treatment of PIP implant resection arthroplasty.[14,19]

Prefabricated orthoses are available, but care must be taken to see that they are adapted specifically for each patient. The availability of low-temperature plastics allows a custom fit directly on the patient. A variety

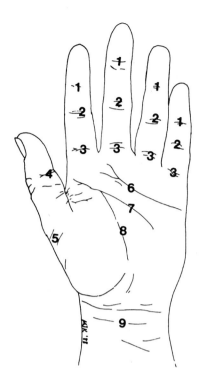

Fig. 18.1. The surface anatomy or creases of the hand often set the boundaries of a splint. Crossing a segmental crease often prevents motion at a joint, whereas clearing the crease allows motion. *1,* Distal creases; *2,* distal middle creases; *3,* distal proximal creases; *4,* distal thumb creases; *5,* proximal thumb creases; *6,* distal palmar crease; *7,* proximal palmar crease; *8,* thenar crease; *9,* wrist crease.

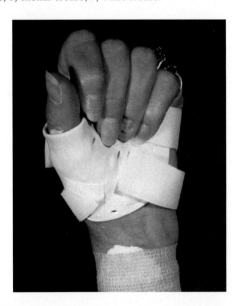

Fig. 18.2. On the thumb, the splint is extended as far as possible to the distal thumb crease to immobilize the MP joint, yet clears the crease to allow thumb interphalangeal joint motion.

of materials are now available to the physician and therapist. Regardless of what material or prefabricated splint is used, the principles of proper fit, construction,

mechanics, and design must be understood. The reader is encouraged to refer to other chapters to gain further insight into these fundamentals. Many of the principles are not within the scope of this chapter. The fabrication of an orthosis is also an art that is learned through experience. The beginner should seek the resources of an experienced orthotist/therapist whenever possible to develop his or her skills.

The application of an orthosis in the treatment of arthritis is a highly individualized undertaking. Some orthoses are often used by the clinician and are presented here. In all of these orthoses, the wearing time is individualized to meet the needs of each patient. Orthoses need to be evaluated for proper fit and usage after a trial application period. Adaptations are made as necessary in conjunction with close follow-up with the orthotist. As with most situations in medicine, patient education is of utmost importance to ensure compliance. An orthosis is of no value and can be harmful if it is worn incorrectly. To avoid the problems that occur secondary to incorrect orthosis use or to disuse, effective instruction is essential. Melvin[10] has outlined important educational objectives to be taught to the patient: (1) the purpose of the splint, including the advantages and disadvantages; (2) when and for how long the splint should be worn; (3) what exercises to do in conjunction with the splint; (4) how to put the splint on and take it off; (5) how to determine if the splint is positioned correctly; (6) how to care for and clean the splint; and (7) how to check the skin for pressure areas.

SURFACE ANATOMY AND ARCHES OF THE HAND

It is necessary to have knowledge of surface anatomy and of the structures that are represented by it when fabricating an orthosis. The surface anatomy of the hand often sets the boundaries of the orthosis. Crossing these boundaries often prevents motion at a joint, whereas clearing these boundaries allows motion and prevents stiffness of the adjacent joints (Fig. 18.1)[6,9,10] For example, Moberg[11] has referred to a line proximal to the transverse fold of the palm, or distal palmar crease, as a life line of the hand. If the orthosis is extended distally, it limits range of motion of the metacarpophalangeal (MP) joints and impairs circulation by decreasing the pumping system. In cases where immobilization is needed, the splint should be extended as far as possible to the next segmental crease to provide adequate support (Fig. 18.2). It is important that the structures to be protected are adequately supported and those that are to be left free for motion are allowed to move completely.

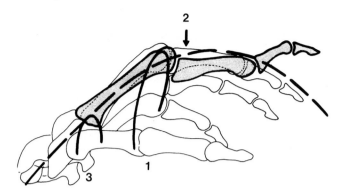

Fig. 18.3. Arches of the hand. *1*, Distal transverse arch; *2*, longitudinal arch; *3*, proximal transverse arch.

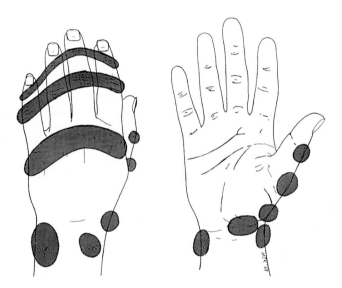

Fig. 18.4. Bony prominences of the hand. Splints must be contoured to prevent pressure over bony prominences. Pressure over bony prominences can result in skin breakdown.

Proper orthotic fabrication and application depend on the understanding of the skeletal arches of the hand. The palm of the hand is concave and is formed by three skeletal arches.[16] The distal transverse arch is deepened by the mobility of the first, fourth and fifth metacarpals around the stability of the second and third metacarpals (Fig. 18.3). This mobility is necessary for coordinated grasp and opposition. The longitudinal arch extends from the wrist to the tip of the third digit and is deepened by the composite flexion of the digits. This mobility is also necessary for grasping. The third arch is the proximal transverse arch, which is located at the wrist. It is formed by the carpal bones and the ligaments. The flexor tendons, nerves, and vascular structures fill this cavity. The longitudinal and distal transverse arches must be maintained in orthotic application to prevent flattening of the hand into a nonfunctional position. Orthotic application must be contoured to prevent pressure over bony prominences. Pressure points and skin breakdown can result from an improperly fitted orthosis (Fig. 18.4).[5,9]

WRIST ORTHOSES

The wrist is a key joint in proper hand function. The wrist joints and surrounding soft tissues are frequently affected by rheumatoid arthritis. In the arthritic state, the wrist can become acutely inflamed, as in acute extensor synovitis in the rheumatoid patient, or it can become chronically involved with problems of deformity, instability, or collapse. This may significantly interfere with the function of the hand. Rheumatoid arthritic changes of the wrist include erosion of the articular surface and involvement of midcarpal and radiocarpal joints resulting in collapse, fusion or fibrosis, and stiffness and ulnad shift of the carpus on the radius resulting in radial deviation of the hand, which then exacerbates the ulnar drift of the fingers resulting in classic zigzag deformity.[16] Palmar subluxation of the carpus on the radius can occur, and occasionally ulnar dislocation of the carpus off the radius would result in pronounced instability and serious loss of hand function.

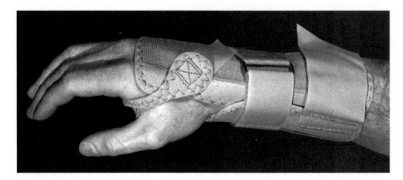

Fig. 18.5.   A simple wrist cockup splint should allow full motion of the digits by clearing the thenar eminence and the distal palmar crease of the hand.

The distal radial ulnar joint is often involved in the arthritic process as well. The ability to supinate and pronate the forearm is affected by its arthritic involvement. Forearm rotation is an important function in positioning of the hand for maximum use. Destructive synovitis produces distal radial ulnar joint instability with dorsal subluxation of the ulna on the radius and palmar subluxation of the extensor carpi ulnaris tendon resulting in pain, weakness, and decreased range of motion.[16] Position of the wrist influences the relative power of the extrinsic muscles of the hand. Extension of the wrist relaxes the extensors and increases the mechanical advantages of the flexor muscles. The opposite is true for flexion. This concept must be understood when preparing orthoses for specific arthritic conditions of the wrist.

Wrist orthoses (WOs) may be used in acute stages of rheumatoid arthritis to decrease pain, assist in proper wrist positioning to increase maximum function, and provide stability to the wrist.[10] The most commonly used WO is the wrist cockup splint. It is a simple, static orthosis that immobilizes the wrist and allows full MP flexion and thumb opposition. This simple WO positions the wrist in approximately 10 to 30 degrees of extension to allow maximum function. It stabilizes the wrist by preventing flexion and extension of the carpus but does not immobilize the distal radio ulnar joint, allowing the patient pronation and supination (Fig. 18.5). If supination and pronation prevention is desirable, as in distal radioulnar joint disease, the orthoses can be made to extend across the elbow a short distance. This allows some flexion and extension of the elbow, while blocking forearm and wrist rotation. The wrist cockup splint is applied volarly extending from the proximal third of the forearm ending just proximal to the palmar crease to allow full MP flexion and thumb opposition. The function of the splint is to immobilize the radio carpal joint, providing rest and stability and allowing reduction of inflammation and pain. It also protects the extensor tendons, which may be at risk for rupture in the rheumatoid patient. The simple volar

splint may also be used to stabilize the wrist in a proper position after flexor synovectomy and carpal tunnel release preventing medial nerve and flexor tendon bowstringing while allowing full finger flexion.

The orthosis may be appropriate for use preoperatively in a patient with severe wrist instability and a patient who is a candidate for wrist arthrodesis. It provides stability and lets the patient feel what it is like to have an immobile wrist. It is important for the WOs to be avoided during active MP synovitis. Wrist immobilization may increase the deforming stresses to the MP joints.[10] In these cases, a resting hand splint may be more appropriate.

The authors use the WOs routinely postoperatively after wrist implant resection arthroplasty or in limited radiocarpal fusion, after cast removal for an additional 6 to 12 weeks. The patient is then encouraged to use the wrist immobilizer thereafter when performing strenuous activities such as lifting. Wrist implant arthroplasty is indicated in case of arthritic or traumatic disability resulting in instability of the wrist from subluxation or dislocation of the radiocarpal joint.[19] Wrist reconstruction should usually be performed before surgery of the finger joints in the rheumatoid. Some believe that wrist implant resection arthroplasty is contraindicated in workers performing heavy manual labor. In this patient population, a wrist fusion would be a better alternative.

Postoperatively the extremity is elevated for 3 to 5 days in a voluminous conforming hand dressing. A short arm cast, keeping the wrist in a neutral position, is applied and worn for 4 to 6 weeks thereafter. If MP joint arthroplasties are performed simultaneously, the outrigger from a high-profile dynamic extension splint may be incorporated in the cast at that time. During the period of plaster immobilization, the patient is encouraged to carry out active exercises for the MP and the interphalangeal (IP) joints. Isometric gripping exercises of the forearm muscles are started in 2 to 3 weeks after surgery. The senior author has developed an isometric grip device (Grip-X) used for this purpose. It is shaped to maintain proper anatomic position of digits

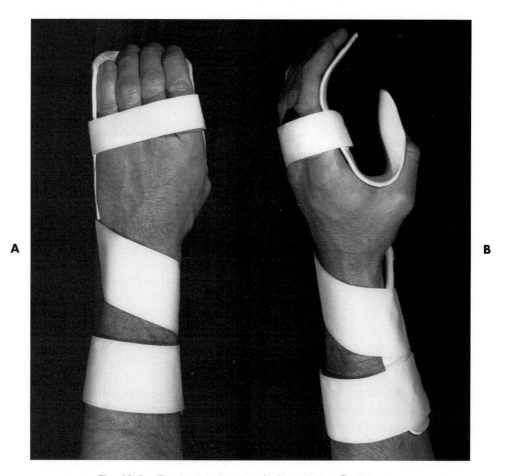

Fig. 18.6.   Resting hand splint. **A,** Dorsal view. **B,** Side view.

and arches of the hand. Following cast removal, wrist exercises are progressively instituted. Flexion and extension exercises are carried out while the forearm is supported on a firm surface. Pronation/supination exercises for the forearm are begun as well. A good ratio of stability to mobility is sought because a joint that is too loose may be unstable. About 50% to 60% of normal flexion and extension movements is ideal after wrist implant resection arthroplasty. Three months after surgery, the active range of motion should approximate 30 degrees of flexion to 30 degrees of extension and 10 degrees of radial and ulnar deviation. The patient is cautioned against any activity such as heavy labor or certain sports that could produce repetitive stresses at the level of the wrist joint, and the patient is encouraged to wear a WO if unable to avoid these activities.[19]

The senior author has developed titanium carpal bone implants that can be used as spacers following resection of the thumb CMC joint, scaphoid, or lunate. These implants can satisfactorily maintain joint space and alignment after bone resection.[14] Adequate capsuloligamentous support around carpal implants is essential for early and late stability. Adequate ligamentous repair must be obtained intraoperatively. The implant

and the wrist capsule must be kept in an anatomic position during the healing period so that encapsulation becomes secure. Once the operative procedure is completed, the hand is elevated in a voluminous dressing 3 to 5 days postoperatively. In scaphoid implant arthroplasty, a long arm thumb spica cast is applied postoperatively, after 3 to 5 days, with the wrist in 20 to 30 degrees of extension and slight radial deviation. In lunate implant arthroplasty, a short arm cast with the wrist in slight extension is applied. The cast is worn for 6 to 8 weeks. The cast is removed after 8 weeks, and a cockup wrist splint is applied for the next 4 to 6 weeks, allowing the patient to remove it for range-of-motion exercises.

The resting pan hand orthosis (Fig. 18.6) provides static positioning to the wrist and digits. It is used in acute rheumatoid arthritis to decrease pain and to align the joints in a normal anatomic position to avoid the zigzag position.[13] It immobilizes the wrist, fingers, and thumb of the arthritic patient. It is applied volarly and extends from the proximal one third of the forearm out to the ends of the fingertips, positioning the hand in a functional position of 20 degrees of wrist extension and 5 degrees of ulnar deviation of the wrist with the thumb in an abducted position. The fingers are placed in slight flexion and radial deviation. In the rheumatoid hand, the MP joints need only a few degrees of flexion, in contrast to "the safe position" of splinting used in the nonarthritic hand. Because of MP joint instability, extension helps prevent palmar subluxation of the MPs without the usual worry of collateral ligament shortening.

The resting pan orthosis is also used in a postoperative program after MP implant resection arthroplasties. Full-time wear of a dynamic MP splint is usually discontinued 6 weeks postoperatively, and a resting pan orthosis can in some cases be used after 6 weeks postoperatively as a night splint to assist in maintaining proper digital alignment. Generally the splint is worn at night, preoperatively as well as postoperatively. It may be used during the day, however, for additional rest during periods of acute inflammation. Care should be taken with the resting pan orthoses to prevent joint stiffness. Night wear is often preferred in cases of acute rheumatoid arthritis, but if it is worn during the day, it should be removed for pain-free range-of-motion exercises. It is important to achieve a balance between rest and activity in the rheumatoid hand.

When correcting MP ulnar deviation in the pan splint, the therapist must be concerned with the wrist position. If the digits align without correcting for the usual radial deviation found in the rheumatoid wrist, the wrist may be pulled into further radial deviation in the resting pan splint. The goal of splinting the zigzag deformity in the resting splint must also include correction of the wrist deformity. Straps can be applied to the resting pan splint to pull the wrist into ulnar deviation while keeping the fingers aligned in radial deviation, thus correcting the zigzag deformity.[2]

ULNAR DEVIATION ORTHOSES IN RHEUMATOID ARTHRITIS

Deformities of the MP joint are usually manifested by increased ulnar drift and palmar subluxation. The MP joint becomes unstable when normal muscle balance is lost and the collateral ligaments are disrupted from the inflammatory process. The MP joint differs from the IP joints in that its movements are not simply flexion and extension but also involve some degree of rotation, abduction, and adduction. Because of this, the MP joint is subject to greater stresses. Palmar and ulnar displaced flexor and extensor tendons produce deforming forces that exacerbate the ulnar drift. The extrinsic muscles, which form a bridge between the extensor and the flexor systems, provide direct flexor power across the MP joint, which can become deforming elements once the restraining structures of the MP

joint have been lengthened by the rheumatoid disease. The intrinsic muscles then further aggravate the tendency toward volar subluxation of the MP joint and toward ulnar drift of the digits. Once the ulnar deviation and palmar subluxation have occurred, muscle pull and forces that develop in functional activities further accentuate the deformity.[16] The ulnar deviation orthosis provides support to the MP joints, which restricts flexion and may assist in proper alignment by pulling the fingers radially out of ulnar deviation. The IP joints are left free to encourage proximal IP flexion during activities. This flexion may be beneficial if patients develop swan-neck deformities. It also prevents further intrinsic tightening. The orthosis can include the wrist when it is involved as well. The orthosis is indicated in the acute stages of rheumatoid arthritis to decrease pain at the MP level and help prevent further deformities. Postoperatively, it is used after MP joint synovectomy to maintain flexor and extensor tendon alignment. The ulnar deviation orthosis may also be used as a night splint starting 6 weeks postoperatively after MP implant resection arthroplasty to assist in maintaining joint alignment (Fig. 18.7, A and B).

The ulnar deviation orthoses may be fabricated in a variety of ways. All of the MP joints may be supported by a single platform or may be supported by individual finger separators. The splint may be applied to the palm and fingers only, if the wrist is not involved. Another use of the splint is to treat swan-neck deformities that occur in conjunction with MP joint deformity. The splint supports the MP joints in near neutral position while allowing the flexion of the PIP and DIP joints, providing repetitive stretch to the tightened intrinsic muscles.[10]

THUMB SPICA ORTHOSIS

The thumb spica orthosis may be hand or forearm based (Fig. 18.8, A and B). It provides support and positioning to the thumb CMC and MP joints. Indications may include acute rheumatoid arthritis or osteoarthritis of these joints to decrease pain and provide stability.[10] During fabrication, the thumb should be positioned in abduction to be used as an oppositional post for the fingers. The patient should be instructed to wear the orthoses during daily activities to reduce pain and enhance function. It may be used at night to rest inflamed CMC and MP joints and provide better positioning. The orthosis may also be used postoperatively in patients who require additional stability after cast removal after trapezium or scaphoid implant resection arthroplasty. Following cast removal usually at 6 weeks, the splint is worn full-time except for bathing and gentle range of motion for 4 to 6 additional weeks.

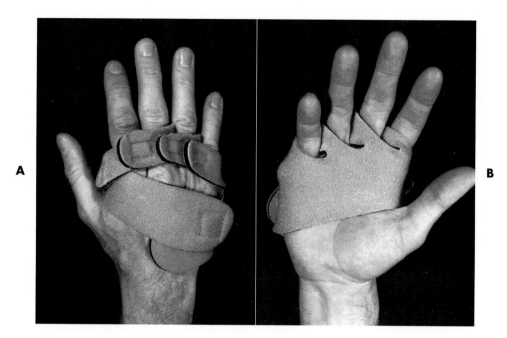

Fig. 18.7. **A,** Hand-based ulnar deviation splint (dorsal view). **B,** Hand-based ulnar deviation splint (volar view).

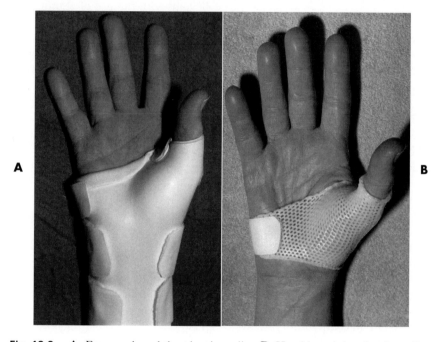

Fig. 18.8. **A,** Forearm-based thumb spica splint. **B,** Hand-based thumb spica splint.

Pathomechanics of the thumb ray in rheumatoid arthritis include most commonly two longitudinal collapse patterns: the boutonnière, which primarily involves the MP joint, and the swan-neck deformity, which primarily involves the CMC joint. The most common collapse deformity of the thumb is the boutonnière. Initially the joint capsule and the extensor apparatus around the MP joint are stretched out by a synovitis process. The extensor pollicis longus tendon and adductor expansion are displaced ulnad. The at-

tachment of the extensor pollicis brevis to the base of the proximal phalanx is lengthened and becomes ineffective. The ability to extend the MP joint is decreased and results in a flexion deformity of the proximal phalanx. The long extensor tendon then applies all of its power to the distal joint, which produces a hyperextension deformity of the distal joint. Pinch movements further accentuate the deformity, and a cycle is established (Fig. 18.9). Severe boutonnière deformities are usually treated with an MP joint fusion in the rheuma-

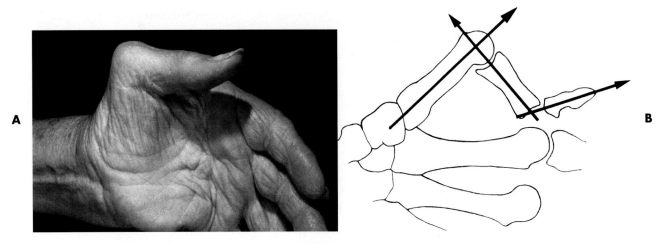

Fig. 18.9. Boutonnière deformity of thumb. **A,** This deformity is a common occurrence in rheumatoid arthritis and starts as synovitis of the MP joint. **B,** Pinch movements of functional adaptations accentuate the deformity, and a cycle of deformity is established.

toid patient; however, deformities can be stabilized with a thumb spica orthosis when they are mild, or the orthosis may be used preoperatively for protection of the early fusion.

The swan-neck deformity of the thumb is usually initiated by synovitis of the CMC joint followed by stretching of the joint capsule and radialward subluxation of the base of the metacarpal. Thumb abduction becomes painful, and a degree of adductor muscle spasm occurs. This imbalance of forces results in an adduction deformity of the metacarpal with contracture of the adductor pollicis muscle. As abduction of the thumb becomes more difficult, the joints distal are used to compensate for lack of motion. This results in hyperextension of the IP joints, more frequently of the MP joint with resulting further adduction of the first metacarpal.[16] A self-perpetuating cycle of deformity ensues. Further hyperextension of the MP joint aggravates the adduction tendency of the first metacarpal.

The swan-neck deformity can be treated in its mild cases or preoperatively by a long thumb spica orthosis (Fig. 18.10). This orthosis provides a stable post for opposition of the other fingers to the thumb, increasing function. In the case of a boutonnière deformity where the MP joint is mostly involved, this can be treated with a small, short thumb spica splint, which does not immobilize the CMC joint by being thumb based only (see Fig. 18.8, *B*). Immobilization of the MP joint of the thumb often improves function by providing more stable base to pinch.

THUMB INTERPHALANGEAL JOINT ORTHOSES

Instability and pain of the thumb IP joint may occur in isolated deformities or in association with collapsed deformities such as swan-neck or boutonnière deformity, as discussed. This may result from osteoarthritis or rheumatoid arthritis of the hand.[17] Immobilizing the IP joint with the use of aluminum and foam splint or small fabricated thermal plastic orthosis (Fig. 18.11) provides both stability and protection to the joint, allowing continued pinching activities without leading to stretching of the supporting soft tissue and instability of the joint, which would make pinch difficult. The thumb IP orthosis may also be used in cases of pain and instability or when patients are considering an IP joint fusion to simulate the postoperative condition.[7] Postoperatively the splint may be used with IP joint fusions for protection following K-wire removal, usually at 6 to 8 weeks for an additional 2 to 6 weeks of immobilization.

PROXIMAL INTERPHALANGEAL JOINT ORTHOSES

The PIP joint collateral ligament system consists of two parts, an oblique and a vertical component. The oblique component connects the middle and the proximal phalanges by a ligament from the head of the proximal phalanx to the side of middle phalanx. The vertical component, frequently called the accessory collateral ligament, is mainly a system for suspension of the palmar plate and the flexor tendon sheath. The extensor apparatus consists of the central tendon, which inserts into the dorsal capsule in the base of the middle phalanx. It is flanked bilaterally by tendons of the intrinsic muscles. These structures are all intimately involved with common deformities seen in rheumatoid arthritis. The deformities include the swan-neck and boutonnière deformities.

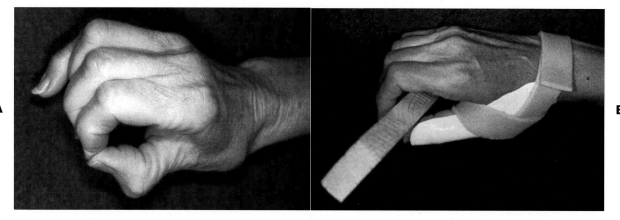

Fig. 18.10.   **A,** A typical thumb swan-neck deformity is shown with first metacarpal adduction, CMC subluxation, hyperextension of the MP joint, and hyperflexion of the IP joint. **B,** A long dorsal thumb splint applied to correct MP and CMC deformities can provide the patient a stable base for pinch.

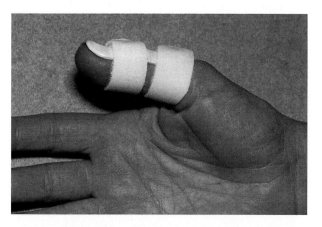

Fig. 18.11.   Dorsal thumb IP splint.

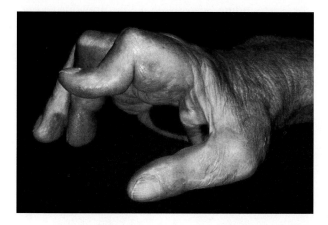

Fig. 18.12.   Boutonnière deformity.

The boutonnière or buttonhole deformity (Fig. 18.12) usually occurs in rheumatoid arthritis through the bulging of hyperplastic synovium between the central and lateral extensor tendons. The central tendon becomes weakened, and relative lengthening of it occurs. The transverse fibers that connect the lateral bands to the central tendon are lengthened by the synovial invasion allowing the tendons to dislocate in a palmar direction. The lateral tendons become relatively shortened in their displacement, and there is increased pull on the distal insertion of the distal phalanx resulting in a hyperflexion deformity of the PIP joint. Once this collapse is established, it becomes self-perpetuating, and the joints become stiff because of contracture of associated soft tissue structures. The DIP joint becomes hyperextended in the process, resulting in further dysfunction.[16]

The swan-neck deformity (Fig. 18.13) is characterized by hyperextension of the PIP joint and flexion of the distal joint. It is caused primarily by synovitis of the flexor tendon sheath with restriction of PIP joint flexion. The main function of the long flexor tendon is to flex the IP joints. When there is flexor synovitis, the patient tends to concentrate most of his or her flexor power on the MP joints, facilitating pull of the intrinsic muscles to the central tendon. Failure of PIP joint flexion therefore leads to greater intrinsic muscle imbalance resulting in a cycle of hyperextension at the PIP joint and hyperflexion of the DIP joint. Hyperextension at the PIP joint causes stretching in transverse fiber ligament and dorsal subluxation of the lateral bands with stretching of the oblique retinacular ligaments. Lengthening of the oblique retinacular ligament causes DIP flexion. Failure of flexor tendons to flex the PIP joint results in permanent joint stiffness and further destruction.

Preoperatively a static orthosis may be fabricated to prevent swan-neck or boutonnière deformities from becoming fixed and to improve hand function.[7] A commonly used orthosis for this situation is the figure-of-eight ring orthosis (Fig. 18.14, *A*) or tripoint finger splint (Fig. 18.14, *B*). The orthosis applies pressure at three points on the finger, providing a correcting force opposite to that of the deformity. For example, in splinting the swan-neck deformity, the pressure is applied dorsally, proximally, and distally, to the PIP joint and volarly over the center of the joint, resulting in a flexion force at the PIP joint, thus preventing PIP hyperextension and allowing active PIP flexion. This splint may be used preoperatively as well as after the deformity is surgically repaired. It is not recommended in the immediate postoperative period because of swelling. A dorsal PIP splint is better immediately postoperatively because it is less constricting (see later). Prevention of hyperextension by splinting in flexion allows structures volar to the PIP joint to shorten and help prevent return of the deformity.[10] For the boutonnière deformity, the orthosis is applied opposite that of the swan-neck deformity with pressure over the central aspect of the PIP joint dorsally and proximal and distal to the PIP joint volarly resulting in an extension force preventing PIP flexion contractures.

Postoperatively, after PIP joint implant resection arthroplasty or surgical correction of PIP deformities, a dorsal orthosis may be used for protection and proper positioning between exercise periods. The orthosis may be fabricated from low-temperature plastics or be of padded aluminum. For surgical treatment of swan-neck deformity, a flexed orthosis is used for postoperative protection of the flexed PIP position after der-

madesis, PIP fusion, sublimis tenodesis, or PIP manipulation (Fig. 18.15). A dorsal straight orthosis (Fig. 18.16) maintaining PIP extension is used for postoperative protection of boutonnière repair.

Implant resection arthroplasty has been used extensively over the last 30 years by this institution for the treatment of MP and PIP joint deformities. Implant resection arthroplasty can be indicated for isolated involvement of the PIP joint not associated with MP joint involvement in the presence of the following: (1) stiff arthritic PIP joint, (2) joint destruction with PIP lateral deviation,[19] (3) boutonnière deformity with joint destruction, and (4) swan-neck deformity with joint destruction. The splinting programs for each of the aforementioned categories are addressed individually. The orthoses described may be taped in place, but velcro closures should be applied for the ease of patient application when range-of-motion exercises are initiated postoperatively.

STIFF PROXIMAL INTERPHALANGEAL JOINT

When implant arthroplasty of a stiff PIP joint does not require reconstruction of the collateral ligaments or central tendon, active movements of flexion and extension should be started within 3 to 5 days after surgery. An orthosis is applied 2 to 5 days after surgery. It is worn continuously except for exercise sessions for 4 to 6 weeks. The orthosis protects the joint while it is healing. The greatest challenge in postoperative rehabilitation of finger joint arthroplasty is maintaining a proper balance between good healing of the surrounding scar tissue while applying proper movements of tension across the scar to obtain the desired range of motion. The ideal ranges of motion after this surgery are from full extension to 45 degrees of flexion in the index finger, 60 degrees in the

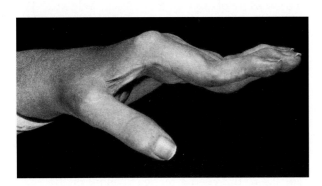

Fig. 18.13. Swan-neck deformity.

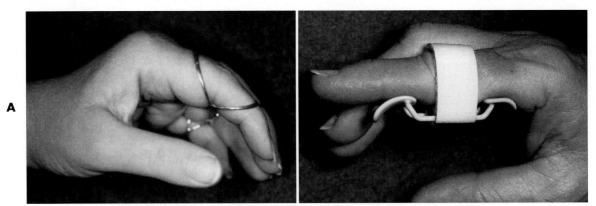

Fig. 18.14. **A,** A figure-of-eight ring splint prevents PIP joint hyperextension in a swan-neck deformity. **B,** A tripoint finger splint is positioned for correction of a boutonnière deformity.

long finger, and 70 degrees in the ring and little fingers. An orthosis to hold the digit in extension is worn mainly at night but may also be worn continuously for several weeks postoperatively depending on the degree of extensor lag present. A dynamic flexion orthosis may be applied three to five times daily for 10 to 20 minutes if flexion is limited (Fig. 18.17). Nighttime extension splinting usually continues for a total of 3 months postoperatively.

Several orthoses have been developed for the postoperative rehabilitation of the PIP joint. Passive and active exercises of the PIP joint should be done, always taking care to support the MP joint in extension. This can be done with the use of a reverse lumbrical bar that supports the proximal phalanges and eliminates motion of the MP joints during flexion exercises. The senior author has developed a finger crutch that functions similarly to the Bunnell wood block and supports the proximal phalanx during flexion exercises (Fig. 18.18, *left*). The Grip-X maintains finger alignment during gripping exercises (Fig. 18.18, *right*).

PROXIMAL INTERPHALANGEAL JOINT WITH LATERAL DEVIATION

In addition to implant resection arthroplasty, these patients require soft tissue reconstruction of the collateral ligaments and central slip; therefore, the orthosis and postoperative program need to incorporate stability and proper alignment techniques. The dorsal splint is placed laterally (Fig. 18.19) to correct any associated radial or ulnar deviation tendency postoperatively. Active range-of-motion exercises are usually delayed 7 to 14 days or longer at the index digit, which requires greater stability for pinch activities. The buddy taping system is used when active range-of-motion exercises

are initiated to maintain alignment during motion (Fig. 18.20). The buddy system is applied only during exercise sessions, five to eight times a day, with the lateral extension orthosis in place the rest of the time. Day wear of the orthosis is usually discontinued after 6 weeks. Nighttime wear continues for 3 months postoperatively.

SWAN-NECK DEFORMITY

After reconstruction of the PIP joint for a swan-neck deformity, it is important to achieve a 20- to 30-degree flexion contracture of the PIP joint. The orthosis is fabricated to keep the PIP joint in 30 to 40 degrees of flexion and the DIP in extension. The joint is immobilized for 3 weeks postoperatively. After 3 weeks, active range of motion is initiated, and the splint is used to block extension. The distal strap of the splint is re-

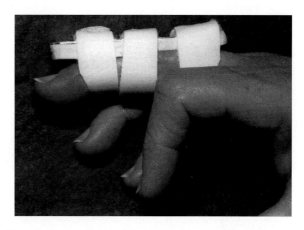

Fig. 18.16. Splinting the boutonnière deformity in extension postoperatively using an aluminum and foam splint with velcro straps for easy adjustments.

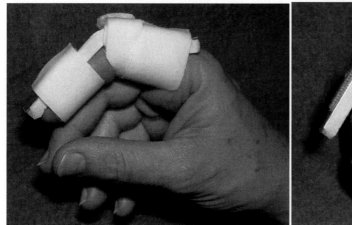

A

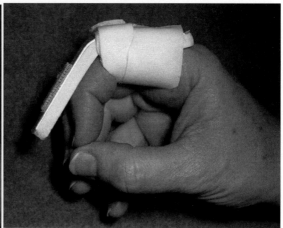

B

Fig. 18.15. **A,** The swan-neck deformity is splinted postoperatively with a flexed padded aluminum orthosis. **B,** The distal velcro strap may be removed for range of motion.

moved four to six times a day for active range-of-motion exercises for 10 to 20 repetitions each (see Fig. 18.15). The orthosis is worn day and night for the first 6 weeks. Nighttime splinting continues for 3 months postoperatively.

BOUTONNIÈRE DEFORMITY

After PIP joint reconstruction for boutonnière deformity, it is important to maintain maximum PIP joint extension, yet allowing DIP flexion. Therefore, an orthosis, taped in place 2 to 5 days after surgery, keeps the PIP joint extended and ends proximal to the DIP joint. The patient is instructed in hourly DIP active range-of-motion exercises. Active range of motion of the PIP joint is initiated usually at 2 to 3 weeks

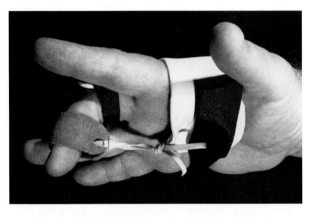

Fig. 18.17. A dynamic flexion splint can be applied three to five times daily for 10 to 20 minutes to increase range of motion if needed after PIP joint implant resection arthroplasty for a stiff joint.

postoperatively. The orthosis is replaced after each exercise session. The use of Velcro straps simplifies the removal and application of the splint (see Fig. 18.16). Daytime PIP joint splinting is usually discontinued after 6 to 8 weeks, but nighttime extension splinting may continue for 3 to 6 months postoperatively to maintain maximum PIP joint extension.

DYNAMIC METACARPOPHALANGEAL JOINT ORTHOSES

The MP joint is a key joint in the normal functioning of fingers. Movement of this joint occurs not only in the AP plane of flexion and extension, but also in the lateral plane of abduction and adduction and involves some passive axial rotation. The index finger normally tends to supinate to 45 degrees during pinch. The MP joint is subjected to great stresses during constant movements in everyday function and is commonly affected by rheumatoid arthritis.

Deformities of the MP joint in rheumatoid arthritis are usually manifested by increased ulnar drift and palmar subluxation (Fig. 18.21). The deformity often begins with the flexor tendons, which enter the fibrous sheath at an angle and exert an ulnad and palmad pull that is resisted in the normal hand (Fig. 18.22, *A*). When the rheumatoid process progresses, normal muscle balance is lost, and if the restraining structures of the ligament system are destroyed by the rheumatoid disease, resistance to the gradual deforming pull of the long flexors is lost, and the tendons are displaced distally, ulnar, and palmar (Fig. 18.22, *B*).[13] The intrinsic muscles, which form a bridge between the extensor and flexor systems and provide direct flexor

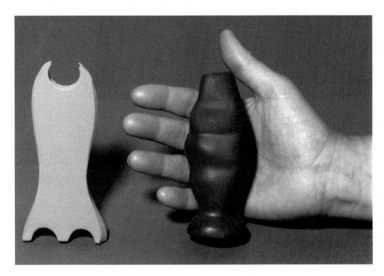

Fig. 18.18. Shown to the left is a finger crutch to help support the proximal phalanx in extension during PIP flexion exercises. On the right is a Grip-X used for postoperative grip strengthening.

power across the MP joint, also become deforming elements once the disease has lengthened the restraining structures of the MP joint and extensor tendon hood. The extensor tendons are then weakened by

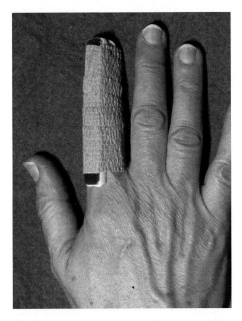

Fig. 18.19. The dorsal splint can be applied slightly laterally to correct any residual deformity.

their ulnad displacement, resulting in loss of balance between intrinsic and extrinsic muscles. The normal mechanical advantage of the ulnar intrinsic muscle is greatly increased once the deformity is established. This creates a cycle resulting in a continued ulnad and palmad dislocation.[16]

Pronation deformity of the index finger is a common disability of the rheumatoid hand. In the normal hand, the pinch mechanism between the thumb and the index finger requires slight supination of the index finger so that the palmar surfaces can meet. In a pronation deformity, the less useful lateral surfaces are opposed. During pinch, the pronation deformity results in an ulnar-directed stress applied to the radial collateral ligaments of the MP joints. This further aggravates ulnar drift and MP subluxation. The many anatomic and pathologic entities that play a role in creating the deformities in the MP joint are summarized by Swanson.[16]

MP joint deformities may significantly impair finger function. Deformities of this joint caused by inflammatory arthritis are best treated in their severest form by flexible implant resection arthroplasty. Flexible implant resection arthroplasty of the MP joints is indicated in rheumatoid or posttraumatic disabilities when (1) the joints are fixed or stiff, (2) radiographic evidence of joint destruction or subluxation is present, (3) ulnar

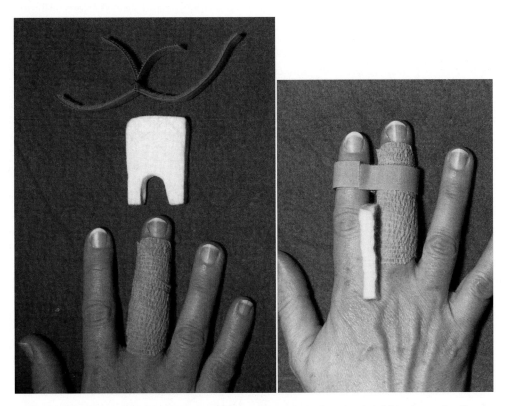

Fig. 18.20. The buddy system is used when active range of motion is initiated, usually after 2 weeks, following implant resection arthroplasty in patients with preoperative PIP joint deviation. Here the middle finger has received the implant and is aligned to the index digit. This allows protection of the collateral ligaments while allowing motion.

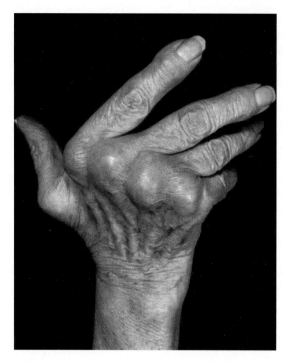

Fig. 18.21. Most common deformities occurring in rheumatoid arthritis are ulnar drift and palmar subluxation at MP joints.

drift is not correctable by soft tissue surgery alone, (4) the intrinsic and extrinsic musculature and ligament systems are contracted, and (5) associated stiffness is found in the IP joints.[17]

Flexible implant arthroplasty of the MP joint as developed by the senior author has become the gold standard for MP arthroplasty. It has stood the test of time and meets the goals of providing a pain-free, mobile, stable, and durable joint.[8] The basic concept of flexible implant resection arthroplasty can be summarized as follows:

$$\frac{\text{Bone}}{\text{Resection}} + \text{Implant} + \text{Encapsulation} = \frac{\text{Functional}}{\text{Joint}}$$

The flexible implant acts as a dynamic spacer, maintaining internal alignment and spacing of the reconstructed joint and supporting the neocapsule that develops around it. The joint is thus rebuilt in a healing phenomenon called the *encapsulation process.*

One of the most important functions of a flexible implant is to maintain internal alignment and spacing of the reconstructed joint, while early motion is started, with the implant acting as a dynamic spacer. Early guided motion is essential in promoting the development of a new functionally adapted fibrous capsule. The basic concept that collagen formation and development can be guided in a controlled postoperative rehabilitation program must be understood by surgeons

and therapists who treat rheumatoid patients. If motion is restricted during the healing phase, there is poor mobility of the joint; therefore, the host tissue or collagen reaction must be used advantageously by training it postoperatively.

A dynamic extension orthosis was designed by the senior author to facilitate early postoperative motion in finger joint resection arthroplasty cases.[14] It is also adaptable for many other conditions requiring MP or PIP extension assistance. It is of high-profile design, meaning the main outrigger for dynamic extension of the MPs is situated directly over (high above) the proximal phalanges to allow for a straight line of pull (Fig. 18.23), in contrast to the low-profile design, which has a smaller outrigger that functions as a pulley (Fig. 18.24). Use of a dynamic extension orthosis following MP implant resection arthroplasty involves a good understanding of the splint, splinting techniques, and postoperative rehabilitation principles. The dynamic extension orthosis has three major functions: to provide complete, adjustable correction of residual deformity; to control motion in the desired plane and range; and to assist flexion and extension power ensuring an adequate alternation of complete extension and flexion ranges of motion in the joint.[7] The high-profile orthosis is made up of many parts (Fig. 18.25). It is adaptable for both the right and the left hands and can be reused for later surgeries, if needed. It is available in three sizes, which are determined by forearm measurements.

Following MP joint resection arthroplasty, the dynamic extension orthosis is applied 2 to 5 days postoperatively. The splint is assembled and applied in the following manner. The base of the brace is applied over a quarter-inch felt pad, trimmed to the correct length and distally shaped over the heads of the metacarpals to account for the descending angle of the phalanges. Lambs wool padding is applied to the middle and proximal straps as well as the radial aspect of the distal strap to provide even pressure distribution. The flexible dorsal wrist splint can then be conformed to the extremity with particular attention to avoid pressure at any bony prominences, incisions, and splint or strap edges. The wrist is placed in near neutral postion. The straps are secured so that the splint is snug enough to prevent rotation or sliding on the extremity, but not too tight to cause pressure or constriction. A palmar pad is passed through the dorsal volar strap and should be located in the palmar arch proximal to the distal palmar crease. It should clear the thenar eminence and conform to the transverse arch of the hand. The outrigger or longitudinal bar is tightly screwed to the splint. The transverse bar is secured to the longitudinal bar with a wing nut at the appropriate location to obtain a 90-degree line of pull when the finger slings are applied to the proximal phalanges. It is also angled to account for

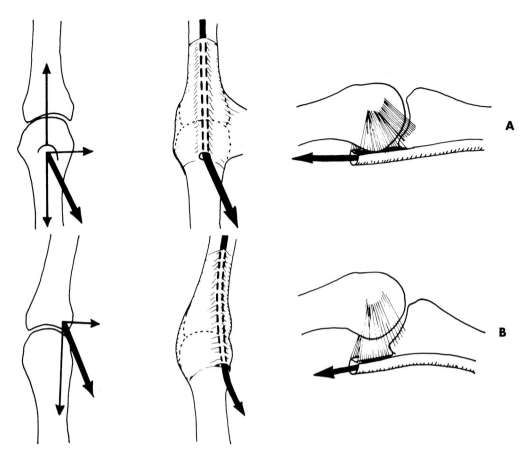

Fig. 18.22. **A,** Common flexor tendons enter the fibrous sheath at an angle, and forces produced by their action have ulnar and palmar components *(left).* In a normal stable MP joint, the ulnar component has little or no displacement effect *(middle)* and resistance of capsule and ligaments prevents displacement of sheath inlet *(right).* **B,** When capsule and ligaments of the MP joint are distended and weakened by rheumatoid process, resistance to these deforming forces is lost. The point of reflection of the sheath is displaced distally, ulnar and palmar *(left).* The ulnar component of the force produces ulnar deviation *(middle)* and palmar subluxation *(right)* of the proximal phalanx. This mechanism is especially deforming at the level of index and middle fingers.

the lateral descending angle of the proximal phalanges. A lateral outrigger is attached to the radial side of the transverse bar, in most cases, to provide for additional radial pull, which is used in index finger supination (see Fig. 18.23). The lateral outrigger is secured at an appropriate angle to achieve a 90-degree line of pull on the radial side of the middle phalanx of the index finger. Additional outriggers (see Fig. 18.23) may be needed initially or later, and they include a thumb outrigger to keep the thumb abducted to avoid lateral pressure on the digits during active flexion and a small finger outrigger used to pronate the little finger and allow range of motion.

The goal of the dynamic brace is to support the fingers in slight radial deviation and to encourage extension without hyperextension. The tension of the rubber band should be tight enough to guide the digits in a desired plane of motion while allowing 70 degrees of active flexion at the ring and little fingers. The

response to dynamic splinting is rapid during the first few days. Initially the therapist may need to adjust the dynamic splint two or three times a week to prevent overcorrection or to increase gradually tension of the slings to facilitate MP joint extension. Placement and adjustment of the slings vary with the situation presented by each finger. The index finger often has a tendency toward pronation deformity preoperatively. The patient then tends to use lateral pinch, which further exaggerates the ulnar deviation of the digits. The index finger must be supported in supination after surgery using the concept of the *force couple.*[19] A force couple is defined as two equal and opposite forces that act along parallel lines and is obtained by applying a second outrigger to provide a supinatory torque (see Fig. 18.23). The index finger needs greater stability and less mobility at the MP joint to perform prehensile activities. In most cases, a string is used instead of a rubber band at the index finger to place the digit in the proper position and limit flexion for at least 2 to 3 weeks to achieve the goal of 0 extension and 45 degrees of flexion.

In most cases, the long finger requires only a sling on the proximal phalanx to maintain a slight radial alignment. An additional lateral sling may be applied to the middle phalanx, if additional radial pull is needed or if correction of pronation tendency is required. The requirements of the ring finger are similar to those of the long finger with the exception that the rubber band tension may need to be reduced to allow 70 degrees of active flexion. The little finger may have weak flexor power, and rubber band tension may need to be reduced accordingly. In some cases, a buddy sling is applied to allow active assisted motion with the ring finger. This buddy sling needs to take into account the

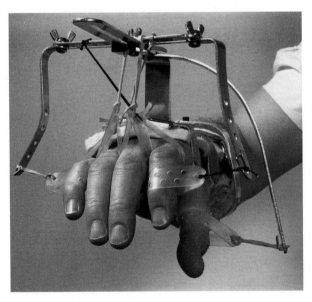

Fig. 18.23. The high-profile hand splint with all outriggers in place to: supinate and stabilize the index finger with a string instead of a rubber band; pronate the little finger and allow motion through use of rubber bands; and abduct the thumb to avoid lateral pressure on the digits during active flexion.

transverse arch to allow proper digital flexion. If the little finger has a supination tendency or tucks under the ring finger, the proximal phalanx sling can be placed radially to facilitate pronation. If further rotation is required, an additional outrigger is used to support a sling pulling ulnarly on the middle phalanx according to the force couple principle (see Fig. 18.23).

The importance of good patient education cannot be overstressed. The exercises are carried out for a short duration but frequently during the day to train the new joint capsule in proper alignment. It is important that the exercises are carried out with the extremity elevated to reduce edema. Active flexion exercises of all MP joints are carried out for 5 to 10 repetitions. These exercises are then repeated five times for each MP joint individually. Patients who have good motion at the PIP joints may have difficulty isolating MP flexion. In these cases, a dorsally padded aluminum splint or molded low-temperature plastic splints are taped to immobilize the PIP joints, thus allowing localization of the flexion force at the MP joints. These splints can be secured with straps for ease of removal. The range-of-motion goals at the MP joints after implant resection arthroplasty are: index finger, 0 to 45 degrees; long, 0 to 60 degrees; ring, 0 to 70 degrees; small, 0 to 70 degrees. If these goals are not reached with active exercises, passive range of motion is initiated. A force no greater than 2 lb of pressure is applied to the proximal phalanx at each MP joint individually for five repetitions (Fig. 18.26). The surgeon may also wish to limit MP flexion in cases where greater stability is desired in the presence of good PIP motion. In this case, the rubber band is replaced with a dacron strap to provide a static sling arrangement. The lumbrical bar, available with the high-profile orthoses, can be used also to immobilize the MP joints.

The reconstructed joints start tightening up during the second postoperative week and are quite tight by the end of 3 weeks. If the desired range of motion has not been obtained by 4 weeks, it is difficult to gain

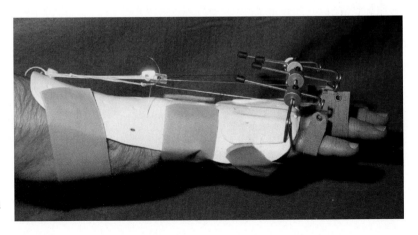

Fig. 18.24. Low-profile dynamic extension orthosis.

further improvement in motion. If at 3 weeks the patient has good MP joint extension with poor flexion, dynamic flexion techniques are used. The therapist should be cautious with dynamic flexion devices because extension is usually more difficult to achieve. Passive flexion is achieved with finger slings on the proximal phalanges attached volarly to the flexion outrigger, which is secured to the base of the brace (Fig. 18.27). The slings should be placed so that the line of pull is directed toward the scaphoid bone. A figure-of-eight elbow strap may be needed to prevent distal migration of the splint during dynamic flexion. Dynamic flexion should be applied for only 20 minutes at a time, three to six times a day or more frequently if

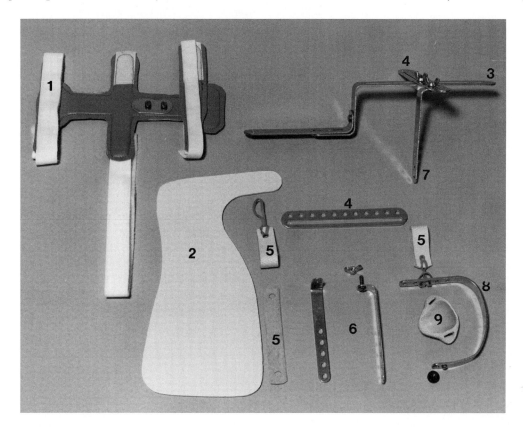

Fig. 18.25.   High-profile prefabricated dynamic splint parts. *1*, Dorsal prefabricated wrist splint; *2*, thermal plastic wrist splint; *3*, longitudinal bar outrigger; *4*, transverse bar; *5*, finger loops; *6*, finger rotation outrigger bars; *7*, thumb outrigger bar; *8*, finger flexion outrigger bar; *9*, palmar pad.

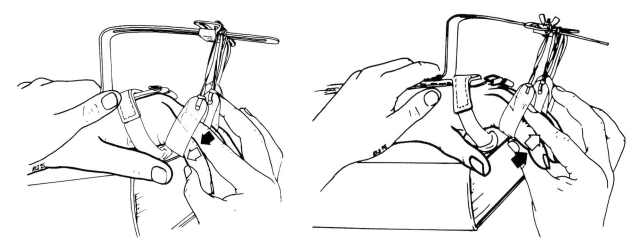

Fig. 18.26.   Passive range-of-motion exercises are shown being performed with the wrist supported. A force no greater than 2 lb of pressure is applied to the proximal phalanx of each MP joint for five repetitions each.

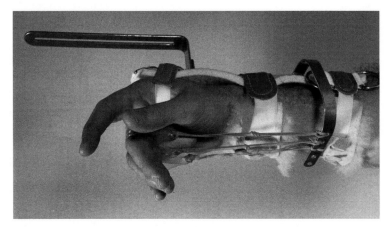

Fig. 18.27. Passive flexion is achieved with slings on the proximal phalanges attached volarly to the flexion outrigger, which is secured to the base of the high-profile hand splint. Passive flexion is applied for only 20 minutes at a time, usually three to six times daily in patients demonstrating flexion limitation.

flexion limitations persist. At the sixth postoperative week, the extension portion of the splint is usually worn at night only for another 3 weeks. If there is persistent extensor lag or tendency for flexion contracture or deviation of the digits, part-time support by this orthosis must be continued for several more weeks or even months.

The patient should follow a prescribed rehabilitation program including active and passive exercises for at least 3 months after surgery to maintain desired range of motion. The range of motion is regularly measured to assess progress. Because collagen maturity, scar contraction, and tendon deficiencies vary from patient to patient, careful attention by the hand surgeon and therapist is required throughout the postoperative period. The patient's response to the rehabilitation program varies with the severity of preoperative deformities; the surgical procedure; the patient's physical and emotional state, ability to understand, and ability to cooperate; and individual collagen and scar tissue production. The program must be carried out with these variables in mind, realizing that some patients reach their goals more rapidly than others. Properly applied therapy can provide a much better result for the patient.

Many types of dynamic extension orthoses are available for postoperative MP therapy. Both the high-profile dynamic orthosis and the low-profile[4] design are commonly used as well as custom-fabricated outriggers. There is considerable debate about the advantages and disadvantages of the high-profile dynamic orthosis versus the low-profile design. The advantages of the low-profile design are better cosmesis and ease of patient dressing. The authors have compared the high-profile versus the low-profile orthosis and have demonstrated an increased amount of force necessary to flex the digits in the low-profile orthosis. Also the high-profile dynamic orthosis provides for more supination at the index finger, which is crucial for pad-to-pad opposition with the thumb.[3] The authors now recommend the use of the high profile dynamic orthosis for the

postoperative management of implant resection arthroplasty in the following cases: for patients demonstrating weak flexion strength, the high-profile splint requires less force to initiate and maintain motion; in patients requiring index supination because of pronation deformities, the high-profile *force couple* design provides greater index finger supination during range of motion.

In short, the postoperative dynamic orthosis serves a variety of purposes. It provides adjustable tension to control alignment of the MP joint during the healing phase, while it limits motion to the desired plane and range during active exercises. It also assists flexor and extensor power to encourage desired finger motion following implant resection arthroplasty. The splint is generally worn day and night for about 6 to 8 weeks with night wear continued through 12 weeks.

SUMMARY

The success of using an orthosis in the treatment of arthritic hand deformities depends on many factors. The patient must understand the purpose of the orthosis, have acceptance of the benefits that the orthosis can provide, and have the proper knowledge and ability to use the orthosis appropriately. The therapist must be skilled in patient evaluation and orthotic fabrication techniques, have a knowledge of the disease process and treatment principles, and develop a good rapport with the patient. The physician must determine the treatment goals of the orthosis and refer the fabrication of the orthosis to the appropriately trained orthotist or learn these techniques himself or herself. When selecting the proper orthosis, the principles outlined by Bennett[1] must be understood:

(1) The device must serve a real need. Applying unnecessary apparatus can be as dangerous as not applying necessary apparatus. (2) The device prescribed must be of a design that can be constructed and, as necessary, repaired by a good orthotist. (3) The device must be as lightweight as possible but capable of standing up under expected

wear. (4) The device must be reasonable in cost. (5) The device must be sufficiently simple that it can be applied by the patient or his or her family. (6) The device must be acceptable in appearance. (7) The device must in no way endanger the structural security of bodily segments through its use.

It is only by adherence of these principles that optimum benefit for the patient with an arthritic hand lesion can be achieved.

REFERENCES

1. Bennett RL: Orthotics for function, Phys Ther Rev :36, 1956.
2. Boozer J: Splinting the arthritic hand. J Hand Ther Jan:46, 1993.
3. Boozer JA, et al: Comparison of the biomechanical motions and forces involved in high-profile versus low-profile dynamic splinting, J Hand Ther 7:171–182, 1994.
4. Colditz JC: Low profile dynamic splinting of the injured hand, Am J Occup Ther 37:182, 1983.
5. Fess EE, Phillips CA: Hand splinting principles and methods, St. Louis, 1987, CV Mosby.
6. Flatt EA: Care of the arthritic hand, St. Louis, 1983, CV Mosby.
7. Grisser RW: Splinting the rheumatoid arthritic hand. Current concepts in orthopaedics: A diagnosis related approach to splinting, 1984, Roylan Medical Products.
8. Kirchenbaum D, et al: Arthroplasty of the metacarpophalangeal joints with use of silicone-rubber implants in patients who have rheumatoid arthritis: Long-term results, J Bone Joint Surg 75A: 3–12, 1993.
9. Malick MH: Upper extremity orthotics. In Hopkins, Smith, editors: Willard and Spackman's Occupational Therapy, Philadelphia, JB Lippincott.
10. Melvin JL: Rheumatic disease: Occupational therapy and rehabilitation, Philadelphia, 1982, FA Davis.
11. Moberg E: Circulatory impairment in splinting: Splinting in hand therapy, New York, 1982, Thieme-Stratton.
12. Phillips CA: The management of patients with rheumatoid arthritis. In Hunter, et al, editors: Rehabilitation of the hand, St. Louis, 1990, CV Mosby.
13. Stack HG, Vaughan-Jackson OJ: The zig-zag deformity in the rheumatoid hand. 3:67, 1971.
14. Swanson AB: Flexible/Implant arthroplasty in the hand and extremities: Consideration for postoperative bracing and rehabilitation for flexible implant arthroplasty of the finger, St. Louis, 1973, CV Mosby.
15. Swanson AB: Pathogenesis of arthritic lesions. In Hunter, et al, editors: Rehabilitation of the hand, St. Louis, 1995, CV Mosby.
16. Swanson AB: Pathomechanics of deformities in hand and wrist. In Hunter, et al, editor: Rehabilitation of the Hand, St. Louis, 1995, CV Mosby.
17. Swanson AB: Reconstructive surgery in the arthritic hand and foot. Clinical symposium, Summit, NJ, 1979, CIBA Pharmaceutical Company.
18. Swanson AB, deGroot Swanson G, Leonard J: Postoperative rehabilitation program in the flexible implant arthroplasty of the digits. In Hunter, et al, editors: Rehabilitation of the hand, St. Louis, 1995, CV Mosby.
19. Swanson AB, et al: Upper limb joint replacement. In Nickel VL, editor: Orthopedic Rehabilitation, New York, 1982, Churchill Livingstone.

Splinting in Peripheral Nerve Palsy

Timothy S. Loth
William W. Eversmann

Recent trends in orthotic treatment of peripheral nerve palsies have favored the lightest and least complicated splints that can accomplish the desired rehabilitation goal(s). To accomplish the primary therapeutic goals of prevention of contractures and enhancement of hand function, splint design should be kept user-friendly (i.e., it should not interfere with intact hand functions [those not affected by the nerve palsy]) and should be lightweight, low profile, and easy to apply. Excessively elaborate splints, although impressive in appearance and ingenious in design, are often not worn because of violation of these principles and result in therapeutic failure through lack of patient compliance.

Although some orthoses are helpful in improving function, most splinting efforts are directed to prevention of predictable deformities secondary to motor imbalance from nerve injury. Orthotic wear must be combined with a conscientious program of patient education and intermittently monitored therapy to assure that the patient maintains full passive upper extremity range of motion. In this manner, once nerve regeneration is complete or tendon transfers have been performed, the extremity function is not compromised by joint contractures. Care must be taken when splinting sensory-deprived areas to avoid the development of pressure sores. Patient education and frequent monitoring are necessary until return of protective sensation to the extremity has occurred.

The orthotic management of established contractures is discussed elsewhere in this book. This chapter focuses on splinting techniques to prevent contractures and to enhance function. There are many orthoses available that can effectively perform the same rehabilitation tasks for each of the clinical conditions discussed subsequently, so it is impractical to illustrate all of them. Instead, a few examples are given to illustrate a general approach to nerve palsies, which can be modified to meet each patient's specific rehabilitation requirements.

MEDIAN NERVE PALSIES

Although a number of motor functions are affected in this injury, the effective minimal splinting replacement for functional purposes consists of a first web spacer, or carpometacarpal opposition splint to facilitate thumb opposition positioning and maintenance of the first web space (Fig. 19.1). Conscientious occupational therapy is essential to maintain passive range of motion to the digits while awaiting nerve regeneration or pending tendon transfer in high median nerve palsies.

RADIAL NERVE INJURY

The key deficit in this palsy is loss of wrist extension, which results in a significant reduction in digital performance, grip strength, and coordination.

The most efficient splinting in a radial nerve palsy consists of a cock-up splint maintaining the wrist in 20 to 40 degrees of dorsiflexion (Fig. 19.2). This wrist position facilitates improved grasp/release activities, enhancing hand function. Individuals unable to comply with routine rehabilitation programs to maintain digital flexibility often benefit from a long dorsal outrigger splint, which provides passive extension to the metacarpophalangeal (MP) joints and abduction/extension to the thumb (Fig. 19.3).

ULNAR NERVE INJURIES

Muscle imbalance primarily from the loss of ulnar intrinsic motors results in losses of strength and hand

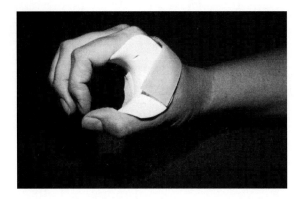

Fig. 19.1.   Median nerve palsy splint. First web spacer.

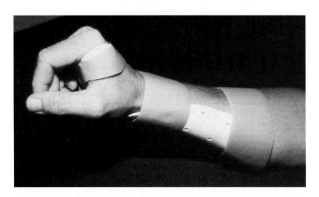

Fig. 19.2.   Radial nerve palsy splint. Wrist cock-up splint.

coordination. If these imbalances are not addressed through therapy and orthotic treatment, fixed claw deformity of the ring and small fingers often develops. Of the involved motors, the most critical for augmentation through splinting are the interossei and lumbri-

cals, which are responsible for MP joint flexion and interphalangeal (IP) joint extension of the ring and small fingers.

There are many MP joint extension block splint designs that transfer the power of the extrinsic extensors of the MP joints to produce extension of the IP joints and yet allow full flexion of the ring and small fingers (Figs. 19.4 and 19.5). This splint's principal function is the prevention of contractures through maintenance of full, active IP range of motion. Another less intrusive way to prevent flexion contractures is through the application of PIP extension gutter splints at bedtime (Fig. 19.6).

COMBINED NERVE LESIONS

Because of their proximity in the medial arm, combined median and ulnar nerve injuries occur frequently with lacerations to the brachium. The same philosophy and technical considerations apply for splinting of multiple peripheral nerve injuries in the upper extremity as for the previously discussed single nerve deficits. The absence of sensation in both the ulnar and the median nerve distributions is devastating to hand function and can lead to splinting problems because of insensate skin. In addition to a conscientious program of active and passive range of motion to maintain joint mobility, an extension block splint of the MP joints of all of the fingers and a first web spacer can prevent IP joint clawing and first web contractures (Fig. 19.7). Dynamic flexion splints for the digits can be useful for patients having difficulty maintaining passive range of motion through exercise alone.

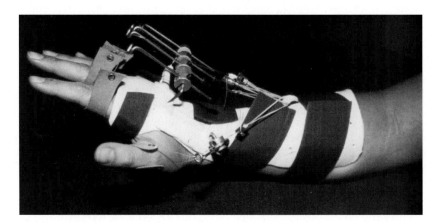

Fig. 19.3.   Radial nerve palsy splint. Long dorsal outrigger with thumb abduction/extension outrigger.

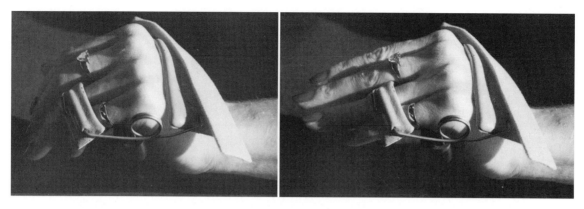

Fig. 19.4. Ulnar nerve palsy splints. Prefabricated Wynn-Perry splint demonstrates active ring and small finger IP joint extension produced through extension blocking of the MP joints. See Fig. 19.5.

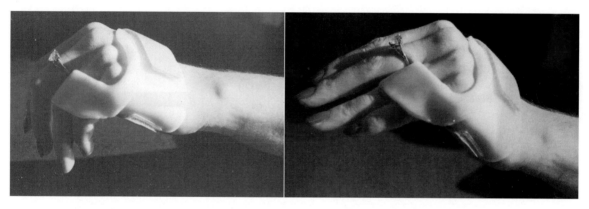

Fig. 19.5. Ulnar nerve palsy splints. Custom-made hand-based MP extension block splint demonstrates active ring and small finger IP joint extension produced through extension blocking of the MP joints. See Fig. 19.4.

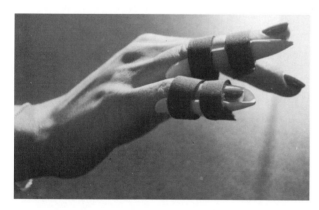

Fig. 19.6. Ulnar nerve palsy splints. PIP extension gutters for ring and small fingers.

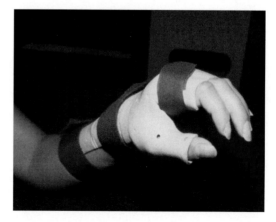

Fig. 19.7. Combined median and ulnar nerve palsy splint. MP joint extension block splint (20 to 40 degrees of MP flexion) for all fingers combined with a first web spacer.

BIBLIOGRAPHY

Cannon NM, editor: Diagnosis and treatment manual for physicians and therapists, ed 3, 1991.

Fess EE, Pillips CA: Exercise and splinting for specific problems. In Hand splinting principles and methods, St. Louis, 1987, CV Mosby.

Mackin EJ, Byron PM: Rehabilitation following nerve repair. In Gelberman RH, editor: Operative nerve repair and reconstruction, 1991.

Orthoses for Brachial Plexus Injuries

Robert D. Leffert
Colleen Lowe
John Snowden

GENERAL CONSIDERATIONS

Many of the concepts used in rehabilitation programs for clients with brachial plexus injuries have come from the experience with poliomyelitis.[5] There are important differences between the two entities, however, that must be considered before attempting to apply these ideas to individuals with brachial plexus injuries.

Polio patients often have lower extremity weakness that imposes a requirement for assistance in transfer and ambulation. Although some victims of polytrauma may also fall into this category, the vast majority of patients with plexus injuries are otherwise healthy individuals in whom one arm only has been affected. Consequently, unless disabled by pain, they generally remain active and able to carry out activities of daily living, albeit one-handed. Because a paretic lower limb may preclude ambulation, the polio patient is more likely to accept a clumsy or unsightly orthotic device to avoid crutches or a wheelchair. This imposes a higher standard for the success and acceptance of any assistive device that may be provided as an aid to the upper limb. The plexus-injured patient may simply prefer to use the sound side and remain one-handed.

The issue of sensibility is one that does not concern the polio patient, because his deficit is confined to motor function. Not only must the plexus-injured patient contend with being deprived of sensory feedback from skin, muscles, and joints, but the possibility of breakdown of insensate skin must be considered in the prescription and wearing of any orthosis that comes in contact with it or that allows it to be used in an unrestricted fashion.

The general principles of bracing of the upper extremity have been articulated by Schottsteadt and Robinson[5] as follows:
1. To prevent deformity.
2. To fix position to obtain maximal function.

3. To correct deformity.

To these ends, the orthosis may be used in the following circumstances:
1. To supplant lost upper extremity function completely.
2. To assist or supplement lost upper extremity motor power.
3. To supplement surgical reconstruction.

To these should be added:
1. To prevent or treat edema of the limb.
2. To maintain bimanuality during the period of recovery.
3. To ease pain caused by traction on unsupported nerves and vessels.[4]

PRESCRIPTION

The prescription of all devices should be according to practical considerations of the needs of the particular patient. It should not be forgotten that most patients are independent with one sound hand. Nevertheless, consideration must be given to the question of whether there are special bilateral activities that must be facilitated. Before proceeding with fabrication of the orthosis, the patient must be informed about the options, if there are any. If possible, the device, or one closely resembling it, should be seen and handled. One should be realistic about what functional gains are possible. The patient's "gadget tolerance" should be assessed because this has a significant influence on the ultimate functional result that is obtained. The device should meet the needs of the patient and not interfere with remaining functional capacity. If it cannot be applied and removed independently, it is of much lesser value. Along with all of these criteria, the cost must also be considered against the anticipated time of use and potential for real benefit. Both the patient and the caregivers should have a realistic estimate of how long

Table 20.1.   Levels of neurologic impairment

LEVEL OF INJURY	MOTOR DEFICIT	SENSORY LOSS	FUNCTIONAL NEED
C5-6	Shoulder abduction and flexion; elbow flexion; wrist extension	Lateral arm, forearm, thumb, and index	Support shoulder, prevent subluxation; flex elbow
C5-6-7	As above, with wrist, finger and thumb extension weakness; weakness of elbow extension	As above and middle finger	As above; wrist support, finger and thumb extension, and thumb extension
C8-T1	Wrist, finger, and thumb flexors; finger and thumb extensor	Little and ring fingers and medial forearm	Wrist stabilization; finger flexion (extension), intrinsic function
C5-T1	Flail arm (+/− scapula)	Total forearm lateral arm entire hand	Support and protect limb; functional splint?

the orthosis will be worn. In some cases, this is a relatively short time as the patient's clinical picture evolves with recovery, whereas in others it may be on a permanent basis.

The written prescription should include the client's diagnosis and reasons for use of the orthosis. It is often beneficial to discuss the prescription with the Certified Orthotist or occupational therapist in advance so that costly and time-consuming revisions are avoided. Finally, the wearing schedule and specific precautions for use should be clearly stated in writing and reiterated to the client.

When applying these principles to the prescription and fabrication of orthoses for brachial plexus palsy, it is useful to categorize the different types of injuries according to the levels of neurologic impairment because this allows for orderly consideration of the requirements that must be met. Each level has specific motor and sensory distributions, and these in turn have unique problems and concerns (Table 20.1). The comments and recommendations for each level should be considered as general guides and modified accordingly for patients with partial lesions.

CLINICAL CATEGORIES OF INJURY AND SPECIFIC PRESCRIPTIONS

C5-6

There is no orthosis that provides normal functional control of the shoulder. The Rancho Los Amigos orthosis attempts to gain a modicum of control with a full shoulder flexion-extension and rotation joint in addition to other supports and assists for the remainder of the limb.[1,4,5] Other variations of these functional devices are custom-designed for the individual's needs.

Unless there is only partial loss of function and tendon transfer is possible, or there is complete loss and fusion is done, the orthotic problem is one of support and prevention of inferior subluxation of the glenohumeral joint. The commonly available sling has the inconvenience of transferring the weight of the limb to the back of the neck, where it soon becomes irritating. In addition, the limb is held in adduction and medial rotation, which, if unrelieved, ultimately results in contractures at shoulder and elbow. To offset these problems, there are several other solutions.

The hemisling with humeral cuff and shoulder saddle spares the neck irritation because the weight is borne on the shoulder girdle (Fig. 20.1). The use of bilateral humeral cuffs and an adjustable strap across the back is a variation on this design and is available as the Biomet hook hemiharness. These devices have the advantage of supporting the ptotic scapula as well as the glenohumeral joint. Maximal support of the limb may be obtained with a pelvic support orthosis, the gunslinger splint (Fig. 20.2).[2] This orthosis has the advantage of reducing traction on the neurovascular structures and can materially diminish pain attributed to traction on them. It also can be an effective device for reduction of edema, in which case the arm and hand would be more elevated than is seen in this illustration.

Because the innervation of the abductors and lateral rotators of the humerus is the same as that of the elbow flexors, patients with C5-6 lesions almost invariably have both deficits. If there is a disparity and the elbow flexors recover, these devices can be employed as individual need dictates.

With the reverse situation of a shoulder under voluntary control and a flail elbow, a number of remedies are possible. These include an elbow orthosis with

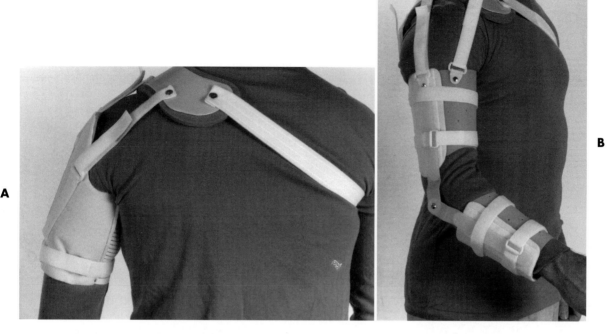

Fig. 20.1. **A,** The basic humeral cuff and shoulder saddle may be worn beneath the clothing. **B,** This appliance may be used to suspend additional orthotic components.

cable-activated elbow lock for manual control and positioning or one that is body-powered for cable control of flexion and lock (Fig. 20.3, *A* and *B*). An elbow orthosis may be constructed with external power, but the indications for this device are both narrow and expensive.

C5-7

These patients have, in addition to the lack of shoulder and elbow control as in the C5-6 group, further loss of extension at elbow, wrist, fingers, and thumb. There is no question that active extension of the elbow is important for activities of daily living. This is particularly evident when pushing open a door, using the limb overhead, or when steadying an object that is being manipulated by the other limb. If elbow extension is lacking bilaterally, such activities as turning over in bed or getting up from a chair are compromised. Fortunately, brachial plexus injuries are usually unilateral. Most orthotic efforts are expended in attempting to supplement active elbow flexion power, and elbow extension, when the patient is in the vertical position, is left to the effects of gravity.

The subtraction of C7 innervation from a patient with a C5-6 lesion adds the equivalent of a radial palsy, with deficits of extension at wrist, fingers, and thumb. The approach to improving function is that employed in treatment of a peripheral radial nerve lesion. The wrist is maintained in a static position of 5 degrees of dorsiflexion by a volar orthosis. The fingers are supported dynamically to produce extension at the metacarpophalangeal (MP) joints by elastic slings from either a low-profile or conventional high-profile outrigger. Finger flexion takes place actively from this starting position. The low-profile device is preferred by most patients because it is considerably less bulky and allows the hand to access narrow spaces such as a pocket (Fig. 20.4). Whether or not the thumb is to be included in the orthosis depends on the degree of weakness as well as the range of motion of the thumb joints. In some patients with free joint motion and sufficient supplementary active control because of intact intrinsics, there is no need to incorporate the thumb. As with most such devices, less is definitely better, and the less of the patient's hand that is constrained or covered, the greater the chance of habitual use of the limb and orthosis. Because of sensory loss in the thumb and index and middle fingers, the wearer initially has to check periodically to ascertain the condition of the skin that is in contact with the dynamic slings. In addition, the patient must remember that if the sense-deficient fingers are used without reservation, they may be injured without the warning that intact sensibility conveys.

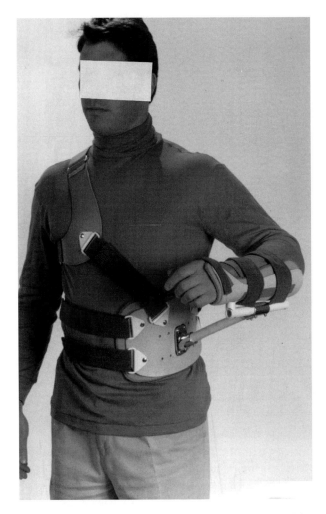

Fig. 20.2. The gunslinger splint is a static orthosis used for total support of the limb, particularly for control of pain. It is rarely used long-term.

Some patients prefer to have only the wrist supported and allow the fingers free range of motion despite the lack of active extensor power. In this case, the wrist is supported in 20 to 30 degrees of extension, and the client extends the MP joints by hooking the fingers around the object to be grasped (Fig. 20.5).

C7-8, T1

It is unusual to see a patient with a pure lesion of the lower trunk of the brachial plexus. This lesion results in loss of all hand intrinsics and weakness of the finger flexors, thus robbing the hand of grasp. The two radial wrist extensors are preserved. If there is no involvement of C7, the ulnar wrist, fingers, and thumb extensors are usually intact. There is adequate wrist control so that this joint usually does not have to be supported, and a hand-based orthosis may be used. Its purpose is to

prevent adduction collapse of the thumb into the plane of the palm and the development of a fixed claw deformity of the fingers because of the muscle imbalance of intrinsic loss. Hyperextension of the MP joints is prevented by a dorsally placed outrigger that extends to the level of the proximal interphalangeal joints (Fig. 20.6). Some extension of the interphalangeal joints is possible because of the pull-through of the long finger extensors. If C7 function is absent, the problem is made considerably more complicated because all three motor components of hand function are lost. With loss of the wrist flexors, the finger flexion tenodesis must be powered by wrist extension (Fig. 20.7, A and B). In the absence of intrinsic muscles, the grasp is less functional than it would be if the intrinsics were present to prevent clawing.

For all of these categories of neurological deficit, allowances and modifications of design are indicated to accommodate and facilitate incomplete or recovering degrees of motor loss.

Flail, anesthetic upper limb (C5-T1)

For these patients, the benefits from orthotic fittings are limited. Protection of the limb, support to minimize pain from traction, and prevention or treatment of edema are the general indications. The pelvic support, gunslinger splint, from Rancho Los Amigos Hospital[2] is useful for these purposes, although it is somewhat cumbersome.

Some patients simply desire to have the paralyzed limb out of the way during work or play, and for these activities, often a simple sling suffices. The hand should be supported in a resting splint to immobilize the wrist and digits in a balanced position. This prevents tendon or joint contracture, particularly if the limb is held in a sling with the hand and wrist conforming to the curve of the abdomen. Some patients have more specific needs (Fig. 20.8).

The question of whether or not such patients should be fitted with a functional arm splint is quite controversial. There have been numerous advocates and designs. Perry and colleagues[4] in 1974 at Rancho Los Amigos Hospital reported that in a group of seven patients with total plexus injuries the indication for fitting was pain, and when patients believed that maximum benefit had been derived from the brace, it was discarded. In this group, the longest period that the brace was worn was 2.5 months. The authors' experience is that few patients continue to use the devices habitually for any length of time after fabrication. The braces are essentially prostheses that are made to surround and protect the limb, usually having the same options and problems of power and control, but with the added weight of the limb still present. They

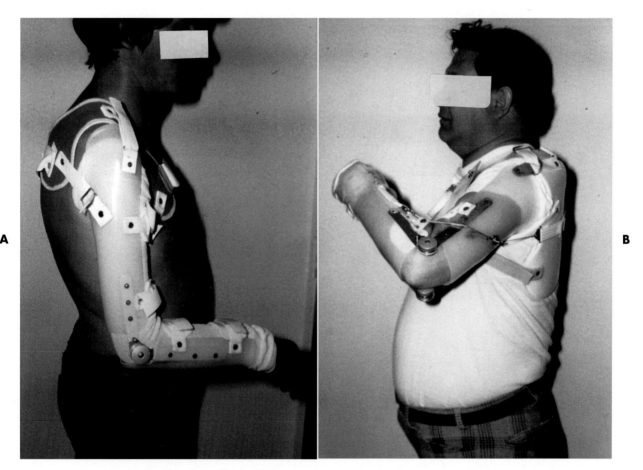

Fig. 20.3.   **A,** This orthosis has a spring-assisted elbow to facilitate flexion. **B,** A more elaborate variant with a cable-powered elbow flexion assist.

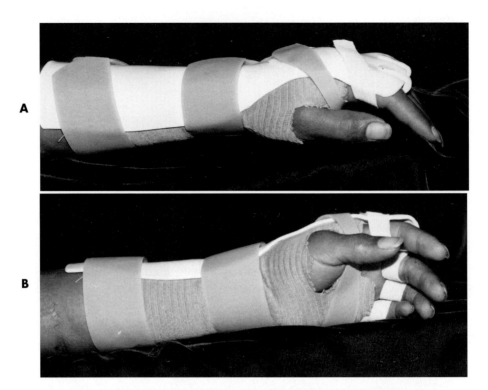

Fig. 20.4.   Low-profile MP extension orthosis. This device is worn during the day.

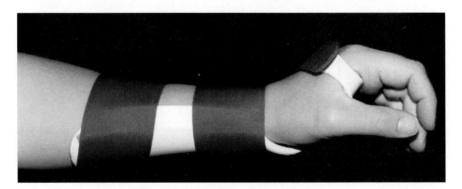

Fig. 20.5.   Volar wrist cock-up splint.

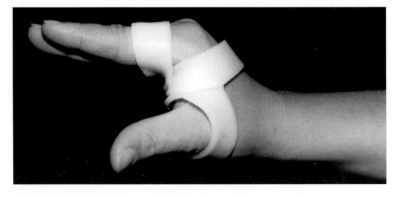

Fig. 20.6.   Hand-based extension block splint with thumb post.

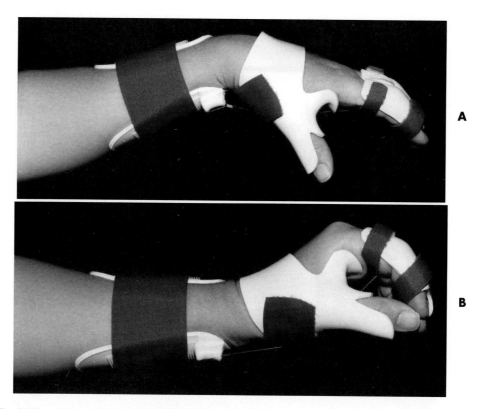

A

B

Fig. 20.7. The tenodesis splint allows index and middle finger flexion when the wrist is actively extended. The finger part is connected to the wrist portion by a cord that is tightened when the wrist extends. **A,** Passive flexion of the wrist allows MP extension through tenodesis effect of the finger extensor tendons. **B,** Active wrist extension brings the fingers to meet the thumb tip that is held in static position. The splint may be used when the wrist extensors are grade 3+ or better. Remember, these patients have normal sensibility in thumb and index finger because C5 and C6 are spared.

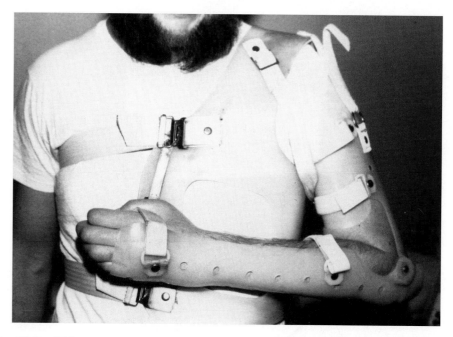

Fig. 20.8. This person was a landscape gardener who wanted his flail-anesthetic arm both supported and protected during the course of his heavy work. *(From Leffert RD: Brachial plexus injuries, New York, 1985, Churchill Livingstone.)*

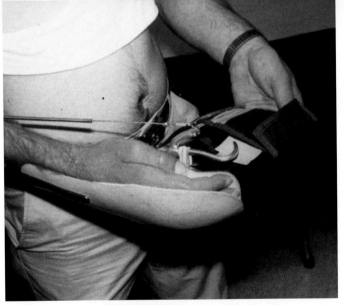

Fig. 20.9. Three views of a static device that this person, who is a missionary, has worn for 10 years since a brachial plexus injury rendered his dominant arm flail and insensate. The shoulder is static, but the elbow and terminal device are cable controlled by forward shrug of his sound shoulder girdle. The elbow lock is manually controlled from the sound side as well. He finds that the brace provides him with a useful assist in prehension.

may or may not include pelvic support, depending on the needs of the patient (Fig. 20.9). This option can be discussed with appropriate patients, who should see and try on the device if at all possible before a commitment is made to supply one. For patients with partial but diffuse lesions of the brachial plexus, the functional orthoses must be designed with reference to the retained function and needs of the patient incorporating all of the aforementioned principles.

REFERENCES

1. Barber LM: Combined motor and peripheral sensory insufficiency: II. Use of orthoses in treating brachial plexus injuries, Phys Ther 58:287–294, 1978.

2. Hoffer MM, et al: Functional recovery and orthopaedic management of brachial plexus injuries, JAMA 264:2467–2470, 1981.

3. Leffert RD: Conservative management of patients with brachial plexus injuries. In *Brachial plexus injuries*, New York, 1985, Churchill Livingstone.

4. Perry J, et al: Orthoses in patients with brachial plexus injuries, Arch Phys Med 5:134–137, 1974.

5. Schottsteadt ER, Robinson GB: Functional bracing of the arm: Part 1, J Bone Joint Surg 38:477–499, 1956.

Functional Bracing of Upper Extremity Fractures

Thomas J. Moore
John Dorris
Scott Calhoun

Functional bracing of extremity fractures was introduced by Sarmiento in 1963. The effectiveness of functional bracing relies on the compressibility of soft tissues resulting in a pseudohydraulic environment that maintains fracture stability and alignment. With the early application of a functional brace after an upper extremity fracture and the initiating of range of motion of the shoulder and elbow joints, stresses are applied on the fracture extremity before fracture healing. This controlled motion at the fracture site with functional bracing promotes early osteogenesis, primarily in the periphery of the fracture. This peripheral callus provides initial enhanced biomechanical stability to the fracture. In the fractures treated with rigid osteosynthesis (i.e., dynamic compression plate), primary callus forms, which is biomechanically inferior to the peripheral callus that forms with controlled motion. The initial stability of a fracture stabilized with rigid fixation is largely dependent on the implant.

The controlled motion at the fracture site with functional bracing occurs even with low levels of load. The compressed soft tissue envelope from the functional brace provides the elastic foundation, which allows the fragments to return to their original position after cessation of the axial load. Functional bracing does not "correct" unacceptable shortening of a fracture at the time of application but does maintain the fracture position with no further shortening. The mechanism of increased osteogenesis that occurs with controlled motion of functional bracing is not entirely known, but thermic, mechanical, electrical, chemical, and vascular factors probably play a role.

HUMERAL SHAFT FRACTURES

Diaphyseal fractures of the humeral shaft represent approximately 1% of all fractures. Nonoperative treatment of humeral shaft fractures has become the treatment of choice because the union rate is satisfactory, and acceptable cosmesis and function occur with nonanatomic reduction. Nonoperative methods of humeral fracture immobilization include U-shaped splints, hanging arm casts, and swing and swath (Fig. 21.1). Complications with these methods of fracture immobilization include adhesive capsulitis of the shoulder, malunion, elbow stiffness, transient inferior glenohumeral subluxation, and axillary skin maceration. Operative stabilization, including plate osteosynthesis and intramedullary nailing, has been advocated for diaphyseal humeral shaft fractures. Complications associated with surgery for humeral shaft fractures include nerve or vascular injury, sepsis, and nonunion.

Functional bracing for diaphyseal humeral fractures was initially described in the mid-1970s. With the exception of proximal humeral fractures, more appropriately treated as shoulder fractures, and intra-articular distal humeral fractures, functional bracing is applicable for most diaphyseal humeral fractures. Unlike femoral and tibial fractures, it is less important to achieve anatomic reduction in humeral shaft fractures. Because of muscle insertions, the untreated diaphyseal humeral fracture is usually in varus, as the unopposed deltoid muscle abducts the proximal fragment. In addition, shortening of the humerus occurs secondary to pull of the biceps, corticobrachialis, and triceps muscle. Cosmesis and shoulder and elbow function are not affected by significant angulatory deformities of humeral shaft fractures. Up to 30 degrees of varus malalignment, 20 degrees of apex anterior angulation, and 1 inch of shortening are readily tolerated with humeral shaft fractures. Surprisingly, transverse noncomminuted fractures of the humeral shaft with initial anatomic reduction are more prone to develop angulatory deformities with functional bracing than comminuted fractures.

There are several relative contraindications to functional bracing for humeral shaft fractures. Fractures

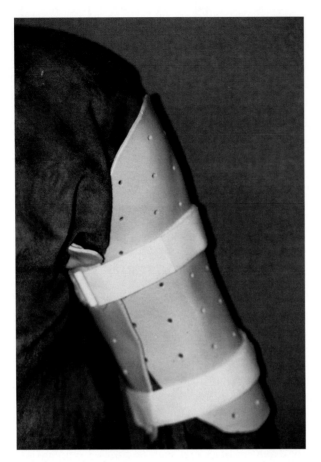

Fig. 21.1. A humeral fracture treated with a functional orthosis.

proximal to the deltoid insertion should be treated as shoulder fractures. Intra-articular fractures of the distal humerus are best treated with open reduction and internal fixation to achieve optimal reduction and stability, thereby allowing early motion, which enhances hyaline cartilage repair. In patients with a brachial plexus injury and concomitant humeral shaft fracture, functional bracing is relatively contraindicated, as the denervation of the muscles decreases muscle contraction and results in decreased fracture motion necessary for fracture healing. In patients with radial nerve injury occurring immediately after the humeral fracture (as opposed to radial nerve palsy occurring at the time of fracture manipulation), functional bracing can be effectively done. In distal one-third humeral fractures, which have the highest incidence of radial nerve palsies, 100% of patients with acute radial nerve palsy treated with functional bracing for humeral shaft fractures had resolution of the radial nerve injury on fracture healing. In humeral shaft fractures with significant soft tissue injuries, sufficient healing of the soft tissue injury before functional bracing is necessary to ensure the compressibility of the soft tissue envelope for functional bracing. In open humeral fractures with

significant bone loss, other methods of fracture treatment, such as initial external fixation and subsequent bone transport, may be necessary. In patients with traumatic brain injury and concomitant humeral shaft fractures, the spasticity and impaired cognition usually preclude functional bracing, and operative stabilization is required.

In patients with spinal cord injury or lower extremity paralysis or in patients with significant pelvic or lower extremity fractures, operative stabilization of humeral shaft fractures may allow more rapid upper extremity weight bearing for transfers or crutch ambulation. In patients with a concomitant humeral shaft fracture and both bone forearm fracture (floating elbow), operative stabilization of at least the humeral fracture is necessary. In patients with a humeral fracture and associated vascular injury, internal fixation is usually necessary to protect the vascular repair. Patients with bilateral humeral fractures usually function better with internal fixation because greater initial mobility is obtained with operative stabilization. Finally, some pathologic fractures may not heal in a functional brace, and operative stabilization, often with cement augmentation, is required.

In the patient with an acute humeral shaft fracture, initial treatment should be a well-padded coaptation splint. After the swelling associated with the acute injury has reached its maximal point, the functional brace can be applied. This period of time averages about 1 week. Once the functional brace is applied, a collar and cuff should accompany the brace initially. Many authors recommend using a commercially available prefabricated brace, whereas others advocate custom-fitted braces. Either type is acceptable as long as there is equal circumferential compression of the arm. The arm should be well padded using web roll. The brace should be of a lightweight material and preferably perforated to enhance ventilation and patient comfort. Polyethylene is the most frequently used material for the orthosis. Proper molding of the soft tissues by the fracture brace should compress the extremity to achieve soft tissue compression, which prevents shortening of the fracture through the incompressible fluid effect. Medially the brace should extend from 2.5 cm below the axilla to 1.5 cm above the medial condyle of the humerus. Laterally, it should extend from a point just below the acromion to distally slightly above the lateral epicondyle. The brace must allow complete range of motion in the shoulder and elbow. The optimal fracture orthosis for humeral shaft fractures should be adjustable by means of anterior and posterior interlocking shells. The anterior component should have a bicipital contour to facilitate suspension, whereas the posterior component should be flat to mold the triceps and provide compression. Velcro straps are recommended for frequent adjustment of the brace as the extremity swelling subsides. As the initial stages of healing occur, manipulation of angular deformities as determined radiographically is usually done during the early weeks of treatment. The patient is encouraged to discard the collar and cuff once pain subsides. Early extension of the elbow is recommended to prevent elbow flexion contractures. Pendulum passive range of motion of the shoulder should be done as soon as the patient can tolerate it.

The union rate with functional bracing of humeral shaft fractures is greater than 90% in series of humeral shaft fractures treated with functional bracing. In a series of 85 distal one-third humeral shaft fractures treated with functional bracing (15% with open injuries and 18% with peripheral nerve injuries), 96% of the fractures healed with satisfactory range of motion of both the shoulder and the elbow and satisfactory alignment (81% of the fractures healed with varus <9 degrees). All peripheral nerve injuries in this series resolved by the time of fracture healing. Fracture healing with functional bracing of humeral shaft fractures clinically can be determined by the ability actively to abduct the arm 90 degrees. In a large series of humeral shaft fractures treated with functional bracing, radiographic union occurred in 9.5 weeks with closed fractures and 13.6 weeks with open fractures.

ISOLATED ULNAR SHAFT FRACTURES

Isolated fractures of the ulnar shaft are often caused by a direct blow to the forearm and are commonly referred to as nightstick fractures. The most common mechanism of injury is a direct fall on the extremity. The fracture pattern may be oblique, transverse, or comminuted. The treatment for isolated ulnar shaft fractures varies from Ace bandage to rigid internal fixation. Regardless of the method of treatment, the emphasis for treatment of isolated ulnar shaft fractures should be rapid restoration of function with a limited period of immobilization.

Initial series of functional bracing of isolated ulnar fractures had nonunion rates of less than 5% with angulatory deformities of less than 5 degrees with no functional loss of pronation or supination of the forearm. In studies, functional bracing has shown good to excellent results in fractures of the ulna. Functional bracing with a prefabricated brace was found to be superior to treatment with a long arm cast in fractures of the distal two thirds of the ulna. In addition, there was a more rapid return to work and satisfactory range of motion.

The strong interosseous membrane connects the radius to the ulna from the elbow to the wrist. As long as the proximal and distal radial ulnar joints are intact, isolated fractures of the ulna are inherently stable because of the interosseous membrane holding the ulnar fragments to the intact radius. Angular stability of the ulna can be improved by soft tissue compression with a functional brace directed toward the interosseous membrane. The brace should consist of two interlocking shells with a molded interosseous groove. There is an unacceptable amount of ulnar angulation toward the radius with a one-piece wrap design because this design may force the radius and ulna together.

Bracing of the ulna works best for those fractures located in the distal two thirds of the shaft. There have been reports of poor results with bracing the proximal one third of the ulna because proximal fractures may have greater angulation with a resultant loss of forearm rotation. Fractures with more than 10 degrees of angulation may result in unacceptable range of motion of the forearm. Contraindications of functional bracing of isolated ulnar fractures include Monteggia fracture dislocation, intra-articular (olecranon) fractures, and angulation greater than 10 degrees at the time of brace application. If angulation greater than 10 degrees exists, either closed reduction and plaster immobilization for 2 weeks and then functional bracing can be done, or open reduction with internal fixation can be done. An additional relative contraindication to functional bracing of isolated ulnar bracing is concomitant traumatic brain injury, which causes increased callus formation with fractures and possible resultant decreased forearm rotation.

At the time of injury, angulation of the ulna should be assessed. If angulation is greater than 10 degrees, reduction is necessary. If angulation is less than 10 degrees, reduction is not necessary, and a long arm cast is applied with the forearm in neutral rotation, the elbow at 90 degrees flexion, and the interosseous space well molded dorsally and volarly. If the fracture is nondisplaced or has minimal angulation, a fracture brace may be applied directly over cast padding. The patient is encouraged to elevate the extremity to avoid swelling.

Within 1 to 2 weeks, repeat radiographs are obtained. If the reduction is still satisfactory (<10 degrees of angulation), the cast is removed, and the prefabricated brace is applied. Seldom does fracture alignment become worse in the functional brace. At this time, active range of motion of the hand, forearm, and upper extremity is allowed. After 1 week, repeat radiographs are again checked. If still satisfactory, the brace can then be removed once daily for hygiene purposes. The patient is followed at 3- to 4-week intervals for radiographs. The brace is discontinued when clinical union is achieved. In ulnar fractures, clinical union occurs several weeks before radiographic union. Early radiographs may suggest development of a nonunion. Subsequently, however, peripheral callus bridges the fracture.

In several series of functional bracing of ulnar fractures, the mean time to healing was 45 to 57 days. Angulation averaged 5 degrees and was less than 10 degrees in all patients. Nonunion rates were less than 2%. Functional results were satisfactory, including range of motion and pain relief.

ISOLATED RADIAL FRACTURES

Functional bracing in isolated radial fractures has a limited role. Most of these fractures occur from a fall on an outstretched hand, and distal radial ulnar instability occurs. With isolated radial fractures, it is critical to maintain the length of the radius. A decrease in length of only 4 to 6 mm can compromise wrist function. Although not without complications, operative stabilization of isolated radial fractures provides the best functional outcome. Functional bracing, however, may be used in treatment of some fractures of the radius. If there is no distal radial ulnar abnormality (Galeazzi) and the fragments are in stable satisfactory alignment, functional bracing may be considered. Such functional bracing should prevent pronation and supination of the forearm while permitting flexion and extension of the wrist and limited elbow motion.

PROXIMAL RADIUS

Radial head fractures are relatively common, constituting 5.4% of all fractures and 33% of elbow fractures. Radial head fractures have been divided into three types: type I, nondisplaced; type II, displaced; and type III, comminuted. The treatment of type I and type III radial head fractures is generally agreed on. Type I fracture should be treated with short-term immobilization and subsequent early motion. Type III radial head fractures should be treated with a short period of immobilization followed by early active motion. If limitation of motion occurs, excision of the radial head can be done. The treatment of type II fractures is controversial. Type II radial head fractures can be treated with closed treatment with early motion, radial head excision, or open reduction and internal fixation. In a study of 26 patients with type II fractures, open reduction with internal fixation was compared to closed treatment. The group with operative treatment had better functional results as well as less radiographic evidence of radiohumeral arthritis. Other series reported satisfactory results with nonoperative treatment of type II radial head fractures. In general, functional

bracing for radial head fractures has limited indications. The treatment of radial head fractures involves initial long arm plaster immobilization and subsequent range of motion, surgical excision of the radial head fracture, or open reduction and internal fixation.

DISTAL RADIAL FRACTURES

Distal radial fractures are common, accounting for about one sixth of all emergency department visits for fractures. There is a large number of eponyms for distal radial fractures, which in the past has led to difficulty in comparing outcomes with treatment of distal radial fractures. A Colles' fracture is a fracture within 2 cm of the distal radius with dorsal angulation of the distal fragment. A Smith's fracture is a fracture within the distal 2 cm of distal radius with volar displacement of the distal fragment. A Barton's fracture is a distal intra-articular fracture of the radius with either volar or dorsal radial carpal instability. More useful than these eponyms is an anatomic classification of distal radial fractures, such as the Frykman classification.

The normal anatomy of the distal radius is an average of 23 degrees of radial angulation in the anteroposterior plane, with a normal radial length of 12 mm from the tip of the radial styloid to the ulnar head. In the lateral plane, there is normal volar tilt of the distal radial articular surface. There is variance in these numbers, however, and an x-ray film of the nonfractured wrist is best used to determine adequacy of reduction of distal radial fractures. Regardless of the method of treatment of distal radial fractures, restoration of normal anatomy is the best predictor of satisfactory functional outcome. The sequelae of malunion of distal radial fractures (dorsal angulation >20 degrees, shortening of the radius >6 mm, or reversal of the normal volar tilt of the distal radius) may lead to carpal instability or posttraumatic arthritis. Median nerve neuropathy can occur with significant dorsal angulation of the distal radial fragment because carpal tunnel impingement of the median nerve may occur.

Treatment of dorsal radial fractures involves cast immobilization (either long arm cast or short arm cast), external fixation, percutaneous pin fixation, internal fixation, or functional bracing. Sarmiento suggests that long arm cast immobilization for distal radial fractures be done with the forearm in supination, to decrease the deforming force of the brachioradialis or the distal fragment. No significant difference in functional outcome with the forearm immobilized in either pronation or supination, however, has been demonstrated. Therefore, because the hand is most functional in neutral forearm rotation or slight pronation, this is the preferred position for long arm cast immobilization of distal radial fractures. In addition, the wrist should be in ulnar deviation with only slight flexion because immobilization of the wrist in excessive wrist flexion can lead to median neuropathy.

External fixation has been used for distal radial fractures, primarily for either intra-articular fractures or significantly comminuted fractures. The theory of external fixation is distraction ligamentotaxis, which aligns the metaphyseal radial fracture. Oftentimes the intra-articular displacement is not adequately reduced with external fixation and supplemental fixation with K-wires can be used. Complications associated with external fixation include wrist stiffness, pin tract sepsis, and superficial radial nerve irritation. Percutaneous pin fixation has been advocated for distal radial fractures, either with concomitant external fixation or with plaster immobilization. A nonprospective study, comparing percutaneous pinning versus external fixation of distal radial fractures, showed better functional outcome with the group treated with percutaneous pin fixation. Occasionally, internal fixation with plate osteosynthesis has been used for intra-articular fractures, usually volarly displaced distal radial fractures (Smith's fractures).

Functional bracing was initially advocated for distal radial fractures by Sarmiento. As with functional bracing with other upper extremity fractures and lower extremity fractures, the emphasis with functional bracing of distal radial fractures is function. The orthosis or cast is trimmed proximal to the proximal wrist palmar crease and trimmed around the base of the thumb to allow finger motion. Molding is applied to gain three-point fixation of the fracture. Range of motion of the elbow and shoulder is encouraged during immobilization of the forearm. Functional bracing has been used in conjunction with external fixation for severely comminuted or open fractures. A short period of external fixation is used followed by functional bracing with good end-functional result. In general, however, functional orthoses have not been necessary for distal radial fractures because plaster immobilization is as effective and more cost-efficient.

BIBLIOGRAPHY

Ark J, Jupiter J: The rationale for precise management of distal radius fractures, Orthop Clin North Am 224:205, 1993.

Balfour G, Mooney V, Ashby M: Diaphyseal fractures of the humerus treated with ready-made fracture brace, J Bone Joint Surg 64A:11, 1982.

Bone J: Fractures of the shaft of the humerus. In Chapman M, editor: Operative orthopaedics, ed 2, Philadelphia, 1993, JB Lippincott.

Brien W, et al: Management of fractures of the humerus in patients who have an injury of the ipsilateral brachial plexus, J Bone Joint Surg 72A:1208, 1990.

Chapman M, Gordon J, Zissimos A: Compression plate fixation of acute fracture of the diaphysis of the radius and ulna, J Bone Joint Surg 71:159, 1989.

Charnley J: The closed treatment of common fractures, Baltimore, 1961, Williams & Wilkins.

Christenson S: Humeral shaft fractures: Operative and conservative treatments, Acta Chir Scand 133:455, 1967.

Collins D: Management and rehabilitation of distal radius fractures, Orthop Clin North Am 24:365, 1993.

DePalma AF: The management of fractures and dislocations, Philadelphia, 1970, WB Saunders.

Depedro J, et al: Internal fixation of ulnar fractures by locking nail, Clin Orthop Rel Res.

Gebuhr P, et al: Isolated ulnar shaft fractures, J Bone Joint Surg 74B:757, 1992.

Herndon J: Distal radius fractures: Nonsurgical treatment options, Instruct Course Lect 42:67, 1993.

Horne J, Devane P, Purdie G: A prospective randomized trial of external fixation and plaster cast immobilization in the treatment of distal radius fractures, J Orthop Trauma 4:30, 1991.

Khalfayan E, Culp R, Alexander A: Mason Type II radial head fractures: Operative versus nonoperative treatment, J Orthop Trauma 6:283, 1992.

Knight P, Purvis G: Fractures of both bones in the forearms in adults, J Bone Joint Surg 31A:755, 1949.

Lange R, Foster R: Skeletal management of humeral shaft fractures associated with forearm fractures, Clin Orthop 192:173, 1985.

Latta L, et al: The rationale of functional bracing of fractures, Clin Orthop Rel Res 146:28, 1980.

Ledingham W, et al: On immediate functional bracing of Colles' fracture, Injury 22:197, 1991.

LeFerte A, Nutter P: The treatment of fractures of the humerus plaster cast—"hanging cast," Ann Surg 114:919, 1941.

Leung J, et al: An effective treatment of comminuted fractures of the distal radius, J Hand Surg 15A:11, 1990.

Leung J, et al: Ligamentotaxis for comminuted distal radial fractures modified by primary cancellous grafting and functional bracing: Long term results, J Orthop Trauma 5:265, 1991.

Mast J, Speigel P, Harvey J: Fractures of the humeral shaft: A retrospective study of 240 adult fractures, Clin Orthop 112:254, 1975.

McMaster W, Tiunon M, Waugh T: Cast brace for the upper extremity, Clin Orthop 109:126, 1975.

Mih A, Cooney W, Lewallen D: Long term follow up of forearm bone diaphyseal plating, Clin Orthop Rel Res 29:256, 1994.

Oberlander M, Seidman G, Whitelaw G: Treatment of isolated ulnar shaft fractures with functional bracing, Orthopedics 16:29, 1993.

Parrish F, Murray J: Surgical treatment of secondary neoplastic fractures: A retrospective study of 96 patients, J Bone Joint Surg 52A:655, 1970.

Sarmiento A: Functional fracture bracing: An update, Instruct Course Lect 36:311, 1987.

Sarmiento A, Latta L: Closed functional treatment of fractures, Berlin, 1981, Springer-Verlag.

Sarmiento A, Zagorski J, Sinclair W: Functional bracing of Colles' fractures: A prospective of immobilization in supination versus pronation, Clin Orthop 146:175, 1980.

Sarmiento A, et al: Functional bracing for comminuted extra-articular fractures of the distal third of the humerus, J Bone Joint Surg 728B:283, 1990.

Sarmiento A, et al: Functional bracing of fractures of the shaft of the humerus, J Bone Joint Surg 59A:596, 1977.

Sarmiento A, et al: The role of soft tissues in the stabilization of tibial fractures, Clin Orthop 105:116, 1974.

Sarmiento A, et al: A quantitative comparative analysis of fracture bracing under the influence of compression plating versus closed weight bearing treatment, Clin Orthop 149:232, 1980.

Sarmiento A, et al: Colles' fractures: Functional bracing in supination, J Bone Joint Surg 57A:311, 1975.

Sarmiento A, et al: Fracture healing in rat femora by functional weight bearing, J Bone Joint Surg 59A:369, 1977.

Schemitsch E, Richards R: The effects of malunion on functional outcome after plate fixation of fractures of both bones of the forearm in adults, J Bone Joint Surg 74A:1068, 1992.

Solgard S, Buenger C, Solund K: Displaced distal radius fractures, Arch Orthop Trauma Surg 22:197, 1989.

Stewart M, Hurdley J: Fractures of the humerus: A comparative study in methods of treatment, J Bone Joint Surg 52A:655, 1970.

Szabo R: Fractures of the distal radius. In Chapman M, editor: Operative orthopaedics, ed 2, Philadelphia, 1993, JB Lippincott.

Unswoth-White J, et al: The non-operative management of radius fractures: A randomized trial of three treatments, Injury 24:165, 1994.

Winfield J, Miller H, LaFerte A: Evaluation of the "hanging cast" as a method of treating fractures of the humerus, Am J Surg 55:228, 1942.

Zagorski J, Schenkman J: The management of humerus fractures with prefabricated braces, Orthop Trans 7:516, 1983.

Zagorski J, et al: Modern concepts in functional fracture bracing: The upper limb, Instruct Course Lect 36:377, 1987.

Zych G, Zagorski J, Latta L: Treatment of isolated ulnar fractures with prefabricated fracture braces, Clin Orthop 219:88, 1987.

Orthoses for Sport-Related Disorders

Letha Y. Griffin
Joseph B. Chandler

OVERVIEW OF UPPER EXTREMITY SPORT ORTHOSES

This chapter on upper extremity sport orthoses covers apparatus or appliances (i.e., braces, casts, and splints) used to support, align, prevent, or correct abnormalities or to improve function[7] as well as tape and protective padding used for the support or protection of the upper extremity during sport participation. When choosing a protective device for a player, one must consider the following:[2,23]

• The nature of the part to be protected
• The sport position played by the athlete
• The sport rules governing the type of protective device (materials) allowed
• The safety of the opposing players
• If the protective device is being used as a functional or rehabilitation orthosis, the risks of returning the injured athlete, even with protection, to play

For example, a football lineman with a stable fracture of the third metacarpal could return to play with a well-molded, well-padded cast as soon as his acute symptoms had subsided, whereas a basketball player could not return until the fracture had healed and he had regained confidence in the use of his hand. Years ago, collegiate football players could not play in well-padded casts because the NCAA forbade players to play with "hard or unyielding substances on the hand, wrist, forearm, or elbow," no matter how well covered or padded.[20] Therefore, the Duke splint[2] (later modified by the Cleveland Clinic[3]) was devised. This was a custom-made, gauze-impregnated rubber splint using either RTV-11 or RTV-7-00 (Fig. 22.1).

Not only do the rules governing which materials can be worn during play differ for each sport but also they differ for the level of play. That is, the rules are different for professional, collegiate, high school, and recreational players within the same sport and for high schools in different states. In some sports such as soccer,

the final decisions about acceptability of a supportive device (that is, whether it would ultimately cause harm to the player wearing it or to other players in the game) lies in the hands of the referee.[23]

Protective devices frequently used in the upper extremity in sports include custom or prefabricated rigid or semirigid splints, casts, and braces, with rigid or flexible uprights, slip-on sleeves, and supports made of Neoprene or elasticized materials and tape. Rigid splints provide more support for the injured part but must be padded with foam to prevent injuries to others. Rigid materials include plaster of Paris, fiberglass, thermoplastic materials such as Orthoplast and Polyform, and aluminum splints.[23] Semirigid devices include silicone rubber casts, flexible leather splints such as the lion's paw in gymnastics, counterforce braces used to treat lateral epicondylitis, tape and elasticized bandages, and cotton wraps.[23] Cotton-backed, rubber-based white adhesive, one of the most common types of semirigid supports used in sports,[15] is available in a wide variety of widths, but the 1-, 1.5-, and 2-inch widths are the most commonly used. Its strength is determined by the number of threads per inch, with more costly heavier-backed tape having 85 or more longitudinal fibers and 65 vertical fibers per square inch.[1] Good quality tape has the following characteristics:

• Adheres readily and evenly despite perspiration and activity
• Contains few skin irritants
• Tears evenly and easily when applied
• Has an even and constant unwinding tension for smooth application
• Is easily removable

The following is a list of suggested general guidelines for applying tape:[9]

1. Clean, dry, and remove hair from area to be taped.
2. Use tape adherent to insure even sticking of the tape.

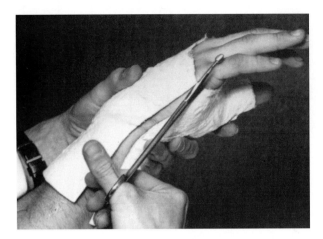

Fig. 22.1. Custom-made gauze-impregnated rubber splint. Figure demonstrates cutting of the splint after it has been formed so that it can be taken off when the player is not playing and exchanged for a well-padded cast but secured with tape to the player while playing. *(From Bassett FH, Malone T, Gilchrist RA: A protective splint of silicone rubber, Am J Sports Med 7:358–360, 1979.)*

3. Apply lubricated pads over bony prominences to protect them.
4. Overlap each tape strip by one-half width to insure uniform pressure.
5. Select tape of a proper size; the more acute angle of the part to be taped, the narrower the tape width needed to fit bony contours.
6. To help prevent skin irritation caused by daily taping, a single layer of underwrap (thin foam) held to the skin with tape adherent can be used between the tape and the skin if desired.
7. Smooth, mold, and properly tension tape as it is applied to insure that it provides support without being constrictive.
8. Allow for muscle contraction and expansion where appropriate.
9. Before taping a joint, place it in the position in which it is to be stabilized.
10. Avoid continuous taping where possible.
11. Start with anchoring strips that circle the part and help to distribute better the tape forces on the skin; the anchor strips also afford a stabilization point for succeeding strips so they are less affected by the motion of the part.

When taping angular areas, linen or cloth tape may be supplemented or replaced with elasticized tape or bandages (Fig. 22.2). Elastic wraps can provide both compression and support. When using elastic wraps or tape, care must be taken to check for vascular compromise after the athlete has warmed up because the part may have swollen, making the previously applied wrap too tight.

Cotton wraps are used less frequently now that reasonably priced, supportive, conforming braces are

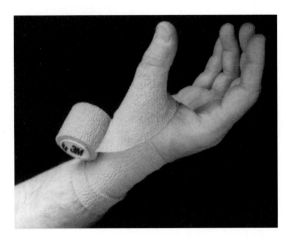

Fig. 22.2. Taping of the thumb with conforming elasticized tape.

available. In the past, because cotton wraps were reusable, they were a more cost-effective alternative to tape. Cotton wraps are still used by some gymnasts and tennis players for finger, hand, and wrist support.

A disadvantage to tape is skin irritability. Tape is occlusive, permitting moisture to collect under it, resulting in softening of the stratum corneum (top layer of skin), a portion of which is then lost when the tape is removed. Moreover, sweat pores are blocked by occlusive tape, resulting in increased bacterial growth, particularly if the tape is worn for several days.

When using thermoplastic materials for splinting, rolls of the material are initially cut to the desired form or pattern, then heated in a water bath at approximately 150 to 160°F or softened with a hot air blowgun. The softened splint is then molded over the stockinette-covered body part that is to be protected. An elastic bandage can then be wrapped about the softened splint to help conform it to the body's curves and arches while it is hardening (Fig. 22.3).

In fashioning splints, one must keep in mind the type of skills required of the athlete wearing the splint as well as the basic anatomy and kinesiology of the part to be immobilized. For example, in making splints for the hand, one must be certain not to flatten the normal gentle curve of the transverse metacarpal arch (Fig. 22.4).[17] One should also be careful in fabricating splints not to restrict motion of uninvolved joints unnecessarily.

PROTECTIVE AND SUPPORTIVE DEVICES FOR THE HAND AND FINGERS IN SPORTS

Sport gloves or grips

Gloves are popular in many sports. They can be used to provide protection, warmth, and increased grip or

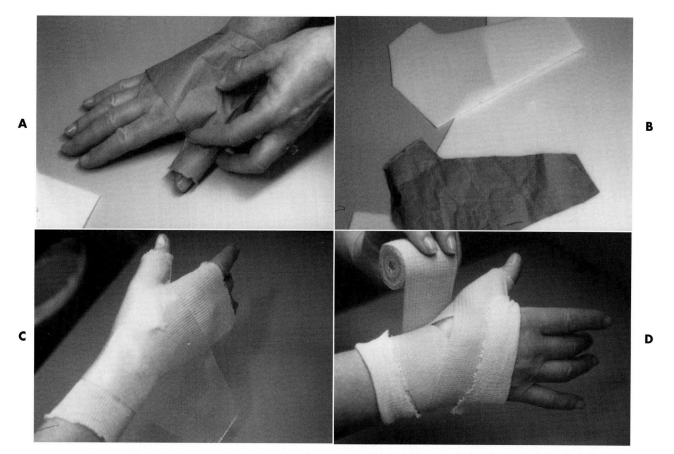

Fig. 22.3. Preparing a custom orthosis. **A,** Fashioning of a paper template to be used to cut thermoplastic materials. **B,** Cutting the material from the template. **C,** The thermoplastic material, once cut, can be heated either in a water bath or by a hot air blower to soften, and the softened splint is then molded on the hand. **D,** The splint can be held in place while hardening with an elastic wrap. Once hardened, it can be secured to the extremity with Velcro straps.

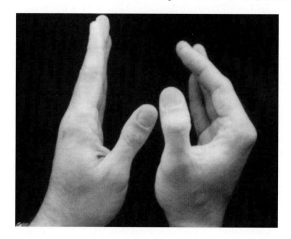

Fig. 22.4. The hand on the left demonstrates a flattened metacarpal arch, whereas the hand on the right demonstrates the normal curve of the metacarpal arch. The metacarpal arch forms a concavity within the palm.

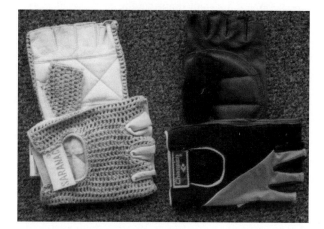

Fig. 22.5. Note the padded palmar surface of cyclist's gloves. The back of the glove frequently is cottony material, such as on the left, or a stretch nylon, such as on the right. Fingertips are generally free, as in these examples.

contact surface. For example, padded gloves (Fig. 22.5) are recommended to help long-distance cyclists avoid cyclist's palsy, or ulnar neuropathy caused by compression of the ulnar nerve as it enters the hand through

Guyon's canal, resulting in the insidious onset of numbness (particularly of the ring and little fingers) and weakness of the interosseous muscles.[5,19] Gloves alone do not protect the cyclist from developing this condi-

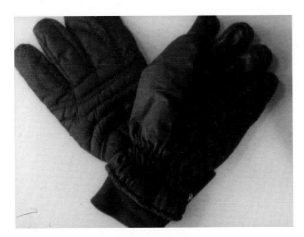

Fig. 22.6. Ski gloves. Note the extension above the wrist on ski gloves to protect the wrist from laceration from the edge of a ski.

tion, which occurs most frequently in cyclists touring or racing long distances. Cyclists should also pad their handlebars with foam wrap, be certain their frame size is correct, and particularly adjust the distance from seat to stem and height of handlebars to fit their body and avoid leaning into the handlebars.[19] In addition, cyclists should change hand positions on the handlebars frequently.[5]

A ski glove called the *Kombi Thumb Saver* has a built-in steel thumb guard and Neoprene pad to protect the thumb from radially deviating on impact, resulting in injury to the ulnar collateral ligament of the thumb. These gloves, though protective, are expensive, costing about $50.00. These gloves can also be used for thumb protection by football linemen and lacrosse players.[23]

Most skiers' gloves lack the steel thumb guard of the Kombi Thumb Saver glove. They typically have a water-resistant outer surface and have sufficient padding for warmth, yet allow enough motion to grasp the pole adequately. Furthermore, such gloves should extend above the wrist to protect the wrist from laceration by the edge of a ski (Fig. 22.6).[6,16]

Volleyball players have begun to use leather gloves with open fingers, particularly during practices, although some players also wear the gloves for match play. The gloves cushion the blow to the hypothenar eminence when diving and landing on the palm, thus helping to avoid not only abrasions in this area, but also direct contusion to palmar nerves and injuries to the ulnar artery, including spasm, thrombosis, and aneurysms. Injuries to the ulnar nerve and artery from sliding on the hand have been reported in baseball, karate, rugby, handball, and lacrosse as well as volleyball.[12]

Various gloves are worn by baseball players. Baseball catchers wear well-padded leather mitts for protection of their palm from the impact of high-speed balls (Fig.

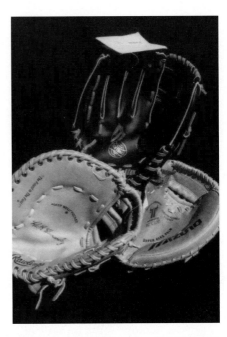

Fig. 22.7. Various baseball mitts. *Left,* First baseman's gloves have a deeper pocket than either infielder's or outfielder's gloves. *Center,* Infielder's gloves have shorter fingers than outfielder's gloves. *Right,* The catcher's mitt is extremely well padded with a deep pocket. Note heavy leather padding in all gloves, however, for shock absorption purposes.

22.7). Sliders' gloves worn by players on base are similar to the leather gloves worn by volleyball players—that is, they are designed to absorb the shock to the palm on ground contact, but many also have extra support for the wrist to keep it from hyperextending. Baseball batters' gloves are designed to provide better traction on the bat. They are leather, generally with fingertips (Fig. 22.8). Frequently, players wear their batting gloves under their fielding gloves for warmth and shock absorption of the ball. Fielders' gloves are padded leather, like catchers' mitts, but have fingers in them for better ball control. Infielders use gloves with shorter fingers, whereas outfielders' gloves have longer fingers. The first baseman's glove is made with a deeper pocket than other infielders' gloves. The fingers of infielders' and outfielders' gloves are sewn together in these grooves to keep the high-velocity ball from breaking through them.

Handball gloves are made for protection of the hand at the time of ball impact (Fig. 22.9). They are generally made of leather and designed to have enough pad to absorb the impact of the ball, which can be traveling at speeds of 55 miles per hour, yet not so much padding that the player lacks "feel" of the ball and loses control in placement of the ball in play.

The gloves used by racquetball and squash players are soft leather on the palmar surface with frequently a breathable material on the dorsal surface (Fig. 22.10). Fingertips are generally included in the gloves. The

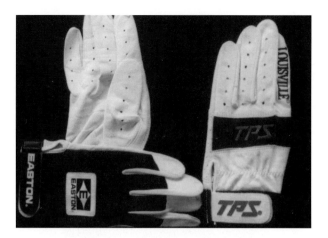

Fig. 22.8. Baseball batter's gloves. The gloves are perforated for better circulation to the hand. They are of soft leather for absorption of sweat on the batter's hand and better traction on the bat.

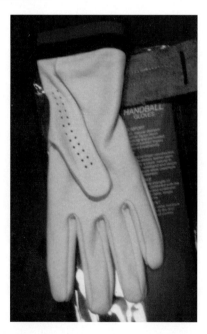

Fig. 22.9. Handball gloves are generally made of leather and have some padding to absorb the impact of the ball.

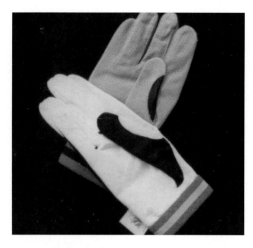

Fig. 22.10. Racquet and squash gloves are made of soft leather so that they absorb the sweat of the player's hand and give the player better traction on the racquet. Some gloves, such as those at the top of the photograph, have a coating placed on the leather to make it tacky for even greater racquet grip.

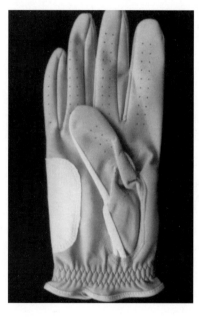

Fig. 22.11. Golf gloves are generally made of soft leather with perforations throughout for better breathability. Frequently they have an elasticized wrist area for easy glove entry.

leather wicks away sweat from the palm, permitting a better grip for the player. The more expensive gloves have a dorsal pad along the metacarpal heads to cushion them at impact with wall surfaces, and often the palmar leather is treated so that it has a tacky surface for better grip.

Golf gloves are made of thin breathable leather with fingertips in or out. Gathers on the dorsal surface allow for midhand expansion with club grip (Fig. 22.11).

Soccer goalies' gloves are of two types. One is a padded leather on the palm, which has a somewhat sticky surface for better ball grip (Fig. 22.12, *right*). Ball grip in the second type is enhanced by a patterned, Neoprene-type material in strips on the palmar surface

(Fig. 22.12, *left*). Some goalies believe that these added strips provide greater ball grip, particularly in rainy or damp weather. Both styles are padded for protection of the goalie's hands against ball impact. These gloves also serve to keep the goalie's hands warm. Most gloves have fingertips included in them, but frequently goalies cut the fingertips out of their gloves to give them a better feel of the ball for control.

Weight lifters use fingertip-free, slightly padded leather gloves to decrease friction across their metacarpal heads and hence prevent blisters (Fig. 22.13). Tape

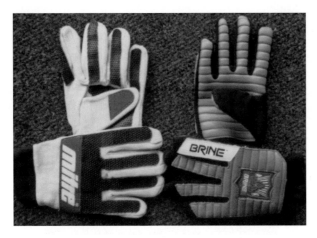

Fig. 22.12. Soccer goalie gloves have padded palmar surfaces. The glove on the left has strips of patterned Neoprene material for added ball grip. The one on the right has "tackified" leather.

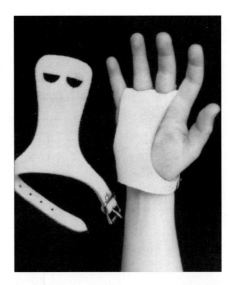

Fig. 22.14. Grips used by gymnasts to protect palmar skin.

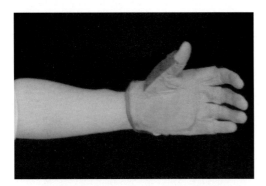

Fig. 22.13. Leather gloves, slightly padded over the metacarpal heads to decrease friction in this area, are used by weight lifters.

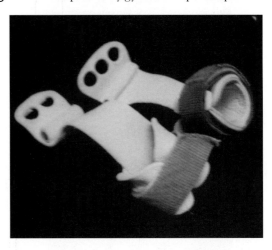

Fig. 22.15. Grips used by men have variable size dowels to accommodate for the apparatus's bar size. Those with the larger dowel are used for rings, the smaller dowel for bars.

can also be used to support and protect the palmar heads of the metacarpals in weight lifters, handball and squash players, and gymnasts in lieu of gloves. Rosin can be rubbed into the tape to make it an even stickier surface in some sports in which this is an advantage, such as gymnastics.

More commonly, however, gymnasts use grips that are leather, straplike supports that help protect the palmar skin from friction when using the bar apparatus (Fig. 22.14). Additionally the men's grips have an added piece of doweling across the metacarpals to enhance grip on bar apparatus. The width of the dowel differs for various apparatus (Fig. 22.15). With the advent of the smaller bar size in the parallel bars for the women, dowels are now becoming more popular with the women gymnasts as well. Gymnasts rub chalk or calcium carbonate dust into their hands to absorb sweat and provide a more reliable grip.

Although boxing gloves were initially designed to provide protection for the hand on impact and therefore decrease injuries such as metacarpal neck fractures,

some now advocate a return to bare-handed boxing.[26] They believe bare-handed boxing would decrease the number of acute and chronic brain injuries seen in this sport, claiming that boxer's gloves, although initially designed for protection, have now become a weapon. The boxer's hand is typically wrapped with a predetermined amount of tape and gauze to hold the knuckles together and make the hand more rigid before it is placed in the glove. Amateur boxers use 10-ounce gloves and professionals 8-ounce gloves, but when the gloves become wet with perspiration or water doused on the boxer between rounds by the trainer, their weight can double.[28] Those who advocate a return to bare-handed boxing believe hooks and roundhouse punches, which have greater knockout power but are more damaging to the brain than jabs or straight punches (due to the torque they produce), would be

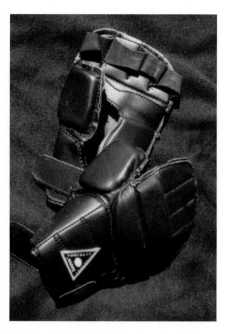

Fig. 22.16. Football linemen's gloves are dorsally padded over the metacarpals and proximal phalanxes. The palmar aspect is unpadded.

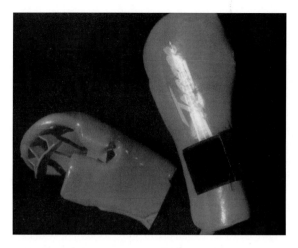

Fig. 22.17. Karate gloves are often made of a foam material and are heavily padded on the dorsal surface with an open palmar aspect.

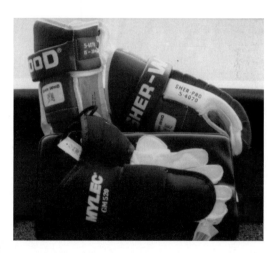

Fig. 22.18. The volar surface of ice hockey gloves is malleable leather, whereas the dorsal aspect of hands and fingers is thickly padded. Goalie's gloves are made of a block of leather on the dorsal aspect of the hand and a thick pad over the dorsal aspect of the thumb.

thrown less frequently if boxers were bare-handed because they result in unequal distribution of force to the metacarpals and, hence, are associated with a greater number of fractures.[26]

Football gloves are generally worn by linemen. They are padded dorsally over the metacarpals and the metacarpophalangeal (MP) joints to provide protection on impact (Fig. 22.16). Other linemen prefer soft-padded, slip-on protective sleeves. Some quarterbacks and receivers have begun to wear gloves designed to provide warmth and increased grip strength in cold and damp weather. These do not have the dorsal padding of the linemen's gloves but instead are made of malleable leather, some with the fingertips free. The palmar surface of receivers' gloves are frequently treated to make them tacky for greater grip strength. Velcro closures at the wrist provide fast entry.

Karate gloves, like football linemen's gloves, are made with protection over the dorsal aspect of the hand to decrease shock and impact. The palm of the hand is, like the lineman's glove, fairly open (Fig. 22.17).

Ice hockey gloves are more padded than either football linemen's or karate gloves. The volar surface is malleable leather, whereas the dorsum of the hand and fingers is thickly padded, and, in contrast to linemen's gloves, the padding extends over the fingertips (Fig. 22.18, *top*). The gloves also extend above the wrist. The goalie's gloves laterally have a block of padding on their dorsal surface with a padded flap over the volar thumb surface (Fig. 22.18, *bottom*).

Finger splints

Efforts continue to be made in each sport to find the ideal glove that provides maximal hand protection without sacrificing dexterity or adversely causing harm to the player or opponent. Finger injuries requiring special protection for early return to sport include the following:

- Extensor tendon avulsions of the distal phalanx (mallet finger)
- Central slip disruption of the proximal interphalangeal (PIP) joint (boutonnière deformity)
- Volar plate avulsion of the PIP joint
- Collateral ligament sprains of the thumb and other finger MP and interphalangeal (IP) joints
- Fractures of the phalanx and metacarpals

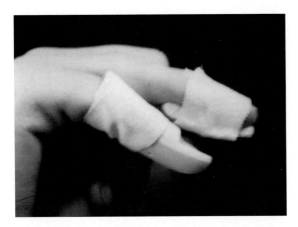

Fig. 22.19. Premolded plastic splint used to treat an extensor tendon avulsion of the DIP joint of the finger is on bottom left. Top right is the aluminum padded splint that can be molded with slight hyperextension at the DIP joint to hold this joint in a protected position until healing of the extensor tendon.

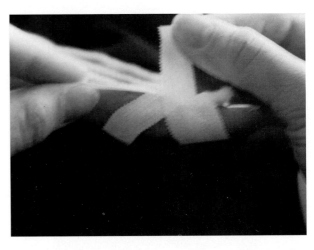

Fig. 22.20. Tape can be used to support the DIP joint after extensor tendon avulsions. This is placed in multiple cross strips for support of the joint. A pad is placed over the dorsal aspect of the skin (for added protection of the skin in this area), and the tape is applied over the pad.

Mallet finger, or rupture of the extensor tendon insertion to the distal phalanx, can be managed with splint protection for early return to many sports, provided that the rupture is not associated with a fracture of greater than one third of the articular surface.[15] Padded aluminum splints placed on the volar surface and allowing free motion of the proximal interphalangeal (PIP) joint, but holding the distal interphalangeal (DIP) joint in mild hyperextension, are commonly used (Fig. 22.19, *top right*). If there is minimal swelling, a premolded commercially available plastic support is available (Fig. 22.19, *bottom left*). These splints must be carefully fitted because if they are too big, they allow the distal phalanx to flex, resulting in inadequate healing of the extensor tendon to the distal phalanx. Custom splints molded from thermoplastic material have the advantage of not having sharp edges, as the aluminum splints do, and can be more form-fitted than the premolded splints. They are, however, more time-consuming to fashion, but in some sports aluminum splints are not permitted because their sharp edges can cause harm to opposing players. Hence, smoothly molded plastic supports offer protection and early return to sport.

Care must be taken with all splints to keep the skin clean and dry beneath them and to ensure that they and the tape used to affix them do not irritate the thin dorsal skin overlying the PIP joint. When removing the splints for cleaning and drying the skin, the DIP joint must be manually maintained in extension because proper healing of the tendon necessitates uninterrupted splinting.[29]

In sports where neither plastic nor metal splints are permitted on the hands, a method for taping the DIP joint in slight hyperextension for protection has been recommended. The tape is applied in multiple cross-strips of spiral tape over the padded, slightly hyperextended DIP joint (Fig. 22.20).[13]

For volar plate injuries of the PIP joint, early active flexion with extension block splinting is frequently possible.[18] In some athletes, the finger splinting from the MP joint distally with the PIP joint in slight flexion for 7 to 10 days is needed to allow swelling to subside. Typically the splint is removed several times a day for gentle motion. Following initial splinting, the finger can then be buddy taped to its adjacent finger (long finger to ring finger, index finger to long finger) for early return to play. When taping the finger, the DIP and PIP joints should be left free of tape for ease of motion. Adhesive tape can be used, as in Fig. 22.21, or there are commercially available Velcro tape supports made for buddy tape purposes. Some of these come with an underlying compressive sleeve to provide compression as well as buddy taping, or one can use a separate compression sleeve with Velcro strips applied over it (Figs. 22.22 and 22.23). Regular adhesive tape, stretchy stockinette, or compressive tape beneath the buddy tape can be used to provide even compression. To avoid vascular compromise, care must be taken with all circumferentially used support after an acute injury.

Collateral ligament injuries of the MP or PIP joints of the finger can be initially splinted in mild flexion at approximately 30 degrees. After several days, the finger can be taped to the adjacent finger to provide support and early return to activity.[4] In collateral ligament injuries, the injured finger should be buddy taped to the finger adjacent to the side of the collateral ligament injury (i.e., a long finger with a sprain of the ulnar collateral ligament of the PIP joint should be taped to the ring finger).

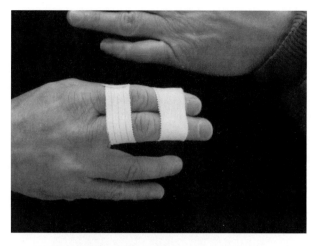

Fig. 22.21. Buddy taping of fingers, which allows for active motion. The tape is placed with joints free.

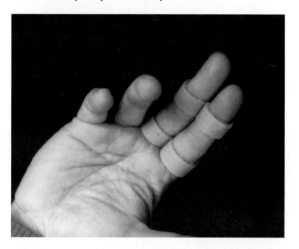

Fig. 22.22. Premade Velcro strips can also be used for this purpose.

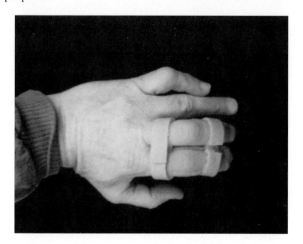

Fig. 22.23. Velcro strips placed over a compressive sleeve.

Players with grade I and grade II ulnar collateral ligament injuries of the thumb can frequently be initially treated in a fiberglass, silicone, or thermoplastic thumb spica splint or cast to allow continued participa-

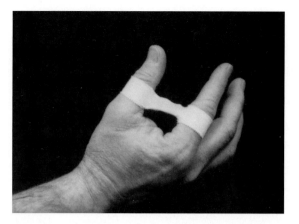

Fig. 22.24. Checkrein tape used to protect the thumb from hyperextension.

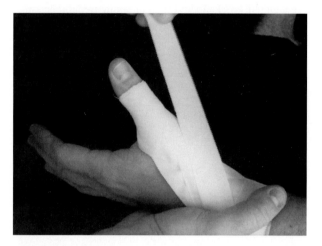

Fig. 22.25. The use of tape applied as a thumb spica to protect the thumb.

tion in sports (e.g., skiing and hockey).[24] After initial stability is achieved, continued protection can be afforded by checkrein or thumb spica taping (Figs. 22.24 and 22.25). For some grade I injuries, taping alone is all that is required to permit early return to sport.[25]

Central slip avulsions of the PIP joint producing a boutonnière deformity, or hyperextension of the MP joint and DIP joint with flexion of the PIP joint, can be managed with splinting of the PIP joint in extension[4] with a well-padded aluminum splint or one of the premolded plastic splints commercially available or a custom-molded thermoplastic splint (Fig. 22.26). Again the same precautions for player safety previously described for mallet finger splints are applicable here.

Hand and wrist splints

Aluminum splints, thermoplastic and custom-molded splints, and silicone rubber playing casts all can be used for the protection of stable fractures of the hand or wrist for early return to play. Similarly, they can be used after open reduction internal fixation of unstable

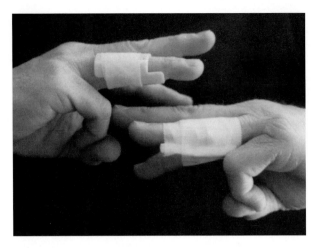

Fig. 22.26. Premolded plastic splint used for protection of PIP joint (*top left*). Padded aluminum splint used for the same purpose (*bottom right*).

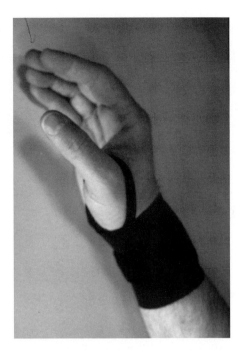

Fig. 22.28. Elasticized wraparound wrist support. Thumb strap aids in preventing migration of the support.

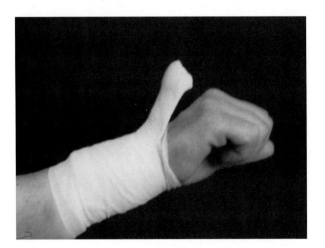

Fig. 22.27. Wrist extension block secured with tape to prevent hyperextension of the wrist.

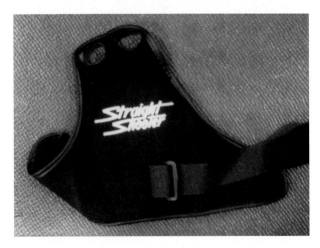

Fig. 22.29. Dorsal wrist splint used by golfers to help stabilize the wrist, perfecting their swing.

fractures to allow participation before the fracture has completely healed. Although rubber splints are effective in providing safe immobilization of the injured part without causing harm to opposing players, they are inconvenient to use because they have to be changed after game play to standard casts or splints because the rubber does not breathe, causing maceration of the skin beneath it, secondary skin lesions, and infection.

PROTECTIVE AND SUPPORTIVE DEVICES FOR THE WRIST AND FOREARM IN SPORTS

Like hand protection, wrist support is commonly sought by athletes to enhance sport participation. In gymnastics, the wrist is transformed into a weight-bearing joint. Compressive loading occurs, most often in the position of wrist dorsiflexion. The so-called lion's paws brace, which is a strap-on, semirigid dorsal support, helps limit dorsiflexion and can be used on the vault, floor, and beam. A dorsal wrist extension block splint made of thermoplastic material secured to the wrist with a wrap and tape was devised for the same purpose (Fig. 22.27).[30] It provides support like the lion's paws splint, but has no thumb strap, so it can be used on bars as well.

Many bowlers use either a dorsal wrist splint (Fig. 22.28) or a combination wrist and hand splint that not only supports the wrist, but also the index and little fingers, to help diminish torsion of the wrist at ball

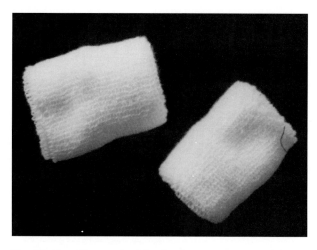

Fig. 22.30. Cotton elasticized wrist support to provide not only wrist support, but also sweat absorption is frequently used by those playing racquet sports.

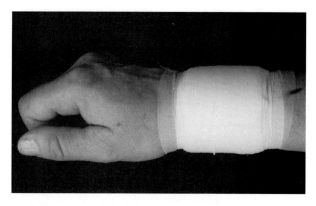

Fig. 22.32. Tape applied in bulk is used to provide not only support, but also to prevent hyperdorsiflexion or palmar flexion.

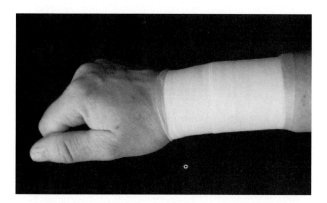

Fig. 22.31. Tape can be used to support the wrist.

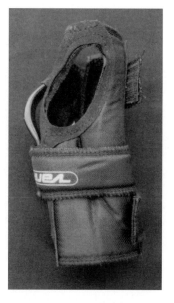

Fig. 22.33. Rigid volar wrist splint used for protection by in-line skaters.

release. A dorsal wrist splint is also used by golfers to stabilize their wrist while practicing their swing (Fig. 22.29).

Wraparound tape, elasticized cotton, and Neoprene wrist supports are frequently used in racquet sports as well as in gymnastics, bowling, and weight lifting (Figs. 22.30 through 22.32), in which support with less restriction of motion is desired. Extra support can be provided by modifications to enhance the radioulnar, dorsal, or volar aspects of the basic tape job. Moreover, if one wraps the wrist, but does so in a bulk-type fashion, this bulk wrist wrap can be used to limit dorsiflexion and palmar flexion and has the advantage over a dorsal splint in leaving the hand completely free (see Fig. 22.32). Some athletes tape or brace their wrists routinely for added protection. Others do so only temporarily after a minor sprain.

Rigid volar splints are recommended for in-line skaters to prevent injury to the wrist when the skater breaks his fall with an outstretched hand (Fig. 22.33).[27] These splints come in colorful decorator designs to

encourage their use. Although not yet popular with ice and roller skaters, their use in these sports may also be desirable, particularly for the novice who is still falling frequently.

Various Neoprene sleeves and padding as needed can be used after contusions of the forearm to allow early return to sport and minimize reinjury (Fig. 22.34).

PROTECTIVE AND SUPPORTIVE DEVICES FOR THE ELBOW IN SPORTS

Elbow injuries are common in both contact and noncontact sports, particularly throwing and racquet sports. Many protective and supportive orthotic devices for the elbow are available for use in sports. The most

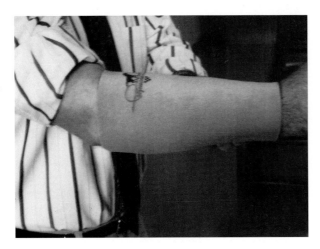

Fig. 22.34. Neoprene sleeve used for protection and support of the forearm.

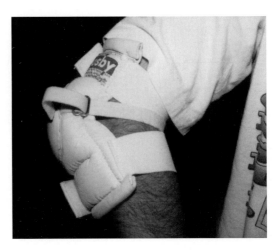

Fig. 22.36. Foam rubber and elastic pad protects the proximal ulna, olecranon, and olecranon bursa.

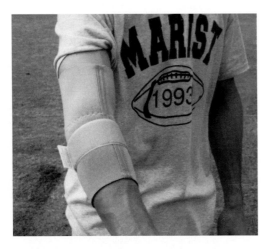

Fig. 22.35. Neoprene elbow sleeve provides compression and warmth to the elbow joint.

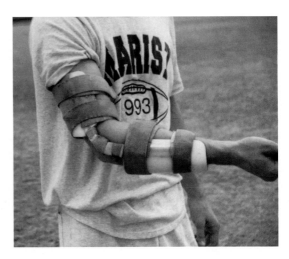

Fig. 22.37. Hinged elbow orthosis is used for the treatment of elbow dislocation.

common of these involves a wraparound sleeve of elastic or Neoprene (Fig. 22.35). Such sleeves offer no true protection or significant support but are used primarily for comfort, affording compression and warmth about the elbow joint.

The use of protective padding about the elbow is popular in many contact sports, providing protection to the proximal ulna, olecranon, and olecranon bursa. Most elbow pads are a combination of foam rubber and elastic (Fig. 22.36). Hard-shell pads are also available or can be fabricated with thermoplastic material. These are designed to provide protection to the proximal ulna, olecranon, and olecranon bursa. Soft elbow pads allow greater freedom of movement but less protection than those with hard shells.

Hyperextension injuries and ligamentous injuries about the elbow (including elbow dislocations) are most commonly encountered in contact sports. Taping can be an effective method of protecting the athlete on

return to participation after mild hyperextension injuries or other ligamentous injuries about the elbow.[22] Hyperextension taping limits elbow extension, and valgus taping limits valgus stress loads. These techniques provide limited support, however, and should be used only in mild elbow injuries.

More severe ligamentous injuries, such as an elbow dislocation, require a more constrained support to allow for earlier return to competition. Such injuries are best treated with hinged elbow orthoses (Fig. 22.37). These may be single-hinged or double-hinged braces and are usually custom-made, although prefabricated products are available. The double-hinged orthosis provides the greatest support to varus and valgus stresses across the elbow joint. Adjustable hinges are preferable so that the degree of motion restricted can be individualized.

The most common orthosis used about the elbow to allow for return from injury is the tennis elbow orthosis,

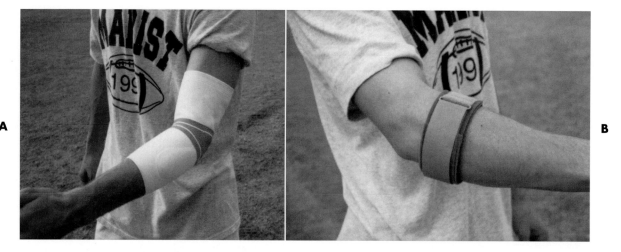

Fig. 22.38. Tennis elbow sleeve (**A**) and tennis elbow strap (**B**) are used for the treatment of medial and lateral epicondylitis.

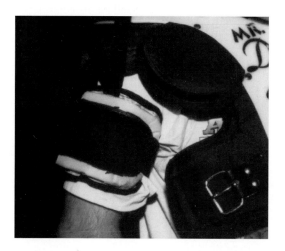

Fig. 22.39. Hard-shell pad protects the upper arm.

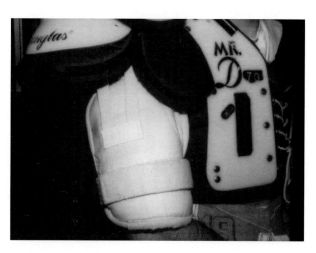

Fig. 22.40. Hard-shell pad functions as an extension of football shoulder pads.

which can be used for medial or lateral epicondylitis.[11] Despite the implications inherent in the term *tennis elbow*, medial and lateral epicondylitis occur frequently in sports other than those involving the use of a racquet, including baseball, bowling, weight lifting, golf, and even cross-country skiing. Tennis elbow orthoses may be of the sleeve type (Fig. 22.38, *A*) or the strap type (Fig. 22.38, *B*). The basic principle behind such orthoses is the counterforce concept,[21] which is applicable to both medial and lateral epicondylitis. The brace applies pressure to the muscle mass distal to its insertion on the epicondyle, either medial or lateral, effectively creating a new origin for the muscle and lessening the force at the injury site of the epicondyle.[10] Tennis elbow orthoses can be helpful in safely returning an athlete with epicondylitis to competition. There is variability in individual tolerance and effectiveness,

however, and finding the right brace for a particular athlete may involve some trial and error.

PROTECTIVE AND SUPPORTIVE DEVICES FOR THE UPPER ARM IN SPORTS

Contact sports often result in contusions to the muscles and soft tissues of the upper arm. Protective equipment for this area is often used both to prevent such injuries and to protect an already injured extremity. The simplest of these protective devices is a padded sleeve made of foam rubber and elastic. Hard-shell pads are commercially available (Fig. 22.39) or can be custom-fabricated with thermoplastic material. For football, such pads are also available as extensions of shoulder pads (Fig. 22.40).

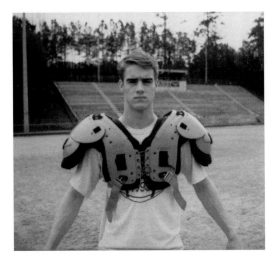

Fig. 22.41.   Shoulder pads cover most of the clavicle, acromion, scapula, and proximal humerus.

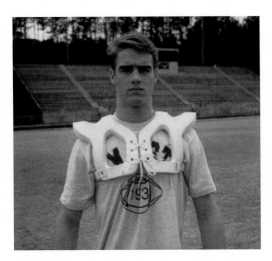

Fig. 22.42.   Spider pads can be used under standard shoulder pads to provide additional protection to an injured acromioclavicular joint (Adams Plastics, Inc., Cookville, Tenn).

PROTECTIVE AND SUPPORTIVE DEVICES FOR THE SHOULDER IN SPORTS

The shoulder is extremely susceptible to injury in contact sports. Many contact sports, most notably football, hockey, and lacrosse, require the use of shoulder pads as a protective device to lessen the risk of such injuries. Shoulder pads protect the shoulders by covering most of the clavicle, the acromion, the scapula, and the proximal humerus (Fig. 22.41). Shoulder pads are sport specific, but even within a specific sport these pads vary by player position and individual requirements. Proper fitting of these pads is essential to insure optimal shoulder protection and yet maintain full range of motion of the upper extremities and neck.[14,22] Many athletes with acromioclavicular (AC) joint injuries may

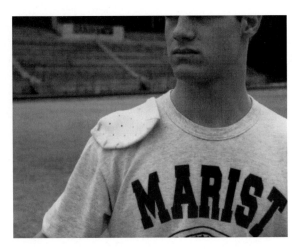

Fig. 22.43.   Rigid orthotic device contains a dome to prevent contact with the injured AC joint.

be safely returned to their sport using various protective orthotic devices. This is particularly true in the contact sports. Various techniques of AC joint taping are available to help stabilize an injured AC joint. Supplemental pads, such as the spider pad (Adams Plastics Inc., Cookville, Tenn.) (Fig. 22.42) can be used under standard shoulder pads to provide additional protection to an injured AC joint. These pads aid in further dispersing the forces about the shoulder. More often, however, a rigid orthotic device is used in a contact athlete returning from an AC joint injury. These rigid orthotic devices are usually custom-made with a thermoplastic material, and a dome of approximately 1½ inches is created in the material to prevent contact with the AC joint (Fig. 22.43). The undersurface of the rigid material is then lined with a soft dispersive medium, and the pad is then held in place with either taping or a strap.

Glenohumeral instability is a particularly challenging problem for sports orthoses to address. Instability of the shoulder joint is a complex entity that no orthotic device can fully prevent. Recurrent anterior instability is the most common type encountered in sporting activities and typically occurs with the arm in the abducted, externally rotated position. Devices designed to prevent anterior instability of the glenohumeral joint must, therefore, restrict this particular motion. The more a brace restricts this motion, the more effective it may be in preventing recurrent instability.[8] Unfortunately, such restricted motion in abduction and external rotation may be incompatible with an athlete's chosen sport or with maximal performance in that sport. Thus, for many athletes in racquet and throwing sports, basketball, gymnastics, and other similar activities, the use of a brace restricting motion of the injured dominant arm is impractical because complete range of motion of the upper extremity is required. Such devices are most commonly used in contact sports,

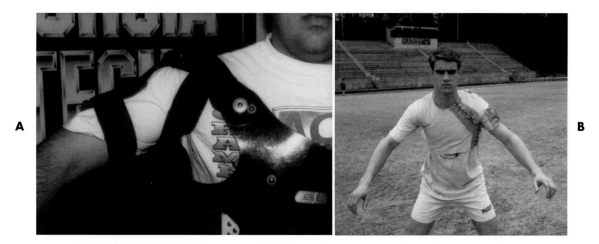

Fig. 22.44.   Shoulder Subluxation Inhibitor (SSI, Physical Support Systems, Inc., Windham, N.H.) (**A**) and CD Dennison-Duke-Wyre shoulder vests (CD Dennison Orthopedic Appliance Co., Baltimore, Md.) (**B**). Both are custom-fitted orthoses that limit anterior glenohumeral instability.

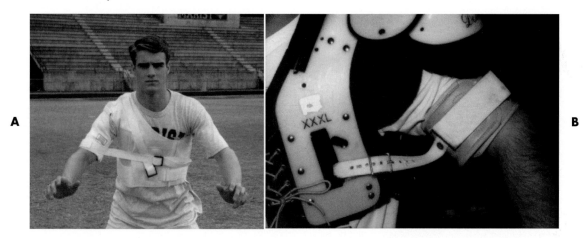

Fig. 22.45.   Alternatives to the custom-fitted devices used to prevent anterior glenohumeral instability are the SAWA Shoulder Orthosis (Brace International, Inc., Atlanta, Ga.) (**A**) and a humeral cuff attached to shoulder pads (**B**).

where restricted motion of the upper extremity is less of an impediment.

Many different types of braces are available to prevent anterior glenohumeral instability.[14,24] Most of these devices are custom-fitted, including the Shoulder Subluxation Inhibitor (SSI, Physical Support Systems, Inc., Windham, N.H.) (Fig. 22.44, *A*) and the CD Dennison-Duke-Wyre shoulder vest (CD Dennison Orthopedic Appliance Co., Baltimore, Md.) (Fig. 22.44, *B*). The SAWA shoulder orthosis, however, is an off-the-shelf device that is less expensive and more readily available (Brace International, Inc., Atlanta, Ga.) (Fig. 22.45, *A*). In football, such a device can also be constructed by using a humeral cuff attached to the shoulder pads, which restricts abduction and external rotation (Fig. 22.45, *B*). The Omotrain (Bauerfeind) (Fig. 22.46) is an off-the-shelf device that allows for significantly more mobility than most, and thus, ath-

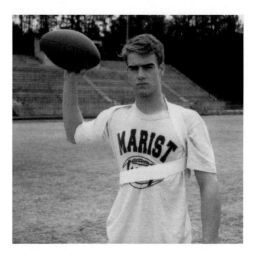

Fig. 22.46.   The Omotrain (Bauerfeind USA, Inc., Kennesaw, Ga.) is used in cases of mild anterior glenohumeral instability.

letes' tolerance of this device seems to be better, but its effectiveness in preventing recurrent subluxation is limited. Therefore, the Omotrain should be used only in mild cases of instability. All of these orthoses are adjustable, attempting to allow free motion in a safe or stable range but restricting the motion beyond which recurrent instability develops. Unfortunately, both athletes' tolerance of these devices and the effectiveness of the devices are variable and unpredictable.

REFERENCES

1. Arnheim DD: Modern principles of athletic training, ed 7, St. Louis, 1989, CV Mosby.
2. Bassett FH, Malone T, Gilchrist RA: A protective splint of silicone rubber, Am J Sports Med 7:358–360, 1979.
3. Bergfeld JA, et al: Soft playing splint for protection of significant hand and wrist injuries in sports, Am J Sports Med 10:293–296, 1982.
4. Brunet ME, et al: How I manage sprained finger in athletes, Phys Sportsmed 12:98–108, 1984.
5. Burke ER: Ulnar neuropathy in bicyclists, Phys Sportmed 9:53–56, 1981.
6. Cabrera JM, McCue FC: Nonosseous athletic injuries of the elbow, forearm, and hand, Clin Sports Med 5:681–700, 1986.
7. Dorland's illustrated medical dictionary, ed 26, Philadelphia, 1981, WB Saunders.
8. Gieck J: Shoulder strap to prevent anterior glenohumeral dislocations, Athletic Train 11:18, 1976.
9. Griffin LY, editor: Athletic training and sports medicine, ed 2, Park Ridge, IL, 1991, American Association of Orthopaedic Surgeons.
10. Groppel JL, Nirschl RP: A mechanical and electromyographical analysis of the effects of various joint counterforce braces on the tennis player, Am J Sports Med 14:195–200, 1986.
11. Harding WG: Use and misuse of the tennis elbow strap, Phys Sportsmed 20:65–74, 1992.
12. Ho PK, Dellon AL, Wilgis EFS: True aneurysms of the hand resulting from athletic injury, Am J Sports Med 13:136–138, 1985.
13. Knight KL: Taping a mallet finger, Phys Sportsmed 13:140, 1985.
14. Konin JG, McCue FC: Taping, strapping, and bracing of the shoulder complex. In Andrews JR, Wilk KE, editors: The athlete's shoulder, New York, 1994, Churchill Livingstone.
15. Kulund DN: The injured athlete, ed 2, Philadelphia, 1988, JB Lippincott.
16. Match RM: Laceration of the median nerve from skiing, Am J Sports Med 6:22–25, 1978.
17. Mayer VA, McCue FC: Rehabilitation and protection of the hand and wrist. In Nicholas JA, Hershman EB, editors: The upper extremity in sports medicine, St. Louis, 1990, CV Mosby.
18. Melchionda AM, Linburg RM: Volar plate injuries, Phys Sportsmed 10:77–84, 1982.
19. Munnings F: Cyclist's palsy, Phys Sportsmed 19:113–119, 1991.
20. National Collegiate Athletic Association: The rules of football, rule 1, section 4, article 5, 1978.
21. Nirschl RP: Tennis elbow, Orthop Clin North Am 4:787–800, 1973.
22. Reese RC, Burrus TP, Patten J: Athletic taping and protective equipment. In Nicholas JA, Hershman EB, editors: The upper extremity in sports medicine, St. Louis, 1990, CV Mosby.
23. Rettig AC, Alexy C, Malone K: Protective devices for hand and wrist injuries in athletes, J Musculoskel Med 9:62–75, 1992.
24. Rovere GD, Curl, WW, Browning DG: Bracing and taping in an office sports medicine practice, Clin Sports Med 8:497–515, 1989.
25. Roy S, Irvin R: Sports medicine, Englewood Cliffs, NJ, 1983, Prentice-Hall.
26. Ryan AJ: Eliminate boxing gloves, Phys Sportsmed 11:49, 1983.
27. Strauss RH: In-line skating: A new path to fitness—and fun, Phys Sportsmed 18:36–38, 1990.
28. The medical aspects of boxing: A round table, Phys Sportsmed 13:57–72, 1985.
29. Vetter WL: How I manage mallet finger, Phys Sportsmed 17:140–144, 1989.
30. Walstead T, Knight KL: Bracing against wrist hyperextension, Phys Sportsmed 13:163, 1985.

SUGGESTED READINGS

Cinque C: Bicycle safety: A balancing act, Phys Sportsmed 17:177–183, 1989.
DeCarlo M, et al: Perfecting a playing cast for hand and wrist injuries, Phys Sportsmed 20:95–104, 1992.
Downhill skiing injuries: A round table, Phys Sportsmed 15:107–114, 1987.
Estwanik JJ, Boitano M, Ari N: Amateur boxing injuries at the 1981 and 1982 USA/ABF National Championships, Phys Sportsmed 12:123–128, 1984.
Fumich RM, Fink RJ, Hanna GR: Offensive lineman's thumb, Phys Sportsmed 11:113–115, 1983.
Garrick JG, Webb DR: Sports injuries: Diagnosis and management, Philadelphia, 1990, WB Saunders.
Grana WA, Kalenak A: Clinical sports medicine, Philadelphia, 1991, WB Saunders.
Hayes D: Reducing risks in hockey: Analysis of equipment and injuries, Phys Sportsmed 6:67–70, 1978.
Lane LB: Acute grade III ulnar collateral ligament ruptures, Am J Sports Med 19:234–238, 1991.
McCue FC: How I manage fractured metacarpals in athletes, Phys Sportsmed 13:83–87, 1985.
Pichora DR, McMurtry RY, Bell MJ: Gamekeeper's thumb: A prospective study of functional bracing, J Hand Surg 14A:567–573, 1989.
Rettig AC: Hand injuries in football players: Getting a grip on fractures, Phys Sportsmed 19:55–64, 1991.
Rettig AC: Hand injuries in football players: Soft-tissue trauma, Phys Sportsmed 19, 1991.
Rettig AC, Wright HH: Skier's thumb, Phys Sportsmed 17:65–75, 1989.
Rovere GD: How I manage skier's thumb, Phys Sportsmed 11:73–83, 1983.
Schelkun PH: Cross-country skiing, Phys Sportsmed 20:168–174, 1992.
Steele BE: Protective pads for athletes, Phys Sportsmed 13:179–180, 1985.
Tucci JJ, Barone JE: A study of urban bicycling accidents, Am J Sports Med 16:181–184, 1988.
Wadsworth LT: How to manage skier's thumb, Phys Sportsmed 20:69–78, 1992.

Orthoses for Cumulative Trauma Disorder

William W. Eversmann, Jr.

The Bureau of Labor Statistics estimated in 1990 that cumulative trauma disorders affected more than 185,000 American workers.[7] This is nine times the number of cumulative trauma disorders that were reported only eight years earlier.[9] Cumulative trauma disorders are a group of health disorders arising from repeated, biomechanical stresses to muscles, tendons, ligaments, and joints and secondarily because of their proximity to the nerves of the forearm and hand.[1,3,4,5] The group of disorders known as cumulative trauma disorders should not be a group of vague, ill-defined, or undiagnosable conditions. Rather, more than 95% of cumulative trauma disorders of the upper extremity distal to the shoulder are embodied in eight separate, distinguishable diagnoses, four of which affect tendons primarily without neurologic concomitance and four of which are more closely related to neurologic conditions, the so-called entrapment neuropathies of the upper extremity.[5] The four tendon conditions include (1) stenosing tenosynovitis of the flexor tendon sheath commonly known as *trigger finger;* (2) stenosing tenosynovitis of the first dorsal compartment, often referred to as *DeQuervain's tenosynovitis;* (3) stenosing tenosynovitis of the second dorsal compartment, which has been termed *intersection syndrome;* and (4) lateral epicondylitis of the elbow involving the extensor origin of the muscle mass at the lateral epicondyle of the elbow.

The four conditions associated with major nerve entrapment syndromes are (1) carpal tunnel syndrome, which is the most common of the cumulative trauma disorders;[4,6] (2) ulnar tunnel syndrome affecting the ulnar nerve at the wrist usually at the level of the wrist flexion crease; (3) cubital tunnel syndrome affecting the ulnar nerve at the elbow most frequently resulting from subluxation of the ulnar nerve out of the ulnar notch; and (4) radial tunnel syndrome affecting the radial nerve in the proximal third of the forearm.

The category of cumulative trauma disorder should not be broadened to include entities such as degeneration of the small joints of the hand and wrist that may be due to repetitive use and osteoarthritic degeneration of those joints.[4] These clinical entities have a different pathophysiologic mechanism than the tendon and nerve conditions outlined previously and should not be included in the term *cumulative trauma disorders.*

Also the vague pain syndromes of the upper extremity that seem to be related to use should not be included in the term *cumulative trauma disorders.* These conditions, sometimes referred to as overuse syndromes or repetitive stress injuries, are ill defined, may have a psychosomatic origin, and do not conform to the rigorous diagnostic criteria of the previously outlined eight musculoskeletal conditions.

WRIST AND FOREARM SYNDROMES

The development of orthotic systems for cumulative trauma disorders by necessity must group the pathomechanics of each of the cumulative trauma disorders to develop an orthosis that protects the extremities from the recurrent biomechanical stresses which seem to be causative. Accordingly, because the pathomechanics of carpal tunnel syndrome, ulnar tunnel syndrome, DeQuervain's tenosynovitis, and intersection syndrome are all related to flexion and extension motions of the wrist, the orthoses that have been developed to be used by the worker affected with these cumulative trauma disorders must protect the extremity from the repeated flexion and extension motion of the wrist. Two general categories of orthoses are appropriate for these conditions. The first, a static orthosis, the most commonly available type of orthosis, is appropriate for the patient to wear during resting hours, particularly while sleeping. The static orthosis in the workplace when flexion and extension of the wrist is required for work activities may be inappropriate because if the worker requires flexion and extension of the wrist to perform his or her usual work and the work cannot be performed without that motion or motion to replace it, additional and even unacceptable stress may be placed on the elbow or forearm if a static orthosis were to remove all motion at the wrist.

Accordingly an orthosis that has some motion at the wrist, although possibly reduced or limited, may be more desirable. The one most preferred by the author was developed by Johnson (Fig. 23.1) and allows a varying amount of flexion of the wrist as is necessary for work but provides a spring mechanism of varying strength to restore the wrist to an extension position so that the worker does not continue in a flexed wrist position for a prolonged period of time while working. The person using this orthotic device generally wears it 4 to 6 hours a day and, if the condition is bilateral, wears the orthosis on only one side at a time, alternating the two sides during the workday. During the resting hours, the patient uses a molded thermoplastic orthotic device referred to as an *ulnar gutter splint* because it contacts the patient's forearm and wrist along the ulnar border of the wrist leaving the midpalmar area of the forearm and wrist uncovered by the orthosis (Fig. 23.2).

Although the cubital tunnel syndrome may be due to compression of the ulnar nerve within the body of the proximal portion of the flexor carpi ulnaris, more commonly repetitive flexion and extension motion of the elbow during work activities, particularly if there has been some increase in the muscle bulk of the medial head of the triceps, causes subluxation of the ulnar nerve as the elbow is brought into flexion at the ulnar notch in cubital tunnel syndrome. In this instance, the ulnar nerve is forced out of its usual anatomic position behind the medial epicondyle by the muscle bulk of the medial head of the triceps or related anomalous muscles, and the retaining ligament of the most proximal portion of the aponeurosis of the flexor carpi ulnaris muscle creates a pressure phenomenon on the ulnar nerve as it attempts to change its position.

In the early stages of this cumulative trauma disorder, the patient experiences some relief from the symptoms of the ulnar neuropathy, usually manifested initially by numbness of the ring and little fingers or along the ulnar border of the distal forearm, with a nighttime, static, resting orthosis applied along the radial border of the forearm and across the elbow that immobilizes the wrist in a straight position as the orthosis is anchored to the base of the thumb and maintains the elbow in a position of 40 to 45 degrees of flexion preventing any further flexion with the position of the orthosis on the flexor radial surface of the forearm (Fig. 23.3). This orthosis is normally worn just during sleeping hours because it interferes with daytime activities to a degree that is unacceptable for most wearers. It relieves the subluxation of the ulnar nerve at the medial epicondyle and by so doing reduces the degree of ulnar neuropathy. The patient often sleeps with the arm on a small or flattened pillow and finds that the orthosis is somewhat difficult to wear initially during sleeping hours. With perseverance, usually over a 3- to 4-week period, a patient begins to tolerate the splint and can rest without the splint disturbing sleep. Some patients cannot tolerate this splint and cannot sleep restfully; in these patients, the splint must be discontinued. In those patients who can tolerate the splint and continue to rest, it is helpful in reducing ulnar neuropathy and may be sufficient conservative treatment to obviate the necessity of operative intervention for cubital tunnel syndrome.

The length of time for the use of the orthoses to obtain an optimal clinical result is 4 to 6 months. Even after this prolonged period of time, gradual removal of the splint over a 3-month period is still necessary to ensure continued improvement.

ELBOW

The long-standing use of an elbow strap around the proximal forearm musculature in patients with lateral epicondylitis or tennis elbow is time honored and yet is associated with swelling of the hand, often numbness of the fingers, and usually a severe constriction of the proximal forearm musculature because wearers must draw the straps so tightly to protect the extensor muscle origin, which pathophysiologically may be torn from the origin of the conjoined tendon at the lateral epicondyle.

Over the last several years, a variety of orthotic devices have replaced the standard constricting strap. Some of the most useful of these devices have been augmented with an elevated felt pad placed against the proximal origin of the extensor muscles, which produces a desired, localized pressure on these muscles, reducing the discomfort of the extensor muscle origin and probably reducing the pull of the extensor muscles with wrist extension. The localizer pad should be elevated by at least 3/16 inch and combined with a circular band of the forearm so that when applied, constriction of the entire forearm does not occur, but maximum pressure is exerted on the extensor muscle origin (Fig. 23.4) The band is worn on the proximal third of the forearm preferably as far proximal as possible, and the localizer pad should be placed directly distal to the most tender area at the lateral epicondyle or distal to the palpable defect if one is found on exami-

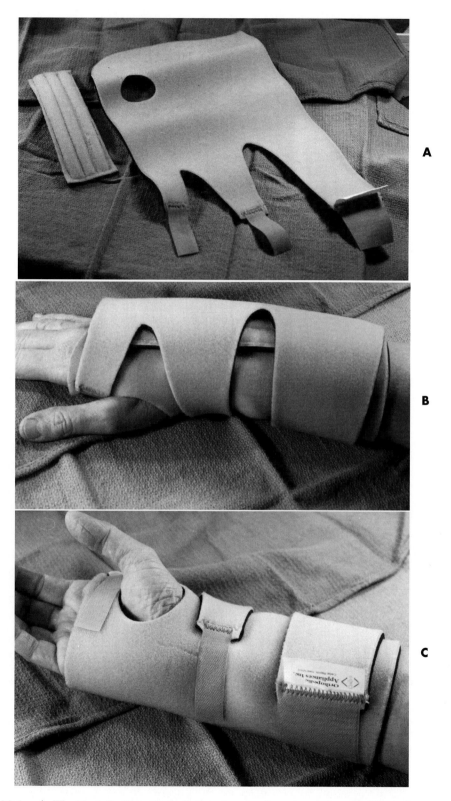

Fig. 23.1.   **A,** The blank for the orthosis designed to permit motion of the wrist. The springs are noted at left and are applied beneath the strapping (**B** and **C**). The orthosis is made of Spenco rubber and provides warmth in addition to soft support.

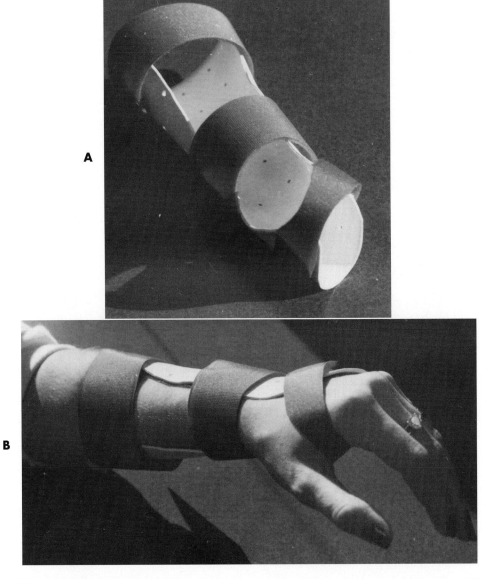

Fig. 23.2.   **A,** The molded thermoplastic orthosis known as the ulnar gutter splint covers 180 degrees of the forearm and hand along the ulnar side. **B,** The patient has applied the orthosis showing its position.

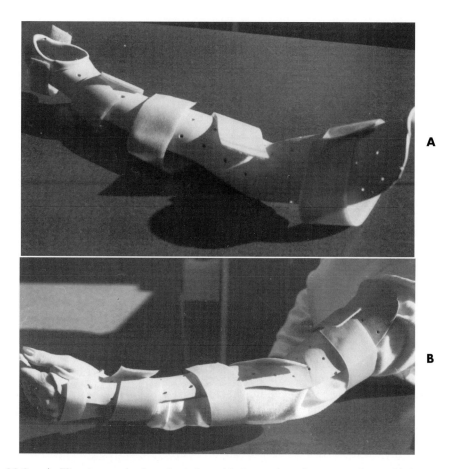

Fig. 23.3. **A,** The thermoplastic orthosis for cubital tunnel syndrome contains multiple straps to hold the orthosis in place. **B,** The orthosis is applied to the flexor surface of the arm and forearm to preclude any possibility of pressure on the ulnar nerve, which the orthosis is designed to protect.

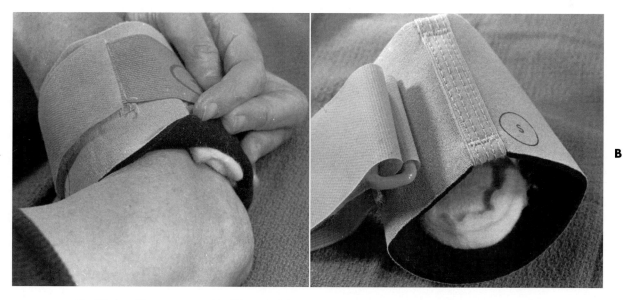

Fig. 23.4. The exaggerated buildup of a felt pad of at least 3/16 inch is placed immediately distal to the painful area of the tennis elbow. This pad, as illustrated in Fig. 23.3, *A,* minimizes constriction of the forearm muscles while providing maximum compression of those muscles distal to the painful lateral epicondylitis.

nation. This localizer pad technique, when it is combined with the elimination of maximum grasp with the elbow in full extension and the wrist in full flexion, can be expected to provide relief over a 3- to 4-month interval when worn during the day only. It should not be worn during sleeping hours. The band, however, should be worn for all activities, not simply work activities during the day. If the patient has required treatment in addition to the orthosis, such as immobilization or injection, the healing period, particularly after injection, is prolonged. A healing period without orthotic treatment can be expected to be in the range of 3.5 to 4 months. If the condition is particularly chronic, continued use of the orthosis for work activities only can be advised. The long-term use can be restricted to workplace activity and need not be continued outside the workplace.

The author has not found a satisfactory orthosis to reduce or minimize the symptoms of stenosing tenosynovitis of the flexor tendon sheath. Nonorthotic treatment of this condition seems generally to be more appropriate.

The orthotic treatment of radial tunnel syndrome, having analyzed the pathophysiology of this condition, requires the extremity to be splinted in full supination with the wrist in extension. Although this position relieves the symptoms of compression of the radial nerve should an orthosis in this position be fitted, it is unlikely that such an orthosis worn by a patient in the prescribed position would allow the patient to have any functionally significant use of the upper extremity. The author has not used this technique for the treatment of radial tunnel syndrome.

REFERENCES

1. Armstrong TJ: Ergonomics and cumulative trauma disorders, Hand Clin 2:553–565, 1986.
2. Armstrong T, et al: Some histological changes in carpal tunnel contents and their biomechanical implications, J Occup Med 26:179–201, 1984.
3. Armstrong T, Chaffin D: Some biomechanical aspects of the carpal tunnel, J Biomech 12:567–570, 1979.
4. Eversmann WW Jr: Advances in operative orthopedics, vol 1, St. Louis, 1993, Mosby-Year Book.
5. Eversmann WW Jr: Entrapment and compression neuropathies. In Green DP, editor: Operative hand surgery, New York, 1983, Churchill Livingstone.
6. Eversmann WW Jr, Ritsick JA: Intraoperative changes in motor conduction latency in carpal tunnel syndrome, J Hand Surg 3:77–81, 1978.
7. Kilborn PT: Department of Labor report: Rise in worker injuries is laid to the computer, New York Times, Nov 16, 1989.
8. Lundborg G, Meyers R, Powell H: Nerve compression and increased fluid pressure: A "miniature compartment syndrome," J Neurosurg Psychiatry 46:119–124, 1983.
9. Millar JD, Meyers MD: Occupational safety and health: Progress toward the 1990 objectives for the nation, Public Health Rep 98:324–336, 1983.

LOWER LIMB ORTHOSES

INTRODUCTION
Thomas J. Moore

This section on lower extremity orthoses examines the multiple uses of lower extremity orthoses. The unique use of lower extremity orthoses for traumatic brain injury, with its accompanying spasticity, is discussed in Chapter 24. Orthoses for spinal-injured patients, with an emphasis on orthotic-assisted ambulation, is discussed in Chapter 25. Chapter 26 reviews the indications and usage of functional braces for lower extremity fractures. The expanding field of orthoses for sports injuries, both therapeutic and prophylactic, is discussed in Chapter 27. Chapter 28 discusses new information about an old disease, anterior poliomyelitis. Chapter 29 discusses the myriad of significant problems in the diabetic foot. Chapter 30 discusses the multiple and variable uses of shoes. Finally, Chapter 31 discusses the complex clinical situation of bracing for unstable total hip and total knee arthroplasties.

Each chapter in this section has been written by a proven expert in the field. A thorough attempt has been made to present current concepts in each chapter. Unproven uses of orthoses have not been included in any chapter. Finally, no author has advocated any commercial product in which he or she has a financial interest.

Orthoses for Brain-Injured Patients

Colin W. Fennell
Arlene N. Yang
Douglas Elson

The use of orthoses is an important adjunct to the management and treatment of the adult with brain injury during both the acute and the chronic stages of rehabilitation. An orthotic device can assist in the rehabilitation program by providing the external support needed to enhance various functional activities. During the acute phase of recovery from brain injury, the primary goal in rehabilitation of the lower extremities is to maintain range of motion of joints and to prevent joint contractures. Orthoses such as splints and casts are therefore used in this stage to prevent contractures caused by spasticity or muscular paralysis. In the subacute and chronic stages of rehabilitation after brain injury, an orthotic device can serve three main functions. First, an orthosis provides lower extremity stability by eliminating excessive joint motion. Second, an orthosis can enhance motion when muscle activity is not adequate in strength, timing, and coordination. Finally, an orthosis can inhibit or decrease abnormal muscle tone or cutaneous and postural reflexes.[13]

PATHOPHYSIOLOGY OF BRAIN INJURY

After a brain injury that is severe enough to affect normal neuromuscular control, there are stages in the return of neuromuscular control. In the first 48 hours, there can be complete flaccidity followed by a gradual increase in tone.[19] As tone increases in the lower extremity, primitive collective patterns of muscle activity and limb positioning become apparent. Increased tone at the hip typically produces hip flexion and adduction. At the knee, the hamstrings typically dominate and flex the knee, although quadriceps spasticity can occasionally lead to an extension positioning. At the ankle, the gastrocnemius-soleus complex dominates, producing an equinus ankle position with the foot

brought into varus primarily by tibialis anterior overactivity but occasionally accentuated by the tibialis posterior.[16]

As the brain injury resolves, neuromuscular control can graduate from primitive patterned movement back to full volitional control, although recovery can plateau at any stage short of normalcy depending on the severity of the brain injury. Cerebrovascular accidents, brain contusion, and penetrating brain injuries typically show the greatest improvement in restoration of neurologic function in the first 6 weeks and plateau in the first 6 to 8 months.

More widespread brain injury,[19,22] such as diffuse axonal injury, which produces axonal shearing in the hemispheres, cerebellum, and brain stem, causes more severe injury and has a more prolonged recovery phase of about 2 years.[2] In general, nonreversible surgical procedures should be avoided during the interim when normal neurologic recovery can occur.

SPASTICITY

Spasticity, which can be defined as an overreaction to the stretch reflex, can be observed in both the acute and the chronic phases of neurologic recovery after brain injury. Perry[14] has shown with the aid of dynamic electromyography studies that the spastic stretch response can present in two forms: either a clonic reaction or a sustained muscle contraction. In addition, the severity of the spasticity was found to be affected by body position, with increased levels of spasticity occurring in the sitting position in comparison to the supine position.

In the acute and subacute phases of recovery, control of spasticity is sought primarily to control joint position to avoid joint contractures from occurring in a nonfunctional position. Initially, this can be accomplished with serial casts,[12] nerve blocks with phenol,[10] or muscle blocks with botulism toxin. In later stages, when weight bearing and ambulation are feasible, rigid devices such as a cast or an ankle-foot orthosis (AFO) may be used to prevent a spastic response and maintain the ankle in neutral position. Rigid devices are preferable because the spastic response rapidly diminishes when the joints are immobile but persists with even the small amount of motion available in flexible devices. In the acute period after a traumatic brain injury, rigid devices such as circular casts should be avoided because desensate limbs and impaired cognition may allow an unrecognized compartment syndrome.

MOTOR CONTROL

Volitional control of movement falls into three broad categories: pattern, selective, and mixed. Patterned volitional movement is an extrapyramidal system, modulated motion that consists of mass extension or flexion occurring in the hip, knee, and ankle simultaneously during movement. This loss of individualized and synchronized movement of the joints substantially impairs gait and can be assisted with orthoses.

Selective motor control implies the ability to flex or extend a joint without triggering a mass extensor or flexion response in the other joints of the same limb. This requires a functioning pyramidal and extrapyramidal system. As neurologic recovery occurs, a mixed pattern of motor control can be present, with selective control being present at the proximal joints and pattern control at the distal joints. Fortunately, because fine motor control is not necessary for all functions of the lower extremity, a mixed pattern of motor control is often sufficient for ambulation. It is these limbs with a mixed pattern of motor control that are typically most aided by the use of orthoses.

SENSATION

As the outflow of stimuli for motor control can be affected by brain injury, so can the inflow of sensory input that affect touch and position be affected. The degree of impairment of sensation affecting proprioception and touch in part determines those individuals that are candidates for ambulation and those that are not. The most extreme version of this phenomenon is hemineglect where the individual is unaware of the affected side.[22] These individuals are not candidates for ambulation but may require orthoses to prevent contractures that may impede transfer activities or even the ability to wear shoes.

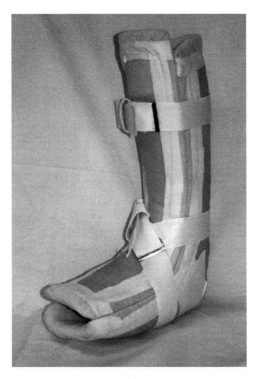

Fig. 24.1. Customized fiberglass below-knee anterior-posterior splint. Note the extra padding and cinch straps used to provide a snug fit and prevent sores from spastic movements.

GENERAL CONSIDERATIONS

After brain injury, the acute management of the lower extremities focuses on maintenance of range of motion and prevention of contractures. Failure to address proper positioning and prevention of contractures may interfere with the eventual functional outcome and may necessitate subsequent surgical procedures.

Customized fiberglass anterior-posterior (A-P) splints (Fig. 24.1) can be used to prevent contracture or to prevent recurrence of contracture in an extremity in which contracture was previously treated with serial casting or a dynamic splint. Anterior-posterior splints can allow a patient after an acute traumatic brain injury to begin early upright activities by supporting the involved lower extremity and can be used as a temporary orthosis while the permanent orthosis is being fabricated or during the interim when normal neurologic recovery can occur.

Foot equinovarus positioning is the most common deformity observed in the lower extremity, and a below-knee A-P splint usually suffices. If knee flexion is also a problem, a long leg A-P splint helps control the knee position and can function as a temporary knee-ankle-foot orthosis (KAFO).

The high-impact nature of the initial injury (i.e., motor vehicle accidents, falls) may cause direct trauma

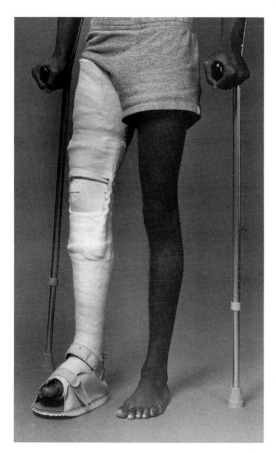

Fig. 24.2. Cast brace made with plaster of Paris provides a secure stabilizing orthosis when knee and foot stability is needed in the confused or noncompliant patient. *(From Hall AJ, Stenner RW: Manual of fracture bracing, New York, 1985, Churchill Livingstone.)*

to the lower extremity. Soft tissue, bone, and joint injuries include ligamentous instabilities and fractures requiring knee orthoses to maintain normal joint alignment and restrict unwanted motion. These orthoses range from a standard canvas knee immobilizer with vertical stays to a knee orthosis with metal uprights attached to various types of joints. The latter orthosis can provide mediolateral stability while allowing variable flexion-extension motion. A confused or noncompliant patient may attempt to remove a knee orthosis. A cast brace (Fig. 24.2) cannot be removed easily by the patient and may be a viable solution to this problem.

As the neurologic recovery progresses, decisions must be made as to which patients are candidates for retraining, how concomitant injuries will have an impact on walking, which assisting devices will be necessary, and whether or not surgery will play a role in correcting deformity before the initiation of gait training. When the neurologic recovery plateaus, the orthosis of choice is one that maximizes function and has the highest degree of compliance in its use.

GAIT ABNORMALITIES

To walk, the brain-injured patient must be able to obtain and maintain an upright position and initiate limb advancement. Before prescribing an orthosis, assessment of the lower extremities during walking should be done if at all possible. Impaired balance, loss of truncal stability, proprioceptive loss, and loss of motor control may necessitate the use of additional supports for walking, such as a platform walker or a quadcane. Once the upright position is achieved and forward motion becomes possible, observational gait analysis can then be used to determine those changes that are detrimentally affecting function. The clinical team, consisting of the physician, physical therapist, and Certified Orthotist, then make the decision as to the type of orthosis based on the patient's gait deviations, motor control, range of motion, sensation, cognitive status, and functional level.

The most commonly prescribed orthosis and the mainstay for management of gait abnormalities after brain injury is the AFO. An AFO acts directly on the ankle joint and indirectly on the knee and hip joints because of their kinematic relationship. KAFOs are used infrequently in this population because of the increased weight factor and greater energy demands with ambulation. Patients with brain injuries have decreased cognitive function, which may affect their ability to use more complex orthoses. Swing phase abnormalities in muscles above the knee, such as scissoring owing to hip adductor activity or knee extension secondary to rectus femoris activity, are seldom managed with an orthosis but may sometimes be improved by surgical release or phenol injections.

The primary indications for use of an AFO for control of gait abnormalities in patients with traumatic brain injuries are as follows:[22]
1. Inadequate dorsiflexion during midswing through terminal swing resulting in a problem with foot clearance.
2. Inadequate dorsiflexion to allow heel-first at initial contact.
3. Mediolateral ankle/foot instability during stance and swing phases.
4. Insufficient tibial control during stance phase.

Inadequate dorsiflexion in swing

In normal gait, the ankle dorsiflexes from 10 degrees of plantar flexion in initial swing to neutral during midswing and terminal swing. Inadequate dorsiflexion during midswing through terminal swing may produce a foot drag and can be attributed to several factors. One factor is dorsiflexion muscle weakness caused by either a central nervous system lesion (brain injury) or a peripheral nerve injury (common peroneal nerve). Another causative factor is the inability of the dorsiflexors to counteract the increased activity (hypertonicity, spasticity, or clonus) of the gastrocnemius-soleus complex.

In addition, decreased dorsiflexion of the foot during swing can be caused by more proximal forces, such as the malalignment of the trunk and lower extremity over the base of support.[5] Malalignments caused by muscle imbalances and movement compensations may occur after a person has sustained a brain injury. Biomechanically, when the pelvis is rotated backward on one side, the femur and tibia externally rotate, which, in turn, plantar flexes the ankle and supinates the foot. This places the ankle and foot in the equinovarus posture. A patient evaluation should include assessment of the distal and proximal muscle groups to determine the primary cause of the equinovarus posture.

When inadequate dorsiflexion in the absence of increased tone is the only gait deviation present, a lightweight flexible plastic AFO is an appropriate orthosis. The advantage of a flexible AFO is that it allows the normal plantarflexion motion to occur during weight acceptance. If inadequate dorsiflexion is the result of overactivity of the gastrocnemius-soleus complex, however, a rigid AFO may be indicated.

Inadequate dorsiflexion in stance

Inadequate dorsiflexion also creates a problem with forward progression by preventing initial contact with the heel. A patient lacking active dorsiflexion contacts the ground with the forefoot or flatfoot rather than the heel. This deviation leads to decreased forward progression of the tibia and decreased shock absorption by limiting knee flexion.[16] To address this deviation, an AFO (rigid or flexible) that positions the ankle in neutral during swing allows for heel-first initial contact. Shoe modifications can be made to decrease the force of loading and to dampen the demands on the quadriceps to counteract the knee flexion moment.

Mediolateral ankle/foot instability

Deviations in the ankle and foot such as varus (excessive inversion) and valgus (excessive eversion) can be observed throughout the gait cycle. The most common deviation is a varus foot, which can be mild (flexible and correctable with weight bearing) or severe (nonflexible). A varus foot with weight on the lateral border becomes an unstable rigid base during weight acceptance. Clinically, patients with mild but persistent varus may benefit from *neurophysiologic* orthoses, such as the dynamic foot orthosis (FO) developed by Utley and Bohman (Fig. 24.3). The dynamic FO is constructed to facilitate eversion and inhibit inversion.[21] The design of the dynamic FO along with other neurophysiologic orthoses is discussed later.

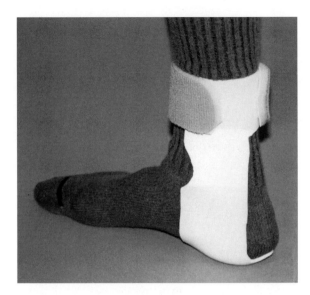

Fig. 24.3.   Dynamic foot orthosis is designed to facilitate eversion and inhibit inversion.

A patient with a strong varus component requires a rigid AFO for maximal support. When severe varus is inadequately controlled by a rigid AFO, additional support may be provided by shoe modifications or shoe inserts. A lateral flare, added to the shoe, increases the base of support and decreases the tendency for the foot to roll out laterally into varus during stance. In some patients, the varus component continues to be a problem even with a rigid orthosis with shoe modifications. The foot may piston out of the shoe or turn inside the shoe. Further assessment is needed to determine the primary source of the varus posturing. The source of the dynamic posturing may be found proximally, such as malalignment or muscle imbalance in the trunk or pelvis. Malalignment of the pelvis can create changes up and down the kinematic chain. If the equinovarus is due to intrinsic foot and ankle spasticity, surgical correction consisting of Achilles' tendon lengthening, toe flexor release, and split anterior tibial tendon (SPLATT) transfer can be done. This correction should be reversed for patients with traumatic brain injury 18 months after the initial injury to allow for normal neurologic recovery.

Tibial instability in stance

Insufficient tibial control during stance manifests itself in two common deviations. A patient with a lack of tibial control owing to weakness in the gastrocnemius-soleus complex may collapse into knee flexion and ankle dorsiflexion during stance phase. Such a patient may benefit from a rigid AFO to maintain a vertical tibia and prevent collapse into excessive dorsiflexion. A second deviation associated with lack of tibial control occurs when the patient thrusts the knee into recurvatum and excessive ankle plantarflexion to achieve a plantigrade foot during weight bearing. This deviation may be due to weakness in the gastrocnemius-soleus complex combined with a plantarflexion contracture, backward rotated pelvis, or a quadriceps weakness.[15] A rigid AFO with a heel lift may be used to maintain a vertical tibia relative to the ground and prevent knee thrust into recurvatum. Even though the AFO crosses only the ankle joint, it plays an important function in controlling the knee because of the biomechanical relationship between the tibia and femur. Therefore, it is not necessary for an orthosis to cross the knee joint to influence knee motion.

POSTOPERATIVE ORTHOSES

In some patients, conservative programs consisting of serial casting, mobilization techniques, and positioning do not alleviate problems with contractures, excessive tone, or spasticity. More invasive medical interventions such as nerve blocks and surgery may be indicated. In choosing appropriate candidates for these interventions, one must take into account the patient's motor control, sensation, cognitive status, and functional level. It is also important to consider the time from onset of injury and goals of the intervention. For example, an anesthetic block to the tibial nerve is used diagnostically to differentiate soft tissue contracture from hypertonicity and spasticity in the gastrocnemius-soleus complex. A nerve block also augments a serial casting program by temporarily reducing the tone and spasticity.[9] After the serial casting program is completed, a rigid AFO is provided to maintain the newly acquired alignment. As the patient undergoes therapy and learns more normal movement patterns, the orthosis is modified accordingly.

An orthotic device plays a critical part in the postoperative management. Common surgical interventions for lower extremity spasticity or contracture after traumatic brain injury include releases of hip flexor muscles for a hip flexion contracture. Hip adduction contracture can be dealt with by selective release of hip adductor muscles with neurectomy of the anterior broach of the obturator nerve. Equinus contracture is relieved by Achilles' tendon lengthening. When the postoperative casts are removed, resting A-P splints are used to protect the transferred tendons, maintain the new joint positions, and prevent recurrence of contractures. Orthoses are prescribed to provide protection and positioning when patients are participating in upright activities and sitting up in wheelchairs. In dynamic equinovarus deformity of the ankle, SPLATT along with release of the toe flexors and lengthening of the Achilles' tendon can be done post-

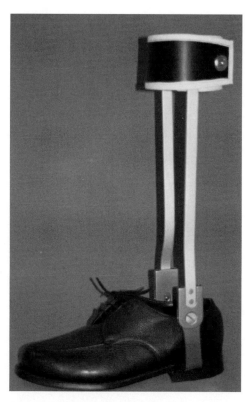

Fig. 24.4. Double adjustable ankle joint AFO. Double uprights with calf band attached to a leather shoe with a steel shank through locking ankle hinges.

operatively, most patients require some form of orthotic support.

Types of orthoses

The prototypical orthosis for management of lower extremity problems of patients with brain injury is the AFO. Various designs of this orthosis accommodate a variety of problems and the stages of recovery.

Double adjustable ankle joint AFO. The double adjustable ankle joint (DAAJ, also known as BiCAAL) AFO (Fig. 24.4) has features that make it the preferred choice in several applications. The ankle joint can be locked in any position from dorsiflexed to plantar flexed or be allowed free motion throughout the range. Dorsiflexion and plantarflexion stops can be used when partial range of motion is desired. Springs can also be used in the posterior channels to assist dorsiflexion.

The orthosis consists of double uprights attached to a calf band with calf cuff and closure, extending proximally to 20 mm below the fibular neck to avoid the peroneal nerve. The closure should be a type that the patient can use independently, with Velcro or a snap type being the easiest to use. The ankle joints are attached at the distal ends of the uprights and articulate with the stirrup, which is attached to the shoe.

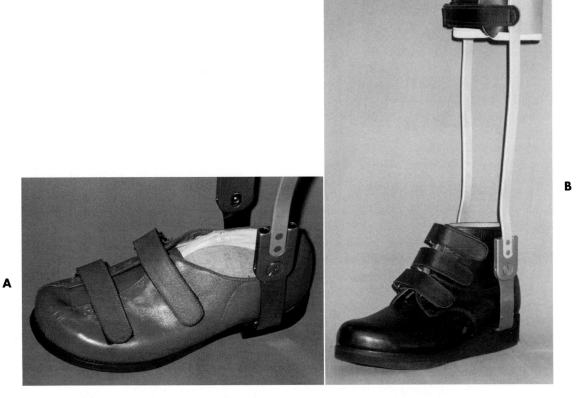

Fig. 24.5. **A,** Modified shoe with wider toe opening to ease entry. **B,** High-top shoe assists in controlling mild varus or valgus deformity.

The shoe should include a leather sole, along with a metal shank extending to the metatarsal heads, to provide secure attachment of the stirrup and increased rigidity and prevent unwanted motion. Because the uprights of the AFO restrict the range normally used in putting on shoes, the Blucher style opening (two flaps that come off the vamp of the shoe) is a preferred type of shoe. As with the calf closure, shoes should be able to be fastened by the patient independently, if possible. Velcro closures or elastic laces are commonly used to facilitate this.

Special shoe features that are appropriate include extra-depth shoes, which can accommodate inserts for corrective or preventive purposes; surgical toe openings for easier donning (Fig. 24.5, *A*), especially helpful after surgery on the foot and ankle areas; and high-top shoes to assist in controlling mild varus or valgus (Fig. 24.5, *B*). The DAAJ AFO is indicated during the initial period of recovery because of its ability to be repositioned and accommodate changes in range of motion as the patient progresses. It is recommended following cast removal after surgery (such as TAL, SPLATT, TFR) when a shoe with a surgical toe is used. For the nonambulatory patient, it provides a stable base of support to lessen the assistance re-

quired for transfers and to prevent contractures at the ankle.

The characteristics of the DAAJ AFO provide advantages when edema or change in girth occurs. The calf cuff closure can be adjusted and calf band widened, and the nonintimate fit also can accommodate changes. Use of heavy-duty stirrups, stainless steel side bars, and more durable shoes with wear-resistant soles can serve the patient who places a high demand on the AFO because of high body weight or heavy use.

An alternative to the DAAJ AFO attached to a shoe that retains most of its advantages but is more cosmetic and versatile is created by substituting a polypropylene footplate that fits inside the patient's shoe (Fig. 24.6). This alternative allows the patient to use different shoes with the same AFO. When the AFO is locked or has dorsiflexion and/or plantarflexion stops, however, some movement can occur between the orthosis and shoe. This can be minimized by using shoes that fully encompass the forefoot and fasten securely.

Plastic AFO. Plastic AFOs are intimate-fitting posterior shells fabricated from polypropylene or similar thermo-forming polymer materials (Fig. 24.7). Prefabricated AFOs are also available but are rarely recom-

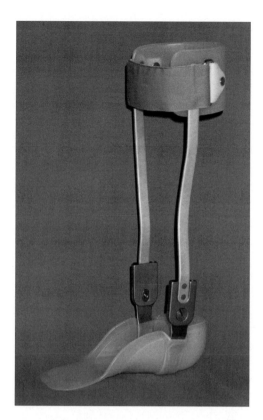

Fig. 24.6. DAAJ AFO with polypropylene footplate allows for a variety of footwear to be used with the same AFO. Increased shoe orthosis motion can occur with this style of orthosis when the ankle is locked or the flexion stops are used and is minimized by using a shoe that fully encompasses the footplate.

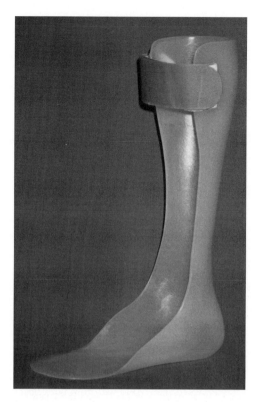

Fig. 24.7. Polypropylene AFO has the advantage of lighter weight and improved cosmesis and accordingly better acceptance in usage.

mended for long-term use because of their generic fit. By varying design characteristics, such as type of plastic, thickness of plastic, trim lines on the AFO, incorporation of reinforcements to the ankle area, and addition of anterior shells to the AFO, the plastic AFO can be made flexible or rigid. This wide range of flexibility allows the plastic AFO to be used in a variety of situations.

Plastic AFOs are more cosmetic, lighter in weight, and more readily accepted by patients. Because of the increased area of contact on the patient, however, those with impaired sensation should be carefully evaluated to determine the appropriateness of their use. Appropriate fitting of plastic orthoses is critical on all patients, including those with full sensation. Areas of pressure can be relieved by heating and reforming the plastic, and padding over bony prominences can reduce the risk of pressure problems. This is especially important when controlling mediolateral motion at the ankle.

For patients requiring a rigid AFO, the heel height of the shoe must be taken into consideration. The heel height must be accommodated when casting the patient with the tibia in the desired position relative to the

floor. For example, an AFO fabricated in neutral (90 degrees) holds the tibia in relative dorsiflexion when used with a shoe with a heel. Patients should be advised that their shoes must have the same heel height as the AFO was intended to accommodate. Otherwise, function is compromised. For those patients lacking only dorsiflexion, a plastic AFO with trim lines posterior to the malleoli provides a dorsiflexion assist during swing phase, while allowing plantarflexion during weight acceptance (Fig. 24.8).

Plastic articulating AFOs. Plastic AFOs incorporating adjustable ankle joints combine the advantages of adjustability, light weight, cosmesis, and mediolateral control of DAAJ AFOs and plastic AFOs (Fig. 24.9). For the patient who requires a rigid AFO, however, it is generally not the orthosis of choice, even though many ankle joint components can be locked. The stress applied at the attachment points of the ankle joints by a vigorous user can sometimes result in fractures of the plastic.

Controlled motion at the ankle joint can be accomplished through the use of components attached to the orthosis. An adjustable plantarflexion stop or dorsiflexion assist spring assembly can be included during fabrication in the posterior where the footplate and proximal section meet. Dacron webbing straps can be used to provide a dorsiflexion stop when attached to the

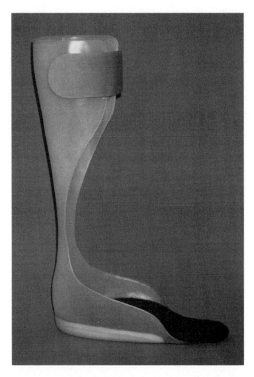

Fig. 24.8.   Polypropylene AFO with trim lines posterior to the malleoli is useful in the patient lacking only dorsiflexion because the increased flexibility allows for a passive dorsiflexion assist during swing phase.

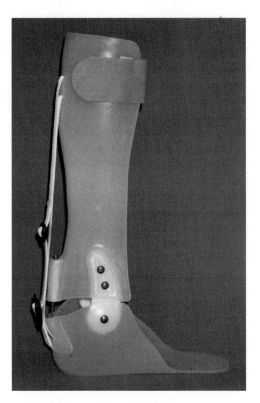

Fig. 24.10.   Polyarticulating AFO with posterior dacron webbing straps to provide a dorsiflexion stop.

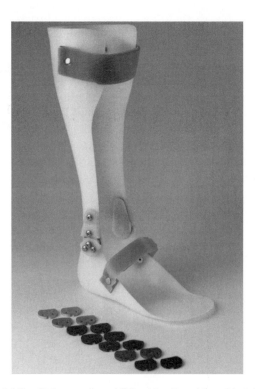

Fig. 24.9.   Polypropylene AFO with adjustable ankle joints. *(Courtesy of United States Manufacturing Company, Pasadena, CA.)*

posterior of the footplate and proximal section and can be adjusted when used with buckles or Velcro (Fig. 24.10).

Shoes

In addition to the special shoes and modifications already discussed, other shoe modifications can be made to improve gait and stability.

For the patient using a rigid AFO and making initial contact with the heel, a knee flexion thrust is produced. This is the result of restricting plantarflexion during weight acceptance. In typical gait, the plantar movement is approximately 15 degrees, with the motion controlled by the eccentric contraction of the anterior compartment musculature.[15] With a rigid AFO, this plantarflexion motion is transmitted to the knee, increasing the demand on the quadriceps to prevent the knee from buckling.

Decreasing the heel lever of the floor reaction force reduces the knee flexion thrust. This can be accomplished by a cushioned heel (Fig. 24.11, *A*) or by beveling (undercutting) the heel (Fig. 24.11, *B*). Although research shows the solid ankle cushion heel to be the most effective,[23] it is not the most durable. Beveling the existing heel is the next most effective method and is more practical. It also can be used to

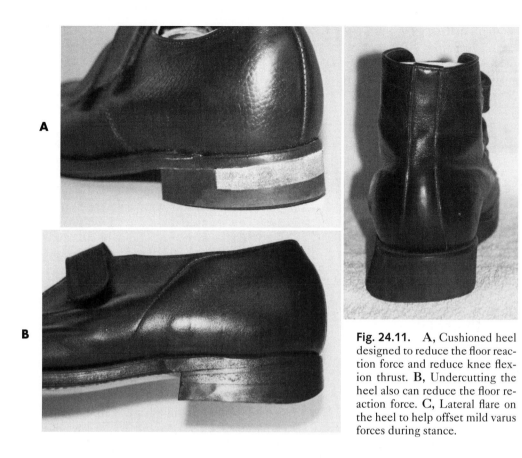

Fig. 24.11. **A,** Cushioned heel designed to reduce the floor reaction force and reduce knee flexion thrust. **B,** Undercutting the heel also can reduce the floor reaction force. **C,** Lateral flare on the heel to help offset mild varus forces during stance.

reduce foot slap because of weak anterior compartment musculature during free plantarflexion.

A flare added to the heel and sole of a shoe increases the base of support on that side and can be an effective method of controlling mild varus forces during stance when applied to the lateral border (Fig. 24.11, *C*). The heel counter and forefoot position in relation to the floor remain unchanged (vertical) during stance because the flare does not add material under the sole or heel. It can be used in conjunction with an AFO or on shoes only.

A wedge of material can be added to the sole and heel of the shoe, either medially or laterally. This wedge positions the shoe into inversion or eversion and is used to counter deforming forces. When used on a shoe attached to a metal AFO, the wedge is placed between the stirrup and the midsole. This changes the position of the shoe without affecting the relationship of the uprights to the floor. Adding a wedge to outside of the stirrup changes the angle of the orthosis in the coronal plane and transmits these unwanted forces proximally, toward the knee. Wedges can be combined with flares on shoes, as needed, and are used to treat varus, often found in this patient group.

T-straps are another method used to attempt to control varus deformities when used with metal upright AFOs (Fig. 24.12). They are not recommended for patients with strong varus because the force required to

counter it can cause skin pressure problems. Surgical intervention is usually indicated in those instances.

Inserts for protection of insensate feet or to provide corrective positioning (medial arch support, lateral wedging) are used in shoes or can be incorporated into plastic AFOs. As previously mentioned, extra-depth shoes should be used when inserts require extra space.

NEUROPHYSIOLOGIC ORTHOSES (TONE REDUCING ORTHOSES)

The concept of neurophysiologic orthoses may be clinically useful even though there are no objective data in the present literature to support it. Orthoses that incorporate designs that inhibit muscle tone are also used in the treatment of patients with brain injuries. Control of the hypertonicity resulting from central nervous system dysfunctions is achieved by these special design principles, which are based on neurophysiological theories.[11]

There are several different methods by which control of the muscle tone is attempted. They include the use of metatarsal pads, positioning the toes in extension, inclusion of pressure points over muscle insertions, static immobilization through a total contact design, and stimulation of antagonistic muscle groups.

Theories of neurophysiologic control differ on design mechanisms, and further research is needed to resolve the differences. The method used on a particular patient is often a collaboration between the orthotist and physical therapist, using the knowledge and expertise from their respective fields to design an orthosis that maximizes function.

Dynamic foot orthosis

The dynamic foot orthosis (FO) is a neurophysiologic orthosis developed by Utley and Bohman based on principles in the neurodevelopmental treatment or Bobath approach (see Fig. 24.3).[21] An appropriate candidate is one who has available ankle/foot range of motion and mild dynamic varus component. By design, the dynamic FO provides medial support at the ankle and holds the calcaneus in a neutral position for better heel contact in initial contact. The major difference between the dynamic FO and the conventional AFO is the facilitatory component of the FO and the stability component of the AFO. The full contact on the plantar surface stimulates the tonic foot reflexes of dorsiflexion and eversion. The flexible material allows for free plantarflexion and dorsiflexion motion. Fabrication materials consist of low-temperature thermo-forming plastic, padding, and Velcro straps.

Toe spreader

Development of the toe spreader (also called toe separator) was based on the neurophysiological principles[21] of inhibition and facilitation and tonic foot reflexes (Fig. 24.13). The toe spreader is used primarily to diminish excessive toe clawing, which may cause pain and impede forward advancement of the lower extremity over the foot. It is designed with two basic premises: (1) Abduction and extension of the toes

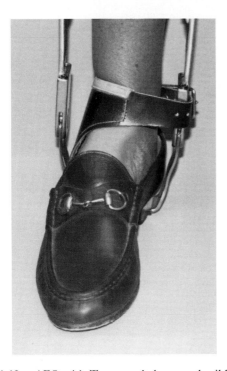

Fig. 24.12. AFO with T-strap to help control mild varus. Not recommended with stronger varus deformity because lateral skin breakdown becomes a concern.

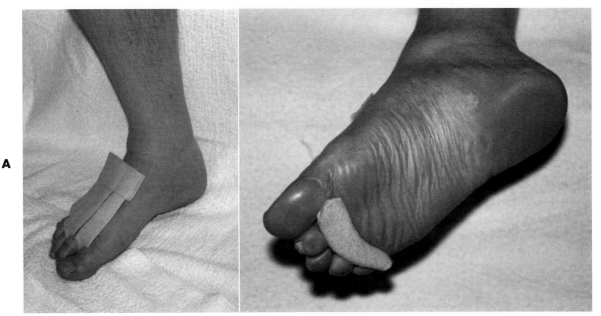

Fig. 24.13. **A,** Plastazote toe spreader incorporates neurophysiologic concepts to inhibit excess tone and reduce the toe grasp reflex. **B,** Plantar view of toe spreader in place.

release intrinsic tone in the toes, and (2) raising the lateral border of the foot facilitates eversion of the foot. The toe spreader is fabricated of compressible foam covered with self-adhesive felt.

Ford et al[6] described a similar orthosis called a toe separator that was found to be effective in inhibiting excess tone and reducing pain in patients with toe grasp reflex. By inhibiting abnormal tone in the toes, the foot becomes a better weight-bearing surface for the body to progress over during stance phase. The toe separator is fabricated from Plastazote with self-adhesive felt cover and toe extensions. Both types of toe orthoses are held in place under the sock.

SUMMARY

The judicious use of an orthosis plays an important role in the successful management of adults with brain injury. The entire team including the patient should work in close collaboration to ensure that the most appropriate orthosis is selected. It is important to consider the patient's cognitive status and goals when choosing an orthosis to ensure compliancy. Once a decision is made, the use of an orthotic device can enhance the patient's quality of life by improving his or her functional status in the home and community.

REFERENCES

1. AAOS: Atlas of Orthotics, ed 2, St Louis, 1985, CV Mosby.
2. Adams JH, et al: Diffuse axonal injury due to non missile head injury in humans: An analysis of 45 cases, Ann Neurol 12:557–563, 1982.
3. D'Astous J, editor: Orthotics and prosthetic digest, ed 2, Ottawa, Canada, 1983, EDAHL Proc.
4. Duncan WR: Tonic reflexes of the foot, J Bone Joint Surg 42A:859–868, 1960.
5. Fisher B, Yakura J: Movement analysis: A different perspective, Orthop Phys Ther Clin North Am 2:1–14, 1993.
6. Ford C, Grotz RC, Shamp JK: The neurological ankle-foot orthosis, Clin Prosthet Ortho 10:15–23, 1986.
7. Garland DE, Rhoades ME: Orthopedic management of brain injured adults, Clin Orthop Rel Res 131:111–122, 1978.
8. Hall AJ, Stenner RW: Manual of fracture bracing, New York, 1985, Churchill Livingstone.
9. Ito C: Casting: Conservative management of joint deformities and dynamic posturing, Orthop Phys Ther Clin North Am 2:25–38, 1993.
10. Khalili AA, Benton JG: A physiologic approach to the evaluation and management of spasticity with procaine and phenol nerve block, Clin Orthop Rel Res 47:97–104, 1966.
11. Lohman M, Goldstein H: Alternative strategies in tone-reducing AFO design, J Prosthet Orthot 5:21, 1993.
12. McCollough NC: Orthotic management in adult hemiplegia, Clin Orthop Rel Res 131:38–46, 1978.
13. Montgomery J: Orthotic management of the lower limb in head-injured adults, J Head Trauma Rehabil 2:57–61, 1987.
14. Perry J: Determinants of muscle function in the spastic lower extremity, Clin Orthop Rel Res 288:10–26, 1993.
15. Perry J: Gait analysis, Thorofare, NJ, 1992, Slack Inc.
16. Perry J, Waters RL, Perrin T: Electromyographic analysis of equinovarus following stroke, Clin Orthop Rel Res 131:47–53, 1978.
17. Rose GK: Orthotics principle and practice, London, 1986, Heinemann Medical Books.
18. Shurr DG, Cook TM: Prosthetics and orthotics, Norwalk, CT, 1990, Appleton & Lange.
19. Twitchell TE: The restoration of motor function following hemiplegia in man, Brain 74:443, 1951.
20. Ummphred DA, editor: Neurological rehabilitation, St Louis, 1985, CV Mosby.
21. Utley J, Thomas C: Orthotics course-lecture and lab material, Downey, CA, 1989, Neurodevelopmental Techniques (NDT) Rancho Los Amigos Medical Center.
22. Waters RL, Garland DE, Montgomery J: Orthotic prescription for stroke and head injury. In AAOS: Atlas of orthotics, St. Louis, 1985, CV Mosby.
23. Wiest DR, et al: The influence of heel design on a rigid ankle foot orthosis, Orthot Prosthet 33:3, 1979.

C H A P T E R
25

Lower Extremity Orthoses for Spinal Cord Injury

James Campbell
Thomas J. Moore

The annual incidence of acute spinal cord injury in the United States is difficult to estimate accurately because spinal cord injury is not a reportable condition, but spinal cord injury occurs at an annual incidence of about 30 per million population of the United States. The causes of traumatic spinal cord injury vary, but in a survey of spinal cord injury patients in trauma centers, 85% of injuries were due to blunt trauma (motor vehicle accidents, falls) and 15% were due to penetrating injuries (gunshot wounds). The majority of spinal cord injuries occur in young men (79% male, average age 33.5 years). The incidence of polytrauma or traumatic brain injury associated with spinal cord injury is significant, and the overall mortality after acute spinal cord injury is 15%.[7]

The care of the patient with acute spinal cord injury has evolved through the decades. In the past, the treatment of acute spinal cord injury often involved long periods of bed rest. Currently, with advances in methods of surgical stabilization of the spine and advances in medical management, the emphasis on the acute care of spinal injured patients is early (once the patient is medically stable) stabilization of the spine to allow early mobilization and to avoid the negative sequelae of bed rest.[11] The effects of early decompression and stabilization in spinal injured patients on eventual neurologic recovery is controversial.[8] It has been shown, however, that high-dose methylprednisone given acutely after a spinal cord injury does enhance neurologic recovery at both 6 weeks and 6 months.[3]

To communicate accurately about spinal cord–injured patients, it is necessary to understand the classification of spinal cord injury levels. Patients with cervical spinal cord injuries usually have both upper and lower extremity paralysis (quadriplegia) or weakness (quadriparesis). Patients with thoracic or lumbar spinal cord injuries have only lower extremity paralysis (paraplegia) or weakness (paraparesis). In describing

spinal cord–injured patients, a functional level is used rather than an anatomic level (Table 25.1). For example, a C6 quadriplegic denotes a patient with a C6 motor functional level (wrist extension functionally present) rather than an injury at the C6 vertebral body level. Grading of muscle strength is done with a uniform scale (Table 25.2).

Each level of spinal cord injury has specific motor (Table 25.3) and sensory physical findings. A spinal cord injury is complete if there is no neurologic function below the physiologic level of injury. Spinal cord injury is incomplete if there is some residual nonfunctional motor or sensory function below the lowest functional level of injury. For example, a C5 quadriplegic is complete if he has grade IV biceps function but no active motor or sensory function distal to the C5 level, whereas a C6 quadriplegic is incomplete if he has grade IV wrist extension but no active motor or sensory function distal to the C6 level with the exception of grade II ankle dorsiflexion and minimally intact perianal sensation. In addition, there are clinical syndromes with spinal cord injuries associated with specific anatomic injuries to the spinal cord. Brown-Sequard syndrome consists of ipsilateral paresis, ipsilateral corticospinal signs, contralateral pain and temperature loss, and ipsilateral loss of vibration and proprioception. A central cord syndrome consists of paresis greater in the upper extremities rather than the lower extremities with patch sensory loss below the level of injury. Anterior cord syndrome consists of complete paralysis after the injury with mild-to-moderate impairment to pinprick and light touch below the level of injury with preservation of proprioception and vibratory sense. Posterior cord syndrome consists of pain and paresthesia in the neck, upper extremities, and trunk with usual symmetric involved mild paresis.

In addition to the obvious motor paralysis and sensory loss that occurs in spinal cord injury, spinal cord–injured patients may have other significant physiologic

Table 25.1. Motor key muscles

C2	—
C3	—
C4	—
C5	Elbow flexors
C6	Wrist extensors
C7	Elbow extensors
C8	Finger flexors (distal phalanx of middle finger)
T1	Finger abductors (fifth digit)
T2	—
T3	—
T4	—
T5	—
T6	—
T7	—
T8	—
T9	—
T10	—
T11	—
T12	—
L1	—
L2	Hip flexors
L3	Knee extensors
L4	Ankle dorsiflexors
L5	Long toe flexors
S1	Ankle plantar flexors

Table 25.2. Grading of muscle strengths

0	Total paralysis
1	Visible or palpable contraction
2	Active movement, gravity eliminated
3	Active movement against gravity
4	Active movement against resistance
5	Active movement against full resistance

Table 25.3. Frankel grades

A	Complete neurologic injury
B	Preserved sensation distal to level of injury
C	Preserved motor nonfunctional
D	Preserved motor functional
E	Normal

problems, including loss of voluntary control of bladder and bowel, impaired sexual function, and, in high quadriplegics (proximal to the C5 level) impaired pulmonary function (because C4-5 innervates the diaphragm). In cervical spine injuries, the autonomic nervous system may be injured, resulting in autonomic dysreflexia (systemic hypertension, usually associated with noxious stimuli such as a distended bladder) or impaired temperature regulation. The sensory loss that occurs in spinal cord injuries often results in loss of

protective sensation. The skin capillary pressure is much less than the pressure over the ischial tuberosities with sitting. Therefore, spinal cord–injured patients must consciously relieve pressure over bony prominences to avoid pressure sores.

The rehabilitation, specifically the orthotic management, of the spinal cord–injured patient should emphasize achievable goals. In theory, a C6 quadriplegic (functional wrist extension) is the highest-level injury compatible with independent living. Independent living for a quadriplegic requires the ability to transfer from bed to wheelchair. Therefore, the primary goal of initial rehabilitation may be independent transfers instead of orthosis-assisted ambulation. Yet the goal of most spinal cord–injured patients, especially in the early rehabilitation period, is ambulation, although the increased energy demands with orthosis-assisted ambulation may preclude functional ambulation. The goal of the lower extremity orthotic management in the spinal cord–injured patient is to prevent contractures in the early period after a spinal cord injury and to enhance function during the later phases of spinal cord injury management.

LOWER EXTREMITY ORTHOTIC MANAGEMENT OF ACUTE SPINAL CORD INJURY

The management of lower extremity musculoskeletal injuries in patients with spinal cord injury, similar to patients with traumatic brain injury, usually requires operative stabilization of fractures.[5] Patients with spinal cord injury, similar to patients with traumatic brain injury, often have desensate limbs, and circular casts or orthoses to treat lower extremity injuries during the acute period after injury should be used with caution because unrecognized compartment syndromes may occur. In addition, significant spasticity in the lower extremity after spinal cord injury may preclude nonoperative treatment of lower extremity injuries, and pulmonary function is enhanced with early operative stabilization of lower extremity fractures.[5]

Spasticity that occurs after spinal cord injury is a significant problem in the immediate period following spinal cord injury. Spasticity that occurs after spinal cord injury is caused by a net reduction of the inhibitory influences on alpha and gamma motor neurons resulting in hyperreflexive peripheral reflexes. Spasticity in the lower extremities after spinal cord injury results in characteristic posturing of the legs, with the foot held in maximal equinovarus. If left untreated, this abnormal posturing leads to permanent contractures in a matter of weeks.[6] The clinical sequelae of contractures may be significant if neurologic recovery occurs (or even if no recovery occurs because an equinovarus contracture may preclude shoewear or independent transfer). Even a relatively small (15 degrees) plantar contracture of the foot results in a cascade of gait abnormalities if the spinal cord–injured patient recovers to an ambulatory state. There is increased weight bearing across the metatarsal heads, compensatory recurvatum of the knee, and even increased strain in the paravertebral muscles of the lumbar spine.[30]

The treatment of acute lower extremity spasticity after a spinal cord injury has usually involved medical treatment (diazepam or baclofen), physical therapy, or inhibitory casts. Usually medical treatment of spasticity is contraindicated in the acute period after a spinal cord injury, and inhibitory casts should be used with caution after an acute spinal cord injury for the same reasons that circular casts should be avoided in the treatment of fractures in desensate limbs.[22] Phenol intraneural motor blocks can be used to decrease spasticity temporarily until either neurologic recovery occurs or definitive surgical treatment can be done.[23]

Well-padded lower extremity orthoses can be used to position the extremity in a position of function. Often a simple ankle-foot orthosis (AFO) with the foot in neutral position is all that is necessary. An orthosis, as opposed to a cast, allows for frequent skin inspection and evaluation for possible compartment syndrome.

ORTHOSES FOR LATE SPINAL CORD INJURY

The major use of lower extremity orthoses in the rehabilitation of patients with spinal cord injury after the acute period of injury is the treatment of spasticity or paresis. An AFO is the most commonly used orthosis for spinal cord–injured patients, and it is used to treat ankle spasticity, impaired ankle dorsiflexion during swing, weak ankle plantar flexion, or impaired proprioception. Occasionally a knee-ankle-foot orthosis (KAFO) is used for weak quadriceps to stabilize the limb during stance and provide a swing-through gait. Often an AFO is used in the spinal cord–injured patient during the period in which normal neurologic recovery can occur (18 months after the acute injury). At that time, definitive surgical treatment for the equinovarus of the ankle after spinal cord injuries can be done (split anterior tibial tendon transfer, toe flexor release, Achilles' tendon lengthening) with uniformly satisfactory functional outcome.[22]

Almost without exception, the question of orthosis-assisted ambulation is encountered with the spinal cord–injured patient. The decision whether to proceed with or abandon consideration of orthosis-assisted ambulation in the spinal cord–injured patient is complex.[42] Although it has been shown that orthosis-assisted ambulation in significantly injured quadriplegics is usually not feasible, it may be useful at least initially to attempt orthosis-assisted ambulation in these patients for psychological reasons.[42]

When these individuals subsequently use primarily wheelchair locomotion, they will have the satisfaction of at least attempting orthosis-assisted ambulation. In addition, orthosis-assisted ambulation has other benefits besides walking. Orthosis-assisted standing can prevent joint contractures, decrease osteoporosis, prevent urinary tract infections, and increase cardiopulmonary function.[9] In the pediatric spinal cord–injured patient, orthosis-assisted standing can enhance the development of trunk and head control.[15]

Although the paraplegia associated with myelodysplasia occurs from a different cause than traumatic spinal cord injury, it is useful to compare functional outcomes in two groups of paraplegics from myelodysplasia, one ambulatory with an orthosis and the other wheelchair-dependent. The group who used orthosis-assisted ambulation had fewer pressure sores and less fractures than the group that was wheelchair dependent.[20,21]

It is necessary to evaluate fully orthosis-assisted ambulation in neurologically injured patients. The end functional outcome both physiologically and psychologically must justify the time and expense of orthosis-assisted ambulation. The psychological benefits from orthosis-assisted ambulation in patients with spinal cord injuries may not be as beneficial as one might predict.[26]

ORTHOTIC DESIGNS FOR SPINAL CORD

Orthoses used to provide swing-through gait

KAFOs. Bilateral KAFOs remain a common prescription for paraplegics and are used to provide stability at the knees and ankles. In addition, many patients who have weakness of the hips and trunk can use KAFOs and achieve a stable upright posture as the hips become stable when the center of gravity falls posterior to them during stance. This is achieved in practice by the patient standing with the hips anterior and by positioning the lumbar spine in lordosis. When crutches are in front of the trunk, stability is achieved by the forces of gravity pulling the hips into extension. After swinging through, the patient is stable with the crutches behind, a lordotic posture is adopted, and the hips are locked by the extension moment that is created by the force line falling behind the hip joint. The specific design of the KAFO used by paraplegics can be variable and mainly is dictated by regional practice.

Paraplegics, using a *swing-through gait,* typically require bilateral KAFOs in the absence of sufficient quadriceps strength to stabilize the knees during stance. Not only must the arms lift and swing the body forward in the swing phase, but also they must provide antigravity support during the stance phase if the hip and trunk extensors are paralyzed. Perry[29] has shown increased energy requirements, with a swing-through gait. As a result, paraplegics who use a swing-through gait compensate by decreasing gait velocity or cease to ambulate at all.

Conventional HKAFOs.   As paraplegics can attain an upright posture and ambulation without a pelvic band, the effect of adding a pelvic band and hip joints was found to be of limited help and should not be prescribed routinely.[44] This conclusion was made after applying an electrogoniometer to the backs of spinal cord–injured patients to estimate the maximal excursion of the lumbar spine throughout the gait cycle. When the patient walked with the pelvic band and locked hip joints, mean stride and center of gravity pathway amplitude were increased. Removing the pelvic band reduced the amplitude of the center of gravity pathway because mobility was increased at the hips, allowing the individual to clear the ground more easily during the swing phase. Another important difference related to donning and doffing time, with an increased time required for the HKAFO variant. The pelvic band did, however, improve standing balance, particularly in the spastic patient. Clinically, it is evident that adult spinal cord–injured patients rarely use conventional HKAFOs because little evidence indicates that walking is significantly improved. The benefit of controlling hip and pelvic motion to allow ambulation must be balanced against the problems associated with the restriction of movement that is vital for the paralyzed individual attempting to be independent in a sitting position.

Orthoses that allow reciprocal gait

Hip guidance orthosis or parawalker.   The hip guidance orthosis (HGO) or parawalker (Fig. 25.1) was developed at the Orthotic Research and Locomotor Assessment Unit (ORLAU) in Oswestry, England.[37]

The essential features of the orthosis are:
1. A rigid body component, which helps maintain the relative abduction of the legs during the swing phase of the gait cycle.
2. A hip joint with a limited flexion/extension range and friction-free operation.

Rose[35–40] outlined the theoretic means by which ambulation might be achieved by paraplegics with stabilized knees and identified the following criteria:
1. The hip must be placed ahead of the foot.
2. One foot must be raised from the ground by a combination of:

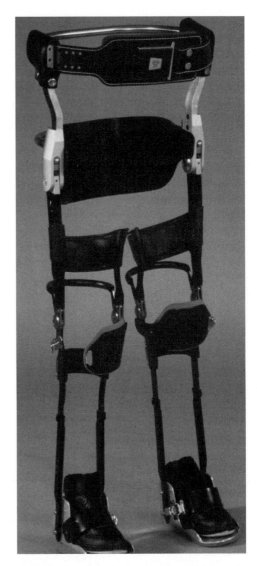

Fig. 25.1.   Hip guidance orthosis/parawalker.

A. Downward pressure by ipsilateral arm and crutch.
B. Body sway to contralateral side.
C. Provision of dihedral wedge under the sole of the contralateral shoe.

In these circumstances, under the influence of gravity, the lifted leg swings forward and can be grounded.

The rigidity of the orthosis as it relates to the capability of the patient to clear the contralateral limb is perhaps the most important aspect of its design. Whittle and Cochrane[47] noted this as probably the most important mechanical difference between the HGO and the reciprocating gait orthosis (RGO). Jefferson and Whittle[13] evaluated a single paraplegic patient with an HGO and found that the legs remain essentially parallel in the coronal plane during swing, giving better ground clearance.

The HGO enables the paraplegic patient to walk independently with a reciprocal gait.[45] This orthosis also provides a form of low energy cost walking because the patient does not have to lift body weight off the ground in swing phase walking. Watkins and coworkers,[45] in a study of almost 200 paraplegics, concluded the HGO works effectively to enable thoracic-level complete paraplegics to undertake therapeutic walking.

A clinical review of 20 adult traumatic paraplegics[43] with neurologically complete lesions C8-T12 demonstrated not only that the HGO is capable of affording reciprocal gait to adult paraplegics, but also the patients continue to ambulate, as 85% of the patients were still using the orthosis at 20 months' follow-up. In addition, patients achieved independent use of the orthosis with low-energy ambulation both indoors and outdoors on a variety of surfaces.

Louisiana State University reciprocating gait orthosis. Douglas and associates[9] described the Louisiana State University (LSU) RGO (Fig. 25.2) as a lightweight bracing system that gives structural support to the lower trunk and lower limbs of the paralytic patient while allowing, through a cable-coupling system, proper hip joint motion for walking.[49] The LSU RGO is designed in such a manner that flexion of one leg results in extension of the other. This is achieved by coupling both hip joints together using two Bowden cables to transmit the necessary forces. It is important to note that the original design used only one cable; however, continual failure resulted in the addition of a second cable. It is believed that the cause of failure in the single-cable systems were kinks and subsequent metal fatigue in the cables that developed as a result of the free hyperextension permitted. Joining the hip joints together also eliminates simultaneous hip flexion, which is one means of differentiating between the HGO and any variant of RGO.

In general, the LSU RGO has been used by children with myelodysplasia who would otherwise be unable to walk, but yet possess sufficient upper extremity strength to use crutches to maintain their balance. Douglas and associates[91] fitted the brace successfully in 138 patients (Table 25.4), reporting that long-term bracing and early ambulation seem to decrease the potential for the recurrence of limb deformity in children, possibly by preventing distortions caused by gravitational positioning of flexed joints. He also reported a series of seven adult paraplegics who were fitted with the LSU RGO who were able to walk 1000 feet with no more than two 30-second rest periods. Average training time in the use of the orthosis was 45 hours.

Functional walking was attained by 40 patients using the RGO,[27] 22 of whom had myelodysplasia. The majority of patients were reported as having thoraco-

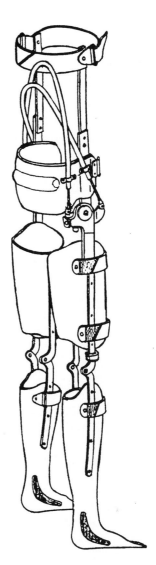

Fig. 25.2. Louisiana State University reciprocating gait orthosis.

Table 25.4. Louisiana State University reciprocating gate orthosis	
CONDITION	**NO. OF PATIENTS**
Spina bifida	95
Paraplegia	18
Muscular dystrophy	15
Cerebral palsy	8
Multiple sclerosis	1
Sacral agenesis	1

columbar or high lumbar lesions. Structural failure was reported in three instances. The LSU RGO has been shown to provide reciprocal gait for both adult and pediatric paraplegics. It is necessary, however, to balance extravagant claims for the LSU RGO and realistic goals for the paraplegic potential ambulator.[28]

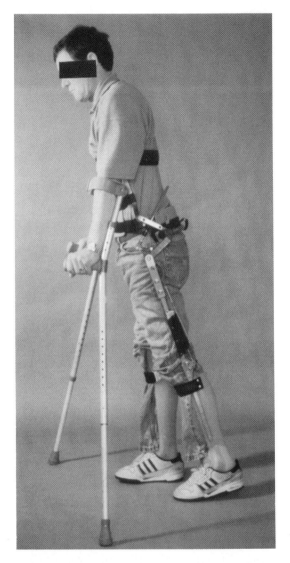

Fig. 25.3. Advanced reciprocating gait orthosis (*Note:* shown over clothes for illustration purposes).

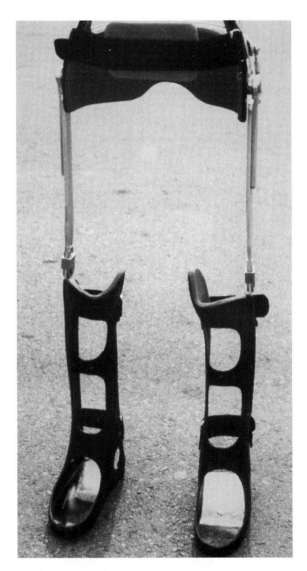

Fig. 25.4. Reciprocating gait orthosis with isocentric bearing; adult version. (*Courtesy of W. Motloch.*)

Steeper advanced reciprocating gait orthoses. The advanced reciprocating gait orthosis (ARGO) (Fig. 25.3) has been developed by Hugh Steeper Ltd, London, and can best be described as a modified LSU RGO. A single *push-pull* cable is used to link the mechanical hip joints; it was hoped by the developers that this mechanism would improve the efficiency of motion as it is transferred from one mechanical joint to another with perhaps a corresponding improvement in performance. The most obvious *improvement* that has been reported by the few investigators who have examined this design is the ease it confers on rising from a sitting position and, conversely, on sitting down again after standing.[13,18] This is achieved in practice by linking the hip and knee joints, via cables, and using the addition of pneumatic struts to assist knee extension. The arrangement allows, and assists, the patient to

stand directly from a sitting position, in which the knees are typically flexed, without prior manual straightening and locking of the knees.

Although the major components of this orthosis are available from the manufacturer, the AFO component must be custom-made. The importance of patient assessment before prescription is emphasised in two published reports,[16,18] and it is suggested that this is best accomplished by employing a multidisciplinary clinic team to determine the feasibility of ambulation with orthotic management.[18]

Isocentric reciprocating gait orthosis. The isocentric reciprocating gait orthosis (IRGG) (Figs. 25.4 and 25.5) is a further modification of the LSU RGO. In this variant, the two crossed Bowden cables are replaced by a centrally pivoting bar and tie rod arrangement. The result of this modification is an orthosis that

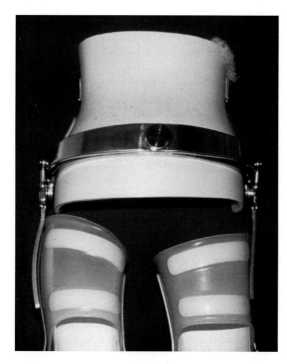

Fig. 25.5. Reciprocating gait orthosis with isocentric bearing; posterior view showing bearing attached to custom-made proximal component; pediatric version.

is much more rigid than the LSU design, while closely resembling the inherent rigidity, and associated advantages, of the HGO. To date, sufficient scientific data do not exist to support this claim; however, it may be that this design, which combines rigidity with a low friction mechanism coupling the mechanical hip joints together, may provide additional advantages.

Comparative studies

The focus of comparative studies has been to compare orthoses in terms of energy expenditure with orthosis-assisted ambulation. Varying designs of orthoses are capable of affording reciprocal gait patterns to both adult and pediatric paraplegics; the important variable is functional outcome, best evaluated by energy-expenditure studies.

Comparing HGO and LSU RGO. Relative oxygen cost (mL/kg/M) was compared in five paraplegic subjects,[2] four children and one adult, while wearing an RGO and HGO while ambulating. An oxylog was used to record oxygen consumption while the subjects ambulated during steady-state. Although all of the subjects trained and used the orthoses for varying amounts of time, the trend from these data shows that the HGO provides a more energy-efficient gait. On the average, the oxygen cost while using the HGO was 27% less compared to the LSU RGO. The reductions in oxygen ranged from 12% to 42%. Following this trend of greater efficiency, the subjects ambulated, on average, 33% faster with the HGO than with the LSU RGO.

These preliminary results indicate that the HGO appears to be a more efficient orthosis for level ambulation in the paraplegic population.

In 1989, the Department of Health and Social Security in the United Kingdom commissioned an extensive comparative trial of both orthoses. The trial took almost 2 years and was completed at the Nuffield Orthopaedic Centre, Oxford, England. Eighteen male and four female paraplegic subjects used each orthosis for 4 months in a crossover study. Clinical, ergonomic, biomechanical, psychological, and economic assessments were performed at appropriate stages on each patient who completed the trial. Fifteen subjects were able to use both orthoses, five were unable to use either, and two succeeded with the HGO and not the LSU RGO. At the end of the trial, 12 subjects chose to keep the LSU RGO, four the HGO, and six neither.[47]

Those choosing the LSU RGO preferred its appearance; those choosing the HGO preferred its speed of donning and doffing. Jefferson and Whittle[13] commented that intersubject differences were much greater than interorthosis differences, but the biomechanical assessments demonstrated that the patterns of movement were not identical in the two orthoses. No children were used in this study, despite the fact that both systems were designed for the pediatric paraplegic patient. It is not therefore possible to draw conclusions relative to either system in the pediatric patient.

Comparing HGO, LSU RGO, and ARGO. Biomechanical analyses were done on three orthoses in terms of general gait parameters and movement of the lower limbs and pelvis.[13] This single case study was of an adult paraplegic who was a proficient user of all three systems. The subject for this study was a 33-year-old man with a traumatic T5 complete lesion. Comparison was made between the HGO, the LSU RGO, and the ARGO.

In terms of general gait parameters, the differences between the orthoses are small; this conclusion was reached using measurements taken from videotape and VICON data. Relative to pattern of movement, this study reported stride length in orthoses to be similar, a smaller range of pelvic motion in the HGO, and a more fluent gait in the HGO. Analyses of hip joint motion in the sagittal plane indicated that the major difference in hip joint motion is the smaller degree of hip extension in the HGO.

Analyses in the coronal plane and the observation that hip abduction in the HGO is greater than that in the RGO is important. In the HGO, the lower extremities remain essentially parallel, making it easier to clear the ground. The pattern of gait was best with the HGO, that with the LSU RGO being slightly better than the ARGO. The main advantage of the ARGO was the greatly improved ease of standing up and sitting down.

This study concentrated on *objective measurement* in a single case study. It is one of few attempts to establish a theoretic base on which to base orthotic prescription for this patient group; the conclusions reached are therefore important.

Comparing LSU RGO and IRGO. A study[46] examined the energy cost of walking in four subjects using the LSU RGO and the IRGO. In this study, the physiological cost index (PCI) was significantly lower during ambulation trials with the IRGO compared to the LSU RGO. This was the only measurement that detected a significant difference between the two designs. Other variables, such as gait velocity, cadence, and step length, were similar in both braces. The methods, testing procedures, and data analysis that were used for this study suggest that PCI can be used as a sensitive indicator of gait efficiency in spinal cord–injured subjects. It would be dangerous, however, to make conclusions that are based on such a small sample size relative to the benefit of one design over another. It is not clear whether the reported advantages related directly to replacing the cables or whether the increased rigidity of the IRGO contributed directly to the reduction in the PCI.

The box at the top of the page lists orthotic designs for spinal cord injured patients.

FUNCTIONAL ELECTRICAL OR NEUROMUSCULAR STIMULATION

The most contemporary means of affording an upright posture and reciprocal gait pattern for a paraplegic patient is through the use of functional neuromuscular, or electrical, stimulation. Functional electrical stimulation (FES) was applied in 50 patients with spinal cord injury in an effort to restore standing and walking.[14] It was reported that all patients in the program with lesions in the range from T4-12 were able to stand by means of FES. Walking using a four-channel stimulator

was accomplished by 25 patients with lesions in the range T4-12. These 25 patients represent approximately 5% of all spinal cord injured patients treated in the authors' rehabilitation facility during this time period. After using the stimulation in a home environment for more than 3 months, the number of patients who continued to use the stimulation for walking declined, and 16 patients remained ambulatory. The discontinuance of FES was mainly because of the time required to put on and operate the FES system and difficulties adapting to a new home environment and living situation.

The use of FES to enable paraplegics to stand is not new or difficult to initiate. There are substantial problems to overcome, however, before such systems can be used routinely by patients without supervision.[10] Patient safety and cost are the most important variables to control in designing FES-orthosis ambulatory. Software to allow closed-loop controlled standing of midthoracic paraplegics using a modified PID controller allowed paraplegics to stand and sit outside the laboratory environment.[5,10]

Marsolais and Edwards[19] compared energy costs of walking and standing with functional neuromuscular stimulation and long leg braces by studying four paraplegic subjects with neurologically complete spinal cord injuries ranging from T4-11. The subjects were implanted with percutaneous intramuscular electrodes in the quadriceps, tensor fascia latae, sartorius, gracilis, semimembranosus, posterior portion of adductor magnus, gluteus maximus and medius, and soleus and tibialis anterior. Subjects followed an outpatient program of electrical stimulation exercise and gait training, which required 15 to 20 hours per week. This study concluded that FES walking was a viable alternative to bilateral KAFOs, and in the future major energy cost reduction should be possible. The main physiologic problem associated with FES are muscle atrophy and muscle fatigue. The main technical problems are providing adequate electrical stimulation, developing sensitive control systems, and protecting the patient in the event of system or power failure. Although FES may eventually prove to be the best system of all, much more research needs to be carried out before it can be considered to be a practical alternative.

FUNCTIONAL ELECTRICAL STIMULATION AND HYBRID SYSTEMS

Neither FES used independently nor FES used in combination with an orthosis (i.e., hybrid system) is currently being used to provide ambulation for the pediatric paraplegic. Both systems are, however, under clinical and scientific evaluation and are being used specifically for the traumatic adult paraplegic in whom typically the lower motor neurone is intact.

Both the HGO and the LSU RGO have been augmented by the addition of FES in an attempt to overcome the shortcomings of both modes of management used independently.[12,24,25,31–34] The hypothesis among researchers is that hybrid systems will afford a more energy-efficient gait.

Hirokawa and colleagues[12] conclude that the FES-powered LSU RGO combines the advantages of a passive mechanical orthosis with those of FES to provide substantial improvements in energy cost, which may provide paraplegic persons with a mode of independent ambulation superior to the wheelchair. Petrofsky and Smith[31] indicated after conducting electromyography studies that the activity in upper body muscles was much higher when walking in LSU RGOs without FES than in LSU RGOs with FES.

Nene and Patrick[25] have indicated through comparative analyses that FES augmentation yields only a small reduction in energy cost. Its long-term physiologic effect could be significant in increasing the aerobic-anaerobic threshold of an individual via recruitment of large muscles such as the gluteus maximus and medius, thereby increasing performance in a sustained activity such as walking.

Andrews and colleagues[1] described a hybrid FES orthosis comprising a rigid AFO, a multichannel FES stimulator with surface electrodes, body mounted sensors, a rule-based controller, and an electrocutaneous display for supplementary sensory feedback. The mechanical component provides stability without FES activation of muscles for standing postures normally adopted by patients. This system featured a control mode to initiate and terminate flexion of the leg during forward progression. Preliminary results of laboratory tests for two spinal cord–injured subjects were presented indicating that by using this combination of FES and AFO, the duration of the cycle of stimulation delivered to the quadriceps was greatly reduced during standing and walking. This avoided fatigue and prolonged the time for which the device could be used. The quadriceps were stimulated in an on/off manner, thus eliminating the need for periodic adjustment of stimulus intensity.

The hybrid approach perhaps shows the greatest potential, and the use of such devices may improve the walking of those already using a purely mechanical system and may extend the use of orthoses to those unable to use them at present. Control of the stimulation may be by a press button on the handle of the walking aid or by some form of automatic control.

SUMMARY

Few areas of orthotic management have attracted as much interest during the past two decades as the development of *improved and advanced* orthoses for the adult patient with a spinal cord injury. Despite this considerable activity and associated expense, research and clinical experience indicate that most paraplegic individuals opt for wheelchair mobility after discharge to the community because this provides a faster, safer, and more practical means of mobility with considerably less energy expenditure.

The *HGO/parawalker* provides better ground clearance, perhaps the smoothest gait pattern; however, mechanical rigidity is possible only with significant cosmetic deficit. The improved cosmesis of the *LSU RGO* is preferred by patients. Its mechanical reliability, however, has been questioned in the literature. The main advantage of the *ARGO* is the reported ease of standing up and sitting down. The *IRGO* attempts to combine the mechanical advantages of the HGO with the cosmetic and therapeutic advantages of other RGOs. *Perhaps the most important finding that is common to all of the comparative studies is that in terms of general gait parameters, the differences between all the contemporary orthotic options are small.*

Most authors agree that the extent to which walking is a practical method of mobility after spinal cord injury depends on the energy costs involved. Therefore, it is difficult to envisage any of the current orthotic options replacing the wheelchair as the principal and preferred choice of paraplegic individuals in the immediate future. The anticipated promise of FES has not been realized because control problems prevent everyday use outside the laboratory setting. Important advantages have been related to hybrid systems that combine orthoses and FES.

Although considerable progress has been made, orthoses for spinal cord–injured patients are bulky, the associated energy expenditure is significant, ambulation is slow, and the perceived physiologic advantages require scientific validation. Because spinal cord injuries are the most devastating injuries to occur in a mostly young population, however, attempts to develop orthoses to allow ambulation will continue.

REFERENCES

1. Andrews BJ, et al: Hybrid FES orthosis incorporating closed loop control and sensory feedback, J Biomed Eng 10:189–195, 1987.
2. Banta JV, et al: Parawalker: Energy cost of walking, Eur J Pediatr Surg 1:7–10, 1991.
3. Barckeu M, et al: A randomized, controlled trial of methylprednisolone or naloxone in the treatment of acute spinal cord injury, N Engl J Med 322:1405–1411, 1990.
4. Beckman J: The Louisiana State University reciprocating gait orthosis, Physiotherapy 73:386–392, 1987.

5. Botte M, Moore T: The orthopaedic management of extremity injuries in head trauma, J Head Trauma Rehabil 2:13–21, 1987.

6. Botte M, Nickel V, Akeson W: Spasticity and contracture: Physiologic aspects of formation, Clin Orthop 233:7–14, 1987.

7. Burney R, et al: Incidence, characteristics and outcome of spinal cord injuries at trauma centers in North America, Arch Surg 128:596–601, 1993.

8. Doerr T, et al: Spinal cord decompression in traumatic thoracolumbar burst fractures: Posterior distraction rods versus transpedicle screw fixation, J Orthop Trauma 5:403–411, 1991.

9. Douglas R, et al: The LSU reciprocation gait orthosis, Orthopedics 6:834–839, 1983.

10. Ewins DJ, et al: Practical low cost stand/sit system for midthoracic paraplegics, J Biomed Eng 10:184–188, 1988.

11. Garfin S, et al: Care of the multiple injured patient with spinal cord injury, Clin Orthop 239:19–29, 1989.

12. Hirokawa S, et al: Energy consumption in paraplegic ambulation using the reciprocating gait orthosis and electrical stimulation of the thigh muscles, Arch Phys Med Rehabil 71:687–694, 1990.

13. Jefferson RJ, Whittle MW: Performance of three walking orthoses for the paralysed: A case study using gait analysis, Prosthet Orthot Int 14:103–110, 1990.

14. Kralj A, Bajd T, Turk R: Enhancement of gait restoration in spinal injured patients by functional electrical stimulation, Clin Orthop Rel Res 233:34–43, 1988.

15. Letts RM, Fulford R, Hobson DA: Mobility aids for the paraplegic child, J Bone Joint Surg 58A:38–41, 1976.

16. Lissens MA, et al: Advanced reciprocating gait orthoses in paraplegic patients, Proceedings of the 7th World Congress of ISPO, Chicago, 1992.

17. Major RE, Stallard J, Rose GK: The dynamics of walking using the hip guidance orthosis (hgo) with crutches, Prosthet Orthot Int 5:19–22, 1981.

18. Marlor JE: The Steeper advanced reciprocating gait orthoses for the spinal cord injured patient: a nineties approach, Proceedings of the 7th World Congress of ISPO, Chicago, 1992.

19. Marsolais EB, Edwards BG: Energy costs of walking and standing with functional neuromuscular stimulation and long leg braces, Arch Phys Med Rehabil 69:243–249, 1988.

20. Mazur JM, et al: Orthopaedic management of high-level spina bifida: Early walking compared with early use of a wheelchair, J Bone Joint Surg 71A:56–61, 1989.

21. Menelaus MB: The orthopaedic management of spina bifida cystica, Edinburgh, 1980, Churchill Livingstone.

22. Moore T: Acquired neurologic disorders of the adult foot. In Mann R, editor: The surgery of the foot and ankle, ed 6, St. Louis, 1993, Mosby.

23. Moore T, Anderson R: The use of open pleural blocks to the motor branches of the tibial nerve in adult acquired spasticity, Foot Ankle 11:219–224, 1991.

24. Nene AV, Patrick JH: Energy cost of paraplegic locomotion with the ORLAU parawalker, Paraplegia 27:5–18, 1989.

25. Nene AV, Patrick JH: Energy cost of paraplegic locomotion using the parawalker-electrical stimulation "hybrid orthosis," Arch Phys Med Rehabil 71:116–120, 1990.

26. Ogilvie C, et al: Orthotic compensation for non-functioning hip extensors, Zeitschnft fur Kindercherungil 2:33–35, 1988.

27. Ogilvie C, Bowker P, Rowley DI: The physiological benefits of paraplegic orthotically aided walking, Paraplegia 31:111–115, 1993.

28. Patrick JH: Developmental research in paraplegic walking, BMJ 292:788, 1986.

29. Perry J: Gait analysis, normal and pathological function, Thorofare, NJ, 1992, Slack, Inc.

30. Perry J: Contractures: An historical perspective, Clin Orthop 219:8–21, 1987.

31. Petrofsky JS, Smith JB: Physiological costs of computer-controlled walking in persons with paraplegia using a reciprocating-gait orthosis, Arch Phys Med Rehabil 72:890–896, 1991.

32. Phillips CA: Functional electrical stimulation and lower extremity bracing for ambulation exercise of the spinal cord injured individual: A medically prescribed system, Phys Ther 60:842–849, 1989.

33. Phillips CA: Electrical muscle stimulation in combination with a reciprocating gait orthosis for ambulation by paraplegics, J Biomed Eng 11:338–344, 1989.

34. Phillips CA, Mendershot DM: Functional electrical stimulation and reciprocating gait orthosis for ambulation exercise in a tetraplegic patient: A case study, Paraplegia 29:268–276, 1991.

35. Rose G: Splintage for severe spina bifida cystica, J Bone Joint Surg 52B:178–179, 1970.

36. Rose GK: Surgical/orthotic management of spina bifida. In Murdoch G, editor: The advance in orthotics, 1976.

37. Rose GK: The principles and practice of hip guidance articulations, Prosthet Orthot Int 3:37–43, 1979.

38. Rose GK: Orthoses for the severely handicapped, rational or empirical choice, Physiotherapy 66:76–81, 1980.

39. Rose GK, Stallard J, Sankarankutty M: Clinical evaluation of spina bifida patients using hip guidance orthosis, Dev Med Child Neurol 23:30–40, 1981.

40. Rose GK, Sankarankutty M, Stallard J: A clinical review of the orthotic treatment of myelomeningocele patients, J Bone Joint Surg 242–246, 1983.

41. Solomonow M, et al: The RGO generation: II. Muscle stimulation powered orthosis as a practical walking system for thoracic paraplegics, Orthopedics 12:1309–1315, 1989.

42. Somers MF: Spinal cord injury, Norwalk, CT, 1992, Appleton & Lange.

43. Summers BN, McClelland MR, Masri WS: A clinical review of the adult hip guidance orthosis (parawalker) in traumatic paraplegics, Paraplegia 26:19–26, 1988.

44. Warren CG, Lehmann JF, Lateur BJ: Pelvic band use in orthotics for adult paraplegic patients, Arch Phys Med Rehabil 56:221–223, 1975.

45. Watkins EM, Edwards DE, Patrick JH: Parawalker paraplegic walking, Physiotherapy 73:99–100, 1987.

46. Winchester PK, et al: A comparison of paraplegic gait performance using two types of reciprocating gait orthoses, Prosthet Orthot Int 17:101–106, 1993.

47. Whittle MW, Cochrane GM: A comparative evaluation of the hip guidance orthosis (HGO) and the reciprocating gait orthosis (RGO), Health Equipment Information No. 192, Longod, National Health Service Procurement Directorate, 1989.

48. Whittle MW, et al: A comparative trial of two walking systems for paralysed people, Paraplegia 29:97–102, 1991

49. Yngve DA, Roberts JM, Douglas R: The reciprocating gait orthosis in myelomeningocele, J Pediatr Orthop 4:304–310, 1984.

Functional Bracing of Lower Extremity Fractures

Thomas J. Moore

The orthopedic world has been divided into the "movers" and the "resters" in the treatment of lower extremity fractures.[29] In the past decades, the resters predominated because it was thought necessary to immobilize fractures, including the joints proximal and distal to the fracture, to insure fracture healing. Before the era of functional fracture bracing and internal fixation of diaphyseal femur and tibial fractures, orthopedic management of these fractures consisted primarily of long-term traction for femur fractures and long leg casts, immobilizing both the knee and the ankle, for tibial fractures.

Partially owing to the realization that joint function is improved with motion rather than immobilization, the movers became preeminent in orthopedics in more recent decades.[29] Advances in operative management of diaphyseal lower extremity fractures, including internal fixation with compression plating, external fixation of severe open fractures, and intramedullary fixation of both femoral and tibial fractures, have allowed early mobilization of joints. The advent of functional bracing of lower extremity fractures in the 1960s has emphasized early weight bearing and early motion of joints in the treatment of lower extremity fractures.[14,31,36,37]

Immobilization of normal joints, even for a relatively short time (3 weeks), leads to intra-articular adhesions and eventual deterioration of hyaline cartilage.[6,28] In experimentally induced damage to hyaline cartilage, immobilization of the joint results in repair of the injured cartilage with fibrous tissue.[28] In contrast, in joints with experimentally induced hyaline cartilage defects, continuous passive motion induces repair tissue superior to the repair tissue that occurs with either immobilization or intermittent motion.[28] Continuous passive motion–mediated repair tissue is superior in structural integrity and is less susceptible to late post-traumatic arthritic changes than repair tissue formed after immobilization or intermittent motion.[28] In addi-

tion, controlled motion has been shown to enhance ligament and tendon healing.[7,39] Although there have not been studies that specifically show enhanced articular function in the joints proximal and distal to a diaphyseal fracture treated with motion of the joints rather than immobilization, it seems reasonable to expect superior function in these joints allowed early motion.

Functional bracing of fractures is a method of fracture care that requires attention to detail as much as operative treatment does. It is a philosophy of fracture management that requires knowledge of the physiology of fracture healing, especially the enhanced osteogenesis that occurs with controlled motion in a functional brace. The basis for functional bracing is that immobilization of adjacent joints in a long bone fracture is not necessary for fracture healing. By use of the soft tissue envelope surrounding a fractured limb, functional bracing achieves fracture stability and controlled motion, which enhances osteogenesis.[34,36,37] The emphasis of functional bracing is early restoration of weight bearing and function in the injured limb to avoid the negative sequelae of immobilization (fracture disease).

Functional bracing uses the compressibility of the soft tissue envelopes surrounding a fractured limb to provide a pseudohydraulic environment that maintains fracture alignment and stability.[36] The intrinsic strength of the soft tissues provides the initial stability of a fractured limb, and the initial shortening that occurs after a fracture remains relatively constant after the initial injury or after stable reduction with functional bracing.[36] Functional braces do not correct shortening in diaphyseal fractures but provide the fracture stability to maintain the initial shortening present after the injury.[33,34] Therefore, if the initial shortening following a tibial diaphyseal fracture is unacceptable, functional bracing and early weight bearing should not be done. Rather, the fracture should be reduced and immobi-

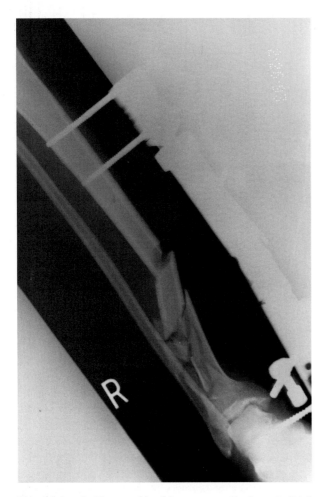

Fig. 26.1. A 25-year-old with an open diaphyseal tibial fracture treated initially with external fixation.

lized in a non–weight-bearing long leg cast to allow soft tissue healing. In some cases, usually open fractures, an external fixator may be used for initial reduction and to gain access for soft tissue reconstruction (Fig. 26.1). After intrinsic stability is gained by soft tissue healing (Fig. 26.2), usually by 3 to 4 weeks, weight bearing and functional activities are begun in a functional brace (Figs. 26.3 to 26.6).

Fracture healing is enhanced by motion.[35] In fractures of bones unable to be immobilized, such as the rib or clavicle, nonunions are rare. The motion at the fracture site that occurs with functional bracing is controlled. There is displacement at the fracture site that occurs with load, but the displacement is recoverable secondary to the elasticity and intrinsic strength of the soft tissues.[33,36,47,49] The mechanism by which increased osteogenesis occurs with this controlled motion is not entirely known, but thermic, mechanical, electrical, chemical, and vascular factors may play a role. The callus that forms with controlled motion of a fracture is biomechanically different than the callus that forms with rigid internal fixation.[33,35]

The fracture callus architecture that forms with controlled motion has enchondral bone formation in the periphery of the callus. In contrast, the callus that forms with rigid fixation of a fracture (dynamic compression plate) is endosteal callus, with minimal peripheral callus. Biomechanically, with bending and torsion, the highest stresses occur in the periphery of the callus, where the callus from controlled motion is the strongest. In animal studies, the torque necessary to refracture limbs treated with either controlled motion or rigid fixation (DCP) was about the same in the acute period after the initial fracture (2 weeks). At 4 weeks, however, the fracture treated with controlled motion had significantly increased resistance to torque in comparison to the fractures treated with rigid fixation.[14,33]

TIBIAL FRACTURES

The tibia is the most frequently fractured long bone. Treatment of tibial fracture has varied through the decades. During the 1970s and early 1980s, the preferred treatment has been closed nonoperative treatment in the major orthopedic textbooks. More recently, there has been a trend of operative treatment of tibial fractures, especially intramedullary nailing.

There has always been significant variances in the criteria for acceptable alignment after a tibial fracture. Satisfactory results in literature has ranged from 10 degrees of varus or valgus malalignment and 20 degrees of malalignment in the antero-posterior plane to anatomic alignment.[10,13,25,26,42,43] Despite the multiple criteria for acceptable alignment in tibial fractures, there are few scientific data about the clinical sequelae of malunited tibial fractures.[8] Ankle impairment, both clinically and experimentally, occurs more frequently than knee impairment with tibial malunions.[15] In long-term follow-up with patients with tibial diaphyseal fractures, greater than 25% had decreased range of motion of the ankle in comparison to the noninjured ankle, whereas less than 3% had decreased range of motion of the knee.[15] Distal one-third tibial malunions increase the likelihood of ankle impairment.[41] Distal one-third tibial malunions decrease tibial talar contact area and increase tibial talar contact pressure, which theoretically leads to degenerative arthritis of the ankle joint.[23,40,41] In contrast, in retrospective studies of healed tibial fractures with long-term follow-up (30 years), there was little correlation between knee pain and radiographic tibial malunion.[13]

The majority of tibial diaphyseal fractures are able to be treated with functional cast bracing. Intra-articular fractures, either tibial plateau or tibial plafond, usually require open reduction and internal fixation. Fractures

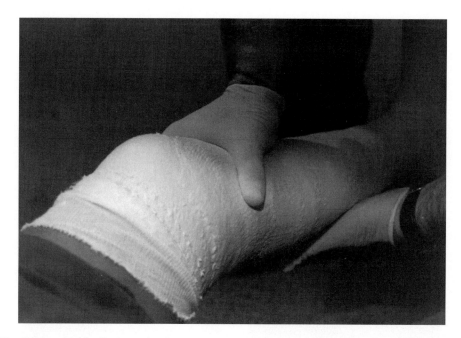

Fig. 26.2. After soft tissue healing (3 weeks after fracture), application of patellar tendon bearing (PTB) cast. It is necessary to apply molding to the cast, especially in the posterior calf and patellar tendon region, to increase the hydrostatic pressure to maintain fracture alignment.

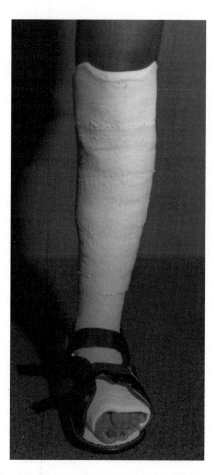

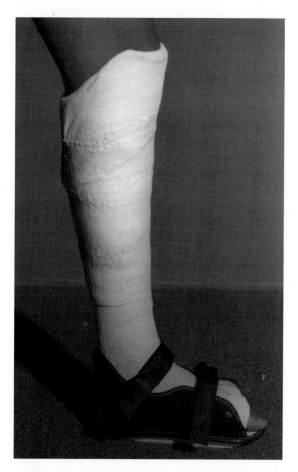

Fig. 26.3. AP photograph of patient in cast. Although it may not be necessary, the proximal extension over the medial and lateral condyles may provide rotatory stability.

Fig. 26.4. Lateral photograph. The cast should be cut in the popliteal space to allow knee flexion of 90 degrees. An alternative to a plaster PTB is either a custom-made or prefabricated PTB orthosis.

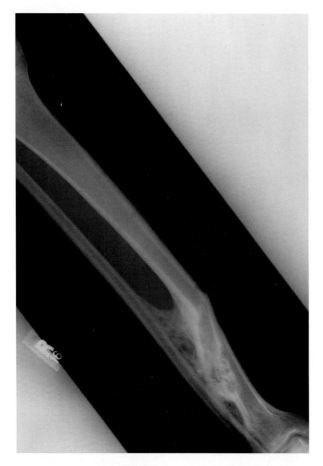

Fig. 26.5. AP x-ray of tibia 17 weeks after fracture with osseous union with satisfactory alignment and function. See Fig. 26.6.

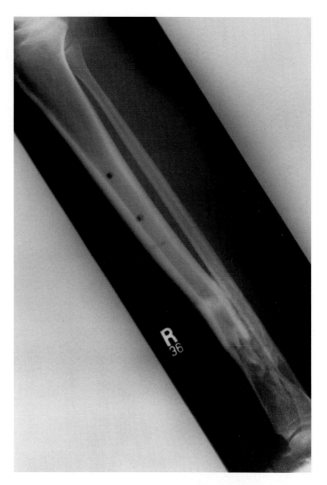

Fig. 26.6. Lateral x-ray of tibia 17 weeks after fracture with osseous union with satisfactory alignment and function. Same patient as in Fig. 26.5.

with significant segmental bone loss or tibial fractures in patients unable to ambulate because of associated injuries are in general not candidates for functional bracing. Open tibial fractures, because of disruption in the soft tissue envelope around the fracture site, are difficult to brace functionally and may require a period of external fixation to allow soft tissue healing before functional bracing. Certain tibial fractures present potential problems with functional bracing. In fractures of the tibia with an intact fibula, varus angulation of the fracture often occurs with weight bearing.[5,34] This complication occurs more frequently with fractures of the proximal one third of the tibia. If the varus angulation becomes too great (>5 degrees), either fibular osteotomy and continued functional bracing or operative stabilization is indicated.

Low-energy tibial fractures with minimal displacement and comminution can be treated with an immediate long leg cast with the knee in extension or slight flexion and weight bearing to tolerance. In comminuted high-energy tibial fractures, rigid circular casts should be avoided in the acute period after the injury to avoid a compartment syndrome. In patients with impaired cognition and decreased lower extremity sensation (such as a patient with a traumatic brain injury), tibial fractures should be initially treated with splints until the acute swelling is diminished to avoid a compartment syndrome. Once the swelling is diminished, the patient is placed in a prefabricated or plaster PTB orthosis. The patient is then encouraged to weight bear to tolerance. The patient is followed at least at monthly intervals, and AP and lateral radiographs, including the knee and ankle, are obtained. If alignment is unsatisfactory (>5 degrees of varus or valgus or >1 cm of shortening), either remanipulation or operative treatment is indicated. Although there has been some discussion about the necessity for the proximal extension of the orthosis over the femoral condyles,[49] the author believes it provides additional rotary and ambulatory stability to a tibial fracture, especially in fractures of the proximal third of the tibia.

In a retrospective, nonrandomized study of tibial fractures treated with either functional braces (Fig. 26.7) or intramedullary nails, overall function and align-

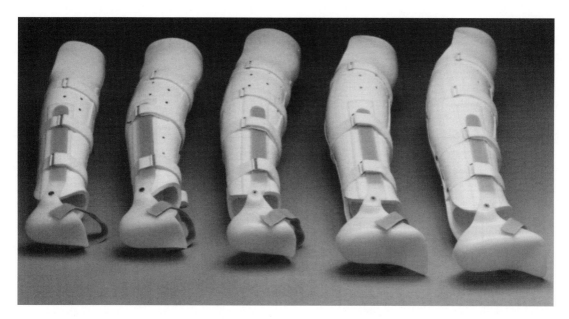

Fig. 26.7. The five sizes of prefabricated functional tibial fracture braces. An anterior and posterior shell are held together and adjusted with Velcro straps. The foot-ankle insert is fastened to the main body of the brace with Velcro straps.

ment were superior in the operative group.[9] In centers experienced with functional bracing of fractures, however, the functional outcome with fracture bracing of tibial fractures has been excellent.[33,34,49] In a study of 780 tibial fractures, both open and closed treated with functional bracing, the union rate was 97.5% at an average of 18.7 weeks with greater than 90% with less than 1 cm of shortening and acceptable alignment.[32]

The goal of treatment of tibial fractures should be osseous union with acceptable alignment, low infection rate, good functional outcome, and reasonable economic cost. In high-energy tibial fractures[21] with significant displacement (even open fractures), treated with unreamed locked intramedullary nails, the union rate, functional outcome, and infection rate have been satisfactory.[1,42,45] In low-energy fractures of the tibia, functional bracing results in acceptable clinical and radiographic results. Functional bracing of tibial fractures requires as much attention to detail as operative treatment. It involves functional activity (weight bearing) by the patient and regular assessment of radiographs to insure satisfactory healing and alignment.

FEMORAL FRACTURES

Diaphyseal femur fractures have been treated in the past with traction and functional bracing (Fig. 26.8) with satisfactory fracture healing. Plate fixation, used primarily in distal femoral fractures, have been used with satisfactory clinical outcome.[30] Plate fixation has been advocated in adult diaphyseal femoral fractures in

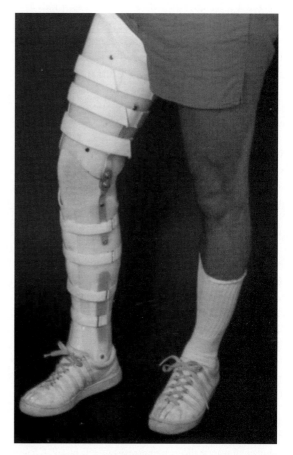

Fig. 26.8. Prefabricated functional femoral fracture brace. It needs to be adjusted regularly so that the snug compression of the soft tissues, which are primarily responsible for maintaining fracture stability and alignment, is not lost.

polytrauma patients and pediatric femoral fractures with associated polytrauma. In rare instances, primarily in contaminated open fractures, external fixation has been used in femur fractures,[2,27] but knee motion is often impaired secondary to quadriceps adhesions from transfixing external fixator pins.[18] In the last several decades, intramedullary nailing has become the predominant method of fixation for diaphyseal femur fractures.[12,40,48]

In the past, successful outcome after femoral fractures consisted of fracture union with satisfactory alignment. Functional outcome, if measured at all, has been defined as satisfactory range of motion of the knee at time of fracture healing. Yet the criteria for satisfactory range of motion of the knee following healing of femoral fractures has ranged from 65 degrees in one study[20] to 117 degrees in another study.[38]

The goal of treatment of femoral fractures should be fracture healing with acceptable alignment and satisfactory function. In the past, when treatment of femoral fractures often involved immobilization of the knee, function has been less than satisfactory.[19] Decreased range of motion of the knee, thigh atrophy, and significant weakness of both the quadriceps and hamstrings are often present long after fracture healing has occurred.[16,17] More recently, closed statically locked intramedullary nailing of comminuted femoral fractures has allowed early rehabilitation of the knee.[12]

Functional bracing of femoral fractures, both diaphyseal and supracondylar, has been done successfully.[3,4] A period of skeletal traction, from 2 to 6 weeks, is necessary before functional bracing and weight bearing. Weight bearing should be gradual, and there should be careful radiographic evaluation for shortening or angulatory deformity. If an unacceptable shortening or angulation occurs, further traction is necessary before any further weight bearing. It is possible to mobilize patients while in traction with roller traction.

Closed functional bracing of femur fractures should be reserved only for those patients who cannot be treated operatively.[11] Several retrospective and prospective studies have shown that pulmonary function is improved with early operative stabilization of femur fractures in polytrauma patients. In addition, shortening and angulatory deformities occur more frequently in patients treated with functional bracing in comparison to those patients treated with statically locked intramedullary nailing.[11]

REFERENCES

1. Alho A, et al: Comparison of functioning bracing and locked intramedullary in the treatment of displaced tibial shaft fractures, Clin Orthop 291:196, 1993.
2. Alonso J, Geissler W, Hughes J: External fixation of femoral fractures: Indications and limitations, Clin Orthop 241:83–96, 1989.
3. Connolly J, Dehne E, LaFollette B: Closed reduction and early cast brace ambulation in the treatment of femoral fractures: Results in one hundred forty-three fractures, J Bone Joint Surg 55A:1581, 1973.
4. Crotwell W: The thigh-lacer: Ambulatory nonoperative treatment of femoral shaft fractures, J Bone Joint Surg 60A:112–123, 1978.
5. DeCoster T, Nepola J, ElRouty G: Cast brace treatment of proximal tibial fractures: A ten year follow up study, Clin Orthop 231:196, 1988.
6. Gausewitz S, Hohl M: The significance of early motion in the treatment of motion on tibial plateau fracture, Clin Orthop 202:135, 1986.
7. Gelberman R, et al: The influence of flexor tendons: A biomechanical and microangiographic study, Hand 13:120, 1981.
8. Green S, Moore T, Spohn P: Nonunion of the tibial shaft, Orthopaedics 2:1149, 1988.
9. Hooper G, Keddell R, Perrny I: Conservative management or closed nailing for tibial shaft fracture: A randomized, prospective comparison, J Bone Joint Surg 73B:83–85, 1991.
10. Johnson K: Management of malunion and nonunion of the tibia, Orthop Clin North Am 18:157–171, 1987.
11. Johnson K, Johnston D, Parker B: Comminuted femoral shaft fractures: Treatment by rollar traction, cerclage wires and an intramedullary nail, or an interlocking intramedullary nail, J Bone Joint Surg 66A:1222–1241, 1984.
12. Kempf I, Grosse A, Beck G: Closed locked intramedullary nailing: Its application to comminuted fractures of the femur, J Bone Joint Surg 67A:709–716, 1985.
13. Kettlekamp K, et al: Degenerative arthritis of the knee secondary to fracture malunion, Clin Orthop 234:159–164, 1988.
14. Latta L, Sarmiento A, Tarr R: The rationale of functional bracing of fractures, Clin Orthop 146:2836, 1980.
15. Merchant T, Dietz F: Long term follow up after fractures of the tibia and fibular shafts, J Bone Joint Surg 71A:599–606, 1989.
16. Mira A, Markley K, Greer R: A critical analysis of quadriceps function after femoral shaft fractures in adults, J Bone Joint Surg 62A:61–71, 1980.
17. Moore T, et al: Knee function after complex femur fracture treated with interlocking nails, Clin Orthop 261:238–243, 1990.
18. Moore T, et al: The results of quadricepsplasty on knee motion following femoral fractures, J Trauma 27:49–56, 1987.
19. Moore T, et al: Complications of surgically treated supracondylar fractures of the femur, J Trauma 27:402, 1987.
20. Neer C, Granthano S, Shelton M: Supracondylar fracture of the adult femur, J Bone Joint Surg 49A:591, 1967.
21. Nicoll E: Fractures of the tibial shaft: A survey of 705 cases, J Bone Joint Surg 46B:373, 1964.
22. Oestern H, Tscherne H: Pathophysiology and classification of soft tissue injuries associated with fractures. In Tscherne H, editor: Fractures with soft tissue injuries, Berlin, 1984, Springer.
23. Olerud C: The pronation capacity of the foot: Its consequences for axial deformity after tibial shaft fractures, Arch Orthop Trauma Surg 104:303, 1985.
24. Pun W, et al: A study of function and residual joint stiffness after functional bracing of tibial shaft fractures, Clin Orthop 267:157, 1991.
25. Puno R, et al: Critical analysis of results of treatment of 201 tibial shaft fractures, Clin Orthop 212:113, 1986.
26. Puno R, et al: Long term effects of tibial angular malunion of the knee and ankle joint, J Orthop Trauma 5:247, 1991.
27. Rooser B, et al: External fixation of femoral fractures, J Orthop Trauma 4:70, 1990.
28. Salter R: The biological concept of continuous passive motion of synovial joints: The first 18 years of basic research and its clinical application, Clin Orthop 242:12, 1989.

29. Salter R: Motion versus rest: Why immobilize joints? Proceedings LeRoy C. Abbott Society, University of California, San Francisco, 124:1–16, 1983.

30. Sanders R, et al: Double plating of comminuted unstable fractures of the distal part of the femur, J Bone Joint Surg 73A:341, 1991.

31. Sarmiento A: A functional below-knee brace for tibial fractures, J Bone Joint Surg 52A:295–311, 1970.

32. Sarmiento A, Gersten L, Sobal P: Tibial shaft fractures treated with functional braces. Experience with 780 fractures, J Bone Joint Surg 71:602, 1989.

33. Sarmiento A, Latta L: Closed functional treatment of fractures, Berlin, 1981, Springer-Verlag.

34. Sarmiento A, Latta L, Sinclair W: Functional bracing of fractures. In American Academy of Orthopaedics Surgeons Instructional Course Lectures, XXV, St. Louis, 1976, CV Mosby.

35. Sarmiento A, Latta L, Tarr R: The effects of function in fracture healing and stability in American Academy of Orthopaedic Surgeons Instructional Course Lectures, XXXIII, St. Louis, 1984, CV Mosby.

36. Sarmiento A, Latta L, Zilioli A: The rose of soft tissues in stabilization of tibial fractures, Artif Limbs, 11:28–32, 1967.

37. Sarmiento A, Sinclair W: Application of prosthetic-orthotic principles of orthopaedics, Artif Limbs 11:28–32, 1967.

38. Seinsheimer F: Fractures of the distal femur, Clin Orthop 153:169, 1980.

39. Takai S, et al: The effects of frequency and duration of controlled passive mobilization on tendon healing, J Orthop Res 9:705, 1991.

40. Tarr R, et al: Changes in tibiotalar joint contact area following experimentally induced tibial angular deformities, Clin Orthop 199:72, 1985.

41. Ting A, et al: The role of subtalar motion and ankle contact pressure changes from angular deformities of the tibia, Foot Ankle 7:290, 1987.

42. Trafton P: Closed, unstable fractures of the tibia, Clin Orthop 230:58–67, 1988.

43. Waddell J, Reardon G: Complications of tibial shaft fractures, Clin Orthop 178:173, 1983.

44. Wagner K, Tarr R, Resnick C: The effect of simulated tibial deformities on the ankle joint during the gait cycle, Foot Ankle 5:131, 1984.

45. Watson J: Current concepts review: Treatment of unstable fractures of the shaft of the tibia, J Bone Joint Surg 76A:1575, 1994.

46. Winquist R, Hansen S, Clawson D: Closed intramedullary nailing of femoral fractures: A report of five hundred and twenty cases, J Bone Joint Surg 66A:529, 1984.

47. Zagorski J, et al: Tibial fracture stability: Analysis of external fracture immobilization in anatomic specimens in casts and braces, Clin Orthop 291:196, 1993.

48. Zuckerman J, et al: Treatment of unstable femoral shaft fractures with closed intramedullary nailing, J Orthop Trauma 1:209, 1987.

49. Zych G, et al: Modern concepts in functional bracing of the lower limb, AAOS International Course Lectures, Vol 36, St. Louis, 1987, CV Mosby.

Orthoses in Total Joint Replacement

Howard S. Hirsch
Paul A. Lotke

Primary total joint replacements of the hip and knee are reliable operations and are usually successful in restoring function to patients with severe arthritic conditions. Although orthoses are rarely needed after these procedures, some external support may be needed in cases involving revision surgery, surgical complications, or unusual primary pathology. This chapter presents a problem-oriented approach to the management of various conditions encountered after hip and knee arthroplasty that may require treatment with an orthosis. Devices useful in the management of these situations are described, and practical suggestions about their use are given.

ORTHOSES AFTER HIP REPLACEMENT

Dislocation

Dislocation of a prosthetic hip is a difficult clinical problem, and an effort to determine its cause is necessary before one can make a reasonable treatment plan. If there is significant malposition of either the femoral or acetabular components, surgical revision is usually indicated. In patients with radiographically satisfactory positioning of the components who dislocate, it is essential to identify the direction of the instability, which may be either anterior or posterior. Posterior dislocations occur with excessive flexion, adduction, and internal rotation and are associated with retroversion of the components. Anterior dislocation occurs with external rotation in extension and often occurs in dysplastic hips with excessive femoral anteversion. Appreciation of the patient's anatomy, the implant position, and the direction of the dislocation is necessary to plan orthotic management.

Once reduced, a total hip can be stabilized with an orthosis until sufficient repair tissue forms a pseudocapsule around the joint. This usually prevents further dislocations, provided that the components are well positioned. In the past, hip spica casts have also been shown to be useful for this purpose.[8] Currently, orthoses offer several advantages over casts: Orthoses weigh less, which makes them easier to tolerate during ambulation. An orthosis may be carefully removed, providing access for wound care and hygiene. In addition, suitable hip orthoses are widely available in adjustable, prefabricated models, which makes application a straightforward process.

The usual orthosis used to treat a dislocated total hip is shown in Fig. 27.1. It has an adjustable pelvic waistband that may be supported, when necessary, by a shoulder strap. A snug-fitting thigh cuff is connected to the waistband by a laterally placed, adjustable, metal hinge, which holds the hip in 10 to 20 degrees of abduction. The hinge may also be adjusted so that flexion and extension can be limited to the desired degree. For posterior dislocation, a range of motion from zero to 60 degrees of flexion usually allows patients to sit comfortably and walk without compromising the joint's stability. In patients with anterior instability, extension should be limited to −30 degrees, whereas flexion to 90 degrees is generally safe. Rotational control is limited because it is provided only by the thigh cuff's grip on the skin. This must be taken into account when fitting and adjusting the brace. Once properly fitted, most patients should be able to ambulate with minimal support and perform most activities of daily living while wearing the brace.

There are no objective criteria to determine how long a brace should be worn. This is determined by many factors, including the intrinsic stability of the joint; the patient's ability to follow *hip precautions*, and the rate of soft tissue healing, which varies among patients. In cases involving early postoperative dislocations of radiographically well-positioned prosthetic hips, the authors' usual practice is to brace patients for 6 to 12 weeks after the initial dislocation. Longer periods of orthotic protection are indicated for patients

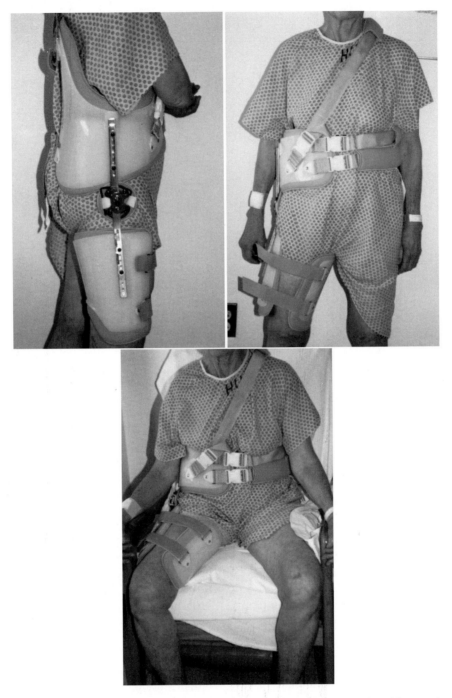

Fig. 27.1.   This patient has recurrent dislocation of the hip. She has been placed in an orthosis that maintains abduction and limits flexion. This orthosis may be worn until soft tissues stabilize.

with impaired soft tissue healing and recurrent dislocations or patients who are noncompliant. Occasionally, permanent bracing is necessary.

Prophylactic bracing should be considered for some hip arthroplasty patients. They may be considered in three broad categories: patients who have undergone revision surgery, those with neuromuscular diseases, and those who are unable to follow the usual

precautions against extreme positions of the hip after surgery.

Revision patients are at increased risk for dislocation and have been shown to benefit from prophylactic treatment with a brace similar to the one described for treatment of a dislocated primary hip.[4] Although some surgeons routinely brace all revision patients, most would use prophylactic bracing only after revisions involving extensive soft tissue dissection or in patients where stability is marginal at the time of surgery.

Patients with neuromuscular disease such as Parkinson's disease, spasticity, or sensory neuropathy may experience recurrent dislocations despite optimally positioned implants. Prolonged bracing should be considered in this population.

The elderly, demented patient treated with an endoprosthesis for a femoral neck fracture is at particular risk for dislocation because of impaired cognition. Although some of these patients may require a hip brace, a knee immobilizer has been shown to be effective in this group. A knee immobilizer locks the knee in extension and prevents excessive hip flexion.[2] The knee immobilizer can be easily removed when the patient is supervised, as in physical therapy, and therefore does not impede rehabilitation.

The usefulness of orthoses for the prevention and treatment of dislocation in total hips has been documented. Thirupathi and Clayton[7] successfully treated dislocations in eight of nine hips using a hip orthosis. Dorr and colleagues[1] reported repeat dislocation in only 2 of 14 hips after brace treatment. Mallory et al noted dislocations in none of 30 primary total hips and in 3 of 37 revisions with the use of prophylactic bracing.[4]

Periprosthetic femoral fractures

These fractures often occur during surgery, particularly during revision procedures and primary implantation of tight-fitting, uncemented devices. In most cases, some degree of internal fixation of the fracture is performed. Therefore, the operating surgeon is best able to judge the stability of the fracture and determine to what degree orthotic protection is needed. In general, orthotic stabilization should be considered for fractures that extend below the distal end of the femoral prosthesis and are associated with insecure fixation or poor quality bone. A similar situation exists when femoral osteotomies are performed in conjunction with hip replacement.

The appropriate brace to stabilize these fractures includes a pelvic band, thigh, and calf cuffs. A hinge with adjustable stops is used at the hip, and a free hinge is used at the knee. The orthosis must cross the knee because rotational loads pose the greatest threat to fracture stability, and even a well-fitted thigh cuff does not adequately control rotation of the lower extremity. Indeed, the authors have occasionally found it useful to extend the orthosis across the ankle to provide more protection from rotational forces. A pelvic band may be omitted in patients who are not obese and whose fractures are located more distally in the femur. Such an orthosis is similar to that recommended for the treatment of some primary femoral fractures.[5] In cases where additional protection from axial loading is deemed necessary, it may be useful to apply an ischial weight-bearing orthosis. This is made by adding a quadrilateral thigh cuff to the usual device.

The duration of orthotic treatment must be determined for each patient based on radiographic and clinical findings that indicate fracture union. External support is usually required for at least 12 weeks but varies according to the fracture pattern, the patient's age and ability to follow postoperative instructions, and other factors associated with fracture healing.

Neurologic complications

Femoral and sciatic nerve palsies are well-known complications of hip replacement surgery. Motor deficits may resolve quickly (in a few days) or may be permanent. Patients whose deficits do not resolve by the time they are ready to leave the hospital usually benefit from an appropriate orthosis, as do those who are believed to have permanent injuries.

Most sciatic nerve injuries are due to surgical trauma. In these cases, the most common finding is a foot drop, which results from injury to the peroneal portion of the sciatic nerve. Decreased ankle dorsiflexion during swing impairs rehabilitation and often makes the patient's gait unsafe. Many orthotic options exist for the management of this problem. In mild to moderate cases, a high-top tennis shoe may be all that is required to support the foot. In more severe cases, an ankle-foot orthosis (AFO) is required. The authors prefer a one-piece, custom-molded device that the patient can insert into various shoes. Other AFOs that may be considered include those with stirrups, calipers, and ankle assists. The selected orthosis should be worn until active dorsiflexion of the foot returns.

Femoral nerve injury weakens the quadriceps, which are the main antigravity muscle group of the knee. Although some patients learn to lock their knee in extension by using their hip extensors while the foot is held in plantar flexion, many remain unable to ambulate well. Those patients with impaired knee extension are best managed in a double upright knee-ankle-foot orthosis (KAFO) with a drop lock knee hinge and a free ankle until the nerve function returns.

Resection arthroplasty

Resection arthroplasty of the hip (Girdlestone procedure) is now performed rarely as a primary reconstructive procedure. Currently, its most common indication is for those patients in whom hip replacements have failed because of infection or severe bone loss and who are not satisfactory candidates for revision total hip arthroplasty. After proximal femoral resection, there is a tendency of the operated extremity to shorten. This may be reduced by placing the patient in skeletal traction for 3 to 6 weeks after surgery. During this

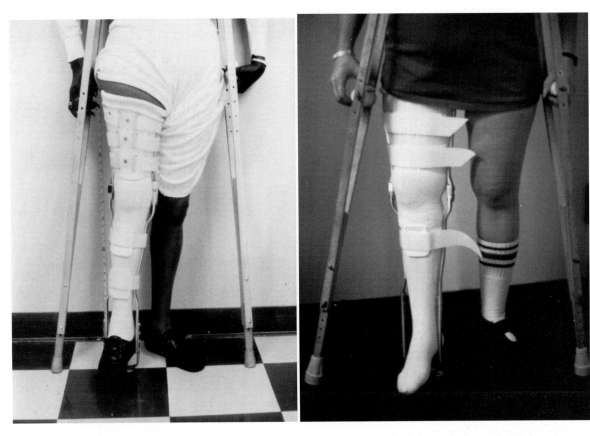

Fig. 27.2. Caliper-type orthosis for Girdlestone patients. This orthosis controls shortening and accepts some ischial weight bearing.

period, scar tissue forms between the resected surfaces of the pelvis and femur. Subsequent protection with an ischial weight-bearing orthosis that suspends the foot with calipers has been recommended to further control shortening. Concomitant use of a contralateral shoe-lift is also necessary. A patient wearing these appliances is shown in Fig. 27.2. An ischial weight-bearing brace with the foot touching the floor may be used as an alternative, but this is not as effective in preventing shortening.[6]

ORTHOSES AFTER KNEE REPLACEMENT

Orthotic support is used less frequently after knee replacement as compared to hip arthroplasty. This may be due to the fact that many surgeons consider the need for long-term bracing to be a relative contraindication to total knee arthroplasty. Nevertheless, there are conditions associated with total knee surgery that are sometimes amenable to treatment with orthotic appliances. The primary examples are weakness or injury of the extensor mechanism (i.e., avulsion of the patellar tendon) and insufficiency of the medial collateral ligament. In addition, salvage procedures for total knee arthroplasty such as arthrodesis or resection arthroplasty

usually require orthotic treatment as part of postoperative management.

Extensor mechanism deficiency

Patients with severe weakness of the quadriceps because of neuromuscular disease and those with mechanical disruption of the extensor mechanism that is not amenable to surgical repair may require bracing to prevent uncontrolled loss of knee extension during the stance phase of gait. This problem can be managed with a KAFO with double upright supports. Two types of hinges may be considered:

1. Droplock hinges are the more secure. They allow the patient to ambulate with a stiff-leg gait but can be released to allow comfortable sitting.
2. A posterior offset hinge is a reasonable alternative. It causes the knee to extend when weight is applied and allows it to bend during the swing phase of gait.[3] More agile patients and those with some residual active knee extension may prefer this to the droplock hinge.

Occasionally the quadriceps tendon or the patellar tendon is disrupted during or after knee replacement. Surgical treatment is usually indicated. Depending on the strength of the repair, protective bracing may be needed. In this situation, a sturdy, prefabricated knee orthosis with adjustable locking hinges is useful. Such a device allows the surgeon to increase the range of motion as healing and extension strength progress.

Collateral ligament instability

Because properly aligned total knees maintain a slight valgus tibiofemoral alignment, the medial soft tissues are under tension. Therefore, a functional medial collateral ligament is essential to the success of all nonhinged prosthetic knees. Even revision total knee implants with highly constrained designs function better with some support from the patient's medial soft tissue. Knees with valgus or varus instability may be treated with a hinged knee orthosis. A locking hinge is unnecessary. Depending on the patient's demands, either a KAFO or a *sports brace* may be used. The latter may be particularly useful in knees that require temporary protection from valgus forces. In the authors' experience, patients (especially the elderly) with chronic collateral ligament instability about a total knee implant do not tolerate an orthosis well. Therefore, the use of such braces should be avoided whenever possible in these patients.

Arthrodesis and resection arthroplasty

In cases of failed total knee implants secondary to sepsis or severe bone loss, it is sometimes necessary to perform a knee arthrodesis. Prolonged casting is indicated after this procedure except when an intramedullary rod is used for internal fixation. The time to union can be prolonged, sometimes as long as 12 months; therefore an orthosis is usually needed after the period of casting. A double upright KAFO is appropriate in this situation. The authors prefer to use a modified device with well-fitted leather cuffs that are secured by Velcro straps. The cuffs are in full contact with the skin, which provides support for the soft tissue. This support is helpful in controlling edema, which can be problematic in these patients. These individuals may stop wearing the device when solid union of the arthrodesis is observed.

Resection arthroplasty is another common salvage procedure after failed knee replacement. Prolonged cast immobilization is needed in the immediate postoperative period. After the soft tissues stabilize, patients usually require permanent bracing with a double upright KAFO with droplock hinges. Total-contact, leather cuffs with Velcro straps are also helpful in providing comfortable support for these patients.

SUMMARY

Orthotic support is occasionally required after total hip arthroplasty, primarily in cases of dislocations with satisfactory implant positioning or in nerve injuries resulting in gait abnormalities. In total knee replacement, an orthosis may be required in cases of significant postoperative instability or in salvage resection procedures for patients who are not candidates for further reconstruction procedures. In both situations, an orthosis is an adjunctive modality to enhance the functional outcome.

REFERENCES

1. Dorr LD, Chandler R, Conaty JP: Classification and treatment of dislocations of total hip arthroplasty, Clin Orthop Rel Res 173:151, 1983.
2. Janecki CJ, Leve AR, Lai LKO: The knee immobilizer as an aid in the prevention of postoperative endoprosthetic dislocations, Clin Orthop Rel Res 168:83, 1982.
3. Kruger LM: Lower-limb orthoses. In American Academy of Orthopaedic Surgeons: Atlas of orthotics, St. Louis, 1985, CV Mosby.
4. Mallory TH, et al: Prophylactic use of a hip cast-brace following primary and revision total hip arthroplasty, Orthop Rev 12:178, 1988.
5. Sarmiento A, Latta LL: Fractures of the femur. In Closed functional treatment of fractures, New York, 1981, Springer-Verlag.
6. Steinberg ME, Steinberg DR: Resection arthroplasty. In The hip and its disorders, Philadelphia, 1991, WB Saunders.
7. Thirupathi RG, Clayton ML: Dislocation following total hip arthroplasty: Management by special brace in selected patients, Clin Orthop Rel Res 177:154, 1983.
8. Williams JF, Gottesman MJ, Mallory TH: Dislocation after total hip arthroplasty: Treatment with an above-knee hip spica cast, Clin Orthop Rel Res 171:53, 1982.

Knee Orthoses for Sports-Related Disorders

Theodore F. Schlegel
J. Richard Steadman

An orthosis by strict definition is a device used to straighten a limb deformity. Historically, knee orthoses (KOs) have been used to correct congenital deformities around the knee. For example, genu varum can be treated using a nonhinged brace to affect the epiphyseal growth at the distal femoral and proximal tibial growth plates. Knee orthoses have also been used to provide knee stability in flaccid paralysis of the quadriceps muscle. For example, in the patient with polio, a single lateral upright knee/ankle/foot orthosis (KAFO) can assist in ambulation. Over time, the applications for knee bracing have been expanded to include use in the athletic population (Fig. 28.1).

Bracing for athletic disorders is a relatively recent phenomenon, dating back to the early 1970s with the introduction of the Lenox Hill derotational brace. These orthoses were designed to protect individuals with functional deficits secondary to disruption of the anterior cruciate ligament. The success of these braces led to the development of both rehabilitative and prophylactic orthoses.

With the expanded indications for knee braces, the traditional definition of a KO is inadequate. A more comprehensive definition was required to improve communication between clinicians and to allow for meaningful research to be conducted on the effectiveness of bracing. For this reason, the Sports Medicine Committee of the American Academy of Orthopedic Surgeons[1] has further classified knee braces into three categories: prophylactic, rehabilitative, and functional.

This chapter reviews the theory behind brace design and fabrication and defines the three categories of knee braces used for sports-related disorders. This chapter also reviews clinical and biomechanical studies related to the effectiveness of each of the three types of braces. With this information, the clinician can make a more informed and intelligent decision concerning which circumstances these orthoses should be prescribed.

BIOMECHANICS OF THE KNEE JOINT

The kinematics of the normal knee joint need to be understood if one is to design an effective knee brace. From anatomic descriptions, the knee has been classified as a diarthrodial or hinge joint. From kinematic studies, however, knee motion is known not to function as a simple hinge but to involve an extremely complex series of movements about variable axes and in three separate planes.[17] Flexion and extension do not occur about a fixed transverse axis of rotation but rather about a constantly changing center of rotation. This polycentric rotation when plotted outlines the approximate shape of the femoral condyle. Motion is therefore achieved by a complex coupled mechanism in which the femoral condyles simultaneously glide and roll back on the tibial plateaus (Fig. 28.2). Strasser[40] showed that the ratio of rolling to sliding varied during flexion and extension. Starting from full extension, the femoral condyle begins to roll without sliding. With increased knee flexion, the sliding movement becomes progressively more important so that at the end of flexion the condyle slides without rolling. The length over which pure rolling takes place varies depending on the femoral condyle. For the medial femoral condyle, pure rolling occurs during the first 10 to 15 degrees of flexion, whereas for the lateral condyle, this rolling takes place until 20 degrees of flexion is reached. Therefore, the lateral femoral condyle rolls far more than the medial condyle during flexion.

In addition to flexion and extension in the sagittal plane, concomitant axial rotation also occurs. Rotation of the tibia occurs automatically in the absence of any voluntary movement. As the knee flexes, there is always an obligatory inward rotation of the tibia. Conversely, as the knee comes to terminal extension, there is an obligatory outward rotation of the tibia. This axial rotation occurs in part for three reasons. First, the

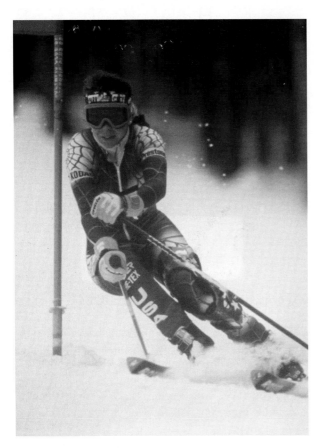

Fig. 28.1.   Downhill skier.

diameter of the lateral femoral condyle's curve exceeds that of the medial condyle. The second reason relates to the shape of the tibial plateaus. The medial femoral condyle recedes only a small amount because it is contained within a concave tibial surface, whereas the lateral femoral condyle slides more freely over the posterior slope of the convex tibial surface. The third reason for rotation of the tibia relates to the direction of the collateral ligaments. When the medial femoral condyle recedes from the medial collateral ligament, it stretches more rapidly than the lateral ligament. These two coupled forces produce a natural axial rotation.

The normal kinematics of the knee joint are guided by the cruciate ligaments. Kapandji[22] described the cruciate ligaments as a four-bar linkage system with the anterior cruciate and posterior cruciate crossing at a 40-degree angle and attaching to the femoral condyle laterally and medially. These ligaments are restraints that create an obligatory motion and are responsible for this complex coupled roll-back and glide mechanism with obligatory axial rotation.

If a knee orthosis is to function properly, it must accommodate the normal roll-back and glide mechanism coupled with the axial rotation of the knee joint. In the uninjured joint, the brace must replicate the normal kinematics of the knee joint. If the brace interferes with the kinematics, motion may be limited or the ligaments can be prestressed leading to chronic laxity. In the ligament-deficient knee, the brace must help prevent abnormal motion and attempt to recreate the normal kinematics of the knee joint.

BRACE DESIGN

All braces are designed on the premise that abnormal translation or motion can be restricted by the application of leverage to the knee joint. Mechanically, this is most easily done when leverage can be applied at a distance from the joint. The further the application of force, the greater the leverage (i.e., longer brace, longer leverage).

The optimal position to apply leverage depends on the function of the knee brace. In prophylactic braces designed to protect the medial collateral ligament, leverage is applied laterally on the femur and tibia to prevent excessive valgus force. With functional knee braces used in patients with anterior cruciate ligament deficiencies, the brace must resist abnormal forward translation of the tibia on the femur. This is most often achieved through a control system that prevents hyperextension. The ability to apply leverage in a controlled fashion depends on several factors. The greatest mechanical consideration affecting brace function relates to soft tissue compliance. The axial soft tissues of the limb serve as the principal mechanical interface between the brace and limb and are the primary factors limiting brace function.[11] Tissue compression and the tendency of the brace to migrate distally on the dependant limb severely limits the brace's effectiveness in applying leverage. In addition, soft tissues have little ability to resist transitional loads, which makes the ability of the brace to control axial rotation of the limb difficult. The design of an effective brace is therefore a challenging problem. Variables such as geometry of attachment, mechanism of attachment, materials of fabrication, and hinge design all influence brace performance.

Geometry of attachment

Maintenance of proper brace position is determined in part by its configuration. Brace fit is achieved by properly contouring the device to the affected extremity. This can be achieved in both off-the-shelf and custom-designed orthoses. Biomechanical and clinical research have shown that both are effective as long as they take into account the shape of the extremity.[6,20,36] This is achieved by approximating the tibial contour below the knee and extending supports across the thigh into the lateral arm. By contouring the brace to the extremity, it is possible to achieve a greater support

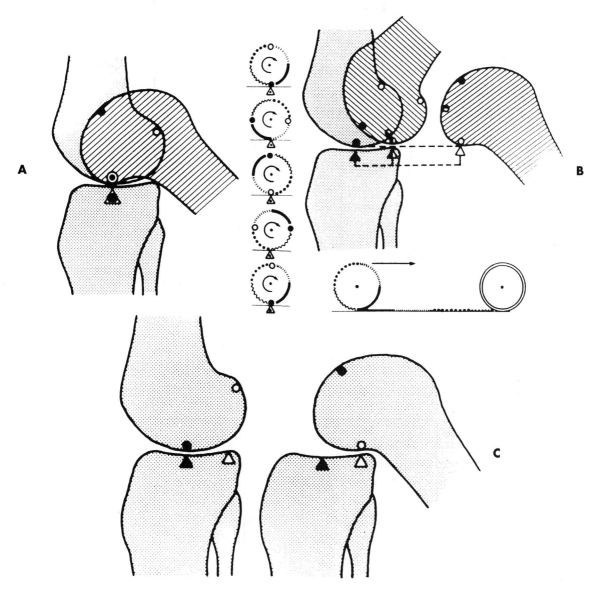

Fig. 28.2. **A,** Pure sliding of the femur on the tibia with knee flexion. Note that the contact point of the tibia does not change as the femur slides over it. Posterior femoral metaphyseal impingement would occur if all surface motion were restricted to sliding. **B,** Pure rolling of the femur on the tibia with knee flexion. Note that both tibial femoral contact points change as the femur rolls on the tibia. The femur would fall off the tibia if surface motion were restricted to rolling. **C,** Actual knee motion involves both sliding and rolling. (From Scott WN: The Knee, St. Louis, 1994, Mosby.)

system to help protect the medial, lateral, anterior, and combined ligament instabilities. The addition of condylar padding also ensures a more precise fit (Fig. 28.3).

Mechanism of attachment

Strapping is one of the most critical features affecting brace performance. Two types of straps exist: elastic and nonelastic. The elastic straps are more comfortable but less effective. Because of soft tissue compliance, leverage is lost with each muscle contraction owing to the flexible nature of the strap. The nonelastic straps are more effective because they function as a shell. This allows for constant leverage to be applied to the extremity. Unfortunately, the nonelastic straps are often constricting and may be less tolerated than the elastic strap.

The number of straps, their arrangement, and how they interface with the hinge brace are all considered important. The number and arrangement of straps determine how load is distributed across the limb. Most braces have at least four straps that secure the orthosis to the extremity. The suprapatellar straps are the most important in maintaining position of the brace because they prevent distal migration of the orthosis. Additional

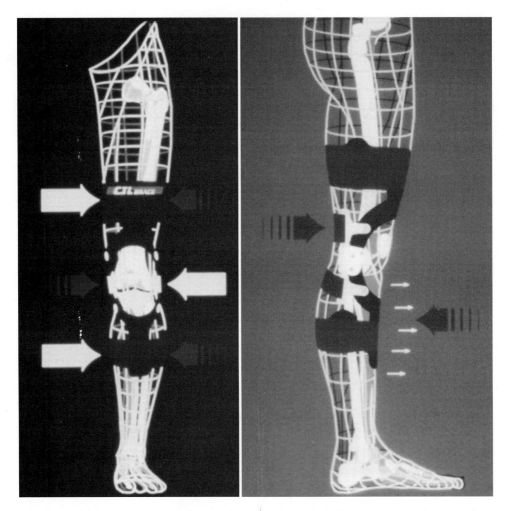

Fig. 28.3. Knee braces are contoured to the extremity to apply leverage, preventing excessive varus/valgus forces and abnormal anterior tibial translation.

straps are often used, particularly in functional knee braces, when added leverage is required. The function of the brace can also be improved by increasing the surface area of the straps. The manner in which the straps secure to the brace is also important. There must be no motion of the strap in relation to the upright bar so that constant leverage can be applied.

Material of fabrication

In the athletic population, brace materials must be lightweight, strong, and durable. Weight is an important factor because it affects performance and an individual's compliance. Strength and durability are necessary to withstand repetitive impact loads in athletic competition. Over the years, brace manufacturers have searched for materials to meet these requirements. The heavy steel braces of the past have been abandoned for lighter-weight material composites. The aerospace industry has provided materials to produce lightweight, strong, durable braces. Lightweight metals alone are not ideal because they have a tendency to bend easily. Composite materials tend to be stronger but are often

brittle and fatigue easily. Combining the two materials, however, creates a strong, durable, lightweight substance. The previous 5-lb steel brace can now be made just as strong and durable with lightweight metal composites that weigh less than 1 lb.

Hinge design

Because the orthosis uses leverage as its principal functional component, the hinge needs to be able to transfer load while allowing for natural motion of the knee joint. The hinge must be able to simulate the rolling, gliding motion of the femoral condyle on the tibial plateau and the obligatory rotational movements as influenced by the anterior and posterior cruciate ligaments. The hinge must be designed not to interfere with the normal kinematics of the knee joint.

There are two basic hinge designs available: a simple unicentric or more complex kinematic hinge. The unicentric hinge assumes that the knee motion is a simple uniplanar hinge and does not account for the normal kinematics of the knee joint. This type of hinge has been most frequently used in prophylactic braces.

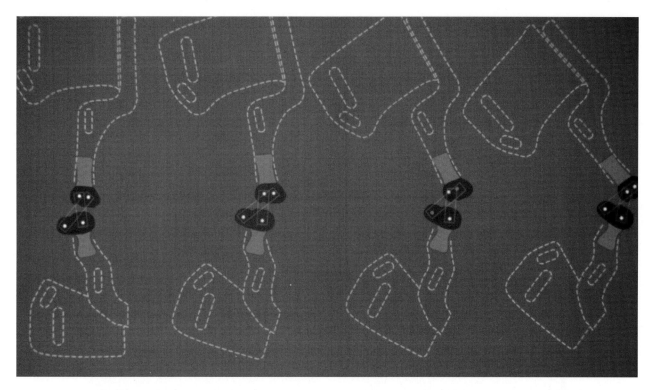

Fig. 28.4.   A kinematic hinge designed on a four bar linkage model to replicate normal knee motion.

In unilateral upright prophylactic braces, the hinge appears less critical. These braces are less likely to interfere with the kinematics of the knee when compared to the functional knee brace.

For functional knee braces, a more sophisticated hinge has been designed based on polycentric kinematics. The kinematic hinge attempts to approximate the relative motion of the tibia and femur while maintaining optimal position of the orthosis on the wearer's leg throughout the knee motion. This design in theory serves to maintain the position of the brace on the tibia and femur helping both to alleviate the common bracing problems of pistoning, migration, and abnormal motion. The kinematics of hinges on external orthoses have been a subject of debate for several years. The predominant opinion favors a hinge that meets the normal kinematics of the knee (Fig. 28.4).[11] Two studies[31,34] have shown, however, that the kinematic design had little effect on knee motion during low loads. These studies also suggested that under physiologic loads the hinge is even less of a factor. For a hinge to replicate accurately the kinematics of the knee, it has to be individualized to fit the geometric shape and size of each knee.

Individual factors affecting brace control

Although the mechanical design is crucial, the final factor affecting brace effectiveness relates to individual compliance. The individual is willing to tolerate only certain mechanical considerations. The individual is not likely to wear the brace if it is uncomfortable or cumbersome. Brace acceptance is strongly influenced by the individual's understanding of why the brace is required.

ORTHOSES RESEARCH

Unfortunately, it can be quite difficult to document the effectiveness of a brace with a controlled experimental model. Brace research is inherently difficult because of the difficulties of obtaining accurate objective measurements in vivo under physiologic conditions. Early published series have been primarily retrospective reviews of brace use. In an attempt to document brace effectiveness more objectively, basic science studies have been completed. These studies have primarily involved biomechanical testing of braces using cadaveric specimens or mechanical surrogate limb models. Both of these models are limited by the lack of active musculature contraction and the difficulties of reproducing the compliance of the soft tissues surrounding the thigh and calf. Both muscle contraction and tissue compliance have been found to influence the measurement of strain on knee ligaments, making analysis of data difficult.[6,19,21] In these models, brace fit is also difficult to assess and reproduce adequately making the results potentially inaccurate.

Clinical studies of the efficacy of knee braces are limited by the challenge that exists to perform direct

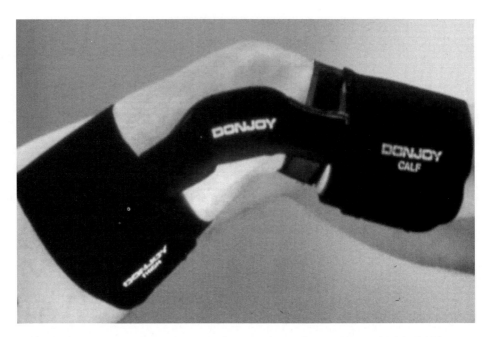

Fig. 28.5. Prophylactic knee brace—single upright unilateral frame with biaxial hinge.

measurements of the tibiofemoral translation and rotation in living subjects under physiologic loads during experimentally controlled conditions. Indirect means of measurement, including devices such as the KT-100, Striker Knee Laxity Test, Genucom, and The Knee Signature System, are inaccurate because of the difficulties in performing measurements with the brace in place. In addition, the low loads that are applied (i.e., 10, 20, and 30 lb) are well below physiologic loads seen during athletic events. Even if testing allowed higher varus/valgus loads to be applied, the data may not be clinically relevant unless concomitant axial loads are applied to the extremity. It becomes readily apparent that both basic science and clinical research projects related to documenting the effectiveness of bracing remains a challenging dilemma. Although past studies have been beneficial in suggesting the effectiveness of braces, further research is required. Future studies need to document in vivo measurements of ligament strain, tibiofemoral translation, and rotation under axial loading of the extremity during physiologic activities.

PROPHYLACTIC KNEE BRACES

Prophylactic or protective knee braces are designed on the premise that they can protect players from sustaining debilitating injuries while not inhibiting knee mobility. The use of these orthoses has been primarily in football and lacrosse to protect the medial collateral and anterior cruciate ligaments from contact injuries. The theory behind protective knee braces is that they can redirect a lateral impact force away from the joint to points more distal on the tibia and femur.[13] This would then limit the force acting on the joint and reduce the strain on the MCL and ACL with contact injuries.

The traditional prophylactic brace design is a single upright unilateral frame with a hinge mechanism (Fig. 28.5). The frame is worn on the lateral aspect of the extremity and secured with a strapping system. The hinge may be either of a single or double joint design. The single hinge design does not accommodate for the normal rollback mechanism and axial rotation of the knee joint. It is designed on the premise that with a unilateral frame system and interposed soft tissues, leverage from the brace is not great enough to affect knee kinematics. The double hinge system attempts to reproduce normal knee motion, preventing the unwanted positioning or prestressing of ligaments, which can potentially result from brace wear.

There is a significant controversy as to whether the brace can actually reduce the number as well as the overall severity of injuries. Several epidemiologic and biomechanical studies on the use of prophylactic braces have had differing results. Epidemiologic studies by several investigators have reported that prophylactic knee braces significantly reduce the number of knee injuries in football.[38,33,39] Sitler and colleagues[39] published a prospective, randomized study completed at the United States Military Academy to determine the efficacy of the prophylactic knee brace in reducing the frequency and the severity of acute knee injuries in football. The athletic shoe, playing surface, athletic exposure, knee injury history, and brace assignment were either statistically or experimentally controlled.

This large study included 1396 cadets who were involved in the intramural tackle football program. All subjects were evaluated for prior knee injuries. ACL-deficient knees or those who had undergone ACL reconstruction were excluded. Brace assignment was made via a table of random numbers. During this 2-year study, 705 subjects served as controls (nonbrace) and 691 subjects wore the Don Joy Orthopedic Protector Knee Guard. This brace is a double-hinged single upright brace, with a no-slip strap and Neoprene thigh and calf strap. This study showed that the unilateral-biaxial prophylactic knee brace significantly reduced the frequency of knee injuries, both in total number of subjects injured and in the total number of MCL injuries. This reduction of knee injuries depended on player position. Defensive players who wore prophylactic knee braces had statistically fewer injuries than the subjects who served as controls. The player's position dependency on knee braces to reduce knee injuries was not attributed to group differences in height, weight, football playing experience, or exposure to injury.

Other epidemiologic studies have contradicted Sitler's results, reporting increases in the total number of knee injuries as a result of prophylactic knee brace wear.[18,37,42] Only Tietz et al[42] reported that the increase was statistically significant. The difference in outcome between these investigators can be attributed to several factors. First, only Sitler et al[39] controlled for prior knee injury. Second, there were differences in the type and number of braces used in each study. Sitler et al used only one brace (Don Joy Orthopedic Protector Knee Guard). Rovere et al[37] and Hewson et al[18] used a different unilateral-biaxial prophylactic knee brace, whereas Tietz et al used four different knee braces, making direct comparisons difficult.

Brace type has been shown to affect results. Grace et al[16] reported that the use of a single-hinged brace resulted in significantly increased number of knee injuries, whereas use of the double-hinged prophylactic knee brace did not. Many of the braces in these studies were of earlier designs and did not accommodate for an individual's normal anatomic varus/valgus alignment. Because of this, there may have existed a prestressing of the collateral ligaments that caused deleterious effects and an increased incidence of injuries. The third factor that could account for differences relates to independent variables. Sitler et al[39] had direct control of athletic shoe wear, athletic exposure, brace assignment, and playing surface, all of which have been identified as important to control for accurate study results. The final factor influencing results has to do with level of play. Sitler's study was completed using players involved in an intramural tackle football program. Although these players were competitive, their intensity most likely falls far below that of the intercollegiate setting in which Rover et al, Hewson et al, and Tietz et al completed their studies, thus possibly partially explaining why these collegiate athletes had a higher incidence of injuries.

An equal amount of disparity exists in the basic science research on prophylactic braces. Several biomechanical studies have been conducted to document the effects of lateral bracing for protection of the MCL. Both cadaveric and mechanical surrogate limb models have been used. France et al[14] tested six different brands on a mechanical surrogate limb model. They found that the unilateral, uniaxial prophylactic knee brace provided the least resistance to lateral impact loads, whereas the Don Joy unilateral-biaxial prophylactic knee brace provided the greatest resistance. These studies have demonstrated that the level of medial collateral ligament protection given by even the best braces was inconsistent and only marginal.[14,32] A more recent study published by Erickson and associates[13] refutes these results. Erickson et al criticized the surrogate limb model as inaccurate because of the misrepresentation of the ligament structures and soft tissue compliance. Using a cadaveric model, the authors performed in vitro measurements of MCL and ACL strain under dynamic impact loading. They found that the brace did significantly reduce the level of impact force at the point of impact as well as reduce elongation of the medial collateral ligament. The braces, however, were ineffective in protecting the anterior cruciate ligament. To confuse matters more, Paulos et al[30] completed a similar study evaluating the effects of six different prophylactic braces on ACL ligament strain under dynamic valgus loads using a mechanical surrogate limb validated against human cadaveric specimens. Medial collateral ligament and anterior cruciate ligament strains were recorded for both braced and unbraced conditions. These tests were conducted to determine whether or not the application of a prophylactic brace might provide protection of the anterior cruciate ligament under valgus loading conditions. This study demonstrated that the braces increased impact duration, which differentially protected the anterior cruciate ligament more than the medial collateral ligament. The study concluded that most of the braces appeared to provide some degree of protection to the anterior cruciate ligament under direct lateral impact. The authors cautioned that these findings needed to be confirmed clinically.

Therefore there still remains some controversy on whether prophylactic knee braces can truly prevent injuries. Epidemiologic studies suggest that the braces may be effective in a certain patient population. The basic science studies demonstrate considerable disparity between results. More research is required before recommending these braces for all athletes.

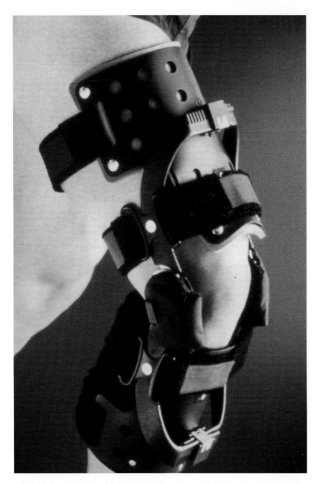

Fig. 28.6. A rehabilitation knee brace is capable of providing rigid immobilization at selected angles or controlled motion through predetermined arcs. The brace is also adjustable for size.

REHABILITATIVE KNEE BRACES

Rehabilitative braces are designed to provide control and protection to the knee after surgery (Fig. 28.6). Their use has become extremely prevalent, and in terms of volume, rehabilitative braces are used more than functional and prophylactic braces combined. Despite this volume, research has focused more on the prophylactic and functional knee braces.

Rehabilitation after any knee injury is aimed at returning the patient to activities in the shortest period of time. This has been achieved by improving surgical techniques and accelerating rehabilitative programs. Although each program is individualized, in most cases after ligament reconstruction, patients are allowed early active range of motion and weight bearing. With these two activities, there is some concern about abnormal tibial translation. At low joint loads in the early postoperative setting, however, these forces are most likely not detrimental to the ligament reconstruction. Of more concern is protection of other healing structures,

such as the patella tendon graft site in ACL reconstruction or the meniscus after repair. The brace needs to allow for a controlled range of motion to prevent excessive force on the weakened patella tendon graft site or meniscal repair.

To achieve this goal, the brace must have the ability to provide rigid immobilization at selected angles of motion. The brace must also be able to permit controlled motion through predetermined arcs. In addition, the brace needs to be adjustable for size so that after the initial postoperative dressing is removed, the brace can be adjusted to maintain an acceptable fit. Adaptability is a necessity to prolong the usefulness of the prophylactic orthosis. Once rehabilitation of the injured knee is almost complete, the long lever of the brace is no longer required, and the brace becomes cumbersome. There may still be the need, however, to control motion or maintain stability in the injured knee. Often an intermediate brace is prescribed while the thigh diameter and strength are returned to preinjury status. In an era where cost-effectiveness is essential, however, the reimbursement process may prohibit this use.

Despite the widespread use of prophylactic knee braces, there have been relatively few objective studies of their efficacy. The interest in postoperative bracing developed out of work done by Krachow and Vetter.[23] In a cadaver study, these investigators found that a well-molded cylinder cast was not able to protect the knee from varus/valgus forces or to reduce anterior translation of the tibia. The concept of a functional cast was introduced in the 1980s to prevent the deleterious effects of long-term immobilization. The theory was to allow for some motion while protecting strain on healing tissues. Gerber et al[15] used an in vivo technique to measure primary translatory motion in the sagittal plane. The authors compared a limited mobilization cast to a specifically modified Lennox Hill derotation brace and found that the latter was more effective in preventing anterior tibial translation during flexion and extension.

Crawley et al[12] designed a testing protocol that mimicked true physiologic loads and allowed for evaluation of postoperative braces under these conditions. With the use of a mechanical surrogate model, these authors evaluated, in detail, a number of mechanical factors that affected the brace. The study demonstrated that orthoses which were integrated and functioned as a single unit were most effective in controlling rotation and translation of the knee. These authors acknowledged that the mechanical surrogate model is not a true physiologic model but did permit comparison of different brace functions.

More research is required to confirm the efficacy of postoperative knee rehabilitation bracing. This re-

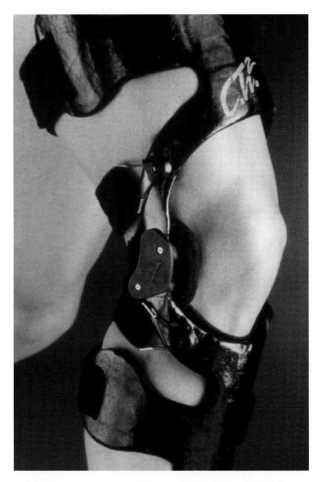

Fig. 28.7. Functional knee brace—rigid shell-type design with a kinematic hinge. Motion stops to prevent knee hyperextension.

search needs to concentrate on in vivo measurements under axial loading during physiologic conditions. With this cost-conscious environment, it is essential that this research be completed to allow for continued use of postoperative braces.

FUNCTIONAL KNEE BRACES

Functional braces are designed to provide stability during sporting activities (Fig. 28.7). They are often used to protect individuals with ligament deficiencies or those who have had ligament reconstructions without impeding performance. The functional orthosis needs to be able to facilitate normal kinematics of the tibiofemoral joint while limiting abnormal displacement or loads that may be detrimental to the injured or reconstructed knee joint.

In the majority of cases, functional knee braces are used for the protection of the individual with an anterior cruciate ligament injury. The brace may be used as an augmentation to treatment in the unstable knee joint owing to an absent anterior cruciate ligament, or it may be worn by the athlete in the later stages of recovery following a reconstructive procedure when returning to vigorous activities.

Despite the common use of these functional knee braces, there is a paucity of data available to support their effectiveness. Several investigators have reported that these braces are effective in protecting healing or damaged tissue and may prevent reinjury.[4,29,44] Other researchers report that "giving-way" continues to occur despite functional bracing.[9,10] Tegner and Lorentzon,[41] in an epidemiologic study, reported that functional knee braces were not effective in preventing knee injuries in Swedish hockey players because serious knee injuries continued to occur even when these athletes were completely rehabilitated.

Clinical evaluation has concentrated on either subjective questioning or indirect objective measurements of brace effectiveness. With regards to subjective satisfaction, several studies have reported that wearers believed that their activity level was improved and that they had less pain, swelling, and giving-way with the use of the functional knee brace.[25,35] Although helpful in determining patient compliance, these studies provide no objective measurements with regards to their effectiveness.

Indirect methods of measurement, including KT-1000, Striker, Knee Laxer Tester, Genucom, and the Knee Signature System, have been used by several investigators.[5,8,29] As previously mentioned, there are several flaws with this form of testing. Understanding these limitations, the studies have been able to demonstrate that translation can be reduced with the use of a brace at low anterior loads (i.e., 15 or 20 lb shear force). At higher loads, the brace was less effective in reducing anterior tibial translation. Unfortunately the magnitude of these loads is small compared with the magnitude of anterior shear loads seen with activities of daily living.[26,27,28] In addition, the tests represent only loading, not dynamic forces. Therefore, these studies all fall short in documenting the effectiveness of the brace under physiologic conditions.

Benynnon et al[6] attempted to quantify more accurately the effect of the functional knee brace on strain of the anterior cruciate ligament through in vivo testing conditions. Using knowledge from a previous cadaveric study[2], the authors attempted to quantify the strain on the anterior cruciate ligament in the presence of normal muscular function when known loads were applied to the knee fitted with a functional knee brace. The authors were interested in determining whether bracing altered the strain detrimentally or beneficially. The braces were tested on subjects who had a normal anterior cruciate ligament and were scheduled for arthroscopic meniscectomy or exploration of the knee under local anesthesia. A Hall-effect strain transducer was applied to the anterior cruciate ligament during the arthroscopic procedure, testing was completed in the operating room suite, and the device was removed at the end of the procedure. Under low anterior shear loads, the brace provided some protective strain-shielding effect. The strain shielding did not occur at higher anterior shear loads, which would be comparable to the high stress activity of athletic endeavors. The brace was not effective in reducing the strain on the anterior cruciate ligament during active ROM or during isometric contraction of the quadriceps. Even though there was no protection with these activities, the brace did not produce any detrimental or adverse affect on the strain of the anterior cruciate ligament. Once again, the data suggest that braces are effective only for low load conditions.

Some clinicians believe that the brace has an ability to improve sports performance either from improved proprioceptive feedback or from potential increase in muscle strength as a result of brace wear. Cook and associates[10] published results of a dynamic in vivo functional analysis of functional knee braces used in athletes with documented ACL deficient knees. Brace effectiveness was tested in running and cutting situations. A footswitch, high-speed photography, and a force plate was used for analysis. Athletes performed straight running, straight cutting, and cross-cutting with and without the brace. Statistical analysis demonstrated that subjectively all athletes reported fewer episodes of subluxation and better athletic performance in the brace. The brace also allowed for significantly better running and cutting performance for the athlete when wearing the brace in the anterior cruciate ligament–deficient knee. These results suggested that improved performance was achieved by proprioceptive feedback of the brace. Branch and colleagues,[7] however, refuted the principle that the brace provided proprioceptive effect by demonstrating that the use of the brace did not alter electromyographic activity or change pattern of muscle firing.

Although there have been ambiguous clinical reports, several basic science studies have been done to determine the effectiveness of the brace in controlling abnormal anterior tibial translations. A number of cadaveric studies have demonstrated that a functional knee brace is effective in controlling abnormal anterior tibial translation.[5,8,9] Similar to the clinical data, however, this appears to be the case only at low anterior shear forces and not with the high loads, which would be indicative of vigorous activities. Wojtys and associates[45] used the Genucom Device as an indirect method of measurement to study the ability of several functional knee braces to control both translation and tibial rotation under rigid mechanical loading. The limbs were tested with and without braces, beginning with an intact knee. This was then followed by cutting the anterior cruciate ligament and repeating the rotation and translation tests at 30 and 60 degrees of knee flexion. The final tests were performed after the medial collateral ligament was divided. Analysis of the data showed that the braces were more effective in decreasing anterior displacement with combined anterior cruciate ligament/medial collateral ligament lesions than with the anterior cruciate ligament lesion alone, even though the absolute value of anterior displacement was greater. The braces were also found to be more effective in decreasing the AP translation than decreasing rotation. Finally, the braces were found to be more effective in decreasing anterior displacement at 60 degrees of knee flexion than 30 degrees of knee flexion. This experiment clearly demonstrated that functional knee braces could prevent anterior tibial translations under certain conditions. Unfortunately the model used indirect means of measurement and lacked muscular contribution during testing, making this less like a real-life situation.

Arms and co-workers[2] attempted to measure more accurately the amount of anterior tibial displacement by performing direct measurements of anterior cruciate ligament elongation using the Hall-effect strain transducer in braced and nonbraced cadaver specimens. The results of this study contradicted findings in other cadaver studies that used indirect methods of measurements of anterior tibial translation. Arms and colleagues showed that when comparing braced to nonbraced cadaver specimens, the brace was not able to protect the anterior cruciate ligament when shear loads were applied across the tibiofemoral joint. In fact, strain on the anterior cruciate ligament was increased when the knee was braced in all positions from 0 to 90 degrees of flexion. This study suggested that a brace may actually cause anterior displacement of the tibia, thus increasing strain on the anterior cruciate ligament. Interpretation of the data suggests that knee braces with a fixed axis of rotation, which are dissimilar to the complex three-dimensional tibiofemoral rotation axis and translatory pathway of the normal knee, may actually constrain the knee joint and produce a deleterious increase in the value of strain on the anterior cruciate ligament. Although this study used a direct means of measurement for anterior tibial translation, the validity of the results remains in question because of the inherent flaws of all cadaveric studies.

The results of the above-noted biomechanical and clinical studies indicate that functional knee braces, at best, are able only to decrease the amount of anterior tibial translation and axial rotation at low shear forces. At higher shear loads, the braces appear to be less effective in reducing abnormal translation and rotation.

Functional braces have also been touted to be able to protect the knee from varus/valgus forces.[11,24] Lunsford[24] used a testing apparatus of an above-knee prosthesis modified to allow for varus and valgus angles much greater than normally seen under physiologic conditions. With this model, it was possible to apply forces and record angular deformation. The ranges of applied torques were studied to represent practical clinical conditions because extreme torques associated with high-level professional sports are unknown. After testing eight braces, the results demonstrated that the brace could resist varus/valgus deforming forces as long as it was a rigid shell-type brace. Baker and co-workers[3] reported similar results in a cadaver model demonstrating that a well-fitted rigid brace could protect the collateral ligament by reducing deforming forces.

All the studies mentioned here are limited by the fact that the limb is not axially loaded during the testing. In daily and athletic endeavors, compressive loads around the knee are produced by body weight and muscle forces. These forces can be difficult to define and control in in vivo situations. During certain activities, the compressive joint loads may produce some restraint to tibial femoral translation and rotation. This represents an important factor in how the brace may ultimately function under normal physiologic conditions.

Research has demonstrated that functional knee braces can protect the anterior cruciate ligament or its replacement at relatively low loads (<100 N) of anterior shear force. This magnitude, however, as previously mentioned, is small compared with the magnitude of anterior shear loads seen with activities of daily living. The weak link in the ability for the brace to provide support exists in the interface between the brace and the soft tissue. Walker and colleagues[43] showed that because soft tissues are interposed between the bone and the brace, it is difficult for the brace to affect the kinematics of the knee joint significantly. Despite these limitations, there may be some role for functional knee braces in the early postoperative period or in the ligament-deficient patient. The brace is capable of providing protection against anterior tibial translation at low shear loads, improving proprioception and muscle force, and, most importantly, preventing hyperextension with the use of a control stop to control detrimental knee motion.

REFERENCES

1. American Academy of Orthopedic Surgeons: Knee Braces. In Derz DJ, editor: Seminar Report, Chicago, 1985, American Academy of Orthopedic Surgeons.
2. Arms S, et al: The effect of knee braces on anterior cruciate ligament strain, Trans Orthop Res Soc 12:245, 1987.
3. Baker BE, et al: A biomech study of the static stabilizing effect of knee braces on medical stability, Am J Sports Med 15:566–570, 1987.
4. Bassett GS, Fleming BW: The Lenox Hill brace in anterolateral rotatory instability, Am J Sports Med 11:345–348, 1983.
5. Beck C, et al: Instrumented testing of functional knee braces, Am J Sports Med 14:253–256, 1986.
6. Beynnon BD, et al: The effect of functional knee-braces on strain on the anterior cruciate ligament in vivo, J Bone Joint Surg 74A:1298-1312, 1992.
7. Branch TP, Hunter R, Donath M: Dynamic EMG analysis of anterior cruciate deficient legs with and without bracing during cutting, Am J Sports Med 17:35–41, 1989.
8. Branch TP, Hunter R, Reynolds P: Controlling anterior tibial displacement under static load: A comparison of two braces, Orthopedics 11:1249–1252, 1988.
9. Colville MR, Lee CL, Cuilli JV: The Lenox Hill Brace: An evaluation of effectiveness in treating knee instability, Am J Sports Med 14:257–261, 1986.
10. Cook FF, Tibone JE, Redfern FC: A dynamic analysis of a functional brace for anterior cruciate ligament insufficiency, Am J Sports Med 17:519–524, 1989.
11. Crawley PW: Post-operative knee bracing, Clin Sports Med 9:763–770, 1990.
12. Crawley PW, France EP, Paulos LE: Comparison of rehabilitative knee braces: A biomechanical investigation, Am J Sports Med 17:141–146, 1989.
13. Erickson AR, et al: An in vitro dynamic evaluation of prophylactic knee braces during lateral impact loading, Am J Sports Med 12:26–35, 1993.
14. France EP, et al: The biomechanics of lateral knee bracing, Part II. Impact response of the braced knee, Am J Sports Med 15:430–438, 1987.
15. Gerber G, Jacob RP, Ganz R: Observations concerning a limited mobilization cast after anterior cruciate ligament surgery, Arch Orthop Trauma Surg 101:291–296, 1985.
16. Grace T, et al: Prophylactic knee braces in injury to the lower extremity, J Bone Surg 70A:422–427, 1988.
17. Gunston FH: Polycentric knee arthroplasty: Prosthetic simulation of normal knee movement, J Bone Joint Surg 53B:272, 1971.
18. Hewson G, Mendini R, Wang J: Prophylactic knee bracing in college football, Am J Sports Med 14:262–266, 1986.
19. Howe JG, et al: Arthroscopic strain gauge measurement of the normal anterior cruciate ligament, Arthroscopy 6:198–204, 1990.
20. Jonnsson H, Karrholm J: Brace effects on the unstable knee in 21 cases. A roentgen stereophotogrammetric comparison of three designs, Acta Orthop Scand 61:313–318, 1990.
21. Kain CC, et al: An in vivo study of the effect of the transcutaneous electrical muscle stimulation on anterior deformation, Trans Orthop Res Soc 12:106, 1987.
22. Kapandji IA: The physiology of the joints, ed 5, London, 1987, Churchhill Livingstone.
23. Krackow KA, Vetter WL: Knee motion in a long leg cast, Am J Sports Med 9:233–239, 1981.
24. Reference deleted in proof. See Chapter 2 of this text.
25. Mishra DK, Daniel DM, Stone ML: The use of functional knee braces in the control of pathologic anterior knee laxity, Clin Orthop 241:213–220, 1989.
26. Morrison JB: Bio-engineering analysis of forced actions transmitted by the knee joint, Biomed Eng 3:164–170, 1986.
27. Morrison JB: Function of the knee joint in various activities, Biomed Eng 4:573–580, 1969.
28. Noyes FR, et al: Biomechanical analysis of human ligament grafts used in knee-ligament repairs and reconstruction, J Bone Joint Surg 66A:344–352, 1984.
29. Noyes FR, et al: The symptomatic anterior cruciate-deficient knee: Part II. The results of rehabilitation, activity modification,

and counseling on functional disability, J Bone Joint Surg 65A: 163–174, 1983.

30. Paulos LE, Cawle PW, France EP: Impact biomechanics of lateral knee bracing: The anterior cruciate ligament, Am J Sports Med 19:337–342, 1991.

31. Paulos LE, Payne FC III, Rosenberg TD: Rehabilitation after anterior cruciate ligament surgery. In Jakson DW, Derz D, editors: The anterior cruciate deficient knee: New concepts in ligament repair, St. Louis, 1987, CV Mosby.

32. Paulos LE, et al: The biomechanics of lateral knee bracing: Part I. Response of the valgus restraints to loading, Am J Sports Med 15:419–429, 1987.

33. Quillian W, et al: Knee bracing in preventing injuries in high school football, Int Pediatr 2:255–256, 1987.

34. Regalbuto MA, Robick JS, Walker PS: The forces in a knee brace as a function of hinge design and placement, Am J Sports Med 17:535–543, 1989.

35. Rink PC, et al: A comparative study of functional bracing in the anterior cruciate deficient knee, Orthop Rev 18:719–727, 1989.

36. Romash MM, Henningsen HJ, Claybaugh J: Knee braces—comparative functional testing, Orthop Trans 13:501, 1989.

37. Rovere G, Haupt H, Yates C: Prophylactic knee bracing in college football, Am J Sports Med 15:111–116, 1987.

38. Schriner J: The effectiveness of knee bracing in preventing knee injuries in high school athletes Med Sci Sports Exerc 17:254, 1985 (abstract).

39. Sitler M, et al: The efficacy of a prophylactic knee brace to reduce knee injuries in football, Am J Sports Med 18:310–315, 1990.

40. Strasser, 1917.

41. Tegner Y, Lorentzon R: Evaluation of knee braces in Swedish ice hockey players, Br J Sports Med 25:159–161, 1991.

42. Tietz C, Hermanson B, Kronmal R: Evaluation of the use of braces to prevent injury to the knee in collegiate football players, J Bone Joint Surg 69A, 1987.

43. Walker PS, Rovick JS, Robertson DD: The effects of brace hinge design in placement on joint mechanics, J BioMech 21:965, 1988.

44. Wellington P, Stother IG: The Lenox Hill derotation brace in chronic post-traumatic instability of the knee, Injury 15:242–244, 1984.

45. Wojtys EM, et al: A biomechanical evaluation of the Lenox Hill knee brace, Clin Orthop 220:179–184, 1987.

Orthotic Management of the Neuropathic and Dysvascular Patient

Richard B. Chambers
Nancy Elftman

Orthotic treatment of the neuropathic foot can prevent or delay the need for limb amputation. Because the loss of peripheral nerve function alone does not cause tissue death directly, the viability of the neuropathic limb is threatened by the delayed recognition of injury to that limb. More extensive tissue damage is more likely to be irreparable. Effective treatment substitutes for the missing link in the body's early warning system. Orthotic devices—shoes, inserts, lower extremity orthoses—in conjunction with the use of substitute warning systems can restore adequate protection to the neuropathic limb. These measures should decrease the need to resort to amputation.

Peripheral neuropathy can produce any combination of loss in the sensory, motor, or autonomic components of nerve function. The clinical result is always the same—skin breakdown, ulceration, or both. The cause of the ulcer is varied. Sensory loss leads to ulceration by virtue of the unrecognized skin trauma. Acute injury from impaling the skin with a tack and chronic injury from a poorly fitting shoe remain undetected for many hours without skin sensation. Charcot joint degeneration, present in some neuropathic limbs, may result in foot deformities. These deformities, when walked on, may lead to ulcers beneath the resultant bony prominences or at the apex of angular deformities. Claw toes, caused by loss of the motor nerve function to intrinsic foot muscles, produce ulcer-prone skin on the plantar surface of the metatarsal heads, the dorsal surface of the proximal interphalangeal joints, and the toe tips. Autonomic nerve functional loss contributes to the skin's vulnerability to breakdown by producing dry, nonelastic skin with the attendant lack of oil and sweat production. Although orthotic devices cannot restore these lost functions, protection of these feet is possible with careful shoe fitting and foot monitoring.

PERIPHERAL NEUROPATHY

Peripheral neuropathy is present when sensation testing reveals that the level of sensation loss is symmetric and equidistant from the spine in both arms and legs (Fig. 29.1). The hands of these patients should be considered in the evaluation process of neuropathy of an insensate foot. Physical signs of upper extremity involvement include *chaeroarthropathy:* when the patient cannot touch the palms together in the prayer position (Fig. 29.2).

Another physical sign of significant peripheral neuropathy is atrophy of the thenar eminence, although there are other causes of thenar atrophy, such as carpal tunnel syndrome. Consideration of the hand deficit must be taken into account for the ability of the patient to don and doff and to close the orthosis and footwear.[4] Little attention has been paid to the "diabetic hand syndrome" or limited joint mobility (LJM) in which the joints of the fingers and wrists become limited. This condition occurs in 30% to 50% of people who have had type 1 diabetes for more than 15 years. One test for LJM is performed by placing hands flat on a table. Persons with severe cases of LJM are not able to flatten fingers onto the table. The skin is thick and can be "tented" on the back of the fingers.[24]

Bilateral testing for sensation is especially important for the unilateral and bilateral amputee to determine areas of insensitivity and progression of the neuropathy. Neuropathy may be present in many disease processes. The neuropathy may be isolated (nerve damage or entrapment), but for most chronic disease processes the effect is peripheral. Any form of peripheral neuropathy can produce the discomfort of paresthesia: prickling, burning, jabbing sensations.[44,47]

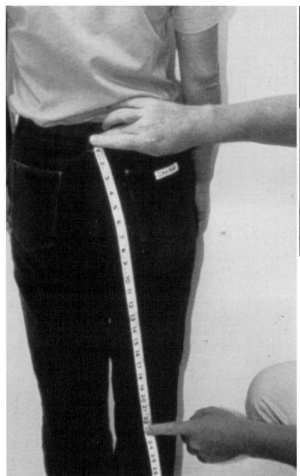

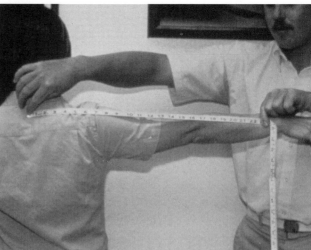

Fig. 29.1. Peripheral neuropathy. Peripheral neuropathy affects limbs symmetrically and equidistant from the spine. The legs and arms are involved beginning with the feet and hands.

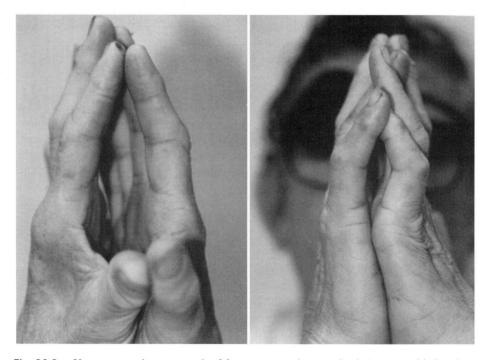

Fig. 29.2. Upper extremity neuropathy. Motor neuropathy seen in the neuropathic hands as *limited joint mobility*.

The most common disease processes resulting in peripheral neuropathy are:
- Diabetes
- Spina bifida
- Hansen's disease
- Lupus
- AIDS/HIV/ARC
- Cancer
- Multiple sclerosis
- Vascular disease
- Charcot-Marie-Tooth disease

The following toxins and syndromes can also cause peripheral neuropathy in the limbs:[8,9,27]
- Alcohol
- Arsenic
- Lead
- Steroids
- Gold
- Uremia
- Vitamin B
- INH use

A high suspicion for neuropathy should be present when examining the feet of individuals with these problems. Diabetes mellitus is the leading cause of peripheral neuropathy in the United States, with 54,000 amputations of the lower extremity occurring yearly in the 14 million diabetics at an annual cost of $14 billion.[3,21,32,36,38,49]

Complaints of numbness, tingling, or burning night pain are common when neuropathy is present. The degree of sensory loss is difficult to quantify. It is important to use an objective method of sensation evaluation for initial detection as well as follow-up. Some researchers have suggested that patients who are unable to detect a monofilament of 5.07 diameter (10 g of force) are at risk for developing ulcerations and require protective shoes and inserts. The use of the Semmes-Weinstein monofilament is the standard to make such determinations. It is important to inspect the insensate foot, looking for areas of vulnerable skin for breakdown, especially the weight-bearing surfaces of the foot. In addition, it is necessary to examine the foot for bony prominences caused by claw toes or fracture malalignment. Signs of concomitant dysvascularity, such as pulselessness, decreased hair growth, gangrene, or decreased skin temperature, add to the risk of eventual amputation if remedial measures are not taken.

Four types of stress can lead to ulceration and destruction of tissue in the neuropathic limb:
1. Ischemic necrosis is caused by moderate pressures (2 to 3 psi) over long periods of time. Local capillary circulation is interrupted leading to skin death and resultant ulceration. This is the mechanism of pres-

sure sores, seen at the sites of shoes that are too narrow.
2. Acute mechanical disruption occurs when direct injury caused by a high pressure ($\geq$600 psi) lacerates the skin. This may also be caused by heat or chemicals that cause acute, rapid skin breakdown. Common injuries include stepping on a foreign object, such as a nail.
3. Inflammatory destruction occurs with many repetitive moderate pressures (40 to 60 psi). Chronic inflammation develops and weakens the tissue, leading to ulceration. Breakdown over bony prominences is an example of this mechanism.
4. Infection (including osteomyelitis) causes the spread of tissue destruction. Once the skin is broken, bacterial invasion may allow surrounding skin to become more vulnerable to even slight pressure rendering it incapable of weight bearing.[11]

The highest incidence of ulceration occurs at sites of previous ulceration and over bony prominences, especially in weight-bearing skin. A newly healed ulcer is covered by thin skin that is more likely to tear with stress. Adherent skin with little subcutaneous padding has poor shock-absorbing or shear-absorbing qualities and is also vulnerable to breakdown. Protection of such skin areas is possible with careful shoe and insert construction.[10,12]

Charcot arthropathy

Charcot joint (Charcot arthropathy) is a relatively painless, progressive and degenerative arthropathy of single or multiple joints caused by underlying neuropathy. The neuropathy can be periosteal and not cutaneous, so the skin surface has intact sensation. There are several theories behind the causes of Charcot joint:
1. Multiple microtraumas to the joints that cause microfractures. These fractures lead to relaxation of the ligaments and joint destruction.
2. Increased blood flow (osteolysis) and bone reabsorption. Patients with Charcot joints can have bounding pulses.
3. Changes in the spinal cord leading to trophic changes in bones and joints.
4. An osteoporosis accompanied by an abnormal brittleness of the bones leading to spontaneous fracture.[17]

Whatever the cause, Charcot arthropathy can lead to radical changes in the shape and stability of the affected joint. The clinical stages of Charcot arthropathy are outlined in Table 29.1. The stages of Charcot arthropathy should be followed and documented carefully to reduce deformity. At each stage, treatment attempts to minimize the effect of deformity, initially with casting in the neutral position. If the Charcot arthropathy

Table 29.1. Charcot arthropathy (Charcot joint)*

STAGE	CLINICAL NOTES	LABORATORY	TREATMENT PROTOCOL
Acute/early stage (duration 1–2 months)	Limb usually painless, swollen, red, and 5–10° F hotter than contralateral	Unhealed fractures often radiographically present	Total contact cast applied. Cast changed in 5–7 days and followed in midstage
Advanced/midstage (6 months–1 year)	Warm with reduced swelling	Extensive bone demineralization and reabsorption	Changing of cast at 1- to 2-week intervals. Casting important for retention of foot shape
Late stage and chronic	Complete bony healing, temperatures equal to contralateral limb	Architectural distortion with shortening and widening of the joint[35]	Accommodate with splint, then shoes/inserts for midfoot to forefoot deformities. Deformities of hindfoot or ankle require neuropathic walker or total contact AFO. Resultant bony deformities may require surgical intervention

*The stages of Charcot joint should be followed and documented carefully to reduce deformity.

becomes quiescent, the foot should then be protected with appropriate shoes and inserts.

Examination

Examination of the neuropathic limb includes a visual and physical examination to determine deformities that may lead to ulceration in the future. The shoes and socks are removed to allow the practitioner to examine for callus, bony prominences, and areas of skin inflammation. The thickening of the skin in the area of callus is preceded by abnormal pressure or friction.[14,46] Dryness of skin is the result of autonomic neuropathy, in which sweat and oil production is decreased and moisture must be replaced. Loss of hair growth may be indicative of vascular impairment. Motor neuropathy distorts skeletal alignment. Charcot arthropathy leaves the foot deformed. All weight-bearing bony prominences must be relieved to prevent excess pressure, which leads to ulceration.

Joint stiffness makes any deformity more ulcer prone, by decreasing normal foot motion during stance, thereby increasing foot-shoe contact. It is important that the ankle has dorsiflexion range of at least 10 degrees to allow ambulation without harm to the great toe.[39] When the heel rises, the forces on the plantar surface of the metatarsal heads and toes can peak to 275% of body weight when running and 80% when walking. With limited motion in the metatarsophalangeal joints, these forces can result in ulceration.[4,42,45]

Toe deformities

Toe deformities may result in ulceration by contact with shoe surfaces or adjacent toes. In the case of claw toe deformity, the toes are dorsiflexed at the metatarsophalangeal joints and plantar flexed at the interphalangeal joints (Fig. 29.3). Such deformities, especially if the joints are stiff, produce shoe contact at their sites.

Soft corns are hyperkeratotic lesions found between toes caused by pressure of opposing toes in a region that is moist.[14] These ulcers between the toes can be relieved with tube foam or lamb's wool (Fig. 29.4).

Hypertrophic nails can be caused by fungus and are common in the diabetic population. The nails tear shoe linings and create areas of rough surface that later abrade the toes.

The great toe should be examined for deformity. An ankylosed interphalangeal joint can cause ulceration that is especially difficult to relieve. Great toe extension can be seen when weight bearing because the person thrusts the toe into extension when ambulating causing callus and discoloration on the distal tip near the nail from shoe contact. Excessive great toe pronation causes a callus seen on the medial/plantar surface of the great toe. Hallux rigidus refers to limited range of motion in the great toe metatarsophalangeal joint and requires a rigid rocker-bottom shoe to allow ambulation without excessive pressure on the great toe. Hallux valgus

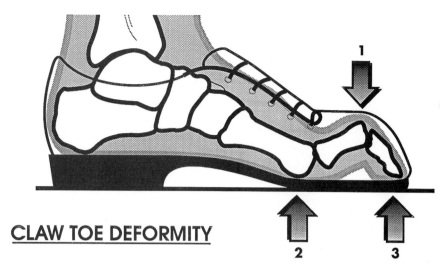

CLAW TOE DEFORMITY

Fig. 29.3.   Claw toe deformity. Clawing of the toe makes skin at the apices of this deformity more vulnerable to ulceration. *1,* Metatarsal heads are increased in their weight-bearing role. *2,* Dorsal callosity indicates increased contact with shoe underlying the toes. *3,* Toe tips become weight bearing leading to nail problems.

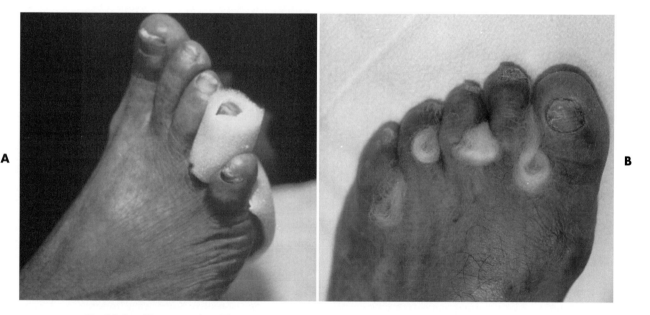

Fig. 29.4.   Toe protection. To prevent maceration and interphalangeal breakdown, the toes can be spaced with tube foam (**A**) or lamb's wool (**B**).

(bunions) is the increased valgus angle of the great toe in relation to the metatarsal, requiring a shoe that can be modified and molded to conform to the medial bunion. Toe amputations may be of single or multiple toes. The distal end of the amputation site, now without a nail, requires protection from trauma.

Complications with neuropathic foot

There are common complications associated with the neuropathic limb. A sinus tract formation results when previous areas of ulceration heal over residual bacteria instead of healing from internal to external tissues. The sinus may be the "tip of the iceberg" with extensive necrosis beneath the sinus.

Another common occurrence in neuropathic feet is burns, caused by either excessive heat or chemicals such as over-the-counter foot remedies. The insensitive foot cannot produce the warning signals necessary to prevent severe burns to extremities.

Dermatological conditions can affect treatment programs until they are resolved. Necrobiosis can be confused with venous stasis disease but does not require or respond to extensive treatment. The round,

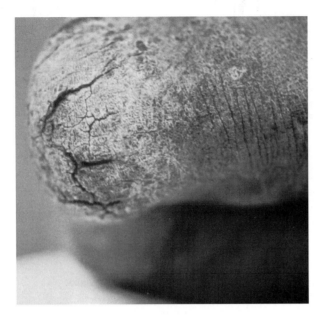

Fig. 29.5. Keratodermia plantaris. Loss of sweat and oil production (autonomic neuropathy) can lead to keratin buildup and deep fissures, predominantly on heels.

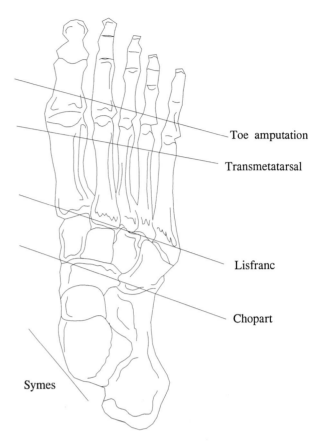

Fig. 29.6. Partial foot amputation. The partial foot amputation leaves a functional limb for weight bearing. The levels of partial foot amputation are distal metatarsal, transmetatarsal, Lisfranc, and Chopart.

firm plaques are reddish brown to yellow and are seen three times more often in women.[35,50] These ulcerations are common along the tibia and require only protective dressings.

Plantar keratoderma (keratin cracks and ulcerations) is caused by the loss of sweat and oil elasticity in the skin (autonomic neuropathy). As keratin builds up, it creates small fissures that allow entrance of bacteria and subsequent infection (Fig. 29.5). The entire sole around the margin of the heel undergoes diffuse thickening and develops painful fissures. Prevention includes reduction of keratin buildup and retention of skin moisture with the use of various creams.[14]

Pseudomonas (a green pigment) is bacterial growth within a moist environment and is treated by allowing the limb to aerate. Many dermatological conditions are discovered by inspection rather than patient discomfort.[50]

Partial foot amputation

Preservation of at least a portion of the foot with the specialized weight-bearing skin surface on the plantar surface generally retains greater ambulatory function than transtibial amputation. Care should be taken to avoid the creation of a residual foot that has unbalanced antagonistic muscle groups (Fig. 29.6). Surgical reconstruction within the foot should also avoid unpadded bony prominences, which make shoe and insert fabrication more difficult and recurrent ulceration more likely. Table 29.2 lists the advantages and disadvantages of some common amputations through the foot.

Sensation

The severity of a neuropathic or potentially neuropathic limb should include assessment of sensitivity. Because sensory loss can have a gradual onset, patient history can be misleading. A more quantitative measure of sensation helps determine the present status and progression of sensory impairment. Several methods have been developed. Use of calibrated monofilaments provides a simple and quantitative method to determine sensory deficit. Semmes-Weinstein filaments can be used to categorize feet into normal sensation (4.17 size: 1 g pressure), impaired sensation requiring protective footwear (5.07 size: 10 g pressure), and no sensation (6.10 size: 75 g pressure) requiring careful foot monitoring in addition to protective shoes and orthoses. The severity of sensory loss is proportional to the ulcer risk.

In 1898 von Frey attempted to standardize the stimuli for testing the subjective sense of light touch by using a series of horsehairs of varying thicknesses and stiffnesses. Weinstein used nylon monofilaments mounted on lucite rods as substitutes for the hairs.[37]

Table 29.2. Levels of foot amputation

LEVEL	ADVANTAGES	DISADVANTAGES
Toe amputation (metatarsophalangeal level and distal)	Little lost function because toe musculature is electrically silent in walking.	If multiple toes are lost, remaining toes become more vulnerable to trauma. Consider transmetatarsal amputation when residual toes number three or less, especially if remaining toes are not adjacent.
Transmetatarsal Lisfranc (short transmetatarsal)	Produces durable, easily shoeable foot, especially if plantar skin is turned up to cover leading surface of foot. Plantar distal corner of bones should be beveled to avoid recurrent skin breakdown at heal-off.	If bones are transected in the proximal shafts, short foot may present problems of shoe suspension.
Chopart	Most proximal level where a formal prosthesis is not required.	May lead to gradual equinus because of stronger plantar flexion of triceps competing with the detached dorsiflexors (anterior tibialis, toe extensors). Weakening plantar flexion by use of tendon Achilles lengthening is possible. The short foot with no leg shortening makes orthotic fitting difficult.
Symes	Distal prosthetic suspension. Most proximal level where plantar skin and subcutaneous tissue are preserved; therefore end weight bearing is possible.	Prosthesis less cosmetic than below knee level because of bulbous distal end.

The Semmes-Wienstein monofilaments can be obtained in elaborate sets for precise measurement, but research at Carville (Hansen's Disease Center, Carville, LA) has consolidated the testing to three sizes of monofilaments for grading the insensitive limb. No patient with protective sensation can ambulate on an ulcerated foot because of pain. Use of the monofilament is not to be confused with the testing for sharp/dull sensation. The monofilament is a single point perception test and requires the examiner to place the monofilament on the skin, press until the monofilament bends (diameter of monofilament controls point of bend), and remove from skin surface (Fig. 29.7). The monofilaments are tested and determined to be reliable at the 95% confidence level.[6]

Temperature

One physical sign that is helpful in detecting areas prone to ulceration is areas of increased skin temperatures (hot spots).[5] These areas of warmth can be caused by local inflammation in the skin and subcutaneous tissue. Once found, a reason for such warmth should be sought. Feeling the surface of the foot should be performed as part of a foot examination.[15] This portion of self-examination should also become part of daily habitual behavior for those with feet at risk for ulcer-

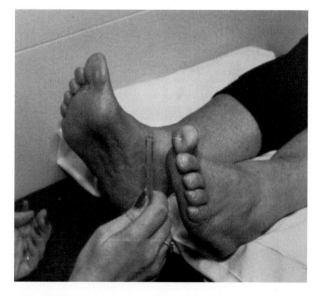

Fig. 29.7. Sensation testing. The Semmes-Wienstein monofilament is placed on the skin, deflected to bending point, and removed to test level of sensation. Sensation decreases at the toes and continues proximally in peripheral neuropathy.

ation. The temperature scanning/mapping can be more reliably measured with several devices from thermocouples to infrared units. The infrared units are fast,

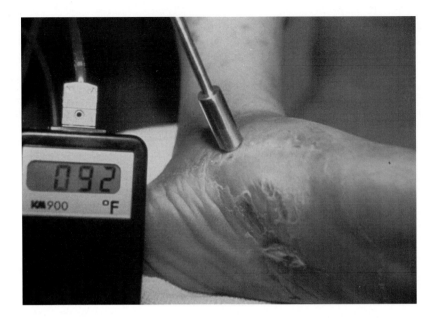

Fig. 29.8.   Temperature testing. Using a surface temperature sensing instrument, temperatures are recorded in predetermined areas and used for objective diagnostic as well as follow-up information.

allowing an examiner to record multiple readings quickly, thus scanning the limbs in question. It should be remembered that the lower limbs normally get colder as one moves proximal to distal.[5]

Using a surface sensing temperature device (thermocouple or infrared), temperatures are recorded in predetermined areas, usually those related to common areas of breakdown. When there is one definite area with temperature 3°F or more higher than adjacent areas, it can be assumed that there is an area of high pressures or stress, including infection (Fig. 29.8). If there is no current breakdown, this area must be relieved of pressure and the pressure distributed over remaining weight-bearing surfaces. Upon follow-up of this same patient, the temperature differentiation should decrease as healing progresses. In comparison to contralateral limbs, vascular impairment should be suspected when one limb is significantly colder or distal portions of the foot show a drop in temperature.[12]

Documentation

Documentation continuity is essential in all patients and requires a standard form to be used for assessment and future follow-up (Fig. 29.9). Tracing the ulceration on transparent film allows for accuracy of detailed healing progression. Providing the patient with a duplicate tracing can improve compliance because the patient can follow his own progress.

Photographs of ulceration sites are important for noting improvement in depth and granulation of ulceration.

Prevention and patient education

It is an important clinical responsibility to teach patients with insensate limbs methods to compensate for the lack of sensory feedback. The sensory-impaired patient must use other intact functions for this self-examination. Loss of sight and impaired hand sensation may limit the accuracy of these examinations. For these patients, more frequent examinations by friends, family members, and medical providers may be required. Self-care begins with daily inspections of feet using mirrors and magnifying glasses. Examination includes footwear and orthoses for wear and foreign objects.

Routine foot care

Patients should wash their feet with mild soap and water and carefully dry, especially between the toes. These hygiene measures aim to maintain skin flexibility and avoid breakdown. Skin that is either too dry or too moist is vulnerable to ulceration. Practices that cause excessive dryness include alcohol-based perfumes, sun lamps, and sun exposure. Direct damage to the skin can result from the use of strong adhesive tape, especially when used repeatedly.

When patients select footwear, they should not only choose the correct size and width but a shoe with no stitching over the forefoot. The stitched areas do not mold to the foot but instead cause breakdown to skin, especially in bony areas. Many foot care products (shoes, lotions, chemicals) should not be used by neuropathic patients. There are occasionally warning labels to this effect but usually in small print.

ORTHOTIC FOOT EVALUATION FORM

PATIENT _____ DIAGNOSIS _____

CODE _____ ORTHOTIST _____ DATE _____

INSENSITIVE FEET WITHOUT ULCERATION

CATAGORY	MONOFILIMENT RESPONSE	FOLLOW UP	PROTECTIVE SENSATION	INSERT	ULCER	DEFORMITY
A	+5.07 (10gm)	12 Mos.	Yes	Cushion	No	Yes/No
B	-5.07 (10gm)	6 Mos.	No	Molded	No	No
C	-5.07 (10gm)	4 Mos.	No	Molded	No	Yes
D	-5.07 (10gm)	3 Mos.	No	Molded	Yes	Yes/No
E	-6.10 (75gm)	2 Mos.	No	Molded	Yes/No	Yes/No

SKIN TEMPERATURE

○ WITHIN ± 3°

⊕ INCREASED TEMP + 3°

◉ INCREASED TEMP > +3°

⊖ DECREASED TEMP

ULCER GRADE

0 INTACT SKIN
1 SUPERFICIAL
2 TENDON OR BONE
3 ABSCESS OR OSTEO
4 FOREFOOT GANGRENE
5 FOOT GRANGRENE

○ DORSAL

○ OTHER

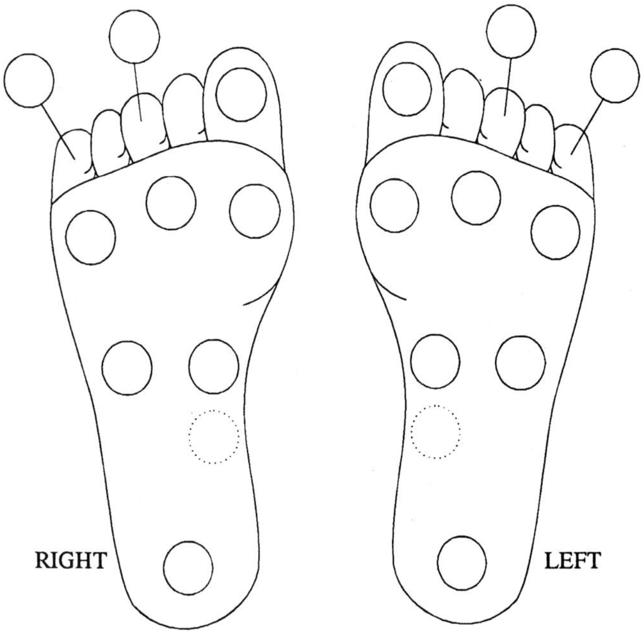

RIGHT   LEFT

Fig. 29.9. Documentation form. A standard documentation form is important for recording sensation and temperature results. Follow-up protocol is determined by results of evaluation.

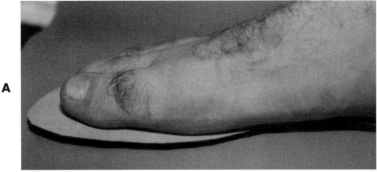

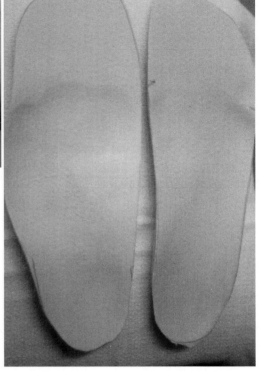

Fig. 29.10.   Prescription by sensation. **A,** The patient with protective sensation is protected by a properly fitting shoe and simple cushioning insert. **B,** The neuropathic patient requires a shoe with depth and custom accommodative insole to protect the weight-bearing surface of the foot.

Exercise programs promote good health, but certain forms of activity may increase the risk of ulceration. High foot impact activities (running, jumping) increase direct forces on the foot to many times the body weight.[20] In patients with insensate feet, safe exercise programs include swimming, cycling, and low-impact dance. In general, walking should consist of slow, short steps.[22]

Orthotic treatment

Foot ulcers.   Use of orthotic devices to prevent or cure foot ulcers in insensate feet should be integrated with other treatment modalities. The major contribution to care is in changing the distribution of forces that impact the foot. For vulnerable but intact skin, forces should be reduced by the shape and hardness of the materials used to fabricate the shoe and insert (Fig. 29.10). For ulcerated skin, maximal pressure relief is desired. An outline of treatment by ulcer is given in Table 29.3. Shoes and inserts serve many deformities, but more severe conditions require enhanced orthotic treatment. Orthotic treatment is appropriate for ulcer grades 0 through 2. Higher ulcer grades imply the need for preorthotic surgery in the form of amputation or operative debridement.[48]

When a patient has no ulceration (grade 0) and no deformity and can sense the 10-g monofilament (protective sensation), he usually does well with a standard shoe of correct sizing with a simple shock-absorbing pad. These patients will sense pain before damage occurs to their feet.

The same patient without protective sensation does not cease ambulating when damage begins to tissues. These patients require extra-depth shoes with a total contact accommodative insert to distribute pressure and reduce forces on areas of potential breakdown. The insert may be molded to the patient or fabricated from a cast. The cast does not have corrective forces added, only accommodation (Fig. 29.11).

Charcot joint.   When the joints of the foot are undergoing Charcot degeneration, the limb is usually painless, swollen, and erythematous. A history of injury resulting in fractures is often present. Radiologically, Charcot limbs may show multiple fractures accompanied by extensive bone demineralization and reabsorption. Later stages reveal architectural distortion of the foot with shortening and widening of the joint.[35]

The foot joints most often involved with Charcot changes are as follows:

Tarsometatarsal	30%
Metatarsophalangeal	30%
Tarsus	24%
Interphalangeal	4%

Charcot arthropathy is frequently misdiagnosed and mistreated and is often confused with joint infection. Untreated Charcot joints may leave the patient with deformities that require further surgical intervention, expensive footwear, or both. In the acute stage the foot is 5 to 10° F hotter than the contralateral foot in the same

Table 29.3.   Foot pathology*

FOOT PATHOLOGY	ORTHOSIS	SHOES/ORTHOSIS	COMMENTS
Claw toes	Accommodative inserts	Depth/leather soft toe box	Severe claw toes may require custom shoes.
Grade 0 foot (with protective sensation)	Cushion insole	Shoes of correct size and width with shock absorption	Patient ceases weight bearing when pain begins, preventing further trauma.
Grade 0 foot (without protective sensation)	Accommodative with reliefs for callus and trauma	Depth shoes	Insert does not have corrective forces, only accommodation and reliefs.
Grade 1 foot (superficial ulcer)	Accommodative insert/relief	ODS splint or healing shoe	ODS splint contains insert that may be adjusted.
		Total contact cast	Cast must be changed in 5–7 days, then every 1–2 weeks.
Grade 2 foot (deeper ulcer—tendon/bone)	Accommodative insert/relief	ODS splint	May require resection of underlying bony prominence to achieve healing to grade 1.
Grade 3–5 foot	Not applicable	Not applicable	Medical/surgical intervention
Chronic heel ulcer or calcanectomy	Neuropathic walker	No shoe required	Relief in heel of integral insert; contralateral shoe lift
	Axial resist AFO	Larger shoe to fit over orthosis	Contraindicated for dysvascular patients

*Evaluation of deformity and correct accommodation. Shoes and inserts will serve many deformities, but more severe conditions require enhanced orthotic treatment.

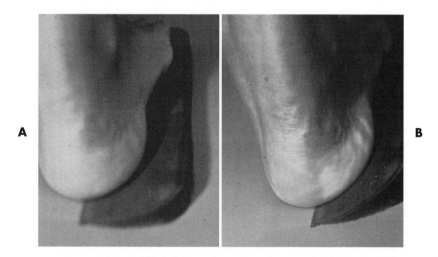

Fig. 29.11.   Accommodation—not correction. Accommodation must be achieved without correction of deformities. **A,** The foot with normal sensation senses a corrective wedge and moves body weight away from the excess force. **B,** The neuropathic foot continues to weight bear over the corrective force because of lack of sensation. The full weight bearing causes breakdown of skin at the site of the correction force.

area. The erythematous, hot, swollen foot usually does not have a skin opening or ulceration (Fig. 29.12).

To maintain bone alignment and to prevent or minimize deformity, Charcot feet should be immobilized in a cast. The duration of Charcot bone destruction, joint dissociation, and eventual recalcification varies with the individual, but average healing times in casts are:

Hindfoot	12 months
Midfoot	9 months
Forefoot	6 months

The process can be monitored by following clinical joint instability on physical examination and by noting the skin temperature over the affected joint (Fig. 29.13) The cast should be continued until temperature returns

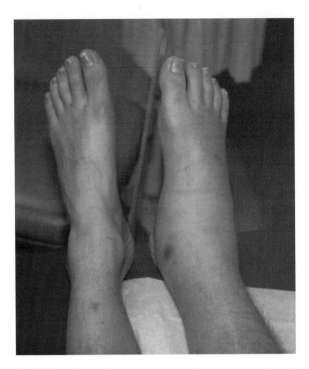

Fig. 29.12.   Acute Charcot joint. On initial examination, the affected foot appears red, hot, and swollen with bounding pulses.

to within 3°F of the uninvolved foot and clinically all affected joints are stable. X-rays show recalcification in the region of the Charcot joint, which implies resolution of the process. With prolonged cast immobilization in a position of neutrality (ankle at 0 degrees dorsiflexion and 0 degrees inversion), a plantar grade, walkable foot is preserved even if little motion is present. Arthrodesis of Charcot joints remains controversial and difficult to achieve. Avoiding residual deformity and gaining joint stability with healing remains the treatment of choice. When midfoot joints are affected, bony prominences may be so severe that the overlying ulcerated skin may not heal unless the prominence is removed surgically.

Charcot joint versus osteomelitis.   The clinical presentation for Charcot foot and osteomyelitis is similar, and the patient should be monitored closely to verify the diagnosis. Laboratory tests may also be similar. The only exception is with an opening in the skin to allow entrance for bacteria to infect the bone. The recalcification does not occur radiographically in the foot with osteomyelitis as in Charcot joint (Fig. 29.14).[2,33]

Total contact cast.   Walking in a total contact cast decreases plantar pressures under specific areas of ulcerated skin by spreading the weight-bearing pressures over the entire plantar surface of the foot. In addition, total contact casts shorten the duration of stance time by forcing the patient to take smaller strides. Total contact casts have been successful as a treatment for plantar ulcerations but require careful application, close follow-up, and patient compliance with scheduled appointments to minimize complications.[31]

The average healing time for ulcerations in insensate feet treated with a healing cast is 6 weeks.[7] This method has been used in patients with and without evidence of severe peripheral vascular disease.[43] Windows in the cast to observe the ulcer should be avoided so that localized window swelling, shear stresses, and eventually a secondary wound do not occur.[10]

Application of the total contact healing cast varies with different institutions. The healing cast was originally designed with minimal padding, but padded variations are used. Most important is to have the cast applied by a skilled health care provider.

The Carville healing cast is applied as follows (Fig. 29.15):

- Ulcer covered with thin layer of gauze.
- Cotton placed between toes to prevent maceration.
- Stockinette.
- ⅛ inch felt over malleoli and anterior tibia.
- Foam padding around toes.
- Total contact plaster shell molded.
- Shell reinforced with plaster splints.
- Walking heel attached.
- Fiberglass roll applied around plaster.

The patient is instructed to ambulate only 33% of usual activity. The initial cast is removed in 5 to 7 days and reapplied. New casts are applied every 2 to 3 weeks.[31] To allow thorough drying, the patient should not stand or walk in the cast for 24 hours.[7]

There have also been attempts to heal ulcers using a cast shoe molded of plaster. This cast must be changed in 3 days and then reapplied every 10 days. Results have reported healing of plantar ulcers in 39 days.[18]

Contraindications for the use of a healing cast include active infection, with significant erythema and drainage. In addition, significantly hypotrophic skin (thin, shiny appearance) or severe peripheral edema precludes the use of a total contact healing cast.[7] There is concern by some health care professionals that the casting procedure does not allow for daily inspections and dressing changes. Use of a total contact cast should be restricted to superficial (grade 1) ulcers when no significant infection is present.

Orthotic dynamic system splint.   The orthotic dynamic system splint (ODS splint) was developed to take advantage of the casting method of a total contact cast with the inclusion of a custom-molded insert that can be removed and reliefs modified (Fig. 29.16). With all the advantages of the total contact cast, the following advantages were added with the ODS splint: daily inspection, regular cleaning/dressings/debridement,

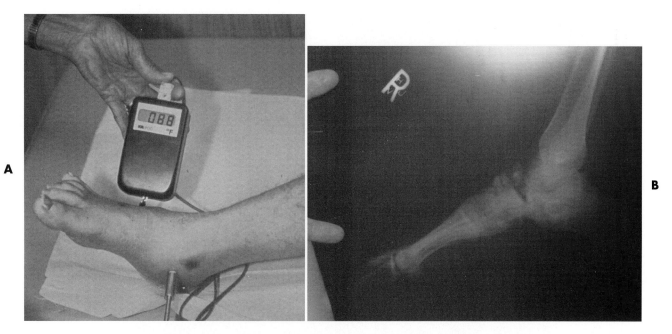

Fig. 29.13. Charcot joint evaluation. **A,** Using the thermometer, the affected foot may be in excess of 5°F hotter than the unaffected side. **B,** Verification by x-ray shows talonavicular Charcot involvement in the acute stage.

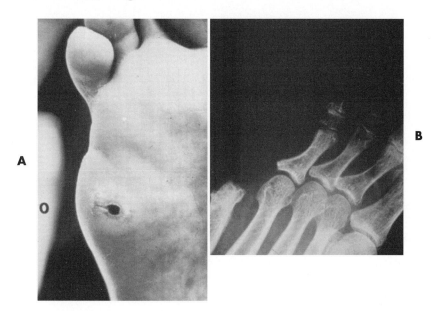

Fig. 29.14. Osteomyelitis. **A,** The obvious skin opening in the area of bony involvement indicates possible osteomyelitis as the diagnosis because of the pathway for infection to begin. **B,** The x-ray shows bony deterioration, indicative of Charcot joint or osteomyelitis.

and adjustments to areas of excessive pressure and/or friction.

The Plastazote/Aliplast insert is first molded to the patient's foot and trimmed to follow the plantar surface with ¼ inch length added beyond toes. A stockinette is placed on the leg, the insert is positioned, and another stockinette is applied to hold the insert in place. A padded total contact cast is applied using fiberglass only. The cast is bivalved, straps are added, edges are

finished, and the insert is removed to relieve the area of ulceration. After insert modification, it is replaced within the splint, and the patient may ambulate with a rocker-bottom cast shoe under the splint (Fig. 29.17). The patient is instructed to control volume with sock thickness. The disadvantage lies with compliancy of the patient. The splint design allows donning and doffing by the patient, thus allowing the patient to remove the cast.

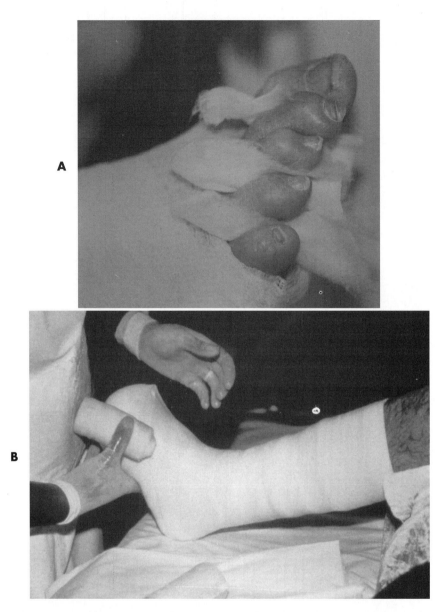

Fig. 29.15.   Total contact casting. **A,** The toes must be spaced with cotton before cast is applied to allow room within the cast and decrease risk of maceration. **B,** In neutral position, the leg is wrapped for the total contact cast.

Shoes.   Shoes for the insensitive foot should be of soft leather that conforms to abnormalities on the dorsal surface and allows for the depth of an accommodative orthosis. Leather gradually adapts to the slope of the foot and retains shape between wearings. Leather breathes and absorbs perspiration.[28] The patient should not depend on the feel of a shoe for correct sizing. The shoe must be full width and girth and allow ½ to ¾ inch space beyond the longest toe to prevent distal contact through the gait cycle. The shoe should have no stitching over the forefoot. Stitched areas never mold to the foot but instead cause breakdown to skin, especially over bony areas.

When properly fit, the instep leather should not be taut. Three tests determine the proper fit of shoes:

1. *Length:* ½ to ¾ inch of space beyond longest toe (Fig. 29.18).
2. *Ball width:* With patient weight bearing, grasp the vamp of the shoe and pinch the upper material; if the leather cannot be pinched, it is too narrow. The ball should be in the widest part of the shoe.[23]
3. *Heel-to-ball length:* Measure the distance from the patient's heel to 1st and 5th metatarsal heads. Bend shoe and repeat measurements on the shoe. They should be close to the same measurements.[30]

Lace shoes give the best control but must be broken in slowly beginning with 2 hours per day and slowly adding time.[10] Caution should be taken with cut-out sandals for the possibility of irritation along the borders of the straps.[7]

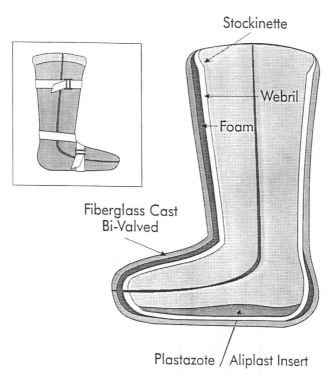

Fig. 29.16. ODS splint. The ODS splint uses the total contact cast with incorporation of a custom-molded insert. The insert is removable and adjustable to assist in pressure relief of affected area.

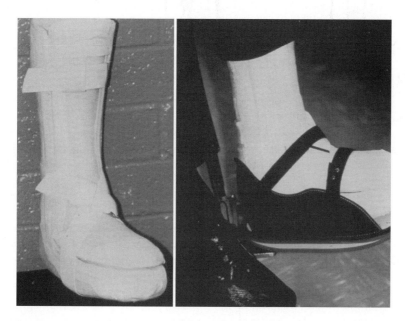

Fig. 29.17. Complete ODS splint. The finished ODS splint is fit with a rocker-bottom cast shoe for ambulation.

Standard modifications of in-depth shoes (Fig. 29.19) for the neuropathic patient include stretching of the soft toe box; padding the tongue; flared lateral (Fig. 29.20) soles to discourage varus instability; and shank/rocker bottom for a partial foot, hallux rigidus, or decreased motion at the metatarsal heads. A rocker bottom should be added to the shoe when metatar-sophalangeal extension is to be avoided.[10] Tapering the heel and toe allows a more natural gait in the standard depth shoe. To protect a healing area in which dressings are to be applied, a healing shoe lined with Plastazote allows greater circumference and adjustability.

Socks for the neuropathic limb should have no mended areas or seams over bony prominences. A

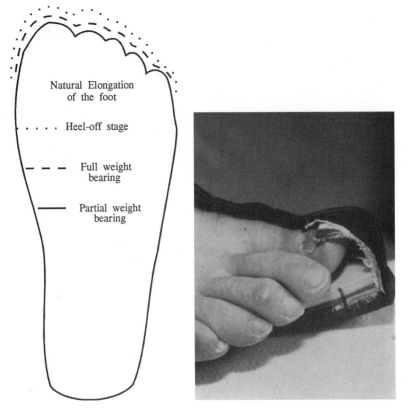

Natural Elongation
of the foot

. . . . .   Heel-off stage

– – –   Full weight
bearing

———   Partial weight
bearing

Fig. 29.18.   Length of shoe. The neuropathic foot requires a shoe that is ½ to ¾ inch longer than the longest toe to prevent distal contact during ambulation.

cotton/acrylic blend assists in the wicking of perspiration away from the foot.[19] The sock should be fully cushioned and have a nonelastic top. The partial foot requires a sock that conforms to the shape without distal prominent seams or excess material at the distal end (Fig. 29.21). For the active patient, socks can be obtained with silicone over high-stress areas to prevent shear for full or partial feet.

Accommodative insert.   The accommodative insert does not apply correction, only filling the spaces between the flat shoe and foot contours (Fig. 29.22). Any rigid corrective force receives full weight bearing, and breakdown may occur. If the addition of metatarsal head pads or scaphoid pads is requested, these pads must be of a soft durometer. Rigid pad additions cause excess pressure and ulcerations. The metatarsal head pads are placed proximal to the metatarsal heads to redistribute the weight from the heads to the metatarsal shafts.

Treatment of the neuropathic foot requires accommodation, relief of pressure/shear forces, and shock absorption. Regardless of materials used for accommodative inserts, the combination of materials must be compressible by one half of original thickness to accommodate for pressure relief through the gait cycle.[12] It is important to evaluate the materials used in the manufacture of inserts. Cellular polyethylene foams such as Aliplast, Plastazote, and Pelite are composed of a mass of bubbles. In closed-cell materials, the gases do not pass freely. Open-cell material has no windows leaving many cells interconnected so gas may pass between cells. Cell walls are not totally impermeable to the flow of gasses. Under sustained load (especially the heavy patient), gasses are squeezed out; when load is removed, gasses are drawn back into the cells.[25] These materials bottom out from compaction of the materials as cells fracture under repetitive stress. The advantages are low-temperature molding, nontoxic substance, water resistant, and washability without absorbing fluid.[28] Plastazote has a limited effective period of about 2 days, with Poron (PPT) remaining effective for 6 to 9 months (Fig. 29.23). The two materials can be combined for their attributes and perform well as a single unit.[40,41]

There are different types of inserts:
- *Soft*— cushioning, improves shock absorption.
- *Semirigid*— some cushion, pressure relief.
- *Rigid*— hard; single layer of plastic, control abnormal foot and leg motion.[29]

The Aliplast/Plastazote insert is an immediate preparation and can be provided within a clinical set-

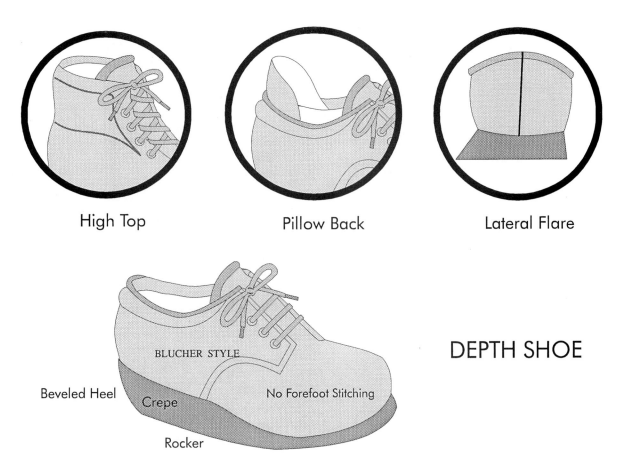

Fig. 29.19.   Modification of shoes. Standard depth shoes without stitching over the forefoot can be modified for the neuropathic foot. Additions include high top, pillowback, lateral flare, beveled heel, rocker sole, and stretching of leather as required.

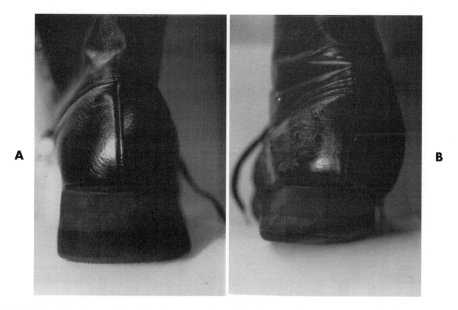

Fig. 29.20.   The lateral flare. **A,** An extension of the lateral sole, not a wedge. **B,** The motor loss at the ankle leads to lateral instability and possible injury without the lateral flare.

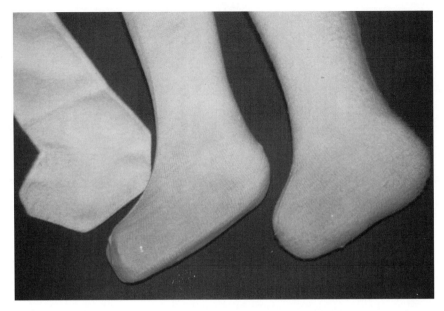

Fig. 29.21. Partial foot socks. The single size partial foot sock accommodates the Chopart amputation as well as distal metatarsal amputation without excess material at the distal end.

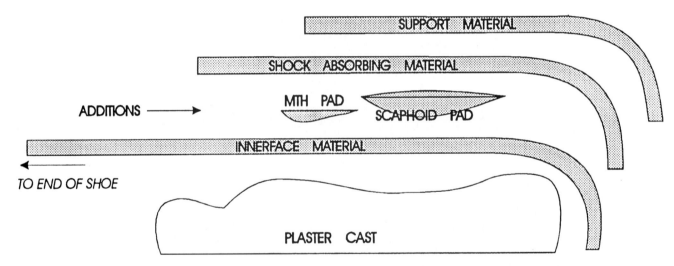

Fig. 29.22. Insert fabrication. With the plaster model, the composite insert is formed by adding the interface material that contacts the foot. The next layer is the addition of soft metatarsal or scaphoid pads followed by a shock-absorbing material. The final base or support material fills the space between foot contours and the plantar surface of the shoe.

ting but has a relatively short life because of compressibility (6 months) (Fig. 29.24). Plastazote is a closed-cell polyethylene foam that can be heated to 280°F and molded directly onto the patient's foot.[10] Care must be taken never to mold the toes or create ridges that the toes will ride over as the patient ambulates. By combining materials over a cast model of the foot, the composite type of insert can achieve all goals of the accommodative insert and provide a life of 1 year minimum (Fig. 29.25).

An insert with Plastazote surface in contact with the foot can be used as an excellent diagnostic tool for future follow-up. The self-molding properties of Plastazote reveal deep sock prints in areas of high pressure. These high-pressure areas should be noted and relieved in future insert design for the patient. Using temperature as a tool for evaluation, the areas of high trauma are noted as increased temperature locations. After the patient has worn accommodative inserts, the temperature differentiation decreases if the proper accommodation has been achieved. If the temperature has not decreased in the area, the relief may require enhancement, or there may be other underlying complications to be investigated. All relief areas are applied

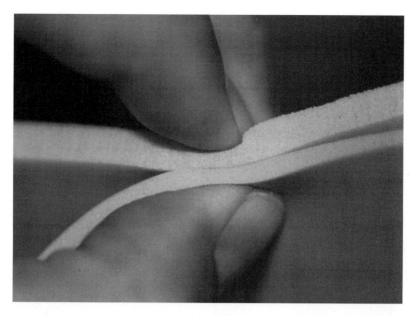

Fig. 29.23. Material compression. The neuropathic foot requires that the combination of materials can be compressed by one half of the original thickness to accommodate weight-bearing bony prominences.

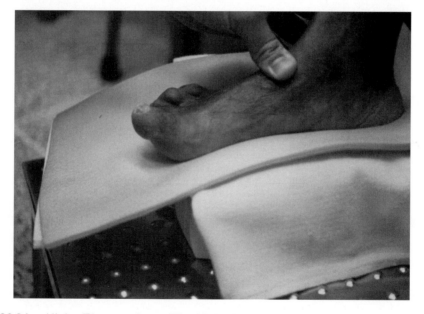

Fig. 29.24. Aliplast/Plastazote insert. The Aliplast/Plastazote insert is molded directly onto the patient's foot. A soft cushion, proximal to the toes, is used to mold the foot contours without leaving toe prints on the surface.

on the underlying surface in contact with the shoe, never in contact with the foot. The surface in contact with the foot is always a solid, uninterrupted surface that does not apply edges for the foot to receive shear forces.

Partial foot blocks.   The partial foot may require a block within the shoe for the area of amputation (Table 29.4). The purpose of a block is to reduce migration of the partial foot and medial/lateral shear for the toe amputation. No block or *prosthetic toe* is

to be used for a central digit amputation. The low pressures applied by a block to central digits cause ischemic ulcerations on medial surfaces. Medial or lateral amputations (first and fifth toes) may require a block to hold the foot in corrected position within the shoe (Fig. 29.26). The forefoot block holds the shoe leather away from the distal end of the foot and discourages distal migration of the foot (Fig. 29.27). All forms of blocks must have space from the amputation site and be an integral part of the insert, not added to an existing orthosis (Fig. 29.28). Forefoot blocks require a rigid rocker sole to prevent ulceration to the distal end.

Neuropathic walker.   The neuropathic walker is a combination of an ankle-foot orthosis (AFO) and custom boot that is individually designed to be total contact for weight distribution (Fig. 29.29). This device is used frequently after initial casting of a Charcot ankle or subtalor joint if inadequate joint stability has not occurred with healing. The ankle is locked to reduce force through the Lisfranc joint or ankle. The design is indicated for the patient with Charcot changes in the tarsal and ankle joints, chronic Charcot recurrence, and chronic ulcerations. The orthosis is easily donned and doffed and fabricated of a copolymer plastic with Plastazote lining. The removable insert may be adjusted to reassign weight-bearing areas on the plantar surface. The insert may also be fabricated to reduce pressure over chronic breakdown areas, such as malleoli, posterior heel, and bunions. The rocker sole allows for easy ambulation, but the contralateral shoe must be adjusted for height.

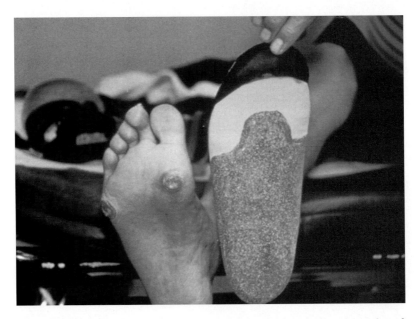

Fig. 29.25.   Reducing specific pressures. The composite insert is designed to reduce forces on vulnerable areas and reduce future callus buildup that can lead to skin breakdown.

Table 29.4.   Orthosis for the partial foot

PARTIAL FOOT	ORTHOSIS	SHOE	COMMENTS
1st or 5th toe amputation	Accommodative insert with toe block	Depth shoe	Toe block reduces shear
Central toe amputation (2, 3, or 4)	Accommodative insert without toe block or spacer	Depth shoe	Constant low pressures create ischemia
Distal amputation of all toes (transmetatarsal)	Accommodative insert	Short shoe	Improves weight-bearing characteristics
	With forefoot block	Full-length shoe	Patients, especially unilateral amputees, prefer for cosmesis.
Lisfranc amputation	Accommodative with forefoot block	Shoe with shank, rocker bottom, and high top	Suspension is a concern for the short foot.
Chopart amputation	Accommodative with forefoot block	Shoe with shank, rocker bottom, and high top	Suspension is a concern for the short foot. The Chopart must be followed carefully.
	Neuropathic walker	No shoe required	Custom AFO/boot
	Total contact AFO	Larger shoe required	
	Limited prosthesis	Standard shoe to accommodate	

The patient must be instructed to check skin for redness and possible breakdown. The patient should be followed and temperatures of plantar surface re-corded for possible adjustment of insert pressures. Sock management is important to continue a snug fit of orthosis and volume control.

Total contact AFO. Similar to the neuropathic walker, the total contact AFO is used for the patient whose resultant leg size is near normal. A shoe is fitted over the AFO rather than incorporating a shoe surface onto the bottom. The orthosis includes a custom removable insert and is lined with Plastazote (Fig. 29.30). The casting procedure is the same as that for the neuropathic walker. The toes are open and the anterior shell terminates at midfoot.

Short leg walkers and orthopedic walkers have been used by some clinics, but they compromise the total contact features. They are traditionally used for acute ligament/muscle and fracture immobilization.

Axial resist (patella tendon bearing orthosis). Patella tendon bearing (axial resist) designs are intended to decrease forces on the plantar weight-bearing surface of the foot (Fig. 29.31). Using this design as a casting procedure, there have been attempts to use it in place of plaster cast immobilization. This design transmits considerable axial forces from the knee region onto the cast but does not offer rotary stability. The results offer little effectiveness in reducing the load from the lower leg.[26]

The PTB design AFO has been used successfully for the calcanectomy, plantar skin graft, and heel ulceration. This orthosis is contraindicated in patients with vascular impairment because of potential excess restriction in the popliteal area compromising arterial flow.

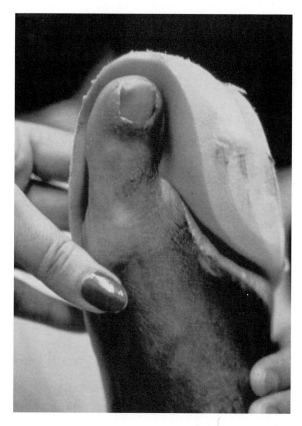

Fig. 29.26. Toe block. The ray resection of 2–5 requires a block to prevent migration within the shoe.

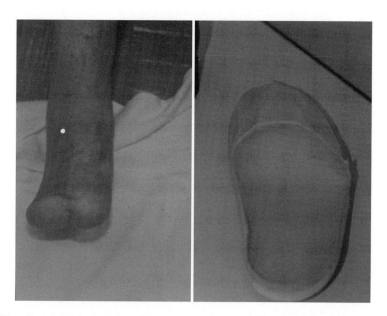

Fig. 29.27. Forefoot block. The transmetatarsal amputation requires a forefoot block to fill the shoe and prevent the shoe from bending at the distal end of the amputation.

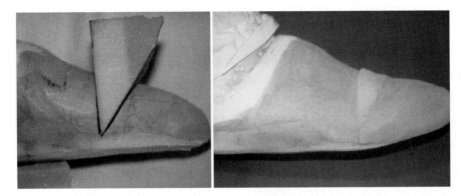

Fig. 29.28.   Toe break in forefoot block. To reduce pressure on the distal end of a partial foot, a soft foam toe break can be added as a wedge in the forefoot block.

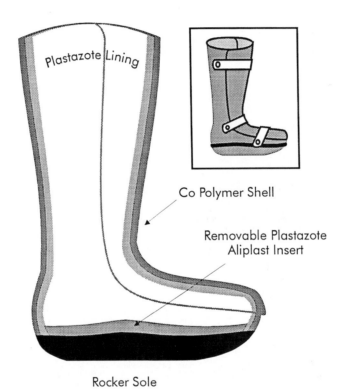

Plastazote Lining

Co Polymer Shell

Removable Plastazote
Aliplast Insert

Rocker Sole

Fig. 29.29.   Neuropathic walker. The neuropathic walker provides total contact to the affected limb with adjustability for chronic plantar surface deformities. The patient with recurrent Charcot joint or ulceration may require this orthosis in place of a shoe.

Prosthosis. The Prosthosis is the orthotic replacement when a patient with a complicated amputation is not a candidate for prosthetic management. The Prosthosis is a useful device for transfers and limb protection. This is always a creative design, with no two the same, unique to the individual and his needs.

PERIPHERAL VASCULAR DISEASE

Peripheral vascular disease is a serious complication affecting millions of Americans. Of the 500,000 annual vascular-related ulcerations in the United States 10% are arterial and 70% are venous ulcerations.

Venous stasis

The venous stasis ulceration has a better prognosis for healing than arterial ulceration. Veins are less elastic than arteries. In venous stasis ulcerations, the valves within veins no longer function to return blood to the heart against gravity, leaving blood to pool in the lower limb (Fig. 29.32). The pooling does not allow new oxygenated blood into the area, and cell walls of the veins begin to break down, allowing extravasation of

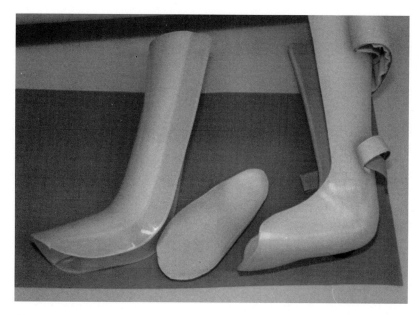

Fig. 29.30.   Total contact AFO. The total contact ankle foot orthosis (TCAFO) combines a lined plastic AFO (anterior and posterior) that is formed over a removable insert. The orthosis must be fit within a shoe.

fluid to occur in the lower limb. Venous stasis ulcerations are commonly located in the anteromedial malleolus area and pretibial area. The ulcerations are irregular in shape, surrounded by bluish-brown skin. Occasionally, these ulcers bleed when abraded.

Arterial ulceration

The intimal wall of arteries is usually smooth, but with atherosclerosis, platelets, calcium, and connective tissue are deposited on the wall. In early stages of atherosclerosis, the patient may experience *intermittent claudication* or cramping in the lower limb with exertion. As the disease progresses, symptoms appear when he is not walking (rest pain).[36] Arterial compromise can be noted by the loss of hair growth, shiny skin, atrophy, and cool skin over toes.[35] Atherosclerosis leads to impaired circulation in legs and is one of the most important causes of gangrene, leading to amputation.[1] Arterial ulcers are located on the tips or between toes, the heel, the metatarsal heads, the side or sole of foot, and above the lateral malleoli (Fig. 29.33). The ulcer looks "punched out" with well-demarcated edges and is nonbleeding. The ulcer base may be deep and pale or be black and necrotic.

In ulcers caused by arterial insufficiency, the initial step in treatment is to determine if the person is a candidate for arterial reconstruction procedures. This may include the use of non-invasive tests, such as segmental Doppler determination of blood flow to the lower extremity, usually compared to the arterial flow in the upper extremity, or transcutaneous P_{O_2} measure-

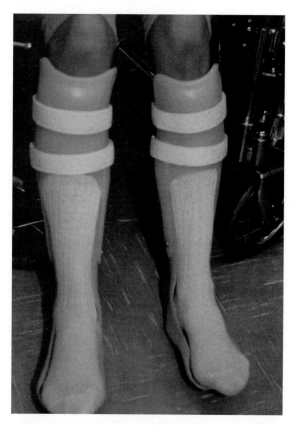

Fig. 29.31.   Axial resist AFO. The axial resist (patella tendon bearing) AFO is preferred when there is a requirement to deweight the heel surface partially. The orthosis is not recommended for dysvascular patients because of high forces in the area of the popliteal artery.

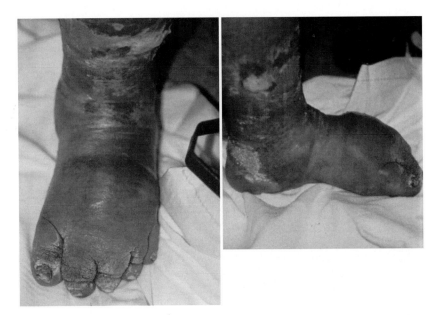

Fig. 29.32.   Lower extremity edema. The venous return system failure is shown with increased edema in the foot and lower limb. Waste products cannot be returned against gravity.

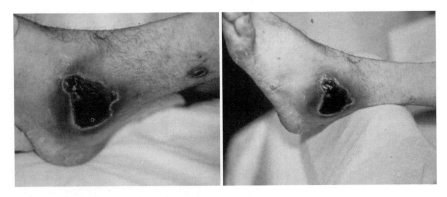

Fig. 29.33.   Arterial ulceration. The arterial system failure shows as dark, well-demarcated regions that are not receiving adequate blood supply.

ments of the ischemic lower extremity. The ultimate treatment of ulcers caused by arterial insufficiency is vascular reconstruction.

Orthotic Treatment

Unna boot.   Treatment of venous stasis ulcerations begins with leg elevation (Fig. 29.34).[16] The limb may be treated with compression bandages or an Unna boot. The Unna boot is a semirigid dressing of gelatin zincoxide (Fig. 29.35). Its application protects vulnerable skin from the weeping exudate, especially below the ulcer site.

The Unna boot is applied wet. When it dries, it forms a nonelastic, nonexpandable, nonshrinkable porous mold that sticks to the skin. This treatment has been used for venous stasis for 100 years. It is a means of controlling edema when it is applied across a joint. The motion of the joint generates a pumping action.[13]

Pressure-graduated stockings.   The lower limb with chronic venous stasis that does not have an open ulceration shows signs of edema that must be controlled. This limb should be treated with pressure-graduated stockings as daily prevention or an Unna boot with Ace wrap for severe edema or periods of breakdown.

Pressure-graduated stockings have a graduated pressure to facilitate venous pumping action, which diminishes lower extremity edema (Fig. 29.36). Antiembolism stockings are not designed for the ambulatory patient and do not supply the pumping action required. In general, antiembolism compression stockings are reserved for the nonambulatory, bedrest patient.

Usually, lower extremity compression occurs in the calf and thigh with compression devices. It is possible to compress the venous system in the foot as a further assist to the venous system. Most patients do well with

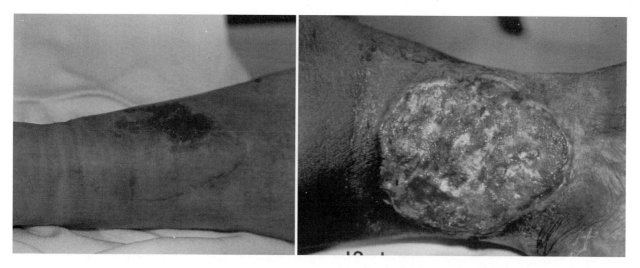

Fig. 29.34. Venous stasis ulceration. The anteromedial malleoli are the common site of ulceration in venous stasis because of the thin skin and close proximity of veins.

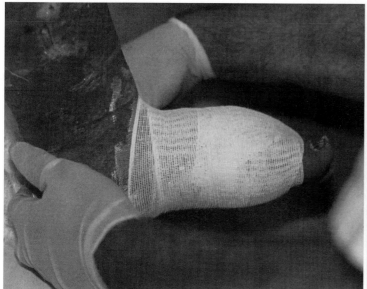

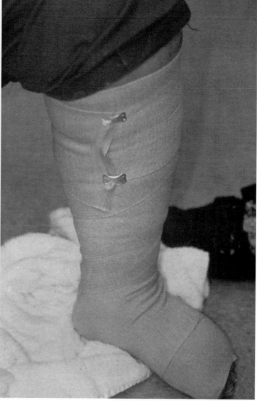

Fig. 29.35. Unna boot application. The venous stasis limb is wrapped with an Unna boot dressing followed by elastic wrap. Tension on the wrap should decrease proximally to promote venous return of fluid.

compression in the range of 30 to 40 mm Hg at the foot and ankle. When using these stockings for the neuropathic or dysvascular patient, it is necessary to avoid both seams around bony prominences and zippers over the malleoli.

The health care practitioner must determine the potential compliancy with the neuropathic, and especially diabetic, patient. These patients do not willfully neglect self-care activities but are simply not aware of the possible dangers of neglect.[42] In addition, most health care providers focus on the immediate problem (i.e., ischemic ulcer) and do not teach prophylaxis adequately. The diabetic may have other complications that compromise compliance in lower extremity care. Many diabetics have impaired vision from retinopathy and impaired smell from autonomic neuropathy, further compromising their ability to detect infection or other potential problems.

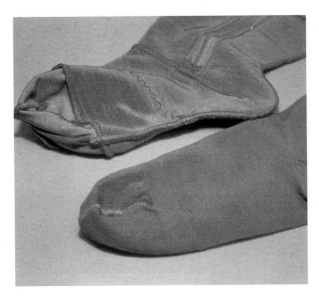

Fig. 29.36.   Graduated pressure stocking. The graduated pressure stocking for the neuropathic limb should not have prominent seams in weight-bearing areas or zippers over susceptible malleoli. Stockings should apply equal pressure in the foot and ankle and decrease proximally.

CONCLUSION

The care of the lower extremity in the neuropathic or dysvascular patient requires the efforts of many professionals. The patient with a plantar ulcer caused by vascular insufficiency should be evaluated for possible vascular reconstruction procedures. The diabetic with a neurotrophic ulcer should be treated with appropriate debridement and antibiotics (usually a polymicrobial infection). The goal of treatment of the neuropathic or dysvascular limb is to preserve the limb to enhance the ambulatory function of the patient. Multiple studies have shown the increased energy demands with prosthetic ambulation, which may preclude ambulation in the diabetic amputee with impaired cardiopulmonary reserve.

Orthotic devices alone do not compensate for lost sensation in the neuropathic limb, but when combined with an educated, compliant patient and early intensive medical and surgical treatment, limbs can escape the need for amputation. The members of the treatment team, which should include the patient, should work cooperatively to compensate for the deficits that accompany the neuropathic or dysvascular limb. Although the principles of treatment are simple and understandable, applying them consistently over a lifetime remains difficult.

REFERENCES

1. Apelqvist J, Castenfors J, Larsson J: Prognostic value of systolic ankle and toe blood pressure levels in outcome of diabetic foot ulcer, Diabetes Care 12:373–378, 1989.
2. Ashbury A: Foot care in patients with diabetes mellitus, Diabetes Care 14 (Suppl 2):18–19, 1991.
3. Bamberger D, Stark K: Severe diabetic foot problems: Avoiding amputation, Emerg Decisions 3:21–34.
4. Barber E: Strength and range-of-motion examination skills for the clinical orthotist, Prosthet Orthot 5:49–51, 1993.
5. Bergtholdt HT: Temperature assessment of the insensate, Phys Ther 59:18–22.
6. Birke JA, Sims DS: Plantar sensory threshold in the ulcerative foot, Bri Leprosy Relief Assoc 57:261–267, 1986.
7. Birke J, et al: Methods of treating plantar ulcers, Phys Ther 71:116–122, 1991.
8. Bowker JH: Partial foot and Syme amputations: An overview, Clin Prosthet Orthot 12:10–13.
9. Bowker JH: Neurological aspects of prosthetic/orthotic practice, Prosthet Orthot 5:52–54, 1993.
10. Brand PW: Management of sensory loss in the extremities. In Management of peripheral nerve problems, 1980.
11. Brand PW: Neuropathic ulceration, The Star May/June:1–4, 1983.
12. Brand P: Insensitive feet—practical handbook on foot problems in leprosy, London, 1977, The Leprosy Mission.
13. Brenner MA: Management of the diabetic foot, Baltimore, 1977, Williams & Wilkins.
14. Cailliet R: Foot and ankle pain, Philadelphia, 1983, FA Davis.
15. Chan AW, MacFarlane IA, Bowsher D: Contact thermography of painful diabetic neuropathic foot, Diabetes Care 14:918–922, 1991.
16. Cherry G, Ryan T, Cameron J: Blueprint for the treatment of leg ulcers and the prevention of recurrence, Wounds Compend Clin Res Pract 3:1–15, 1991.
17. DeJong R: The neurological examination, New York, 1969, Harper & Row.
18. Diamond J, Sinacore D, Mueller M: Molded double-rocker plaster shoe for healing a diabetic plantar ulcer, Phys Ther 67:1550–1552, 1987.
19. Dwyer G, Rust M: Shoe business, Diabetes Forecast June:60–63, 1988.
20. Furman A: Give your feet a sporting chance, Diabetes Forecast April: 17–22, 1989.
21. Fylling C: Conclusions, Diabetes Spectrum. 5:358–359, 1992.
22. Graham C: Neuropathy made you stop, Diabetes Forecast Dec: 47–49, 1992.
23. Hack M: Fitting shoes, Diabetes Forecast Jan: 1989.
24. Huntley AC: Taking care of your hands, Diabetes Forecast Aug: 11–12, 1991.
25. Kuncir E, Wirta R, Golbranson F: Load-bearing characteristics of polyethylene foam: An examination of structural and compression properties, Rehab R D 27:229–238, 1990.
26. Lauridsen K, Sorensen CG, Christiansen P: Measurements of pressure on the sole of the foot in plaster of Paris casts on the lower leg, Int Soc Prosthet Orthot 13: 1989.
27. Letts M: The orthotics of myelomeningocele. In AAOS: Atlas of orthotics, St. Louis, 1985, CV Mosby.
28. Levin M, O'Neal L: The diabetic foot, St. Louis, 1988, CV Mosby.
29. Lockard MA: Foot orthosis, Phys Ther 68:1866–1873, 1988.
30. McPoil TG Jr: Footwear, Phys Ther 68:1857–1865, 1988.
31. Mueller M, Diamond J, Sinacore D: Total contact casting in treatment of diabetic plantar ulcers, Diabetes Care 12:384–388, 1989.
32. Newman B: A diabetes camp for Native American adults, Diabetes Spectrum 6:166–202, 1993.
33. Newman LG, et al: Unsuspected osteomyelitis in diabetic foot ulcers: Diagnosis and monitoring by leukocyte scanning with indium in oxyquinoline, Diabetes Spectrum pp 5:346–347.

34. Oakley W, Catterall RCF, Martin MM: Aetiology and management of lesions of the feet in diabetes, BMJ 27:4999–5003.

35. Olefsky J, Sherman R: Diabetes mellitus: Management and complications, New York, 1985, Churchill Livingstone.

36. Olin J: Peripheral vascular disease, Diabetes Forecast. Oct: 78–81, 1992.

37. Omer GE Jr: Sensibility testing. In Management of peripheral nerve problems, 1980.

38. Pecoraro R, Reiber G, Burgess E: Pathways to diabetic limb amputation: Basis for prevention, Diabetes Care 13:513–521, 1990.

39. Perry J: Normal and pathologic gait. In AAOS: Atlas of orthotics, St. Louis, 1985, CV Mosby.

40. Pratt DJ: Medium term comparison of shock attenuating insoles using a spectral analysis technique, J Biomed Eng 10:426–428, 1988.

41. Pratt DJ: Long term comparison of shock attenuating insoles, Prosthet Orthot Int 14:59–62, 1990.

42. Shipley D: Clinical evaluation and care of the insensitive foot, Phys Ther 59:13–22, 1979.

43. Sinacore D, Mueller M, Diamond J: Diabetic plantar ulcers treated by total contact casting, Phys Ther 67:1543–1549, 1987.

44. Thomas PK: Clinical features and differential diagnosis: Peripheral neuropathy. Philadelphia, 1984, WB Saunders.

45. Thomas PK, Eliasson SG: Diabetic neuropathy. Philadelphia, 1984, WB Saunders

46. Tiberio D: Pathomechanics of structural foot deformities, Phys Ther 68:1840–1849, 1988.

47. Tsairis P: Differential diagnosis of peripheral neuropathies. In Management of peripheral nerve problems, 1980.

48. Wagner FW Jr: A classification and treatment program for diabetic, neuropathic and dysvascular foot problems, :1–47, 1983.

49. Weingarten M: Commentary, Diabetes Spectrum 5:342–343, 1992.

50. Wilson J, Foster D: Textbook of endocrinology, Philadelphia, 1992, WB Saunders.

Orthoses for Postpolio Syndrome

Robert S. Lin
Thomas J. Moore

Orthotic management of the postpolio individual is uniquely challenging from many perspectives. A paralytic motor disorder that keeps the sensory input largely intact can both facilitate orthotic management and, in the case of hypersensitivity, complicate orthotic management.

Although new cases of postpolio are rare outside of Third World populations, the emergence of individuals diagnosed with postpolio syndrome has once again brought this disease to the orthotic forefront. Technologic advancements in materials and components and an enhanced understanding of kinesiology better prepare today's Certified Orthotist to meet the challenges of postpolio pathology. Orthotic design for this population is complex and must incorporate an awareness of the cause, the instability, deformity, and the patient's compensatory movement patterns.

ANKLE-FOOT COMPLEX

The plantar surface of the foot should be carefully examined for weight-bearing or biomechanical stresses. The presence of metatarsalgia or hypercallosities on the plantar aspect of the foot indicates the need for improved weight distribution, absorption of ground reaction forces, or both. Careful attention to the medial longitudinal, lateral longitudinal, and transverse metatarsal arches of the foot is often indicated to improve weight-bearing comfort for this population. Using a viscoelastic interface inside the thermoplastic foot section can enhance comfort and make the application of biomechanical forces more tolerable. Such a soft inlay has similar results in the shoe of a conventional double upright orthotic system.

Because the clinical picture of the postpolio patient varies widely depending on medical and surgical history, generalizations are difficult. There are, however,

guidelines that should be considered when prescribing and designing any orthotic system.

ANKLE-FOOT ORTHOSES

If the proximal joints (hip/knee) are stable, painless, and free from gross deformity, an ankle-foot orthosis (AFO) can be applied with success. When previous surgical intervention has attempted to eliminate motion at the subtalar and talocrural joints (triple arthrodesis), the primary orthotic goals become the absorption of ground reaction forces, the protection of fusion sites from developing pseudoarthroses, and the protection of the midtarsal joint from developing a midfoot break and resultant rocker-bottom deformity of the foot.

In the thermoplastic foot section, medial-lateral control can be achieved with strategically high trimlines that apply forces over as broad a surface area as possible. Reinforcements about the ankle area (carbon graphite or rope corrugations (Figs. 30.1 and 30.2) can provide maximum sagittal plane stability with minimal plastic thickness and bulk.

When useful talocrural motion is present, this should be preserved by the design of the AFO to allow maximum gait efficiency. The articulating AFO permits variable motion at this joint axis through introduction of a variety of mechanical ankle joint designs (Figs. 30.3 to 30.5).

Primary concerns in orthotic joint selection include available range of motion, durability, adjustability, and biomechanical implication on the knee joint axis. Weakness of the pretibial muscles usually results in problems with swing phase clearance. In addition, foot slap at initial loading may occur secondary to the absence of an eccentric contraction of these weakened muscles. Without orthotic assistance, the individual often uses compensatory gait deviations, such as cir-

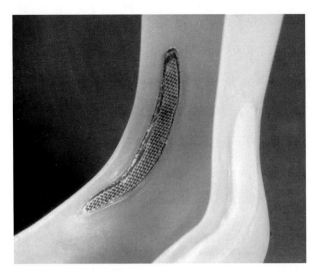

Fig. 30.1. Carbon composite reinforcement incorporated at the ankle to enhance stiffness without undue plastic thickness.

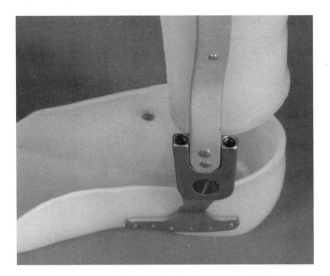

Fig. 30.3. Double-action ankle joint used in conjunction with a thermoplastic foot section allows adjustable plantar/dorsiflexion range of motion.

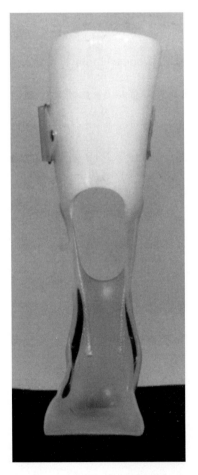

Fig. 30.2. Anterior floor reaction AFO made stiffer by incorporating rope corrugation at the ankle-foot complex.

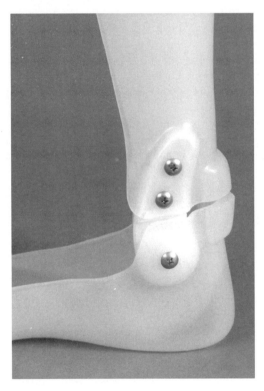

Fig. 30.4. Articulating AFO with plastic Oklahoma joints and 90 degrees plantar flexion stop.

cumduction or hyperflexion at the knee or hip joints. These mechanisms may suffice, but the increased energy cost and risk of stumbling make such compensations undesirable. A posterior leaf spring AFO with proper flexibility can effectively counter the foot slap and swing phase clearance problems seen in this patient group (Fig. 30.6).[2]

Ankle instability in dorsiflexion during stance phase must be addressed through the application of an AFO, which controls anterior tibial motion and prevents collapse of the weight-bearing extremity. A solid ankle

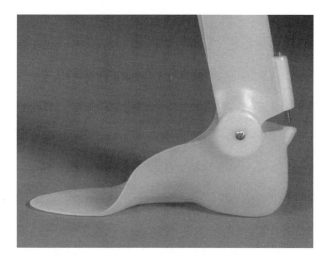

Fig. 30.5. Double overlap plastic articulating AFO with adjustable posterior stop to vary plantar flexion range.

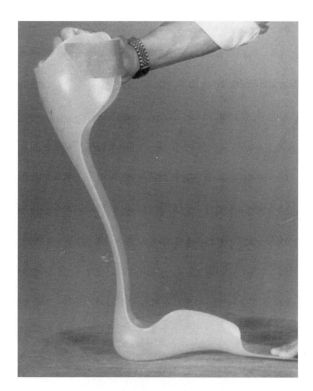

Fig. 30.6. Posterior leaf spring AFO constructed out of polypropylene.

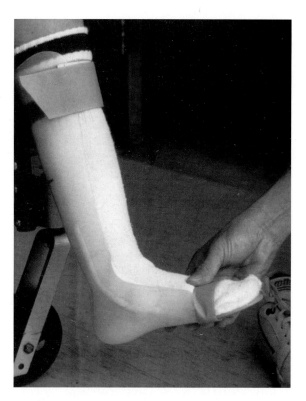

Fig. 30.7. Solid ankle AFO with rope corrugation at the ankle to enhance stiffness.

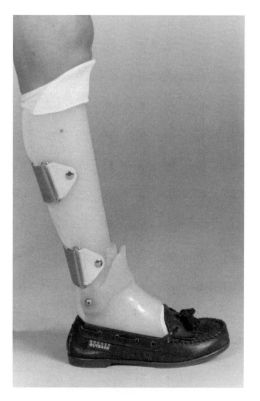

Fig. 30.8. Rear-entry articulating AFO with free plantar flexion and 90 degrees dorsiflexion stop.

thermoplastic AFO set near 90 degrees (neutral) may be used to provide stance phase stability for the ankle foot complex in all planes (Fig. 30.7).

Material selection and reinforcements must be sufficient to tolerate the forces required to resist sagittal plane motion. When swing phase clearance is not a problem, a rear entry articulating AFO can provide maximum resistance to dorsiflexion collapse, while allowing active plantar flexion (or push-off) at terminal stance (Fig. 30.8).

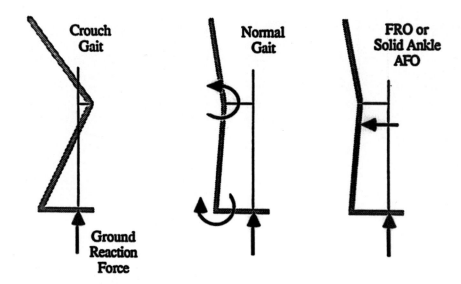

Fig. 30.9. Biomechanics of the anterior floor reaction AFO.

A weakened gastrocnemius-soleus with or without concomitant quadricep involvement can result in an unstable, buckling knee during single support. If the knee is relatively free of transverse plane deformity and recurvatum, an anterior floor reaction AFO design may suffice. It should be noted, however, that if there is a fixed flexion deformity of the knee beyond 20 degrees, the ground reaction force harnessed cannot be passed anterior to the anatomic axis at midstance, thus reducing the knee extension moment (Figs. 30.9 and 30.10).

MANAGEMENT OF THE KNEE

Genu recurvatum is common, secondary to weak quadriceps and the individual's attempt to place his or her body weight anterior to the knee joint. This action provides a biomechanical knee extension moment, often augmented by the classic "hand on the front of the thigh" posture.

Years of repeated knee extension forces can result in progressive recurvatum and potential damage to the posterior joint capsule. The knee often becomes painful, and function is compromised because of the greater flexion range that is required to achieve clearance in swing phase. Orthotic management of this patient group almost always requires a knee-ankle-foot orthosis (KAFO) to control terminal knee extension. This can be achieved via the mechanical stop (knee joint) or posterior check strap (Fig. 30.11). In those patients who have adequate hip musculature (fair or better), the placement of the limb during and after swing is more predictable and weight shift more reliable when the recurvatum is reduced. Whenever possible, it is desire-

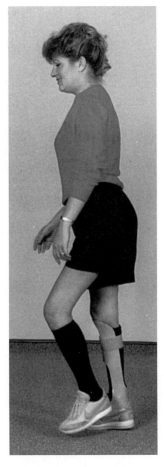

Fig. 30.10.   Stance phase stability is achieved in this patient despite a trace quadriceps femoris. A carbon graphite floor reaction AFO is applied in 90 degrees ankle alignment.

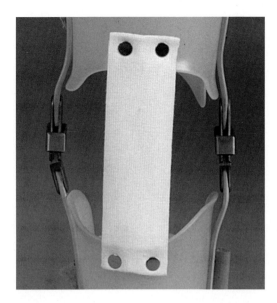

Fig. 30.11. A nonelastic posterior check strap helps resist genu recurvatum when used in a KAFO design.

able to incorporate a posterior offset knee joint to help insure an anterior weight line while allowing free knee flexion in swing (facilitating foot clearance) (Fig. 30.12).

KNEE JOINTS

When severe quadriceps weakness is present, a manual knee lock should be provided. Use of the traditional ring (drop) lock, although affording stability, introduces the added complication of poor clearance in swing and the need to operate a positive locking system. The addition of a spring-loaded mechanism on the lateral knee joint eliminates the need to flex at the hip to engage the lock and provides an automatic locking action at full knee extension (Fig. 30.13). The medial drop lock, however, still requires manual operation. Elimination of this lock is not advised for the active polio patient because too much torque is placed on the single, lateral lock mechanism.

The alternate locking joint is the CAM or BAIL type of lock with vertical/horizontal trigger levers. Such designs provide automatic positive locking upon knee extension, and the strategic connection of the two levers enables dual operation with a single action (Fig. 30.14).

Coronal plane deformities of the knee are commonplace in this group because of muscle weakness about the hip and the resultant positive Trendelenburg gait pattern. Genu valgum is much more common and typically difficult to address from an orthotic perspective. This valgum angulation at the knee places the ankle foot complex further lateral to the weight line and places the gluteus medius at a mechanical disadvan-

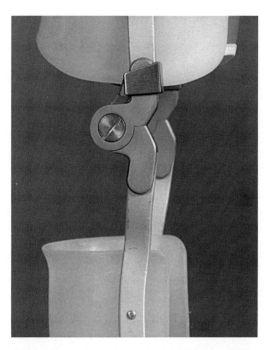

Fig. 30.12. A posterior offset knee joint places the mechanical axis behind the anatomic joint axis and the weight line—shown here with optional ring lock.

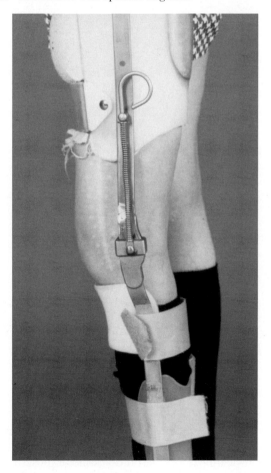

Fig. 30.13. Spring-loaded lateral drop lock provides automatic lock engagement at full extension.

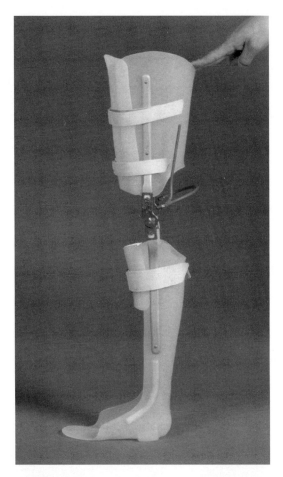

Fig. 30.14. KAFO with Ball/Cam lock. *Note:* Medial lateral lift levers are connected to enable single action function.

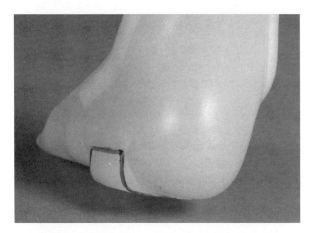

Fig. 30.15. Lateral heel wedge post used to extend lever arm and broaden the base of support.

tage. KAFO design must use the medial tibial flare area as the fulcrum of leverage to address these pathologic weight-bearing forces. In addition, a medial post should be considered at the heel of the AFO section to increase the lever arm length (Fig. 30.15).

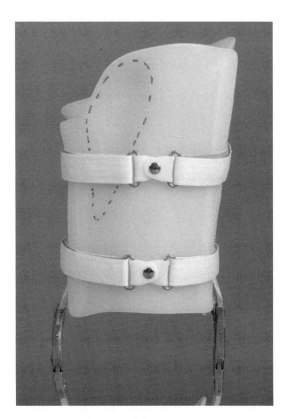

Fig. 30.16. Quadrilateral brim-type femoral section. Note the outlined compression provided in the area of the femoral triangle.

There are two design options available in the thermoplastic KAFO system that can effectively maximize the patient's residual function. The traditional quadrilateral-style brim, which affords anterior-posterior compression, helps the individual assume a hyperextended attitude at the hip and rest against Bigelow's ligament on the posterior proximal wall of the thigh section. The compression at the femoral triangle afforded by the quadrilateral design also helps maximize the initiation of swing by harnessing pelvic motion and hip flexion (Fig. 30.16). If the hip abductors are disproportionately weaker than the hip flexors, the priority shifts to the need to facilitate lateral weight transfer over the base of support. In this case medial-lateral compression along the length of the femur (narrow ML design) helps achieve the desired stability in the coronal plane (Fig. 30.17). If all the muscles about the hip are equally affected, the quadrilateral-style brim should take precedence over the narrow ML design.

GENERAL CONSIDERATIONS

The emergence of postpolio syndrome has brought the challenge of polio management back into the

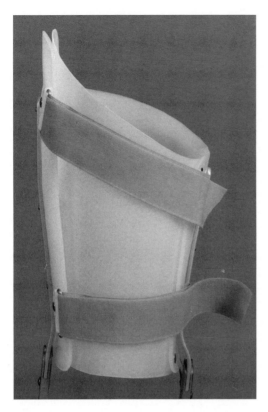

Fig. 30.17.   Narrow ML femoral cuff affords coronal plane compression and maximizes control needed with weak hip abductors.

orthotic arena. The success of new intervention requires the recognition of several key factors:

1. One must recognize that any new orthotic initiatives change the biomechanics of walking that have been habitually used for many years. This can have a profound effect on proximal joints (heretofore unaffected) such as the sacroiliac or lumbosacral joints of the spine.
2. Careful attention must be paid to the need for intimate contact with, but pressure distributed over a broad area because many in this population are markedly hypersensitive and suffer from profound overuse syndromes.
3. The degree in which new ultra-lightweight materials can be incorporated into the orthotic design

provides distinct benefits by reducing energy consumption required for ambulation, which is of critical importance.

4. Any new orthotic initiative must be preceded by extensive discussion with the patient so that he or she is well informed and willing to accept the changes that lie ahead. This step maximizes the chances of acceptance and future satisfaction.

SUMMARY

Epidemiologic studies indicate that nearly one quarter of those diagnosed with antecedent paralytic poliomyelitis develop new symptoms and acquire the designation of postpolio syndrome. This translates to more than 50,000 individuals in the United States alone. In addition, the immigration of polio victims from other parts of the world where widespread vaccination is unavailable or recent results in a significant body of individuals who require new orthotic intervention.[1]

The challenge in the successful management of this population lies in the understanding of the cause of polio, a knowledge of the biomechanics of lower limb deformity, and the appreciation of the typical personality profiles seen in this unique patient group. If successful, new orthotic management can help stem the onset of postpolio syndrome and enable the patient to continue to function at the same (high) level experienced before the onset of new symptoms.

REFERENCES

1. Cashman N, et al: Post polio syndrome: An overview, Clin Prosthet Orthot 11:74, 1987.
2. Clark DR, Perry J, Lunsford TR: Case studies—orthotic management of the adult post polio patient, Orthot Prosthet 40:43–50, 1986.

BIBLIOGRAPHY

Halstead LS, Weichers DO: Introduction. In Halstead LS, Weichers DO, editors: Late effects of poliomyelitis, Miami, 1985, Symposia Foundation.

Maynard FM: Differential diagnosis of pain and weakness in postpolio patients. In Halstead LS, Weichers DO, editors: Late effects of poliomyelitis, Miami, 1985, Symposia Foundation.

Perry J: Orthopedic management of post-polio sequelae. In Halstead LS, Weichers DO, editors: Late effects of poliomyelitis, Miami, 1985, Symposia Foundation.

Foot Orthoses

Kent K. Wu

DEFINITION

A foot orthosis (FO) is a mechanical device used to (1) align and support the foot; (2) to prevent, correct, or accommodate foot deformities; or (3) to improve the overall functions of the foot.

FUNCTIONS OF A FOOT ORTHOSIS

A functional FO should evenly distribute the weight-bearing stresses over the entire plantar surface of the foot; indirectly reduce the stress and strain on ankle, knee, hip and spine; alleviate pain from sensitive and painful areas of the sole; support the various foot arches; provide relief for metatarsalgia of various causes; decrease the amount, degree, and rate of foot hyperpronation during walking and running; improve foot alignments; accommodate congenital or developmental foot anomalies; serve as an addition to an ankle-foot orthosis (AFO); equalize foot length discrepancy; compensate for mild leg length discrepancy; limit the motion and weight-bearing stresses of various painful foot joints; and minimize the pressure and irritation from external (shoe) or internal (bony prominence) sources.

DIFFERENCES BETWEEN A CUSTOM-MADE FOOT ORTHOSIS AND AN OVER-THE-COUNTER FOOT ORTHOSIS

Although an over-the-counter FO can be purchased from drug stores, supermarkets, department stores, sporting goods stores, and surgical supply houses, it lacks many functional qualities a custom-made FO possesses, such as anatomic fit and comfort, unlimited

sizes, unlimited variations in configurations, ease of modification, effectiveness in relieving painful foot disorders, high patient acceptance and satisfaction, excellent shoe fit, and minimal chances of aggravating or creating painful foot disorders. The drawbacks of a custom-made FO include its high cost, limited supply, prescription requirement, inconvenience in acquiring it, and relative difficulty in obtaining good service and repair.

CLASSIFICATION OF FOOT ORTHOSES

Foot orthoses can be classified in accordance with their overall length or intrinsic rigidity. Based on *overall length*, there are four groups of FOs: (1) metatarsal length with the orthosis ending immediately proximal to the metatarsal heads, (2) sulcus length with the orthosis extending to the web spaces of the toes, (3) Morton's extension with a full-length extension under the great toe and the remainder of the orthosis ending at the web spaces, and (4) full length with the orthosis extending beyond the tips of toes (Fig. 31.1).

Based on *intrinsic rigidity*, there are three main types: (1) rigid, (2) semirigid, and (3) soft FOs.

Rigid orthoses

Stainless steel Whitman plate and Shaffer plate, polypropylene UCBL, and acrylic FOs are examples of rigid FOs (Fig. 31.2). They are strong, hard, stiff, and durable and are effective in transferring weight, limiting joint motion, and stabilizing flexible deformities. Rigid FOs are usually made from a single layer of material, such as stainless steel, acrylic, or polypropylene sheet, and are usually metatarsal length. The disadvantages of rigid FOs include poor shock absorption ability, aggravation of bony or soft tissue lesions on the sole of the foot, inability to make fine adjustments on them, and difficulties in working with the tough materials these FOs are made of.

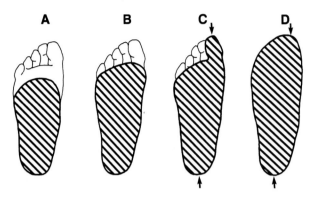

Fig. 31.1.   Four basic types of FOs based on overall length. **A,** Metatarsal length. **B,** Sulcus length. **C,** Morton extension. **D,** Full length.

Semirigid orthoses

Semirigid FOs come in all three lengths and are made of a combination of materials with a wide range of rigidity depending on the functions these materials are designed to perform (Fig. 31.3). The materials used in fabricating semirigid FOs include leather, felt, spring steel (for the steel shank of a FO), natural and rubberized cork, thermoplastic cork, cellular rubber, plastazote, and polyethylene. In comparison to rigid FOs, semirigid FOs are usually weaker, softer, more flexible, less durable, and bulkier. They are more comfortable to wear and can also provide pressure relief, shock absorption, improvement of weight-bearing transfer, and support and stabilization of various foot deformities. Unlike the plastics used in rigid FOs, which require high temperature to make them soft and moldable on the bottom of a cast of the foot, some plastics used in semirigid FOs such as plastazote can be molded directly against the foot after moderate heating. Therefore FOs can be fabricated in a medical practitioner's office, where adjustments and modifications can be con-

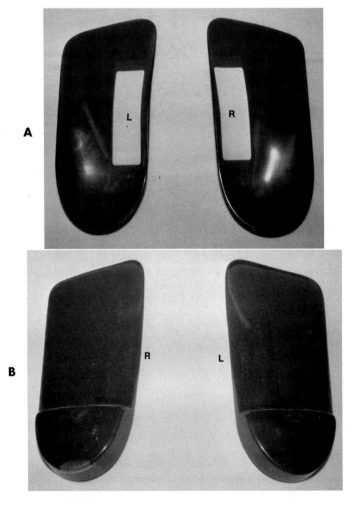

Fig. 31.2.   Top (**A**) and bottom (**B**) views of a pair of metatarsal length rigid acrylic FOs.

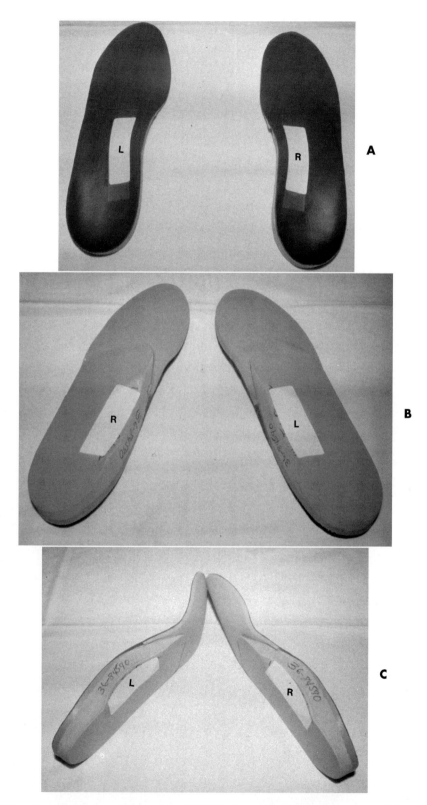

Fig. 31.3. Top (**A**), bottom (**B**), and medial (**C**) views of a pair of custom-made full-length semirigid FOs. They are made of multiple layers of plastic foam materials, and their top covers are made of vinyl.

veniently made to accommodate clients' feet properly without sending these foot devices to distant orthotic laboratories. In addition, semirigid FOs can also be molded against the positive model or cast of the foot.

Soft orthoses

In comparison with rigid and semirigid FOs, soft FOs usually come in a full-length form and are often made of plastazote (Fig. 31.4), polyurethane foam (PPT), polyvinyl chloride foam, or latex foam. They have the best shock-absorbing ability and are quite effective in reducing shear, compression, and tension stresses. These foot devices are comfortable to wear, but they are relatively weak, soft, not durable, bulky, and the least precise in fitting foot deformities. They are often used to accommodate fixed deformities of the feet, especially in clients with neuropathic, dysvascular, and ulcerative disorders of the feet.

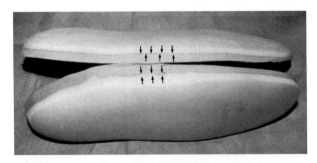

Fig. 31.4. Side and bottom views of a pair of soft plastazote insoles fabricated for a diabetic patient with severe peripheral neuropathy. They are ½ inch thick. The top ¼ inch is made of a soft-density plastazote for cushioning; the bottom ¼ inch is made of a medium-density plastazote for support and to prolong the useful life of this pair of FOs.

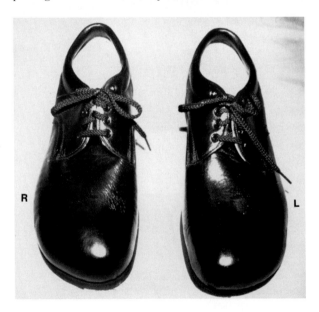

Fig. 31.5. A pair of extra-depth shoes with plain toes, wide and roomy toe boxes and vamps, high lacing, and extended heel counters.

SHOES FOR FOOT ORTHOSES

A pair of extra-depth shoes is usually prescribed for clients who wear custom-made FOs (Fig. 31.5). This kind of shoe can accommodate FOs up to ¼ inch in thickness. Any FO thicker than ¼ inch usually requires a custom-made shoe. A standard shoe for a FO is usually made of leather with a blucher pattern, leather lining, plain toe, high and broad toe box, roomy vamp, high lacing, extended heel counter, broad and low rubber heel, wide and strong shank reinforced with a spring steel shank, and a thick leather or neoprene sole with or without a rocker bar.

Stretching of the shoe's upper

Painful forefoot lesions such as bunion, hammer toe, corn, tailor's bunion, and claw toes are commonly found in people who need FOs for other reasons. In these patients, an orthosis can aggravate these same forefoot disorders by decreasing the available space within the vamp of the shoe. It may be necessary to stretch the various parts of the shoe's vamp before a FO can be worn comfortably. A shoemaker's swan (Fig. 31.6) is a useful tool to stretch the shoe's upper over a painful lesion such as a bunion (Fig. 31.7), a hammer toe (Fig. 31.8), or a tailor's bunion. A leather softening solution is usually sprayed on the shoe leather before the shoemaker's swan is applied. When

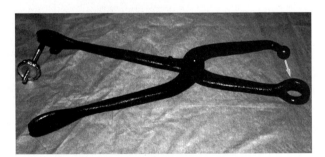

Fig. 31.6. A shoemaker's swan.

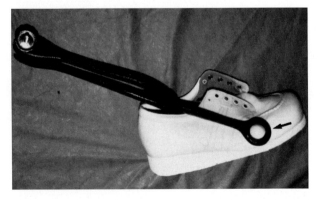

Fig. 31.7. Stretching the toe box over a painful bunion to provide pain relief.

the stretched area is completely dry, the bulge on the shoe's upper usually remains for a long time, and the underlying painful foot lesion is not constantly irritated by the shoe.

Major modifications of the outer sole in association with the use of foot orthoses

Rocker sole. A rocker sole assists the heel-off and toe-off phases of the walking cycle and is therefore quite effective in relieving various causes of metatarsalgia, such as sesamoiditis, hallux rigidus, plantar callosities under the metatarsal heads, hammer toes, claw toes, Morton's neuroma, and metatarsal fractures. For the rocker sole to be effective, the sole of the shoe should be rigid. This rigidity can be achieved by inserting a stiff steel plate between the inner sole and outer sole before constructing the rocker sole (Fig. 31.9).

Medial heel outflare. A medial heel outflare is commonly used to treat a severe flat foot caused by diabetic Charcot's foot, rheumatoid foot, chronic rupture of the posterior tibial tendon, tarsal coalition, or vertical talus. It increases the size of the base of support of the shoe and helps to support the longitudinal arch. A semirigid FO commonly accompanies a shoe with a medial heel outflare (Fig. 31.10).

Lateral heel outflare. A lateral heel outflare is usually used to treat a clubfoot or a varus foot. A 5/16-inch wedge is often inserted into the lateral aspect of the sole and heel in an attempt to pronate the foot or to accommodate the varus foot deformity (Fig. 31.11).

Overcoming leg length discrepancy. When the leg length discrepancy is 1 inch or less, a lift can be placed under the heel of the shorter leg to equalize the leg length. When the leg length discrepancy is much greater, however, lifts should be added to both the sole and the heel. For example, a patient with a cavus foot and claw toes also has a 3-inch leg length discrepancy. A FO with toe filler was fabricated to accommodate the cavus foot, and a 3-inch heel lift and a 1-inch sole lift were added to the sole of the shoe to equalize the length of both legs. A rocker bar was also built into the shoe to facilitate ambulation (Fig. 31.12).

Custom-made molded shoes

Molded shoes are made directly over a plaster cast of a human foot without using a shoe last. They are usually employed to treat severe foot deformities, marked leg length discrepancy, marked foot size discrepancy, congenital absence of various parts of the foot, various forefoot amputations, insensitive foot, dysvascular foot, and weak and severely arthritic foot. The foot cast is best taken in a sitting semi–weight-bearing position with the knee and ankle joints at 90

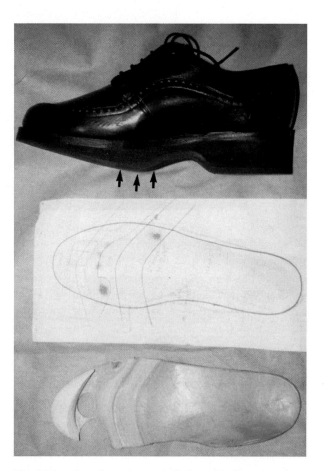

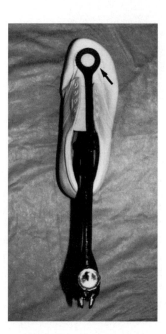

Fig. 31.8. Stretching the toe box over a painful second hammer toe to decrease friction between the dorsal aspect of the PIP joint of the second toe and the toe box.

Fig. 31.9. A rocker sole was built into this shoe to assist a patient with a claw foot, caused by a crush injury to his lower leg, to ambulate better.

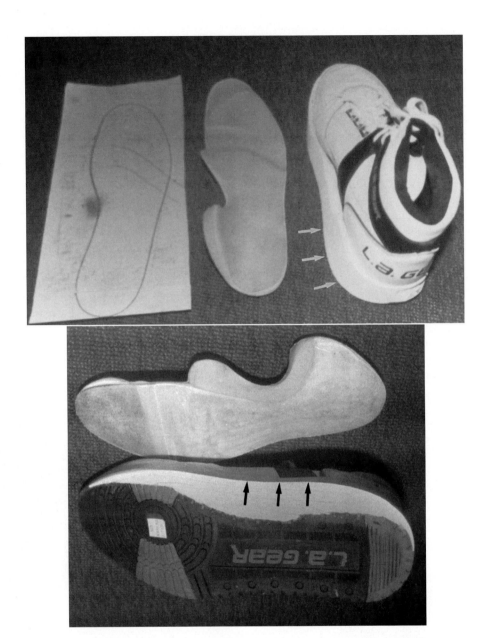

Fig. 31.10. A medial heel outflare was built into this right shoe to provide more medial support for a diabetic rocker-bottom flat foot for which a custom-made FO had been fabricated.

degrees. The foot should be casted in a neutral position when it is flexible. If the foot deformities are fixed, however, casting the foot in a deformed position has to be accepted.

FOOT-CASTING TECHNIQUE

With the client sitting with his or her foot in a neutral position, a wet, fast-setting plaster splint is applied from the plantar aspect of the toes to the posterior aspect of the ankle joint. The soft plaster is carefully molded around the metatarsal heads, the spaces beneath and around the toes to produce a precise toe crest, the longitudinal and transverse arches of the foot, the medial and lateral borders of the foot, the contour of the heel, and the two malleoli (Fig. 31.13, *A*). When the bottom portion of the cast starts to become solidified, a thin layer of Vaseline is applied to the margins of the bottom half of the cast, and another wet fast-setting plaster splint is applied from the dorsal aspect of the toes to the anterior aspect of the ankle. The sides of the second splint are allowed to overlap the medial, lateral, and anterior margins of the first splint, and the second splint should be meticulously molded around the dorsal aspect of each toe and the entire dorsal surface of the foot and ankle (see Fig. 31.13, *B*). When the two halves of the foot cast

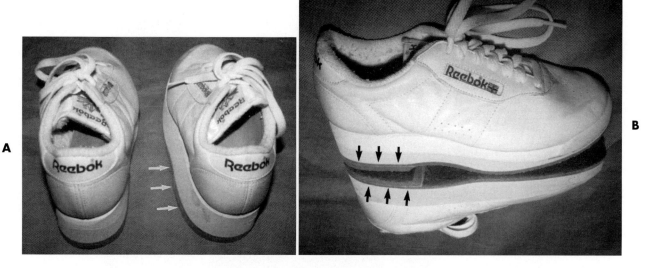

Fig. 31.11. **A,** This left shoe has a lateral heel outflare built into its sole. **B,** By placing the two soles of the same pair of shoes together, the increased area of weight bearing on the lateral of the sole of the hindfoot of the left shoe becomes obvious.

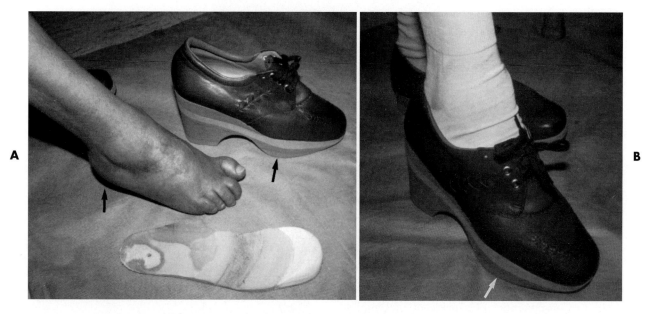

Fig. 31.12. **A,** This patient had poliomyelitis as a child, which produced a smaller right claw foot with a leg length discrepancy of 3 inches. A custom-made FO with a toe filler was made to accommodate the smaller right claw foot, and a 3-inch heel lift and a 1-inch sole lift were added to the shoe to equalize the two legs. A rocker bar was also built into the shoe to facilitate ambulation. **B,** The two legs were now equalized. Her gait and ability to walk longer distances had been significantly improved.

are sufficiently hardened, they can be easily taken apart to free the foot. Later on, they can be securely taped together, and liquid plaster can be poured into this hollow, negative cast to produce a positive cast that is an exact replica of the client's foot (see Fig. 31.13, *C*). A custom-made molded shoe can then be fabricated directly over this plaster foot replica (Fig. 31.14). In addition, FOs can be molded over the plantar surface of this plaster foot cast.

PLASTICS FOR MAKING FOOT ORTHOSES

There are two basic types of plastics: thermoplastics and thermosetting plastics. The thermoplastics are usually rigid in a cooled state and become soft and moldable when heated or reheated. The molecules of these thermoplastics are usually chainlike and may or may not have side chains. When they are heated, segmental motion and sliding of mole-

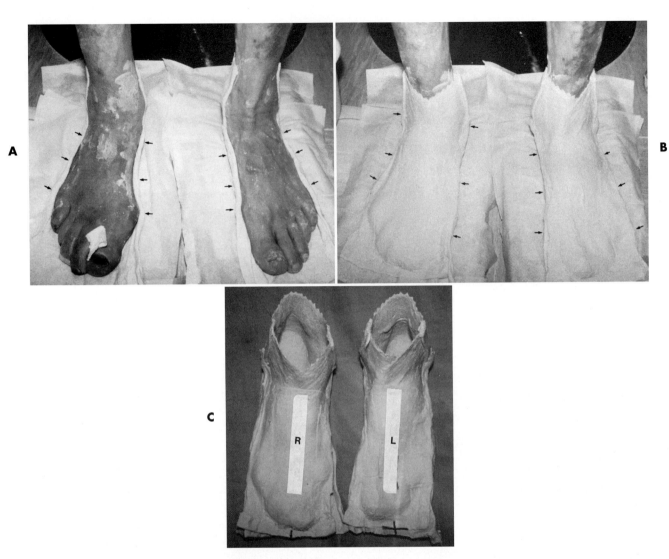

Fig. 31.13. **A,** A presoaked, fast-setting plaster splint has been molded to the entire sole, the heel, and the posterior ankle region of each of the two feet. **B,** Another piece of identical plaster splint has been molded to the dorsal aspect of the foot and ankle of the two same feet. **C,** Two negative casts of the same patient's two feet.

cules over one another allows repeated reheating and reshaping. Consequently, FOs made of thermoplastics can be modified at will by simply heating them to the appropriate temperature. Examples of thermoplastics include polyethylene, polyvinyl chloride, polyester polycaprolatone, cellulose acetate, acrylics, polypropylene, and polycarbonate. In contrast, thermosetting plastics are usually liquids in their original state. They can be transformed from a liquid state into a solid state by adding a catalyst such as benzoperoxide and promoters such as cobalt and aniline. The molecules of thermosetting plastics form highly cross-linked polymers with rigid and irregular three-dimensional molecular structures that cannot be softened or reshaped by reheating. Thermosetting plastics are commonly reinforced with nylon, dacron, cotton, carbon, and glass fibers to make them

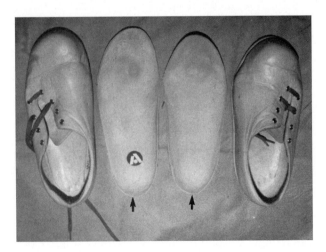

Fig. 31.14. A pair of custom-made molded shoes with two associated full-length soft FOs made of plastazote.

stronger, stiffer, and lighter per unit volume. Polyester resins, epoxy resins, and polyurethane foams are examples of thermosetting plastics.

TECHNIQUE FOR FABRICATING A THERMOPLASTIC FOOT ORTHOSIS

A piece of thermoplastic slightly larger than the plantar surface of the foot replica is heated in an oven until it is completely pliable (Fig. 31.15). It is placed over the plantar surface of the foot replica, and a vacuum suction is used to pull the softened plastic

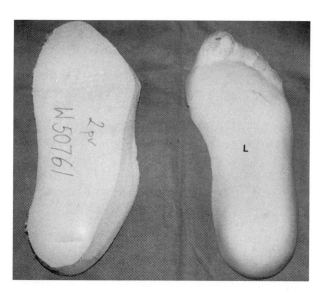

Fig. 31.15. Plantar view of a plaster foot replica with a piece of thermoplastic next to it, which will be heated and then vacuum formed over the foot replica to produce a FO.

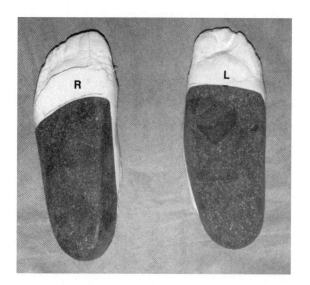

Fig. 31.16. Two pieces of thermoplastic cork have been heated and vacuum formed over the plantar surfaces of two foot replicas to produce two metatarsal length semirigid FOs.

tightly against the sole portion of the foot replica. After the plastic has returned to room temperature, excess plastic from the peripheral edge of the rough FO is carefully ground off until it fits perfectly on the sole of the foot mold (Fig. 31.16). A heel post made of thermomoldable cork, thermoplastic, or hard rubber is attached to the heel portion of the FO to stabilize the FO in the shoe and to adjust for hindfoot varus or valgus by varying the mediolateral sloping of the heel post. Similarly, forefoot posting can also be added to the plantar surface of the distal part of the FO to accommodate or correct forefoot varus or valgus.

FOOT PRESSURE GRAPH

The foot pressure graph is obtained by having a client's foot bear full weight on a foot imprinter (Figs. 31.17 and 31.18). It is the blueprint for the FO to be fabricated because it reveals the outline of the foot; the length, width, shape, and any deformities of the foot; the length and height of the foot arches; the level of the ball of the foot; the longitudinal axes of the toes; and the sites of the talonavicular joint and first tarsometatarsal joint on the medial aspect of the foot (Figs. 31.19 through 31.21). By comparing foot pressure graphs taken at different times, the clinical course of various painful foot disorders can be monitored in an extremely economical and practical manner.

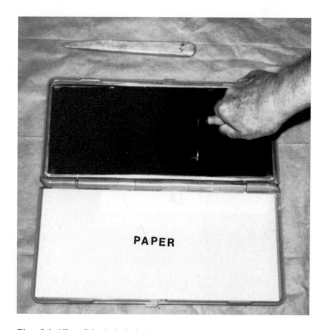

Fig. 31.17. Black ink is being evenly applied to the fine rubber mesh of a foot imprinter in preparation of taking a foot pressure graph.

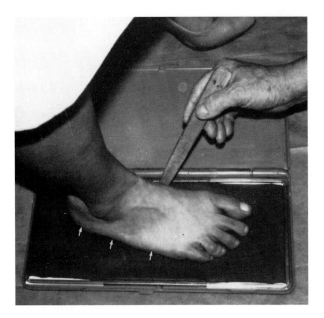

Fig. 31.18. Full weight bearing is being performed by a right foot on a foot imprinter. Various foot parameters can be taken now.

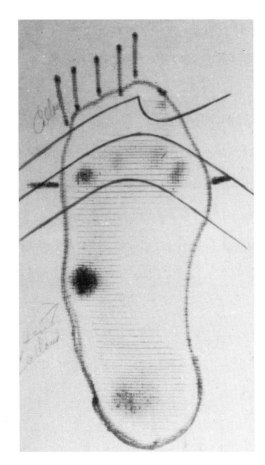

Fig. 31.20. Foot pressure graph of a club foot shows the varus deformity of the foot with a high longitudinal arch and concentration of pressure under the fifth metatarsal head and base.

FOOT ORTHOSIS IN COMBINATION WITH A LEATHER ANKLE CORSET

When a foot has a short transmetatarsal amputation, a Lisfranc's amputation, or a Chopart's amputation, it is often treated with an AFO. The author's experience has demonstrated, however, that a leather ankle corset in combination with a FO can take care of many of these amputations (Fig. 31.22). The leather ankle corset is light, cosmetically appealing, and functionally quite adequate to accommodate these midfoot amputations. When an amputation is performed through the midfoot level, the dorsiflexion power of the anterior tibialis, extensor hallucis longus, and extensor digitorum longus muscles is lost. Consequently the triceps surae pulls the foot into an equinus and slightly varus position, which causes painful callosity and sometimes even ulceration at the end of the amputation stump. To avoid this deformity, the Achilles' tendon should be routinely lengthened when a midfoot amputation is performed. In chronic cases, when the ankle is in a fixed plantar

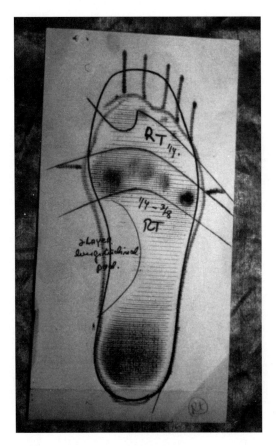

Fig. 31.19. Foot pressure graph of a cavus foot shows a high longitudinal arch and elevated pressure on the five metatarsal heads and the heel.

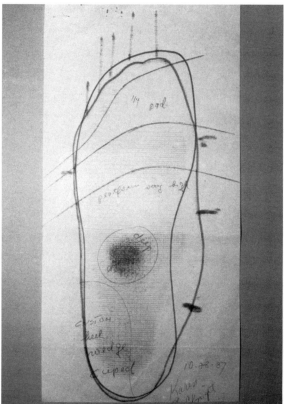

Fig. 31.21. Foot pressure graph of a diabetic Charcot's rocker-bottom flat foot shows a complete absence of the longitudinal arch with bulging of the medial border of the midfoot and a rather large area of increased weight-bearing pressure under the cuneiform.

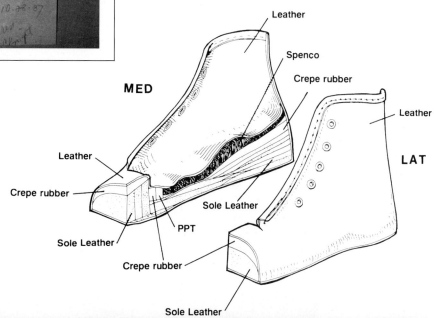

Fig. 31.22. A midsagittal section through an ankle corset to show the various materials used in its construction.

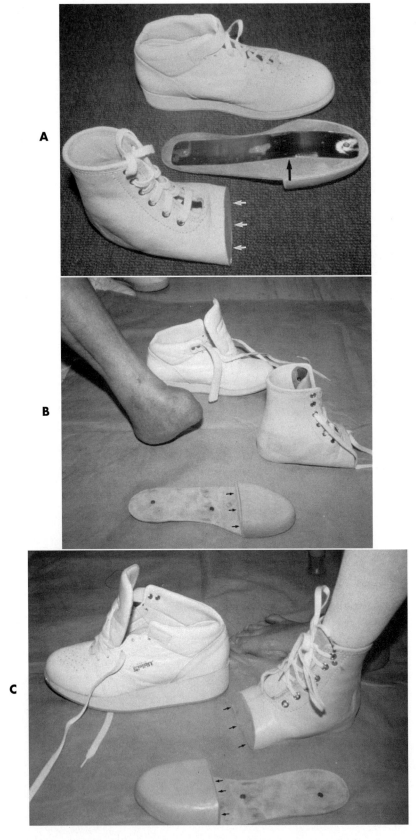

Fig. 31.23.   **A,** The matching FO of an ankle corset shows a strong piece of spring steel has been riveted to the bottom of the FO to provide stability and rigidity for the ankle corset. **B,** A foot with midfoot amputation, a shoe, an ankle corset, and a matching FO with a forefoot filler. **C,** The foot has been securely placed in an ankle corset.

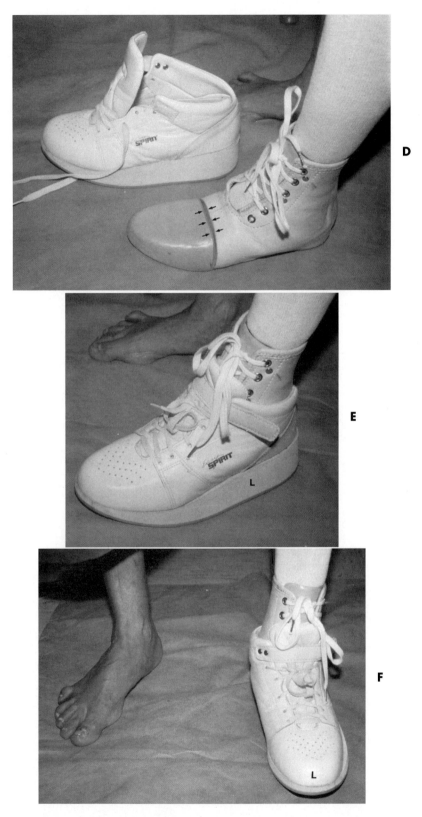

Fig. 31.23, cont'd.   D, The ankle corset has been locked into the FO with a forefoot filler. **E,** This partially amputated foot and its ankle corset and FO have been snugly inserted into a shoe. **F,** Frontal view of the same foot wearing an ankle corset and a shoe.

flexion, in addition to Achilles' tendon lengthening, a posterior ankle joint capsulotomy should be performed to allow the ankle to come to a neutral position. Postoperatively the foot should be casted in this neutral position for a few weeks to maintain the neutral ankle position.

The FO basically consists of a strong leather insole that is reinforced on its plantar aspect with a piece of spring steel running almost the entire length of the insole. A forefoot filler made of plastic is covered with leather, and a groove is created at the proximal and inferior aspect of the forefoot filler. A matching ridge is created at the anterior and inferior aspect of the ankle corset. When the anterior ridge of the ankle corset is slid into the posterior groove of the forefoot filler, the foot prosthesis and the ankle corset become one single unit, which can be easily inserted into a shoe similar to a normal foot (Fig. 31.23).

BIBLIOGRAPHY

Axe MJ, Ray RL: Orthotic treatment of sesamoid pain, Am J Sports Med 16:411–416, 1988.

Bates BT, et al: Foot orthotic devices to modify selected aspects of lower extremity mechanics, Am J Sports Med 7:338–342, 1979.

Brodke DS, et al: Effects of ankle-foot orthoses on the gait of children, J Pediatr Orthop 9:702–708, 1989.

Brown D, Smith C: Vacuum casting for foot orthoses, J Am Podiatr Assoc 66:582–587, 1976.

Doxey GE: Clinical use and fabrication of molded thermoplastic foot orthotic devices: Suggestion from the field, Phys Ther 65:1679–1682, 1985.

Due TM, Jacob RL: Molded foot orthosis after great toe or medial ray amputations in diabetic feet, Foot Ankle 6:150–152, 1985.

Glass MK, et al: An office-based orthotic system in treatment of the arthritic foot, Foot Ankle 3:37–40, 1982.

Helfand AE: Basic considerations for shoes, shoe modifications, and orthoses in foot care, Clin Podiatr 1:431–440, 1984.

Hughes J: The clinical use of pedobarography, Acta Orthop Belg 59:10–16, 1993.

Jahss MH, editor: Disorders of the foot and ankle, Philadelphia, 1991, WB Saunders.

Janisse DJ: Indications and prescriptions for orthoses in sports, Orthop Clin North Am 25:95–107, 1994.

Jones DC: Foot orthoses, Instr Course Lect 42:219–224, 1993.

Lockard MA: Foot orthoses, Phys Ther 68:1866–1873, 1988.

McPoil TG, Schuit D, Knecht HG: Comparison of three methods used to obtain a neutral plaster foot impression, Phys Ther 69:448–452, 1989.

Penneau K, Lutter LD, Winter RD: Pes planus: Radiographic changes with foot orthoses and shoes, Foot Ankle 2:299–303, 1982.

Pratt DJ, Rees PH, Butterworth RH: RTV silicone insoles, Prosthet Orthot Int 8:54–55, 1984.

Riegler HF: Orthotic devices for the foot, Orthop Rev 16:293–303, 1987.

Tomaro J, Burdett RG: The effects of foot orthotics on the EMG activity of selected leg muscles during gait, J Orthop Sports Phys Ther 18:532–536, 1993.

Ward AB: Footwear and orthoses for diabetic patients, Diabet Med 10:497–498, 1993.

Wickstrom J, Williams RA: Shoe corrections and orthopaedic foot supports, Clin Orthop 70:30, 1970.

Wu KK: Surgery of the foot, Philadelphia, 1986, Lea & Febiger.

Wu KK: Foot orthoses, Baltimore, Williams & Wilkins, 1990.

PEDIATRIC ORTHOSES

INTRODUCTION
John R. Fisk

Throughout this atlas, the reader has been made aware of the three overriding principles of orthoses: to support, to protect, and to improve function. In the following chapters, the relationship of these principles to the care and treatment of pediatric conditions is presented. With them come an additional role for orthoses. These chapters discuss the importance of bracing in the care and treatment of specific pathologic conditions in addition to the three traditional functions just listed. Hip abduction orthoses in the treatment of Legg-Calvé-Perthes disease, spinal orthoses in the treatment of scoliosis, and knee-anklefoot orthoses in the treatment of Blount's disease are a few examples. Their impact on these diagnoses may be controversial. Some of the current data surrounding these issues appear along with indications and contraindications for orthotic prescription. The central thrust of this section is that in addition to support, protection, and improved function, when working with children an additional role of disease management needs to be considered. The authors, all professionals working in multidisciplinary clinics, recognize that there are many different approaches to treatment of the specific problem, but in the *Atlas of Orthoses* emphasis is on orthotic use, as the chapter on Myelodysplasia addresses.

It has often been said that a child is not just a small adult. There are many issues of physiology and disease processes where this realization is important. Another area of importance is the manner in which a child presents for care. Rarely are children alone. They come to the clinic with parents and often with grandparents or siblings. The feelings and goals of all of these individuals need to be taken into consideration when planning the best treatment for the child. Expectations will vary. Depending on the severity of the condition that is affecting their child and the timing since diagnosis, family members are in different periods of the grieving process. Kubler-Ross[1] outlined these periods. They apply to children with disabilities just as aptly as they do to the death of a loved one because lost expectations can be equally charged with emotion. The goals we hold for our children begin with the first awareness of pregnancy and grow until delivery, but when that child is born with a disability or when the child acquires a disability later in life, those expectations are lost and we grieve. Where individuals are in that grieving process greatly influences their receptivity and understanding of recommended therapies, especially when that involves placing a device with many preconceived notions on their child. There may be denial leading to noncompliance, anger with outward belligerence directed at health care providers, and depression with its poor follow-through; only later is there acceptance and understanding. The person prescribing and the person fitting a device must be aware of this process and the impact it may be having on their patients and the family's acceptance of recommended treatment.

As we look to orthotic prescriptions to have a therapeutic impact on the conditions we are treating, we must be critical of the information that is available about their effectiveness. All of us are guilty at times of going with our impressions of what works best. Sometimes that is all we have to go on. Many of the conditions we are treating do not lend themselves to randomized, controlled, prospective studies. Nevertheless, many such studies do exist but are ignored. Little needs to be said about the significant expense involved with many of the orthoses today, to say nothing of the physical burden they may place on an individual. Therefore, before we make a recommendation or write a prescription, we must be certain that it will have its desired effect. Is there evidence that a given orthosis will be effective? Is that evidence scientifically valid? Is the recommended device the least expensive one and the most durable one that is available? These are but a few of the questions that need to be answered every time we write a prescription.

Techniques vary widely. The individual writing a prescription needs to be equally aware of the design and purpose of the device they desire as the individual who manufactures the device. To give a slip of paper to a family and then send them across town does not address these concerns. There needs to be a two-way communication between the prescription writer and the prescription filler. Furthermore, the needs of all those involved with the child's care must be addressed. The best format for this is a team clinic, where everyone can come together and arrive at a consensus. Remember too that the most important members of that team are the patient and the patient's family. It is only with this type of a coming together that everyone's needs are addressed and the proper device supplied. It is only after a proper device is delivered that any determination can be made about its effectiveness.

With a clear understanding of the needs of everyone involved with a child's care and a clear knowledge of proper design and construction and the scientific evidence for the effectiveness of an orthosis, we can expand on the original three principles of bracing: support, protection, and improved function. Now we can say that our orthoses prevent and/or correct deformity, provide a base of support, facilitate training, and improve the dynamic efficiency of gait.

REFERENCES

1. Kubler-Ross E: On death and dying, New York, 1969, Macmillan.

Congenital and Acquired Disorders

Alvin H. Crawford
Rita Ayyangar
Gregory L. Durrett

Pediatrics is distinguished by the fact that the child is constantly growing and developing. Growth is an increase in physical measurements, and development is the acquisition and refinement of skills that follow a constant sequence. The rate of acquisition of these skills shows a wide range of normal variation.[47] A knowledge of the patterns of growth and development is important in the management of a child with a physical deformity; it indicates when to introduce an intervention such as an orthotic device so as to potentiate normal development. The best interventions are made with the primary goal of attaining specific skills and maximizing the child's function while encouraging the development of emotional maturity and self-reliance.[2] Orthotic and prosthetic devices are important tools in the habilitation and rehabilitation of children with congenital and acquired disorders of the lower extremity.

CONGENITAL FOOT DEFORMITIES

The foot is an integral part of the lower limb, and this needs to be taken into account when prescribing orthoses for the lower extremity. Humans function as upright animals, and the feet serve a primary role as a weight-bearing surface. It is important to have a plantigrade, painless foot capable of tolerating the body weight and withstanding the various forces generated during stance and gait. The foot is unique in that it is flexible during some phases of activity and rigid during others; it is flexible during swing phase and early stance phase and converts to a rigid lever arm just before toe-off.[45] This flexibility may be affected by structural changes primarily in the foot and by deformities of other parts of the lower limb.

Common pediatric problems of the lower extremities requiring the use of orthoses, such as myelomen-

ingocele, cerebral palsy, and congenital dislocation of the hip, have been covered elsewhere in this book. This chapter discusses the commonly seen congenital foot deformities, which may or may not occur in isolation, and focuses on nonoperative treatment measures, including splints, braces, and shoes.

METATARSUS ADDUCTUS

Metatarsus adductus (MA) is a frequent problem in young children and is the most common musculoskeletal problem in the newborn. Although numerous theories have been proposed, the exact etiology and pathogenesis are unknown. It is a postural deformity, possibly related to *intrauterine packing*. The deformity is present at birth but often not diagnosed until the first year of life. The sole of the foot is described as *kidney-shaped*. MA was described by Henke in 1963.[30]

The incidence is 1:1000 live births.[87] Bilateral involvement is present in over 50% of patients. Hip dysplasia is associated with MA in 10% of patients.[35] A positive family history is found in 10% to 15% of patients.[53]

MA must be distinguished from clubfoot early on. One of the salient features in the differential is the fact that MA usually has the hindfoot in a valgus position as opposed to the varus position of clubfoot, and the clubfoot invariably has a fixed equinus with an inability to dorsiflex the foot. Even though a MA foot may appear to be more deformed than a clubfoot, it is easy to dorsiflex and plantar flex the hindfoot, thus ruling out the possibility of a clubfoot. The main anomaly in MA appears to be in the medial cuneiform/metatarsal joint. Reiman and Werner[58] in the autopsy findings of a newborn infant with MA noted alterations in the size and shape of the first cuneiform bone. There is confusion about the terminology, and the terms *metatarsus*

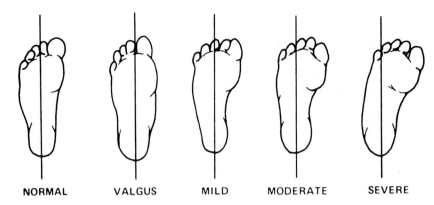

Fig. 32.1.   Heel bisector method defines the relationship of the heel to the forefoot. *Normal—* bisecting between the second and third toes. *Valgus—*bisecting between the great and second toes. *Mild MA—*bisecting the third toe. *Moderate MA—*bisecting between the third and fourth toes. *Severe MA—*bisecting between the fourth and fifth toes. *(Adapted from Bleck EE: Dev Med Child Neurol 24:545, 1982.)*

adductus and *metatarsus varus* are often used interchangeably. Ponseti and Becker[53] refer to mild forefoot adductus as *metatarsus varus* (MV). When heel valgus is also present, the condition is called *metatarsus adductus* (MA).[53]

A good scheme to classify the MA deformity is based on clinical examination, assessment of foot flexibility, and location of the heel bisector. It can also be classified based on radiographic evaluation such as suggested by Berg.[5] A recent study by Cook et al,[13] however, suggests that this method is prone to large differences in intraobserver and interobserver reliability. A method that we use to classify the severity of MA incorporates Bleck's heel bisector (Fig. 32.1).[6] The normal foot shows the weight-bearing surface of the heel to be an ellipse. The major axis tends to determine the center line of the foot and if one were to erect an ellipse on the base of the foot, the center line would tend to bisect between the second and third toes in 85% of normals. If it were to bisect the third toe, one would have a mild deformity; between the third and fourth toes, one would have a moderate MA; and if it were to bisect the fourth and fifth toes or possibly exit lateral to the fifth toe, this would represent a severe MA. Smith and Bleck[68] discussed standing the child on a photo-copying machine to get an impression of simulated weight bearing of the infant's foot (Fig. 32.2). This method usually serves well for children ≤10 years old. It is a permanent record and easy to obtain. Others have used graphite paper. MA can also be classified based on flexibility:[6]

- *Type I*—flexible (abduction beyond the midline of the heel bisector).
- *Type II*—partly flexible (abduction to the midline only).
- *Type III*—inflexible (rigid with no abduction possible).

This can be tested as follows. In the flexibility scale, type I is a foot that corrects with stroking or tickling the lateral foot or leg. A type 2 foot corrects only with passive stretching. A type 3 foot fails to correct with manual stretching.

Nonoperative treatment based on assessment of severity

Treatment of MA is still controversial. Observation and stretching in the less than 6 month old infant with passively correctable deformities usually suffices. When initiated before 8 months of age, manipulation followed by splinting with an orthosis and in more severe cases retention casting has resulted in a better nonoperative outcome. More recently, Farsetti and colleagues[23] in a long-term study spanning over 32 years looked at the outcome of untreated and nonoperative-treated MA. Their study confirmed that classification at the time of diagnosis of MA based on foot flexibility is valid. Feet with mild or moderate deformity that were passively correctable did well untreated. Those with rigid MA responded well to correctly performed serial manipulation plus plaster casting. These authors declare that it is best to start treatment as soon as the deformity has been detected and noted not to be passively correctable. Bleck's large study on MA indicates that age of the patients (range 1 day to 8 months) was the only good predictor for a good outcome.[6,13] Hallux valgus has been reported to be a common outcome of MA.[53]

The treatment of MA can be based on the severity or flexibility of the foot. It is considered to be the treatment of a C foot; that is, the lateral margin of the foot appears to be curved similar to a C. The type I foot generally spontaneously resolves, and simple observation is indicated. For type II deformities, parental

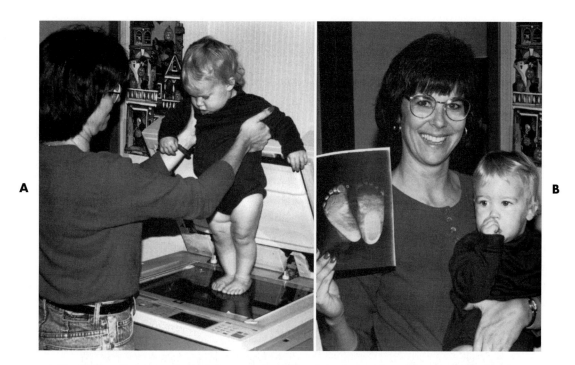

Fig. 32.2. Simple method of documenting MA using photocopies of feet in weight-bearing position. **A,** Mother holding child over photocopy machine. **B,** Permanent copy of child's foot illustrating MA of the right foot.

manipulation and stretching is recommended, approximately 10 times, 4 times a day with the foot held in the corrective position for no less than 6 seconds per repetition. Treatment for a type III foot that fails to correct with passive stretching involves manipulation and serial casting in a long leg cast with the knee flexed and the foot abducted and externally rotated. Overcorrecting the forepart of the foot with the cast should be attempted at 2-week intervals for no less than 6 weeks followed by 23 hours a day in a reverse last shoe for 3 to 6 months.

A small plastic knee-ankle-foot orthosis (KAFO) or ankle-foot orthosis (AFO) with Velcro lacers to prevent forefoot adduction has been heavily marketed for the management of MA (the Wheaton brace) (Fig. 32.3). This polypropylene KAFO/AFO is manufactured in slight hindfoot varus and forefoot abduction. It provides an economical and effective method for MA treatment, especially when minor alterations can be done in the office.

Retention casts are occasionally applied to maintain the passive correction. Serial manipulation and above-knee bivalved plaster holding casts are used to treat MA with a partly flexible or a rigid deformity. Ponseti and Becker[53] noted that MA is often associated with internal tibial torsion (ITT) and therefore advises long-leg, bent knee serial casts allowing simultaneous correction of both the MV and ITT. They oppose the use of the Denis-Browne bar in association with MA because of its tendency to produce correction through the subtalar

joint and thus cause excessive hindfoot valgus in an already predisposed foot. Berg[5] noted an increased incidence of flatfeet in those treated with a Denis-Browne bar. Rarely, children older than 3 years of age may require corrective osteotomies for residual deformities.[31,51]

Moderate MA can be treated by a simple and effective method using straight last and reverse last shoes in sequence. The plantar surface of a reverse last shoe closely resembles that of the Wheaton brace.

Operative Treatment

Rarely, for more severe cases and for older children with delay in diagnosis, surgery may be necessary. Maintenance casts, splints, or special shoes are used after surgery for varying periods of time. Before undertaking forefoot surgery, it is important to ascertain that the heel is not in excessive valgus. If forefoot adduction is corrected in the presence of heel valgus, it results in a severely pronated foot. Surgery is not without complications, and these have been well documented. Complications of tarsometatarsal capsulotomies include (1) a prominence of the fifth metatarsal following the release of the lateral ligament during tarsal metatarsal capsulotomies,[31] (2) prominence of the base of the third metatarsal dorsally, (3) avascular necrosis of the cuneiform secondary to inadvertent total circumferential release, (4) complete division of the metatarsal-tarsal joints leading to instability, and (5) osteoarthritis of the tarsometatarsal joints in the older

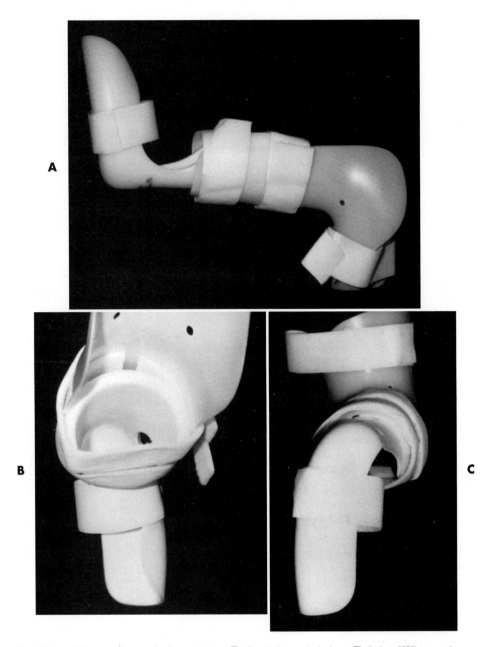

Fig. 32.3.   Wheaton brace. **A,** Lateral view. **B,** Cephalocaudad view. **C,** Sole of Wheaton brace; note similarity to a reverse last shoe.

child. Other complications related to *osteotomies* include excessive shortening, superficial wound sloughs, non-unions, malunions, and epiphyseal growth arrest when the first metatarsal has been approached proximally at its growth plate as opposed to distally.

Needless to say, the treatment of MA is controversial. Long-term studies of the deformity in adulthood are scarce. Farsetti and co-workers[23] demonstrated that the natural history of the disorder fails to show many adult complaints. Only 10% of patients ever require treatment (Fig. 32.4). There are few poor results of treatment, and the average follow-up is usually under 2.5 years. More often than not, the health care providers

treating the disorder more aggressively are podiatrists, pediatricians, and general orthopedists. Most pediatric orthopedists prefer to observe the flexible deformities and treat the severe rigid ones with a series of casts sometimes followed by reverse last shoes.

SKEWFOOT

This foot deformity is characterized by significant forefoot adduction and heel valgus with displacement of the navicular to the lateral aspect of the talar head. It is an uncommon deformity and may represent a spec-

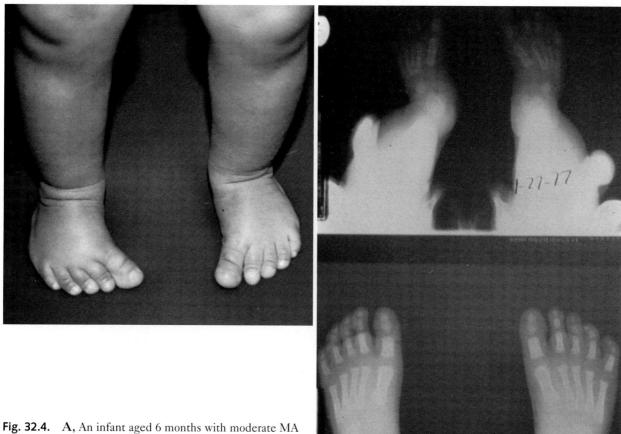

Fig. 32.4. **A,** An infant aged 6 months with moderate MA was treated by close observation only and shows spontaneous correction of the deformity over an 11-month period as noted by x-ray. **B,** Simulated standing AP x-ray at initial presentation. **C,** Standing AP x-ray 11 months later.

trum, with MA being its mildest and more frequent manifestation. It is important to differentiate it from clubfoot. The etiology of skewfoot remains unknown. Skewfoot is not commonly seen in the newborn,[51] and it has been suggested that a skewfoot results from improperly applied casts used in managing simple MA.[46]

The navicular bone is the radiographic key to diagnosis. Unfortunately the navicular does not ossify before age 3 to 6 years (Fig. 32.5). This may explain the low frequency of the diagnosis of skewfoot in the newborn. The talo–first metatarsal angle is significantly increased. On a lateral maximum dorsiflexion view, the talocalcaneal angle is widened to greater than 35 degrees, whereas the clubfoot T-C angle remains locked, does not converge, and is essentially parallel at less than 17 degrees.

Treatment ranges from serial plaster casting and thermoplastic and/or fiberglass splinting to surgical correction, with the objective being a painless, plantigrade foot that is accommodated in a normal shoe. Because this deformity is more severe than MA, it takes longer to reach the sufficient correction. Berg[5] reported

that in milder forms of skewfoot, successful correction can be achieved with serial casting. Petersen,[51] however, notes in his review of the world literature that all the authors found nonoperative treatment to be unsuccessful.

CALCANEOVALGUS FOOT

This is a frequent finding among newborns. Its incidence is 1:1000 live births with a greater occurrence in females.[79] It is thought to be the result of *intrauterine packing* and is common in the firstborn of young mothers. No clear inheritance patterns are known.

The forefoot is abducted and dorsiflexed with its dorsum lying against the anterior leg, and the heel is in severe valgus (banana appearance). In severe cases, the foot cannot initially be plantar flexed much beyond neutral. Overall, however, the foot is flexible, and the heel and forefoot can be passively corrected into varus, as opposed to congenital vertical talus, where the hindfoot is in fixed equinovalgus.

Kite[42] pointed out the association of external rota-

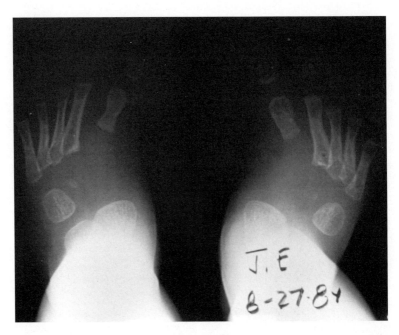

Fig. 32.5. Foot x-rays of a 1-year-old child with skewfoot. Although the navicular bone is the radiographic key to diagnosis, it is frequently not ossified before 6 years of age. The forefoot is adducted; however, the midfoot is shifted laterally, thus differentiating it from a clubfoot.

tion contractures of the hips with calcaneovalgus foot, and Wetzenstein[84] in a large population study noted the increased association of flexible flatfeet in later life with previous severe calcaneovalgus feet. This deformity is perpetuated by sleeping patterns (hips flexed, abducted and externally rotated).

The differential diagnosis includes congenital vertical talus (CVT), congenital posteromedial bowing of the tibia, and low spinal dysraphism with loss of gastrocnemius function. In CVT, the calcaneus is not palpable in the heel pad as it is drawn up out of the heel pad. The heel cord is elongated in the CV foot in contrast to CVT where it is extremely tight.

Treatment

Calcaneovalgus (CV) can be considered an "intra-uterine packing" defect, and the foot begins to correct when it is no longer "packed". Treatment is therefore somewhat expectant because most CV feet correct spontaneously. Passive stretching, retention taping, casting, or molding a thermoplastic AFO with the foot in plantar flexion and adduction are often-used modes.

CONGENITAL TALIPES EQUINOVARUS (CLUBFOOT) (CTEV)

The clubfoot deformity is easily recognized at birth because the foot presents similar to a club on the end of the leg. Its occurrence is 1.24 per 1000 live births.[11] The calf is smaller, and the extremity may be shorter. It is most important that the parents be aware of these differences early on before treatment so that they are not subsequently identified as a complication of treatment.

Clubfoot was depicted in ancient Egyptian tomb paintings, and its treatment was described in India as early as 1000 B.C. The oldest written description of clubfoot and its treatment is ascribed to Hippocrates (460–377 B.C.).[11,83] He stressed the importance of early treatment and gentle manipulation. There were no further reports until the sixteenth century. The exact cause of clubfoot remains unknown, and its pathogenesis is debated.

Clubfoot deformities can occur from abnormalities in the uterine environment such as oligohydramnios and amniotic bands and rings, from drugs such as aminopterin and tubocurarine, and as a part of syndromes inherited in mendelian fashion or produced by cytogenetic abnormalities. It may also be secondary to various neuropathies or myopathies. Idiopathic clubfeet in otherwise normal children are the most common and likely the result of a multifactorial system of inheritance. *Bedsheet clubfoot* is a term used to describe the equinus positioning of the foot occurring from the positioning and force of the sheet across the foot while being tucked into bed. Bedsheet clubfoot does not occur in the normal foot but in the incompletely treated clubfoot and the neurologic foot not splinted by an orthosis.

Pathoanatomy

Commonly agreed on findings of spatial malalignment include medial subluxation of the navicular bone toward the medial malleolus, medial displacement of the cuboid, and medial and plantar deviation of the head and neck of the abnormally shaped talus with external rotation of the body in the ankle mortise. There is debate regarding lateral/medial rotation of the talus in the ankle mortise. Fukuhara et al[24] by histomorphometric and immunohistochemical study of fetuses noted that in severe clubfeet before the third trimester of gestation, myofibroblastlike cells seemed to create a disorder of the ligaments resembling fibromatosis, leading to contraction and resulting in the typical clubfoot deformity. Fukuhara et al[24] and Howard and Benson[34] have noted a dense fibrous knot at the inferomedial aspect of the foot. This supports an intrinsic contractile process as being active in the pathogenesis.

Physical examination commonly reveals a toe-in deformity at birth with a severe medial midfoot crease and a small heel. The forefoot is adducted and supinated. The heel is usually fixed in equinus. The distinguishing feature of a clubfoot versus a severe adductovarus foot is the rigid heel equinus in the clubfoot. The heel in the severe adductovarus foot is supple, and the forefoot can be easily dorsiflexed. If the deformity is unilateral, the involved foot is usually smaller.

The incidence is higher in first-degree relatives at 2.14%. If one child has clubfoot, the chance for a subsequent sibling to have it is 20 to 30 times the baseline incidence.[87] About 50% of cases are bilateral, and 70% of clubfoot occurs in boys.[11] Rasool and co-workers[57] in a study of foot deformities and associated occult spinal abnormalities noted that in these children the foot deformities do not often become apparent until 4 to 6 years of age, as reported by Till in 1969. They also note that atypical clubfeet asymmetry of foot size, trophic ulcers, progressive foot deformities, and recurrences of deformity after foot surgery are clues to a possible associated dystrophic state. The treatment of clubfoot when associated with such conditions as arthrogryposis multiplex congenita, diastrophic dwarfism, and myelodysplasia is extremely difficult and problematic because of the recalcitrance of the soft tissue.

Treatment

Understanding of the pathoanatomy is essential to successful operative and nonoperative treatment. Manipulation, bandaging, and various therapeutic splinting techniques were the mainstay of early treatment. They still play an important role in present-day treatment. Almost 70% of cases, however, require some form

of surgery. Active correction is best obtained by manipulation, taping, casting, and surgery, whereas passive maintenance can be achieved with the use of orthoses, including splints, braces, and shoes. Thometz and Simons[78] have attempted to classify radiographically the calcaneocuboid joint in patients with idiopathic CTEV to help determine appropriate treatment choice.

The first detailed description of an orthosis for treatment of clubfoot was by Antonio Scarpa in 1803. This was an AFO with metal upright bars and cuffs at the proximal calf and the malleoli with a cup gripping the hindfoot. The orthosis produced a pronation and an abduction moment at the forefoot.

Denis-Browne described his special splint for treatment of clubfoot in 1930.[8] This consisted of taping the feet onto a bar to maintain the position obtained by manipulation.

The reverse last shoe is the most commonly used orthosis for clubfoot. The reversed last tends to maintain the abducted position achieved by either surgical or manipulative correction. A lateral T-strap attached to the shoe enhances abduction. The shoes may be combined with a Denis-Browne bar outrigger to maintain external rotation and prevent turning in of the child's feet during sleep (Fig. 32.6). The bar should not be longer than the width of the pelvis to prevent stress on the knees.

Various orthoses are used for the treatment of clubfoot. Most often, an orthosis is used as a holding device after active or passive correction. A child usually sleeps more than 8 hours at night, and this is valuable corrective time that can be used to maintain foot position with a holding device.

A prefabricated orthosis (see Fig. 32.3) is used in some centers following both manipulative and surgical correction of clubfoot. It is more appealing to parents because it permits the use of conventional shoes. The Bebax shoe is used to control the adductus deformity of the clubfoot (Fig. 32.7).

The current philosophy of treatment for this disorder is that of nonoperative treatment until the child is 9 to 12 months of age. When seen in the newborn period or before 4 months of age, the child undergoes a series of manipulations followed by serial casting using plaster of Paris for retention of the corrections obtained by manipulations. This is done at weekly intervals for 2 weeks, biweekly intervals for 2 weeks and 1 month later, at which time a lateral maximum dorsiflexion x-ray view of the foot is taken. If the heel has been brought out of equinus, the child is then placed into reverse last shoes until age 9 to 12 months. If the heel is fixed in equinus on the lateral maximum dorsiflexion view, a percutaneous heel cord release is performed, and the child is manipulated and recasted for another 2

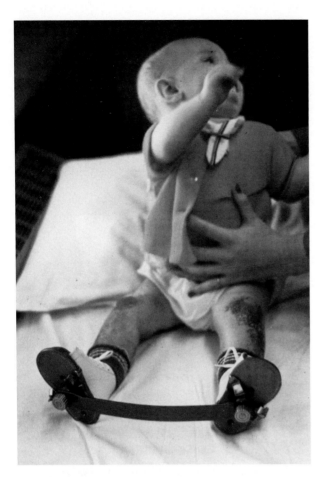

Fig. 32.6. Eleven-month-old child in reverse last shoes and Denis-Browne bar after bilateral clubfoot repair. The combination helps maintain external rotation, the corrected abducted position, and prevents turning in of the feet. The postoperative cast had just been removed, leaving behind thickened, hyperpigmented skin over both legs.

months. This is followed by the application of a reverse last shoe and a Denis-Browne splint with the feet in approximately 30 degrees of external rotation. When the child is approximately 9 to 12 months old, the foot is evaluated for its clinical appearance and its functional attributes. If the child is able to stand comfortably with the foot in the neutral position, continuing orthotic management and shoeing is recommended. If the foot is in equinus or varus or there is "medial spin" where the calcaneus is rotated posterior lateral towards the fibula, a posterior medial lateral release is performed. The posterior medial lateral release is performed through a Cincinnati incision followed by internal fixation of the surgical correction with Steinmann pins. The pins are invariably removed within 6 to 8 weeks, and the child is placed in an above-knee retention cast for 2 months followed by a reverse last shoe and a Denis-Browne bar for approximately 12 months. The decision has to be made at that time as to whether or not the child requires further orthotic treatment.

Conventional AFOs have been used following surgery. Most often, the foot is casted with the forefoot overcorrected in abduction, and the orthosis is thus molded and fabricated.

The authors recommend reversed last shoes with a nighttime Denis-Browne bar for the postoperative treatment of susceptible clubfoot deformities under 5 years of age. We utilize a custom-molded AFO for older children after treatment by lateral transfer of the anterior tibialis tendon.

CONGENITAL VERTICAL TALUS (CONGENITAL CONVEX PES VALGUS) (CVT)

This is an uncommonly occurring rigid flatfoot deformity that requires early identification and aggressive treatment. Serpentine foot, Persian slipper foot, congenital rocker-bottom foot, and congenital convex pes valgus are all terms used for CVT. Tachdjian submitted the term *teratologic dorsolateral dislocation of the talocalcaneonavicular joint*. The etiology is often unknown, but it has a high association with congenital anomalies such as trisomy 13, 14, 15, and 18 and with neuromuscular disorders such as spina bifida, arthrogryposis, and sacral agenesis.

Clinical features preclude a rigid rocker-bottom foot: The heel is in fixed equinus, the forefoot is dorsiflexed and everted, the arch is convex, and the foot is stiff and uncorrectable. The head of the talus is prominent and felt medially in the sole. *Congenital convex pes valgus* is the anatomically correct term. One should use x-rays to differentiate the diagnosis of congenital vertical talus from a congenital rigid flatfoot.[16]

Treatment consists of early manipulation and retention casting to stretch the soft tissue and prepare for complete surgical correction. Orthotic devices, especially AFOs with accentuation of the medial longitudinal arch, are very useful *after* surgery to passively maintain correction. The devices may or may not be articulated at the ankle (Fig. 32.8).

FLATFOOT POSTURE

Flatfoot deformity is physiologic in the newborn and toddler. The toddler may pronate the foot to gain more stability, especially when the toddler starts to walk. Flatfoot deformities are often associated with a generalized ligamentous laxity. There is a tendency to bear weight over the medial column of the foot as opposed to the lateral column.

Flexible flatfoot is a very common disorder in children and in fact has been considered by some to be an anatomical variant of ligamentous laxity that may not need treatment.[73,78]

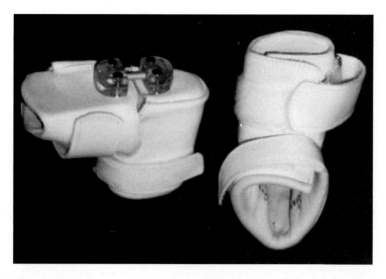

Fig. 32.7. Bebax shoes are designed for progressive and dynamic correction of some congenital forefoot deformities. The multidirectional hinge is designed to permit adjustment of the forefoot in relation to the hindfoot on the horizontal.

A

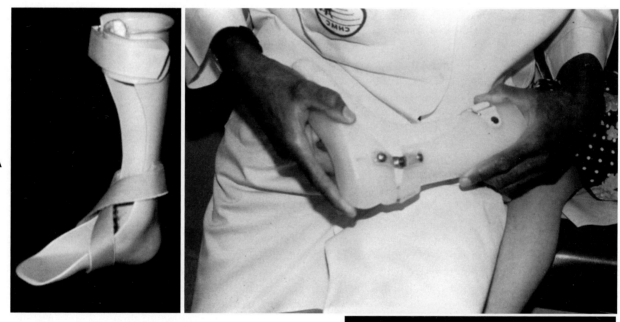

B

C

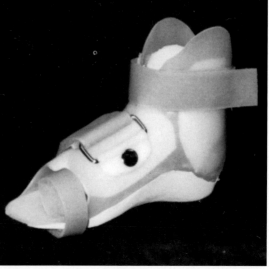

Fig. 32.8. Views of nonarticulated and articulated AFOs and an SMO. **A,** Lateral view of nonarticulated on solid ankle AFO. This functionally equals a double upright AFO. The angle at the ankle influences bending moment at the knee. The solid ankle AFO is useful when the ankle dorsiflexors or plantar flexors are weak. Adjustments in trim lines change their ability to provide mediolateral stability. A flexibly rigid material can provide posterior leaf spring action. **B,** Articulated AFOs are useful when there is some active dorsiflexion ability. The AFO may have a free ankle or incorporate a plantar flexion stop and dorsiflexion assist as necessary. Their lightweight properties and easily adjusted trim lines make them more acceptable than the double upright metal AFO. **C,** Supramalleolar orthosis (SMO) with U cut back provides mediolateral support at the ankle with little limitation in dorsiflexion and plantar flexion. The absence of a longer lever arm makes this less effective if there is significant weakness in the dorsiflexors. If some restriction of plantar flexion and dorsiflexion is desired, a flat cut back may be used instead of a U cut back.

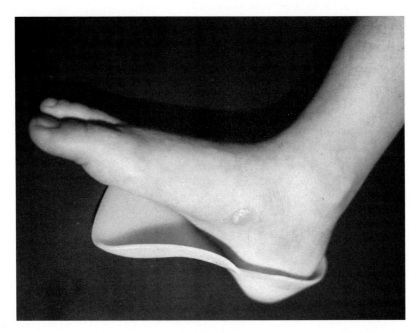

Fig. 32.9. UCBL is often used in the treatment of flexible flatfoot. Note the callosity over the talar head. As with all other orthoses, skin should be monitored for breakdown.

In a large study of 2300 children in a rural population of India, Rao and Joseph[56] noted that the prevalence of flatfoot was higher in the shod foot and was quite low in the unshod foot. The susceptibility of flatfoot among children who wear shoes is higher if there is associated ligamentous laxity. Their study also suggests that closed-toe shoes inhibit the development of the arch more than open-toed shoes or slippers. This is contrary to Kelsey's[40] observation that type of footwear does not influence the occurrence of flatfoot. It appears that the critical age for development of the longitudinal arch is 6 years, and treatment begun after 4 years is less effective than that started earlier.[56,60] There is a natural tendency to improvement in the arch with age as evidenced by the prevalence of flatfoot, which is higher in the 6-year-old than in the 10-year-old.[56]

FLEXIBLE FLATFEET

The flexible flatfoot is characterized by the foot being flat with weight bearing on the medial border when the child is standing (a pronated foot). The longitudinal arch tends to reappear when the foot is suspended and especially with the great toe extended,[59] and this serves as one of the primary differentials between a rigid and a flexible flatfoot. The flexible flatfoot is occasionally seen with tight heel cords. The heel cord contracture may be secondary to a persistent pronated valgus foot. The flexible flatfoot may be seen in an idiopathic toe walker. When one sees a flatfoot, especially a unilateral deformity, a complete neurologic assessment is indicated.

Clinically a flexible flatfoot can be differentiated from the rigid flatfoot by the "tiptoe" test. If the heel is in valgus while the patient is standing with full weight-bearing and then it shifts into varus while standing in tiptoe, it is assumed that the child has a flexible flatfoot.[80]

On the AP view the talocalcaneal angle is invariably increased. On the lateral view the talus appears to be oriented more vertical than normally. The calcaneus and the metatarsus tend to be more horizontal, and there is a talonavicular or naviculocuneiform sag. An axial view of the calcaneus shows the heel to be in valgus.

To help differentiate accurately between the normal foot, the flexible flatfoot and the rigid flatfoot, Aharonson et al used the footprint apparatus that helped them measure the exact amount of abnormal pressure being applied by the middle weight-bearing area. Their method demonstrated that introduction of a wedge of proper height under the medial portion of the heel brought about optimal correction of the calcaneovalgus and restored the normal longitudinal arch.

Treatment of flatfoot is controversial.[63,69] Overall, there is agreement that treatment may be beneficial in symptomatic flatfeet.

For a symptomatic flexible flatfoot, passive Achilles' tendon stretching exercises are recommended. In addition, we recommend a modified UCBL or a heel seat cup to prevent the talonavicular sag (Fig. 32.9). Others have suggested use of the Blake inverted foot orthosis (FO) with various modifications and suggest the medial heel skive technique to enhance the pronation controlling features of FOs.[41] Jay and Schoenhaus[37] have developed a dynamic stabilizing inner sole system that helps offset the calcaneus into about 45 degrees varus within the heel cup, thereby controlling hyperpronation. Surgical treatments include raising the internal arch, calcaneal osteotomies, and subtalar arthrodeses for ankle valgus. Viladot[79] suggests a double approach: raising the internal arch and simultaneously correcting the hindfoot with use of an endorthosis to limit talarcalcaneus mobility.

RIGID FLATFOOT

The rigid flatfoot has no longitudinal arch when the foot is suspended. It is most often associated with some form of pathologic condition. These include inflammatory arthritis such as JRA, occult fractures, tumors, and abnormal tarsal bones to include tarsal coalition, accessory naviculars, etc. When the rigid flatfoot is associated with pain and discomfort of the lateral sinus tarsi and the lateral leg, it is considered to be a peroneal spastic flatfoot. The initial assessment includes ruling out other anomalies such as a tarsal coalition. One should evaluate the severity and assess the degree of subluxation of the talocalcaneal navicular joint. The primary causes of peroneal spastic flatfeet include osteochondral fractures, accessory navicular deformity, avulsion fracture of the fifth metatarsal bone, inflammatory diseases, tumors, and tarsal coalitions.

Tarsal coalition involves partial fusion of the tarsals that is initiated during fetal life. There is a fibrous, cartilaginous, or bony connection of two or more tarsal bones. The incidence of tarsal coalition ranges approximately 1.7% to 3% but has at times been reported to be as high as 6%.[74,83] Tarsal coalition may at times be entirely asymptomatic, so its incidence may be higher than reported. Leonard[44] in 1974 postulated an autosomal dominant gene inheritance of almost complete penetrance. There is no race preference.[53] The etiology of tarsal coalition is varied. Congenital and acquired conditions are implicated.

Onset of symptoms is usually in the second decade around adolescence—12 to 16 years for talocalcaneal and 8 to 12 years for calcaneonavicular[38,61]; however, there are documented cases of symptomatic coalitions as early as 2 years of age.[12] In most, the onset of pain correlated with increase in repetitive organized activities, such as soccer and little league baseball. Subtalar motion is progressively decreased, and valgus deformity of the hindfoot is characteristically noted. Various biomechanical imbalances may occur, and the pain is usually proportionate to activity or may coincide with trauma. Gait analysis has been used to better understand the effects of tarsal coalition and its pathophysiology.[54] Joint pain and muscle spasms or shortening, particularly peroneal muscle shortening, are common,

with a resultant peroneal spastic flatfoot. The foot is frequently held in a fixed valgus position and a nerve block does not correct the deformity. Harris and Beath[29] wrote that EMG shows no true muscle spasm. Other types of coalition may cause inversion spasms of the foot due to involvement of the anterior and posterior tibial muscles.

Clinical diagnosis should be confirmed by radiographic imaging. Anteroposterior, lateral, and 45-degree oblique views of the foot are usually diagnostic in calcaneonavicular coalition. The lateral foot view may show an anterior elongation of the superior calcaneal process "anteater nose sign" found to be diagnostic of calcaneonavicular bar.[49] There may be beaking of the anterosuperior talus on the lateral view with either of the bars. Talocalcaneal coalitions are harder to detect, and CT scan in the axial plane has proven to be clearly superior and accurate in detection.[52]

Symptomatic tarsal coalition can be troublesome to treat. For minor symptoms, a simple medial arch support or a medial heel wedge may be sufficient. Initial treatment should be conservative and aimed at alleviating pain by using splints or casts to support (reduce) subtalar movement or injecting hydrocortisone and local anesthesia into the sinus tarsi. For persistent spasm, manipulation under anesthetic and a short leg walking cast with foot in neutral position for 3 to 6 weeks may be required. Unfortunately, because of a strong tendency for relapse, prolonged splintage for up to 6 months with a carefully molded splint may be required. The orthosis should start by exerting a mild inversional pressure against the deformity and should be gradually increased as the patient is able to tolerate more pressure.[76]

The main indication for surgery is persistent pain. The type of surgery depends on the type of coalition, the age of the patient, and the absence/presence of degenerative changes in the tarsal joints. The primary surgery for tarsal coalition is some form of resection arthroplasty.[48] The resection arthroplasty requires that full subtalar motion be obtained at the time of surgery. Most of the failures are due to inadequate resection of the synchondrosis. The more readily responsive condition is the calcaneal navicular bar where the calcaneonavicular synchondrosis is excised in toto. The extensor digitorum brevis muscle is then released from its origin on the distal calcaneus and placed into the resected space for an interposition arthroplasty. The foot is placed in a below-knee cast in inversion for approximately 10 days followed by active range of motion in and out of a bivalved cast or splint for 3 weeks. A UCBL shoe insert or heel seat cup is used until rehabilitation has been completed.

The talocalcaneal bar is the more difficult and resistant one to manage surgically. The bar is excised from its medial aspect until the cartilaginous interface is identified. At that point, one can insert the fat from the surrounding tissue or split the flexor hallucis longus longitudinally and interpose it into the resection space. There is a difference of opinion about the merits of T-C as opposed to the consistently good results of C-N resection, but studies corroborating resection of talocalcaneal coalition as a worthwhile procedure are being increasingly reported.[54] The post-operative regimen is essentially the same using a cast immediately followed by a UCBL shoe insert or heel seat cup for the remainder of the rehabilitation. The contraindications to surgical correction include degenerative changes in the joints, a pronounced talar beak, a complete ossification of the bar, or multiple coalitions.

ACCESSORY NAVICULAR BONE

Accessory bones are common in the foot. Symptomatic accessory navicular (AN) bone is a common finding with a greater incidence in females. The AN lies on the medial plantar border of the navicular bone. Most often, the symptomatic AN presents as an "overuse" syndrome in young athletes. Specific findings include pain over the medial aspect of the foot over the navicular tuberosity increased by abducting the forefoot. An element of posterior tibial tendinitis is frequently present.

The tendon of the tibialis posterior attaches to the AN as it inserts into the main body of the navicular and the metatarsals. It develops around the second month of fetal life with mineralization occurring at around 9 to 11 years of age. There are three types:

• *Type 1:* AN is separate from the main body.
• *Type 2:* AN is connected to the main navicular body by a fibrous or cartilaginous band.
• *Type 3:* AN demonstrates a bony union to the main navicular body.

AN presents as a prominent extension of the tarsal navicular body, and histopathological changes of chronic injury and repair are noted.

Nonoperative treatment is the mainstay and includes FOs such as the navicular cookie and a heel seat cup to relieve pressure over the navicular body and reduce the pull of the tibialis posterior tendon (Fig. 32.10). For chronic pain symptoms not relieved by orthoses, a simple excision of the separated ossicle through the medial limb of the Cincinnati incision usually provides permanent relief.

CAVUS DEFORMITY

Cavus deformity is characterized by an excessively high arch resulting from a varus deformity of the

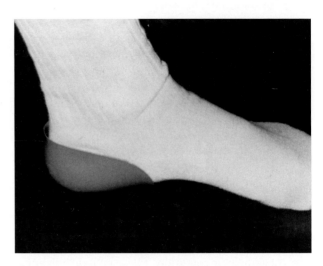

Fig. 32.10.   Heel seat cup provides cushioning of the calcaneus as it helps reposition the calcaneal pad of fat.

hindfoot and a plantar flexed equinus deformity of the forefoot, especially the first metatarsal. Care needs to be taken to insure accurate diagnosis of potential underlying causes.

Shoe modifications and bracing are rarely effective. Invariably the deformity is fairly rigid, and more problems are caused by orthoses than benefits, especially if the cause is neurologic and there is any evidence of a sensory problem. The surgical treatment is based on the rigidity or flexibility of the forefoot and hindfoot as illustrated with the Coleman block test.[76] The surgical procedures may be soft tissue when the lesion is picked up early in young children, whereas bony procedures are required in older children. Watanabe[80] recommends using the metatarsal osteotomy as a simple procedure for correction of the pes cavus deformity in combination with other soft tissue or bony procedures as indicated. It cannot be emphasized enough that all cavus deformities should be thoroughly evaluated and investigated for evidence of neurologic disorders.

ARTHROGRYPOSIS

Arthrogryposis (arthrogryposis multiplex congenita [AMC]) is a nonprogressive congenital syndrome. It is a term derived from Greek meaning "curved joints" and describes the presence of multiple joint contractures at birth with an intact sensory system.

It was first described by Otto in 1841,[50] and its pathogenesis continues to be debated. The incidence is approximately 0.03% of newborns. There are two main forms, neurogenic and myopathic, depending on the primary site of the neuromuscular lesion.[4,7] The former is more common, there is usually no obvious hereditary component, and it presents with fixed flexion/

extension deformities of the limbs. The rarer myopathic form is characterized by muscle changes similar to those in progressive muscular dystrophy with fixed flexion deformities of the limbs and gross deformities of the chest and spine. There is usually a strong hereditary factor. In addition, other reasons cited for development of arthrogryposis include defects of connective tissue and intrauterine packing.[27]

Neurogenic arthrogryposis most frequently is thought to be due to absent/decreased anterior horn cells occurring with a predominance in specific neuronal segments. There is usually no disturbance of sensory function, and the bowel and bladder are usually not affected. Sometimes there may be associated involvement of the brain. Amyoplasia is the most frequent neurogenic form with primary limb involvement, few to no associated anomalies, and normal to high intelligence.[28]

Amyoplasia is characterized by multiple, frequently severe orthopedic deformities but follows a favorable natural course. Many of these patients subsequently ambulate. Predictors for successful functional ambulation[32] include good hip extension and range or crutchability as a substitute (strong shoulder depressors and elbow extension), fair-to-good quadriceps strength and range or KAFO as a substitute, and plantigrade feet.

The orthopedic deformities involving the lower extremity can involve the hip, knee, or foot.[86] The frequency of lower extremity joint involvement increases from proximal to distal segment with foot deformities being most common.[20]

Foot Deformities

Talipes equinovarus deformity was the most commonly occurring foot and ankle deformity, followed by congenital vertical talus.[14] The foot deformities of arthrogryposis are quite rigid and more often than not resistant to conservative treatment (splints, passive stretch). Various surgical procedures have been applied to their treatment, including posteromedial release in combination with talectomy and the less radical Verebelyi-Ogston procedure[26] for correction of hindfoot varus deformities and metatarsal/midtarsal osteotomies for forefoot deformities.[19] Surgical correction of deformities is usually required and is best done at 1 to 2 years of age to promote development of standing and ambulation with postoperative use of appropriate orthotic and prosthetic devices. Casting before surgery helps prepare the soft tissue and promotes maximal correction. Postsurgical retentive splinting must be maintained for many months to years to maintain correction because there is an absence of supportive musculature and thereby an increased risk of recurrence (Fig. 32.11).

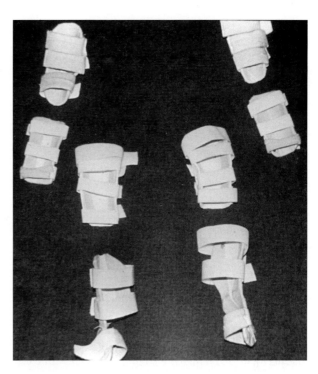

Fig. 32.11. Splints directed at passive correction of the multiple contractures seen in the arthrogrypotic child. Proximal lower limb contractures are generally addressed before distal ones with the goal of correction by 2 years to permit upright ambulation. In the upper limbs, a more functional position is one with one elbow flexed for hand-to-mouth activities and the other elbow extended for greater reach.

Knee deformities

Knee deformities may include muscle and soft tissue contractures, low mobile patella, and dislocation of the knee secondary to extensor contractures. Physiotherapy, accompanied by prolonged casting or bracing, is useful.[64] The flexion contractures are much more resistant to correction. Ambulation is possible using a KAFO with knee locked in extension despite a flexion contracture of up to 15 degrees. For contractures exceeding 15 degrees, an extension osteotomy of the distal femur is often needed.[77]

Hip deformities

The characteristic deformity is a flexion-abduction-external rotation contracture often accompanied by dislocation of the hip.[3,17] The reported incidence of hip dislocations ranges from 14% to 42%.[32,72] Early treatment focuses on passive stretching with physical therapy, splints, or positioning devices. There is consensus that unilateral dislocation should be reduced to prevent pelvic obliquity, leg length inequality, and scoliosis.[72] Long-term night bracing with appropriate positioning is useful in the postoperative period. Bilateral dislocations are not functionally limiting, and surgical treatment is often not indicated.

Spine

Scoliosis, especially a large C-shaped thoracolumbar curve, is a common occurrence in arthrogryposis. Age at onset and patterns of scoliostic deformity are variable. Progressive scoliosis is difficult to control by bracing alone, and operative stabilization may be effective in rigid, progressive curves.[65]

Upper extremities

The aim of upper limb management is to facilitate the individual's independence in self-care activities and activities of daily living. Splinting started early is useful. It is beneficial to maintain one elbow in extension and the other with flexion to permit weight bearing and hand-to-mouth activities. In the severely affected, surgery is often contraindicated, especially when hand function is poor. When surgery is indicated, procedures may be necessary at the shoulder, elbow, and wrist, followed by retentive splinting.[10,85]

Cognitive functioning is often quite well developed in the child with arthrogryposis, and rehabilitation should focus on facilitating cognitive, social, and communicative abilities.

BUNION (HALLUX VALGUS)

Bunions are noted primarily in the adolescent age group. A positive family history is quite frequent (approximately 60% of the time). It presents as an autosomal dominant characteristic. A mother with bunions usually delivers a child with bunions. It is nine times more common in females than in males. The deformity presents psychological problems for young girls. The etiology is somewhat controversial and includes various conditions, such as metatarsus primus varus, ligamentous laxity, hypermobile forefoot, a pronated foot, pes planus, excessive rounding of the first metatarsal head, overtreatment of MA, and excessively long metatarsals and their relationship to shoe style with an inadequate toe box. Although ill-fitting shoes do not cause hallux valgus (HV), they can certainly cause bunion formation from pressure over the medial side of the first metatarsal head. HV is most often accompanied by valgus of the foot, which may be the reason for the toe deformity.

Physical examination usually shows a swelling over the medial aspect of the great toe metatarsophalangeal joint. There is a widened forefoot with a laterally deviated great toe. The pes planus is associated in 56% of cases. It is usually bilateral, although one may be larger than the other. HV in the pediatric age group is usually less frequent than in adults, and there are fewer complaints of pain but more complaints related to cosmesis than in adults. The radiographic evaluation determines whether or not there is a congruous deformity, a deviated joint, or a subluxed metatarsophalangeal joint. The intermetatarsal angle is usually greater than 9 degrees.[9] There is occasionally an oblique orientation of the cuneiform first metatarsal joint, and the hallux valgus metatarsophalangeal angle is usually greater than 15 degrees.[39]

Nonoperative treatment usually is related to relief of shoe pressure on the first metatarsophalangeal joint. The change of the shoe should include a more roomy toebox, a toe bar, and a medial arch support to correct the pes valgus. It is unlikely that the fashion-conscious female adolescent would wear shoes very different from her peers.[64] The current fashion switch to more roomy styles may serve today's child well.

It is extremely important to evaluate the child for evidence of recognizable joint hyperelasticity, the presence of a pes planus, a tight heel cord, or subtle spasticity. Most recently, Groiso[25] has advocated conservative orthotic management of the deformity because this proved quite effective in delaying or stopping the progression of deviation and sometimes even completely correcting the deformity. He used a thermoplastic office-made splint that was custom-molded to the child's foot. The authors have had limited experience with this technique; however, we feel it has several advantages over the surgical treatment of adolescent bunion (Fig. 32.12). There are more than 200 surgical procedures, which include both soft tissue and bony approaches to this deformity, and, needless to say, there is not a consistently good result found with any of the surgical techniques. Surgical treatment includes an osteotomy aimed at correcting the angle of the big toe and reducing the width of the foot and prominence of the head. It is recommended to treat the lesion conservatively until the child has reached skeletal maturity, at which time surgical procedure might be indicated.[3,17,67]

Most cases present with a deformity at the metatarsophalangeal joint but a few are angled at the intermetatarsal joint. The foot valgus rotates the metatarsals. The first metatarsal head rolls medially, thus losing its hold on the sesamoid, which dislocates laterally and upsets the vector forces of all associated muscles. The MP joint medially angulates into valgus. The bunion is a bursa over the medial aspect of the metatarsal head that frequently gets inflamed. The second toe overlaps or underlaps. The anterior arch flattens and leads to anterior metatarsalgia. The valgus slowly increases, and the MP joint subluxes and gets arthritic over time.[15] Juvenile hallux valgus is different from the bunion seen in the adult. Overall the deviation of the toe is less pronounced. The surgical management of adolescent hallux valgus is extremely controversial. Orthotic management is becoming popular, but its results are unknown. We recommend orthoses such as the Groiso

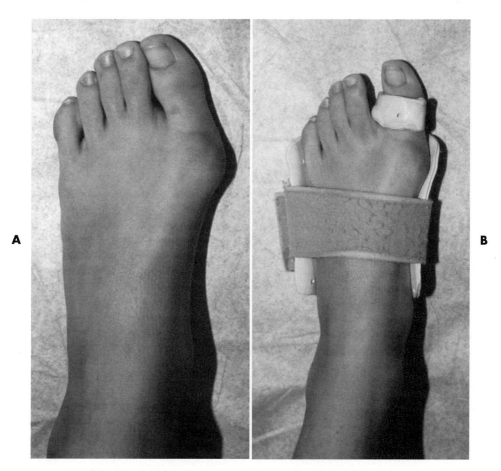

Fig. 32.12. **A,** Foot with hallux valgus and bunion deformity. **B,** Groiso splint demonstrating a medially directed force at the great toe and an improved foot shape.

orthosis or modifications thereof in the initial management of hallux valgus in the preadolescent or before skeletal maturity. This, associated with modifications in the shoe as described earlier, may help delay or alleviate the need for surgical treatment.

BOWLEGS AND KNOCK KNEES

Bowlegs and knock knees (genu varum and valgum) are a common occurrence in infants and children. Bowlegs and knock knees are a part of normal development. Lateral tibial bowing is commonly noted in early infancy. Later in infancy, physiologic bowing involving both the femur and the tibia is seen. This bowing gradually changes to knock knees between 18 months and 3 years. The valgus may be extreme but decreases to 5 to 6 degrees by about 7 years of age.[62]

The terms *varus* and *valgus* are often confused. Fairbank and Fairbank[22] noted that valgus denotes a malalignment in the coronal plane in which the part distal to the site of deformity deviates away from the midline. In varus, the part distal to the deformity deviates toward midline.

Genu varum may occur due to actual angular deformity of the proximal tibia or may be apparent due to external femoral torsion or internal tibial torsion. It may also occur as a result of incurvature of the tibia or be due to pathologic processes such as tibia vara/dysplasia. Similarly, genu valgum may be due to the deformity or may be apparent due to recurvatum at the knee.

Evaluation should include a good history focusing on the family, growth pattern, and diet, and physical examination should include height and weight percentiles, joint laxity assessment, rotational profile, and measurements of the femoral-tibial angle and the intercondylar and intermalleolar distances. Radiographs are indicated if there is suspicion of a pathologic force as when there is a severe deformity, asymmetry, stature below the fifth percentile, or other musculoskeletal abnormalities.

Genu varum and genu valgum often spontaneously improve with growth, and bracing is not usually required before 5 years of age. No particular treatment is required for physiologic bowing where the intercondylar distance (between the knees) is less than 10 cm with the ankles together (Fig. 32.13). Shoe wedges, splints, and special shoes have been used over the years without

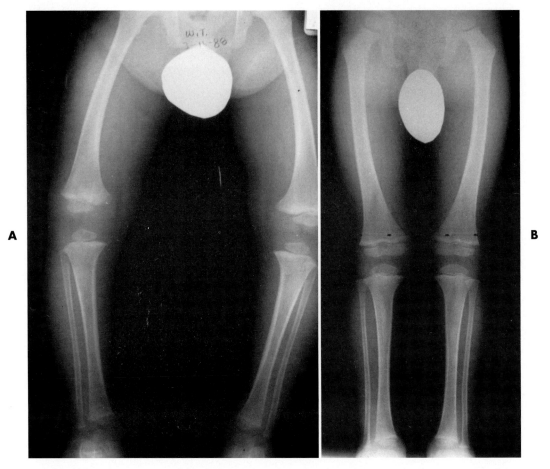

Fig. 32.13.   X-rays demonstrating the spontaneous resolution of bowlegs (genu varum). **A,** An 18-month-old with genu varum. Cosmesis or deviant gait pattern with teasing by peers is often the reason for referral. **B,** Nine months later, the same child shows resolution of genu varum.

particular success. They may in fact cause more harm. If the intercondylar distance is greater than 10 cm with the malleoli approximated, treatment with a nighttime Blount's bowleg brace may be initiated. Surgery or bracing may also be indicated in a progressive pathologic form, such as Blount's disease. Braces in these conditions primarily serve as holding devices because the pressure required for correction must be moderately severe and applied over a long time, making them uncomfortable and difficult to tolerate.

BLOUNT'S DISEASE

Blount's disease characteristically presents as a bowing deformity resulting from disordered growth of the proximal medial physis and metaphysis at the tibia. It goes through stages, including fragmentation of the medial proximal tibia metaphysis.[43] The incidence is greater in black and obese children and is rare in many parts of the world.[83]

Without fragmentation of the metaphysis and a failure of further development of the proximal tibial epiphysis, the diagnosis of Blount's disease cannot be made. Radiographs, bone scan, and tomography are necessary in the older child when a physeal bar is suspected.[70] Once a diagnosis of Blount's disease has been made, depending on the age and stage of presentation, it must be treated directly. In the younger child with minimal involvement, a Blount's brace, A-frame brace, or any type of three-point lateral support can be used for treatment (Fig. 32.14). The aim of bracing is to provide a force at the medial side of the thigh and medial malleolus with an opposing lateral support, while controlling rotation of the leg and flexion of the knee in the brace. Sometimes putting the pressure pads on a swivel so that they rotate with the skin increases toleration. Orthoses, as mentioned previously, are recommended only in the early stages (stages I and II of Langenskiöld[43]) for the treatment of Blount's disorder.[70] Once the disease has started to advance, operative intervention is usually the only treatment for the problem. In the advanced stage of Blount's disease, there are alterations of the proximal tibia metaphysis as well as the proximal tibia epiphysis. This may result in permanent shortening of the involved site. Most often,

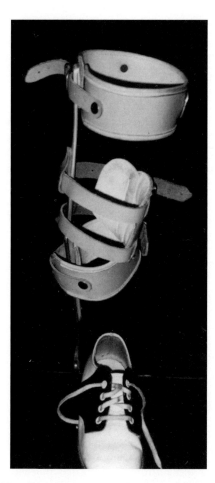

Fig. 32.14.   A bowleg brace may be used to aid in correction of genu varum. The brace continually exerts a medially directed force on the lateral aspect of the knee during standing or walking. The child is expected to wear the brace at least 8 hours a day.

true Blount's disease presents as a unilateral deformity. One should make every effort to treat Blount's disease aggressively when first diagnosed and before the appearance of a physeal bar. Once a physeal bar has presented on the medial aspect, the treatment invariably requires surgery, and more often than not multiple surgeries are required to correct both the angular rotational and the subsequent length problems that are created by this deformity. The newer methods of lengthening, especially the lengthening achieved with a ring configuration, have brought some advances to treatment of this condition.

TIBIAL BOWING

Lateral tibial bowing

Lateral tibial bowing is a normal physiologic variation during the first year of life. It reaches its maximum angulation between 18 and 36 months. Treatment is usually by observation to rule out Blount's disease. It is usually mild, is bilateral, and shows spontaneous reso-

lution. In the more persistent cases, a three-point lateral support, A-frame, or Blount's brace may be used.

Anterior bowing

Anterior bowing may be associated with an absent/ hypoplastic fibula, and the main problem here is tibial shortening. Dimpling of the skin of the anterior leg usually identifies more fibular involvement. This shortening often requires correction by a limb-lengthening procedure.

Posteromedial bowing

Posteromedial bowing is associated with a calcaneus foot deformity, triceps weakness, extension contracture of the ankle, and anisomelia. Spontaneous improvement of the angulation occurs with growth, and correction should be delayed. Limb shortening is a problem and is often progressive. At maturation, shortening may be significant, exceeding 2.5 cm. Occasionally, epiphysiodesis of the proximal tibia is usually necessary. Casting into plantar flexion, ROM exercises, and AFOs have been tried, but their effectiveness is still unclear.

Anterolateral bowing

Anterolateral bowing of the tibia is a prepseudarthrotic lesion and is a dangerous form of bowing. It may be a precursor to and associated with pseudarthrosis of the tibia. The fibula is often affected with narrowing, angulation, and an occasional pseudarthrosis. If fibular pseudarthrosis occurs independent of the tibia, there is shortening of the fibula with proximal displacement of the lateral malleolus to produce ankle valgus. Orthotic management should be initiated as soon as the diagnosis is confirmed to prevent fracture. Postfracture treatment includes excision of soft tissue and the lesion, intramedullary rodding and placing an onlay bone graft over the defect, free fibular vascularized bone graft, and distraction histogenesis using the Ilizarov frame. Anterolateral bowing of the tibia can result in fracture and pseudarthrosis. Therefore, bracing should be tried as a preventive measure. For the young infant, a nonarticulated plastic KAFO is prescribed. The older infant and young child are treated with an articulated KAFO, whereas in the older child a high AFO may suffice.[70] Osteotomy for angular deformity is contraindicated because primary healing is rare, and it is better to avoid formation of a pseudarthrosis.

BALL AND SOCKET ANKLE

The ball and socket ankle is a developmental abnormality in the shape of the ankle joint, in which there is a domed shape of the talus and a corresponding cup configuration of the distal tibia-fibular complex. The cause remains unknown. When talocalcaneal coalition is rigid at birth, the result is a ball and socket ankle.[75] The deformity is usually a part of a lower extremity deletion syndrome, such as a congenitally short femur, absence of several rays of the foot, or congenital tarsal coalition,[70] or may be an adaptive change providing inversion and eversion secondary to loss of subtalar motion. When one considers a lower extremity deletion syndrome, it is not uncommon to find the association of a congenitally short or bowed femur, deficiency of the lateral femoral condyle, deficiency of the anterior cruciate ligament, deficiency of the proximal fibula, some shortening of the tibia, a ball and socket ankle, a tarsal coalition, and deficiency of the lateral rays of the foot.

The true incidence of congenital ball and socket ankle may never be determined. The ankle deformity itself is totally asymptomatic, and it is suspected that many never come to medical attention. There are, however, significant associations with other deformities in the ipsilateral lower extremity that certainly do lead to orthopedic observation and/or intervention. Those associations include tarsal coalition in more than 50% of the cases, absent lateral foot rays in more than 50% of cases, partial absence of the fibula, short bowed tibia and fibula, congenitally short femur, absence of the cruciate ligaments, and deficiency of the lateral femoral condyle.

On occasion we have seen children with a ball and socket ankle with a deficiency of the lateral rays of the foot who have instability of the ankle. For these children we usually recommend an articulated custom-molded AFO or supramalleolar orthosis (SMO) (see Fig. 32.8, C). The single action hinge tends to give them the stability that they lack and usually allows them to participate freely in athletic activities. One has also to consider a shoe spacer orthosis in that more often than not the symptomatic children are those with an absence of the lateral rays of the foot, and suspension of the foot in the shoe becomes a problem.

Radial clubhand

Radial clubhand is an autosomal dominant inheritable condition characterized by partial or complete absence of the radius. There may or may not be complete development of the ulna ray (this includes the lateral structures of the forearm, wrist, and hand). There is occasionally an associated thrombocytopenia described as a TAR baby (thrombocytopenia absent radius). Children with radial clubhand tend to have their hand laterally or radially deviated. Occasionally, there is a bursa over the end of the distal ulna epiphysis when the hand has subluxated or translated radially. The lesion presents with variations from partial to total absence of the radius. The management of this problem has been cyclical, and there does not appear to be as many proponents of early centralization and surgery (centering of the hand off the distal ulna) as there once

was. More often than not, once the child is noted to have the deformity after birth, an occupational therapist is called on and usually applies a thermal labile orthoplast splint. This is successively adjusted into more ulnar deviation as the child grows (Fig. 32.15).

Considerable discussion and counseling of the child and the family have to be carried out before determining whether or not these children should be treated surgically. They tend to function quite well, although the cosmesis of the hand coming off at approximately a right angle to the forearm is somewhat unsettling. When the condition is noted bilaterally, it is safe to perform centralization on one side and let the child determine whether or not he or she would like the other side done. It is extremely important that one counsels the parents about the amount of flexibility and function the child achieves with a flexible wrist as opposed to a rigid wrist following centralization, even though the hand is more cosmetically positioned. We strongly recommend a thermal labile orthosis for the growing child in an attempt to maintain the hand in as much of a neutral position as possible.

FOOT GEAR/SHOES

The commercial shoe is the standard means of protecting and supporting the normal foot in both childhood and adulthood. A normal arch will develop without shodding.[71] In cases of foot and ankle deformity, shoes may help relieve abnormal pressure, especially with weight-bearing conditions. A shoe is considered to be corrective when internal or external modifications are added, such as a Thomas heel, medial heel wedge, lateral sole wedge, or navicular cookie. An "orthopedic shoe" was considered to have any or all of the aforementioned with either straight or reverse last or high-top quarters. The shoe may not correct the deformity but may help to relieve symptoms or prevent further deformity (i.e., a reverse last shoe following clubfoot surgery; see Fig. 32.6).

To understand which type of shoe is best for a child, one must take into account the demands of the modern-day world and growth and development of the foot and child. It is important to note, however, that there are numerous studies suggesting that forefoot deformities such as hallux valgus and progressive narrowing of the exterior portion of the foot are more frequent in the shod foot.[21,33] Sim-Fook and Hodgson,[66] in a prominent comparative study of shod and unshod feet in a Chinese population in 1953, noted that the unrestricted foot in its natural form is mobile and flexible without static deformities, whereas the foot restricted by use of stockings and shoes is altered, and static deformities and complaints of pain are encountered. It may be appropriate to state that whenever possible wearing

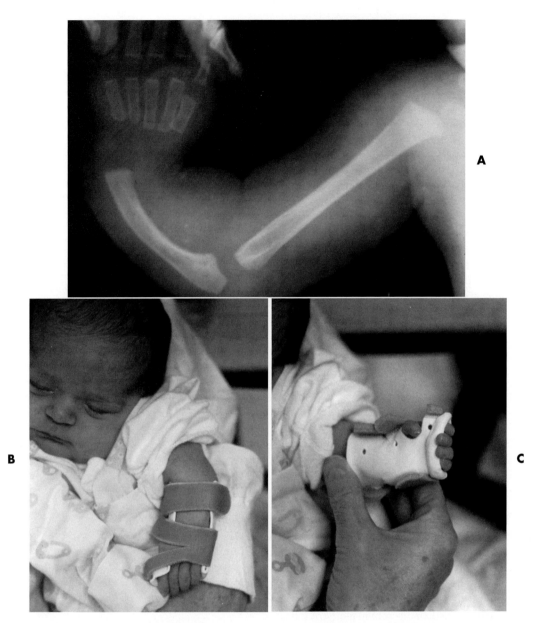

Fig. 32.15. Radial clubhand. **A,** X-ray demonstrating absence of the radius. Differential growth of the medial aspect of the forearm and wrist causes lateral deviation of wrist and hand as seen. Sometimes there may be associated incomplete development of the ulna. This child has five fingers. **B** and **C,** A thermolabile forearm wrist orthosis is used in the growing child to maintain the extremity passively in a neutral position so it can participate in functional tasks.

shoes should be avoided in childhood to preserve and strengthen natural functions of the feet. The foot, however, does need to be protected from lacerations, punctures, and infections, and well-made shoes serve a protective function while minimizing the inevitable foot changes.

Suggestions for a good shoe

1. *Proper fit:* The shoe should simulate the shape of the foot it covers as closely as possible.[83] The shape of the shoe is dependent primarily on the last or mold on which the shoe is made. It is particularly important to have a snug fit around the heel, allow ad-equate width across the ball of the foot, and have at least ⅜ to ½ inch between the end of the shoe and the longest toe.[26]

2. *Rigid shank:* The area of the shoe from back of the heel to the area where it bends the ball of the foot should be rigid to enable the foot to act as a proper lever for locomotion. Since 1972, a soft sole simulating a bare foot has been advocated.

3. *Heel height:* For infants heel height should be 3/32 inch and it should be up to ⅝ inch for older children. It can gradually be elevated up to 1 inch for males and 1⅓ inch for females to maintain slight plantar flexion at the ankles.

4. *Proper material:* Quality of shoe material and construction is important. Porous material (i.e., leather or canvas) should be used because these permit aeration of the foot and reduce irritable dermatologic conditions of the foot.

5. *Arch area:* The arch area should be molded well to prevent the foot from excessively pronating.

Pedorthists currently measure the length and width of a child's foot using a Ritz stick with the child weight bearing on both feet. Wenger and colleagues'[82] study of foot growth in children documents that growing children should have their shoe size checked frequently.

Children may be started to wear shoes as soon as they start to weight bear. These shoes should have a mild arch (inflare) to conform to the foot and should be flexible at the ball of the foot. A stiff compressive shoe may cause deformity. Leather is one of the finest materials for good shoe-making because of its flexibility, porosity, and ability to absorb moisture. It is therefore ideal for shoe uppers.[36] Canvas works equally well.

"Corrective shoes" is a misnomer. There is no such thing as a corrective shoe.[81] The main function of a shoe is as a protective covering to prevent injury and infection to the foot. It therefore fits or does not fit and is either a correct shoe or not. Merchandising "corrective shoes" is harmful to the child, expensive for the family, and discredits the medical profession.

SUMMARY

The more common congenital and acquired nontraumatic deformities of the extremities in children and adolescents not covered elsewhere in this book have been presented in this chapter. Mainly, deformities of the foot that use orthotic devices in management have been covered. Miscellaneous conditions affecting the upper extremity, such as radial clubhand have also been included.

Orthotic devices incorporated in the management of the discussed conditions are supportive and used in an attempt to enhance or preserve a functional extremity with the goal of potentiating normal growth and development. The process of growth and development is dynamic and a continuum. Orthotic devices and surgical treatment both play a necessary role in the period of active growth with a varying emphasis during the course. We would not consider surgery to be more radical than orthoses or vice versa. At times, it may be more conservative to operate on the child, maintaining the correction in orthoses, and at other instances more radical to maintain the child in orthoses until a time when correction could be surgically achieved, as a final step in an effort to maximize function. Close interactions between various caregivers, including the pediatrician, orthopedist, physical and occupational therapists, orthotist, and parent, is crucial to providing the best care.

REFERENCES

1. Aharonson Z, et al: Foot-ground pressure pattern of flexible flatfoot in children, with and without correction of calcaneovalgus, Clin Orthop Rel Res 278:177–182, 1992.
2. Alexander MA: Orthotics, adapted seating, and assistive devices. In: Pediatric rehabilitation, Baltimore, 1985, Williams & Wilkins.
3. Ball J, Sullivan JA: Treatment of the juvenile bunion by Mitchell osteotomy, Orthopaedics 8:1249–1252, 1985.
4. Banker Q: Neuropathologic aspects of arthrogryposis multiplex congenita, Clin Orthop Rel Res 194:30–43, 1994.
5. Berg EE: A reappraisal of metatarsus adductus and skewfoot, J Bone Joint Surg 68A:1185–1196, 1986.
6. Bleck EE: Metatarsus adductus: Classification and relationship to outcomes of treatment, J Pediatr Orthop 3:2–9, 1983.
7. Brown LM, Robson MJ, Sharrard WJW: The pathophysiology of arthrogryposis multiplex congenital neurologica, J Bone Joint Surg 62B:291–296, 1980.
8. Browne D: Talipes equinovarus, Lancet 2:969–974, 1934.
9. Can CR, Boyd GM: Correctional osteotomy for metatarsus primus varus and hallux valgus, J Bone Joint Surg 50A:1353–1367, 1968.
10. Carlson WO, et al: Arthrogryposis multiplex congenital—a long term followup study, Clin Orthop Rel Res 194:115–123, 1985.
11. Carrol N: Clubfoot. In Morrisey RT, editor: Lovell & Winter's pediatric orthopedics, ed 3, Philadelphia, 1990, JB Lippincott.
12. Cohen AH, Laughner TE, Pupp GR: Calcaneonavicular bar resection: A retrospective review, J Am Podiatr Med Assoc 83:10–17, 1993.
13. Cook DA, et al: Observer variability in the radiographic measurement and classification of MA, J Pediatr Orthop 12:86–89, 1992.
14. Corridera KJ, Drennan JC: Foot and ankle deformities in arthrogryposis multiplex congenita, Clin Orthop Rel Res 194:93–98, 1985.
15. Coughlin MJ, Mann RA: The pathophysiology of the juvenile bunion, Instruction Course.
16. Crawford AH, Gabriel KR: Foot and ankle problems, Orthop Clin North Am 18:649–666, 1987.
17. Creissele AE, Stanton RP: Surgical treatment of adolescent hallux valgus, J Pediatr Orthop 4:32–38, 1984.
18. Crould N: Shoes and shoe modification. In Jahss MH (ed): Disorders of the foot and ankle, Vol III, Philadelphia, 1991, WB Saunders.
19. Dias LS, Stern LS: Talectomy in the treatment of resistant talipes equinovarus deformity in myelomeningocele and arthrogryposis, J Pediatr Orthop 7:39–41, 1987.
20. Drummond DS, Cruess RL: The management of the foot and ankle in arthrogryposis multiplex congenita, J Bone Joint Surg 60B:96–99, 1978.
21. Elmslie M: Prevention of foot deformities in children, Lancet 2:1260–1263, 1939.
22. Fairbank TJ, Fairbank JCT: The crooked semantics of valgus and varus, Clin Orthop 185:6–8, 1984.
23. Farsetti P, Weinstein S, Ponseti I: The long-term functional and radiographic outcomes of untreated and non-operatively treated MA, J Bone Joint Surg 76A:257–265, 1994.
24. Fukuhara K, Schollmeier G, Uthoff HK: The pathogenesis of clubfoot, J Bone Joint Surg 76B, 1994.

25. Groiso JA: Juvenile hallux valgus: A conservative approach to treatment, J Bone Joint Surg 74A:1367–1374, 1992.
26. Gross RH: The role of the Verebelyi-Ogston procedure in the management of the arthrogrypotic foot, Clin Orthop Rel Res 194:93–98, 1985.
27. Hall JG: An approach to congenital contractures, Pediatr Ann 10:249–257, 1981.
28. Hall JG: Arthrogryposis, Am Fam Pract 39:113–119, 1989.
29. Harris RI, Beath T: Etiology of peroneal spastic flatfoot, J Bone Joint Surg 30B:624–634, 1948.
30. Henke W: Contractur des metatarsus, Zeitschr Rationelle Med 17:188–203, 1863.
31. Heyman CH, Herndon CH, Strong JM: Mobilization of the tarsometatarsal and intermetatarsal joints for the correction of resistant adduction of the forefoot of the foot in congenital clubfoot or congenital metatarsus varus, J Bone Joint Surg 40A:299–310, 1958.
32. Hoffer MM, et al: Ambulation in severe arthrogryposis, J Pediatr Orthop 3:293–296, 1983.
33. Hoffman P: Conclusions drawn from a comparative study of the feet of barefooted and shoe-wearing peoples, Am J Orthop Surg 3:105–136, 1905.
34. Howard CB, Benson MKD: Clubfoot: Its pathological anatomy, J Pediatr Orthop 13:654–659, 1993.
35. Jacobs JE: Metatarsus varus and hip dysplasia, Clin Orthop 32:500, 1960.
36. Janisse DJ: The art and science of fitting shoes, Foot Ankle 13:257–262, 1992.
37. Jay RM, Schoenhaus HD: Hyperpronation control with a dynamic stabilizing innersole system, J Am Podiatr Med Assoc 82:149–153, 1992.
38. Jaykumar S, Cowell HR: Rigid flatfoot, Clin Orthop 122:77, 1977.
39. Kalen V, Brecher A: Relationship between adolescent bunions and flat feet, Foot Ankle 8:331–336, 1988.
40. Kelsey JLP: Epidemiology of musculoskeletal disorders, New York, 1982, Oxford University Press.
41. Kirby K: The medial heel skive technique, J Am Podiatr Med Assoc 82:177–188, 1992.
42. Kite JH: The treatment of flatfeet in small children, Postgrad Med 15:75, 1954.
43. Langenskiöld A, Riska EB: Tibia varus (osteochondrosis deformans tibiae): A survey of 23 cases, J Bone Joint Surg 46A:1405, 1964.
44. Leonard MR: The inheritance of tarsal coalition relationship to spastic flatfoot, J Bone Joint Surg 56B:520–526, 1974.
45. Marr RA: Biomechanics of the foot. In AAOS: Atlas of orthotics—biomechanical principles and application, St. Louis, 1975, CV Mosby.
46. Meehan P: Other conditions of the foot. In Morrissey RT, editor: Lovell and Winter's pediatric orthopedics, ed 3, Philadelphia, 1990, JB Lippincott.
47. Molnar GE, Kaminer RK: Growth and development. In Molnar G, editor: Pediatric rehabilitation: Rehabilitation medicine library. Baltimore, 1985, Williams & Wilkins.
48. Morgan RC Jr, Crawford AH: Surgical management of tarsal coalition in adolescent athletes, Foot Ankle 7:183, 1986.
49. Oestreich AE, et al: The "anteater nose": A direct sign of calcaneonavicular coalition on the lateral radiograph, J Pediatr Orthop 7:709, 1987.
50. Otto AW: A human monster with inwardly curved extremities—a translation, Clin Orthop Rel Res 194:4–5, 1985.
51. Petersen HA: Skewfoot, J Pediatr Orthop 6:24, 1986.
52. Pineda C, Resnick DL: Diagnosis of tarsal coalition with CT, Clin Orthop 208:282–288, 1986.
53. Ponseti IV, Becker JR: Congenital MA: The results of treatment, J Bone Joint Surg 48A:702–711, 1966.
54. Pontious J, et al: Talonavicular coalition: Objective gait analysis, J Am Podiatr Med Assoc 83:379–385, 1993.
55. Rankin EA, Baker GI: Rigid flatfoot in the young adult, Clin Orthop 104:244–248, 1974.
56. Rao UB, Joseph B: The influence of footwear on the prevalence of flatfoot, J Bone Joint Surg 74B:525–527, 1992.
57. Rasool MN, et al: Foot deformities and occult spinal abnormalities in children: A review of 16 cases, J Pediatr Orthop 12:94–99, 1992.
58. Reimann I, Werner HH: Congenital metatarsus varus: A suggestion for a possible mechanism and relation to other foot deformities, Clin Orthop 110:223–226, 1975.
59. Rose GK: Pes planus. In Jahss MH, editor: Disorders of the foot, Philadelphia, 1982, WB Saunders.
60. Rose GK, et al: The diagnosis of flatfoot in the child, J Bone Joint Surg 67B:71–78, 1985.
61. Salamao O, et al: Talocalcaneal coalition: Diagnosis and surgical management, Foot Ankle 13:251–256, 1992.
62. Salenius P, Vankka E: The development of the tibiofemoral angle in children, J Bone Joint Surg 57A:259–261, 1975.
63. Scheffler NM, et al: Letters to the editor, J Bone Joint Surg 72A:470–473, 1990.
64. Scranton PG Jr, Zuckerman JD: Bunion surgery in adolescents: Results of surgical treatment, J Pediatr Orthop 4:39–43, 1984.
65. Shapiro F, Specht L: The diagnosis and orthopedic treatment of childhood spinal muscular atrophy, peripheral neuropathy, Friedreich ataxia and arthrogryposis, J Bone Joint Surg 75A:1699–1714, 1993.
66. Sim-Fook LR, Hodgson AR: A comparison of foot forms among the non-shoe wearing Chinese population, J Bone Joint Surg 40A:1058–1062, 1958.
67. Simmonds FA, Menelaus MB: Hallux valgus in adolescents, J Bone Joint Surg 42B:761–768, 1960.
68. Smith JT, Bleck EE: Simple method of documenting MA, J Pediatr Orthop 11:679–680, 1991.
69. Smith MA: Flatfeet in children, BMJ 301:942–943, 1990.
70. Staheli LT: The lower limb. In Morrisey RT, editor: Lovell & Winter's pediatric orthopedics, ed 3, Philadelphia, 1990, JB Lippincott.
71. Staheli LT, Chew DE, Corbett M: The longitudinal arch, J Bone Joint Surg 69A:426–428, 1987.
72. Staheli LT, et al: Management of hip dislocation in children with arthrogryposis, J Pediatr Orthop 7:681–685, 1987.
73. Tachdjian MO: The child's foot, Philadelphia, 1985, WB Saunders.
74. Tachdjian MO: Pediatric orthopaedics, ed 2, Philadelphia, 1990, WB Saunders.
75. Takakura Y, et al: Genesis of the ball and socket ankle, J Bone Joint Surg 68B:834–837, 1986.
76. Tax H: Podopediatrics, ed 2, Baltimore, 1985, Williams & Wilkins.
77. Thomas B, et al: The knee in arthrogryposis, Clin Orthop Rel Res 194:87–92, 1985.
78. Thometz JG, Simons GW: Deformity of the calcaneocuboid joint in patients who have talipes equinovarus, J Bone Joint Surg 75A:190–195, 1993.
79. Viladot A: Surgical treatment of the child's flatfoot, Clin Orthop Rel Res 283:34–38, 1992.
80. Watanabe RS: Metatarsal osteotomy for the cavus foot, Clin Orthop Rel Res 252:217–229, 1990.
81. Wenger DR, et al: Corrective shoes and inserts as treatment for flexible flatfoot in infants and children, J Bone Joint Surg 71A:800–810, 1989.
82. Wenger DR, et al: Foot growth rate in children age one to six years, Foot Ankle 3:207–210, 1983.

83. Wenger DR, Rang M: The art and practice of children's orthopedics, New York, 1993, Raven Press.

84. Wetzenstein H: The significance of congenital pes calcaneovalgus in the origin of pes planovalgus in childhood, Acta Orthop Scand 30-64, 1960.

85. Williams PF: Management of upper limb problems in arthrogryposis, Clin Orthop Rel Res 194:60–67, 1985.

86. Williams P: The management of arthrogryposis, Orthop Clin North Am 9:67–87, 1978.

87. Wynne-Davies R: Family studies and the course of congenital clubfoot, talipes equinovarus, talipes calcaneovalgus and metatarsus varus, J Bone Joint Surg 46B:445, 1954.

Pediatric Spinal Injuries

Cathleen S. Van Buskirk
James C. Drennan
John F. Ritterbusch

Spinal injuries in children and adolescents are relatively rare. Nonetheless, awareness of mechanism of injury, pattern types, and potential complications can lead to improved recognition and management of pediatric spinal trauma. Orthoses play an important role in the acute and long-term treatment of spinal injury in children. Knowledge of specific indications, effectiveness, and possible complications of orthotic use is essential for appropriate decision making.

OVERVIEW

Etiology

The leading causes of spinal injury in children are motor vehicle accidents (MVAs) and falls from a height. Other causes include diving accidents, sports injuries, motorcycle accidents, bicycle/motor vehicle collisions, all-terrain vehicle accidents, firearm injuries, birth injuries from difficult breech and forceps deliveries, and child abuse. Causes differ according to age. McGrory et al[18] showed the two most common causes of spinal injury in children less than 11 years of age to be falls and MVAs, whereas children 11 years and older were more likely to be injured in sports and MVAs. Patients with spinal cord injury without radiographic abnormality (SCIWORA) by plain radiographs and computed tomography are generally younger than patients whose spinal cord injury has an accompanying radiographic abnormality.[16,25] The absence of fracture is attributed to the fact that immature spinal ligaments and disks have greater elasticity than the spinal cord, which is tethered by the segmental nerve roots and dentate ligaments.

Frequency and gender

The gender ratio of children with SCIWORA is nearly equal (1:1), whereas the male-to-female ratio of children with spinal cord injuries with radiographic abnormality is about 5:1.[25] Overall, more children in the 11 years and older group have cervical injuries than the group younger than age 11.[18]

Level of injury

It is well documented that young children have a propensity to injure the craniocervical region (defined as the base of the skull, atlas, and axis), whereas adolescents tend to injure the lower cervical spine (C3-7).[6,18] The fulcrum of normal cervical spine motion in children under 8 years of age is located at C2-3; C5-6 serves as the fulcrum in adults, and trauma occurs in a more adultlike fashion over the age of 8.

Neurologic injury

Neurologic deficits occur in 29% to 43% of children with spinal injury.[6,16,18] Furthermore, Pang and Wilberger[21] found that 52% of children with SCIWORA had delayed onset of paralysis up to 4 days. Younger children without radiographic abnormality are more inclined to have complete neurologic deficits than older children with fracture.[16,25] McGrory et al[18] also found that younger children with neurologic deficit had a five times greater relative risk of death because of cervical injury than older children with neurologic deficit.

Associated injuries

Associated injuries are common in spinal injured patients. These include head injuries, extremity fractures, chest and abdominal injuries, superior vena cava syndrome, and brachial plexus injuries.[6,16] Flexion-distraction type spinal injuries (Chance fractures,[4] seat belt fractures) are injuries of the middle and posterior columns under tension and are occurring more frequently with the general public's improved adherence to seat belt laws. There is a 15% to 80%[8,10,22] rate of concomitant abdominal injuries requiring laparotomy. Furthermore, the recognition of spinal injury in patients with abdominal injury is often significantly delayed. Green et al[10] reported that the diagnosis of spinal injury was delayed an average of 13 days (range, 6 to 23 days) in patients suffering both abdominal injuries and flexion-distraction injuries, compared to a 3.5-hour average (range, 0 to 16 hours) in patients with isolated spinal injuries. This high association between flexion-distraction injuries and abdominal injuries should alert the physician that when one type of injury is identified, the other should be searched for.

ACUTE MANAGEMENT

Care of an acutely injured child focuses on maintenance of airway, breathing, and circulation. Spinal stability and support are also of paramount importance when a spinal injury is suspected. Young children have disproportionately large heads in comparison with the rest of their bodies, and this can result in a flexion posture of the neck when positioned on a standard backboard. Herzenberg et al[11] demonstrated this cervical position radiographically and have recommended either raising the chest with a pad or double mattress or lowering the head through an adjustable cut-out in a modified backboard. As a general rule of thumb, the external auditory meatus should be aligned with the shoulders during transport and radiography. The immediate goal is stabilization to prevent further spinal damage. This can be accomplished by means of either external orthotic devices or surgical intervention, depending on the nature of the injury. In general, injuries that are primarily ligamentous are better treated with surgical fusion because torn ligaments heal by fibrous scar tissue, which is often not strong enough to prevent abnormal mobility. Injuries that are mainly bony often heal well with adequate external immobilization. Additional considerations in initial treatment are specific location of injury, instability, and concomitant injuries.

Cervical spine

Cervical spine injuries in children that are considered stable and nondisplaced with or without neurologic deficit can be immobilized with a cervicothoracic orthosis (CTO). Injuries to the cervical spine that are unstable, displaced, or dislocated are appropriately treated initially with skull traction (halo or Gardner-Wells tongs). Traction is used both to immobilize the acutely injured spine and to aid in closed reduction of deformities.

Thoracic spine

Thoracic spinal injuries (T1-10) inherently have increased stability secondary to the strong ligamentous attachment of ribs to the vertebral bodies. Acute thoracic compression fractures are stable and were found to be the most common spinal column injury in a pediatric study by Mann and Dodds.[16] More severe injuries, such as rare burst fractures, are a result of extreme force, can be unstable, and are difficult to stabilize by orthoses alone. The Milwaukee brace is often used in stable thoracic injuries above T8.

Thoracolumbar spine

Thoracolumbar injuries (T11-L2) are generally unstable and are caused by a combination of flexion, compression, and rotation forces. Flexion-distraction injuries mainly occur at the thoracolumbar junction and lumbar spine. If these are treated nonoperatively, initial recumbency followed by a custom-molded bivalved thoracolumbosacral orthosis (TLSO) fabricated in extension is usually employed.

Lumbar spine

Lumbar spinal injuries are difficult to immobilize by external orthoses because of the short distance between fixation points on the pelvis. Halo-femoral traction, however, can provide adequate external fixation.

Sacral spine

Sacral injuries in children have received little attention, perhaps because of their rarity. These fractures are often associated with pelvic injuries or thoracolumbar fractures. They are generally treated with progressive weight bearing as tolerated and usually do not require orthoses.

LONG-TERM MANAGEMENT

Long-term management of spinal injuries in children focuses on promotion of bony healing and prevention of progressive spinal deformity. Multiple studies have demonstrated a high incidence of progressive spinal deformity at or below the level of injury in children with spinal injuries of the cervical and thoracic spine. Progressive spinal deformity generally does not occur with lumbar or sacral injuries.[5,17] Spinal deformity results from gravity, chronic postural effects, and unbalanced muscle pull. It is most commonly seen as scoliosis but can also be kyphosis, lordosis, or combinations thereof. Preadolescent children, generally defined as girls less than 12 years old and boys less than 14 years old, are at a much higher risk for progressive spinal deformity than mature patients, although they, too, are at increased risk overall. Dearloff and associates[5] demonstrated a 97% rate of spinal deformity in preadolescents and a 48% rate in mature patients, which is consistent with other studies.[2,3,17] Additionally, they established that the rate of curve progression if no treatment was instituted in preadolescents was twice

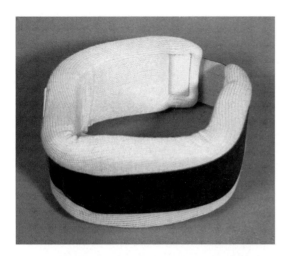

Fig. 33.1. Prefabricated soft cervical collar. Children less than age 7 often require a custom-made soft collar using an open cell foam, stockinette, and Velcro. Infants have short necks and cannot use cervical collars. They can benefit from use of craniothoracic shells or gravity positioning.

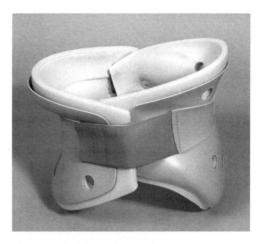

Fig. 33.2. Philadelphia collar consists of overlapping anterior and posterior shells secured with Velcro straps. Chin piece can be lined with moleskin to avoid skin irritation.

that of the mature group (10.6°/yr vs. 5.4°/yr).[5] Yngve et al[25] reported that patients with complete neurologic deficits have a higher incidence of spinal deformity than those with incomplete deficits.

Bracing patients with spinal injury serves multiple purposes. It improves sitting balance, frees the upper extremities for activities other than trunk support, and slows the rate of spinal deformity, thereby, it is hoped, delaying the possible need for surgery in preadolescents until longitudinal growth of the spine is more complete. Bracing possibly prevents the need for surgery in both preadolescents and mature patients.

ORTHOSES IN PEDIATRIC SPINAL INJURIES

A multitude of orthoses for control of spinal injuries is available. The type of injury and treatment goals should guide orthotic decision making.

Cervical spine

Cervical orthoses can be categorized into four groups: collars, poster-braces, CTOs, and skeletal external fixation.

Collars. Soft collars are prefabricated and are made from foam rubber covered with cotton stockinette and have a Velcro closure (Fig. 33.1). Soft collars are recommended for the treatment of cervical muscle spasms or minor ligamentous injury. They usually serve as a gentle support and remind the child to restrict neck motion. Johnson and colleagues[12] have shown that this type of collar reduces flexion-extension of the entire cervical spine by 26%, rotation by 17%, and lateral bending by 8%. Philadelphia collars are also prefabri-

cated and are made from a stiff molded polyethylene foam (plastazote) reinforced with plastic in front and back (Fig. 33.2). They are recommended for use in treating muscle spasms and atlantoaxial rotary subluxation.[24] Philadelphia collars reduce flexion-extension of the entire cervical spine by 71%, rotation by 56%, and lateral bending by 34%.[12]

Poster braces. Poster braces control the head by using padded mandibular and occipital supports, which are connected to either two or four metal rods attached to a thoracic support (Fig. 33.3). Use of these braces is becoming increasingly rare. They are recommended for flexion or extension injuries of the midcervical region, especially at C4-5.[12,13] The four-poster brace limits flexion-extension of the entire cervical spine by 79%, rotation by 73%, and lateral bending by 54%.[12]

Cervicothoracic orthoses. Examples of cervicothoracic orthoses (CTO) include the Minerva, Yale, and sterno-occipitomandibular immobilizer (SOMI). They are similar to the poster braces but provide increased stability by extending more caudally over the trunk. The SOMI is a prefabricated CTO consisting of a rigid metal frame that rests on the anterior chest, padded metal straps that pass posteriorly over the shoulders, and adjustable uprights that extend to the occipital and mandibular components (Fig. 33.4). The mandibular support is removable and can be temporarily replaced with a headband support to allow the child to eat. It is easy to fit, and most children find it comfortable to wear. The SOMI is recommended for C1 fractures without subluxation, stable hangman's fractures (traumatic subluxation of C2 on C3), and flexion injuries C3-5.[12,24] The SOMI brace restricts flexion-extension of the entire cervical spine by 72%, rotation by 66%, and lateral bending by 34%.[12]

The cervicothoracic brace (rigid CTO) is the most effective conventional brace. It is similar to a four-

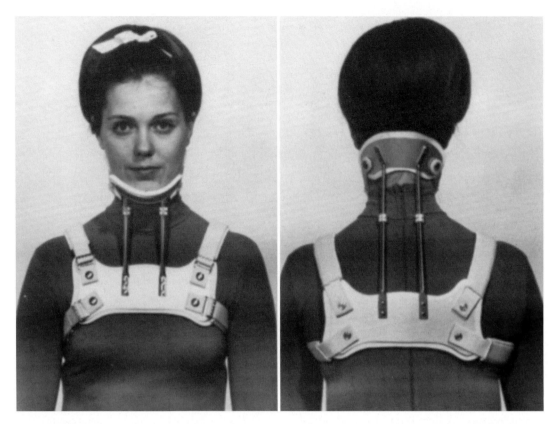

Fig. 33.3.   Four-poster brace made with anterior and posterior metal uprights, which are height adjustable.

poster brace but extends further down the trunk. It is made of a closed cell foam with Velcro straps securing the anterior and posterior components. There is a circular opening anteriorly over the neck for a tracheostomy in patients who require one (Fig. 33.5). This brace is considered quite uncomfortable. They are recommended for flexion injuries C5-T1 and extension injuries C3-5.[24] CTO braces restrict flexion-extension of the entire cervical spine by 87% of normal, rotation by 82%, and lateral bending by 49%.[12]

Minerva.   The Minerva is made of kydex or a blend of polypropylene and polyethylene and includes anterior and posterior aluminum bars for stability. The entire posterior skull is enclosed, and a band straps across the forehead. Velcro straps are used for closure (Fig. 33.6).

They are recommended for flexion or extension injuries of the cervical spine. Ogden[20] specifically recommends its use in the treatment of C1 ring fractures. Additionally, they can be used effectively in unstable hangman's fractures (defined as >3 mm of forward displacement of C2 on C3). Benzel and colleagues[1] showed a thermoplastic Minerva jacket to restrict flexion and extension better than a halo jacket at all individual cervical intervertebral segments except C1-2. Its overall flexion-extension restriction of the

entire cervical spine was, however, the same as the halo. Analysis of the limitation of rotation and lateral bending has not been reported with the Minerva.

Skeletal fixation.   Skeletal traction devices include the halo and Gardner-Wells tongs. These provide rigid fixation of the head via pins that pierce the outer table of the skull and attach to a metal ring. Both can be used as traction devices in the acute management of spinal injured patients. The halo, however, has the advantage of allowing attachment to a plastic vest or cast at a later time to permit ambulation or wheelchair activities.

Gardner-Wells tongs are spring-loaded and have two pins that are placed just above the ears, which is also just below the widest diameter of the skull. An outer semicircular metal frame is attached to the skull pins, then traction is applied. Of concern are children younger than 18 months of age in whom the cranial bones may not be sufficiently thick to support the Gardner-Wells tongs, which may penetrate the inner table of the temporal bone.

The halo apparatus consists of pins placed in the outer table of the skull in carefully selected locations under local or general anesthesia. The pins are secured to the halo ring by appropriate lock nuts or set screws. The halo ring can then be attached through metal bars

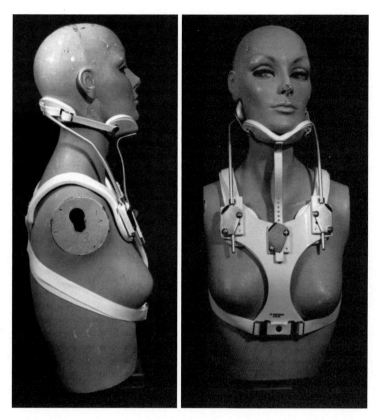

Fig. 33.4. SOMI has aluminum uprights and shoulder straps that are radiolucent but not MRI compatible.

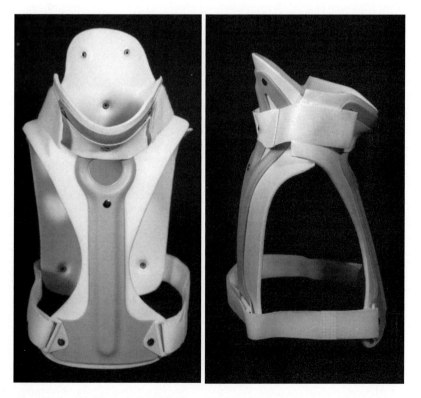

Fig. 33.5. Prefabricated CTO. Note the opening suitable for a tracheostomy.

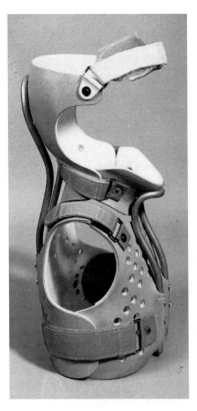

Fig. 33.6. Custom-molded Minerva encompasses the entire posterior skull and must not extend anterior to the temporal bone or the visual field is impaired.

to a cast jacket or molded plastic body jacket. The prefabricated plastic jacket is well padded, fits relatively loosely, and is ideal for children with insensate skin, such as quadriplegics (Fig. 33.7).

Garfin and associates[7] studied the skull thicknesses of pediatric patients ages 1 to 12 using computed tomography to determine optimal halo pin site placement. Considerations including skull thickness, cranial sutures, temporal muscles, and the frontal sinus resulted in the recommendation to place pins in the anterolateral and posterolateral portions of the skull. Furthermore, they recommended using six pins rather than four in young children (2 to 5 years of age), with a torque of 4 to 6 inch-lb. Mubarak and co-workers[19] have described a low-torque, multiple-pin technique for application of the halo in children less than 2 years of age. They recommend insertion of 10 to 12 pins tightened to 2 inch-lb of torque.[19] The halo jacket is recommended for Jefferson fractures (C1 four-part burst fracture) with rupture of the transverse ligament, odontoid fractures, unstable hangman's fractures, and extension injuries C3-T1.[24] The ability of the halo coupled with a plastic body vest to limit all motions of the cervical spine is superior to all other orthoses; however, no device has been shown to restrict all motion. The halo prevents 96% of flexion-extension throughout the cervical region, 99% of rotation, and 96% of lateral bending. Regarding individual interver-

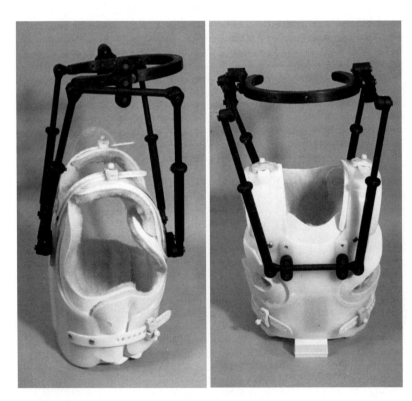

Fig. 33.7. Halo jacket. Current models, as shown here, have a titanium ring and suprastructure, which are MRI compatible. Sheep skin is used to line the jacket.

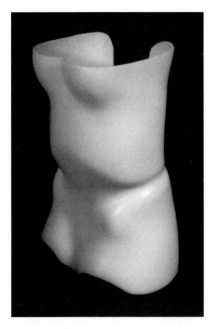

Fig. 33.8. Univalved custom-molded TLSO. Note the well-molded region superior to the iliac crests and inferior to the costal margin.

tebral cervical joints, the halo is the most effective orthosis in limiting all motion from C1-3.[12]

Thoracic and lumbar spine

The most common orthosis for thoracic and lumbar injuries is a custom-molded univalved or bivalved TLSO (Fig. 33.8). The two pieces of a bivalved TLSO must overlap to prevent pinching of the skin. This is a removable underarm plastic brace with Velcro straps for closure. A thigh cuff may be added and is an extension of the TLSO down one or both thighs. It is used to prevent pelvic rotation and to preserve lumbar lordosis. When placing a thigh cuff, the hip should be held in 30 degrees of flexion. TLSOs provide total contact, yet the foam padding inside makes them relatively comfortable. Proper fit of a TLSO is of utmost importance. In general, the anterosuperior edge should lie below the sternal notch and should not contact the clavicles. The anterosuperior pressure should be lateral to the sternum and medial to the deltopectoral groove. The axillary region should be trimmed to comfort or, in insensate patients, well below the axillary crease. The anteroinferior edge should never impinge upon the symphysis pubis. The posteroinferior edge should terminate proximal to the chair seat when the patient is sitting in a good upright position. Therefore, the TLSO crosses the iliac crests and superior aspect of the gluteal muscles. To prevent cephalad migration of a TLSO, it must be well molded in the region just superior to the iliac crests and inferior to the costal margin. The bivalve permits diligent skin inspection.

Ensuring complete patient and family compliance is of monumental importance given that deformities may progress if a TLSO is not worn faithfully. Depending on the specific injury, TLSOs can be molded appropriately to resist further deformity. For example, TLSOs are often fabricated in hyperextension for compression, burst, and chance fractures. Hyperextension TLSOs use a long anterior shell that acts as a lever arm and a shorter posterior shell that acts as a pivot point at its superior border. For example, an L2 burst fracture can be treated with a hyperextension TLSO having its superior border of the posterior shell at L2, thereby creating a pivot point at the level of injury to enhance healing in a hyperextended position and to prevent an increasing kyphotic deformity. Overall, pediatric thoracic and lumbar fractures heal well with orthotic immobilization. Flexion-distraction injuries present a unique problem. In general, isolated bony injuries resulting from flexion-distraction forces are treated with a hyperextension cast or brace, whereas ligamentous injury is an indication for surgery. Glassman and co-workers,[9] however, demonstrated successful bracing of all types of flexion-distraction injuries and found that an initial kyphosis at the level of injury of less than 20 degrees resulted in successful bracing in all cases, whereas initial kyphotic deformities of greater than 20 degrees failed bracing in all cases. Associated abdominal injuries that require laparotomy or ostomy can be accommodated by making a window in the TLSO to allow for close inspection of the wound or stoma. Window edema, however, is a concern, and the window should be replaced in its proper position at a lower than normal pressure.

Maintenance of orthoses. Compliant orthosis use usually causes perspiration, which can be uncomfortable and cause skin irritation. To avoid this, one should always try to place an absorbent material between the patient and the orthosis. Sheepskin is often used to line halo plastic jackets, cotton T-shirts are worn under TLSOs, and stockinette or a cotton handkerchief can be used creatively to line most cervical collars.

Rubbing alcohol or soap and water can be used to clean closed cell foam orthoses, such as the Philadelphia collar. Closed cell foam does not absorb fluid but must be completely dry before reusing or skin irritation is likely to ensue. Open cell foam orthoses, such as a soft cervical collar, absorb fluid and therefore cannot be washed. It is common practice to give the patient two orthoses of the same type if they are made of open cell foam, so that their use can be alternated.

Orthoses making. Casts are used to create a mold to make custom-made orthoses. These include the Minerva, TLSO, and some custom-made CTOs. The halo plastic vest requires obtaining specific measurements, which are then used to mold the plastic vest correctly without the use of a preliminary cast. Orthoses that are prefabricated include the SOMI, poster-braces, and cervical collars. It has been the authors' experience that children less than 7 years of age generally require custom-made orthoses for proper fit.

Complications of orthotic use

Orthotic use is not without potential complications, a number of which are preventable. The most dangerous problem is inadequate treatment of the injury because of inappropriate selection of orthoses. Children with spinal trauma and loss of protective skin sensation are at considerable risk for developing pressure sores. Any orthotic device can cause pressure sores, but the halo jacket and TLSOs are most frequently cited. Frequent position changes and skin inspection cannot be overemphasized in these patients. Halo plastic vests are better tolerated than casts in children with insensate skin or limited respiratory reserve. Halo casts can also cause visceral compression and cast syndrome. Halo pins also have well-defined risks, including perforation of the inner table of the skull during pin placement. Additionally, pin tract infection, aseptic loosening, and supraorbital or supratrochlear nerve injuries can occur.

CONCLUSION

Spinal injuries in children, although uncommon, have identifiable patterns and outcomes. Young children are more likely to injure the upper cervical spine, whereas older children tend to injure the lower cervical spine. Younger children are also more likely to incur SCIWORA. Almost all preadolescent patients with spinal injury develop a progressive spinal deformity, which may be slowed by the use of orthoses. Orthotic use is the mainstay of treatment for numerous pediatric spinal injuries. Thorough familiarity with the available spinal orthoses, their indications, efficacy, and complications is necessary in the treatment of children with spinal injury.

REFERENCES

1. Benzel EC, Hadden TA, Saulsbery CM: A comparison of the Minerva and halo jackets for stabilization of the cervical spine, J Neurosurg 70:411–414, 1989.
2. Brown JC, et al: Late spinal deformity in quadriplegic children and adolescents, J Pediatr Orthop 4:456–461, 1984.
3. Campbell J, Bonnett C: Spinal cord injury in children, Clin Orthop 112:114–123, 1975.
4. Chance GQ: Note on a type of flexion fracture of the spine, Br J Radiol 21:452–453, 1948.
5. Dearolf WW, et al: Scoliosis in pediatric spinal cord injured patients, J Pediatr Orthop 10:214–218, 1990.
6. Evans DL, Bethem D: Cervical spine injuries in children, J Pediatr Orthop 9:563–568, 1989.
7. Garfin SR, et al: Skull osteology as it affects halo pin placement in children, J Pediatr Orthop 6:434–436, 1986.
8. Gertzbein SD, Court-Brown CM: Flexion-distraction injuries of the lumbar spine: Mechanisms of injury and classification, Clin Orthop 227:52–60, 1988.
9. Glassman SD, Johnson JR, Holt RT: Seat belt injuries in children, J Trauma 33:882–886, 1992.
10. Green DA, et al: Flexion-distraction injuries of the lumbar spine associated with abdominal injuries, J Spinal Disord 4:312–318, 1991.
11. Herzenberg JE, et al: Emergency transport and positioning of young children who have an injury of the cervical spine, J Bone Joint Surg 71A:15–22, 1989.
12. Johnson RM, et al: Cervical orthoses: A study comparing their effectiveness in restricting cervical motion in normal subjects, J Bone Joint Surg 59A:332–339, 1977.
13. Johnson RM, et al: Cervical orthoses: A guide to their selection and use, Clin Orthop 154:34–45, 1981.
14. King AG: Spinal column trauma, Instr Course Lect 35:40–51, 1986.
15. Kostuik JP: Indications for the use of the halo immobilization, Clin Orthop 154:46–50, 1981.
16. Mann DC, Dodds JA: Spinal injuries in 57 patients 17 years or younger, Orthopedics 16:159–164, 1993.
17. Mayfield JK, Erkkila JC, Winter RB: Spine deformity subsequent to acquired childhood spinal cord injury, J Bone Joint Surg 63A:1401–1411, 1981.
18. McGrory BJ, et al: Acute fractures and dislocations of the cervical spine in children and adolescents, J Bone Joint Surg 75A:988–995, 1993.
19. Mubarak SJ, et al: Technique: Halo application in the infant, J Pediatr Orthop 9:612–614, 1989.
20. Ogden JA: In Skeletal injury in the child, Philadelphia, 1982, Lea & Febiger.
21. Pang D, Wilberger JE: Spinal cord injury without radiographic abnormalities in children, J Neurosurg 57:114–129, 1982.
22. Smith WS, Kaufer H: Patterns and mechanism of lumbar injuries associated with lap seat belts, J Bone Joint Surg 51A:239–254, 1969.
23. Rogers LF: The roentgenographic appearance of transverse or chance fractures of the spine: The seat belt fracture, Am J Roentgenol Radium Ther Nucl Med 111:844–849, 1971.
24. Wilberger JE: Orthotic devices for children. In Spinal cord injuries in children, New York, 1986, Futura.
25. Yngve DA, et al: Spinal cord injury without osseous spine fracture, J Pediatr Orthop 8:153–159, 1988.

Hip Disorders

John A. Reister
Robert E. Eilert

Orthotic applications in children's orthopedics are common. Almost every day in clinics a new prescription or periodic evaluation of a child's orthosis is done. In children's orthopedics, the majority of orthotic applications can be classified as disease specific.

This book has successfully evolved away from the rote thinking that a specific diagnosis requires a specific orthotic prescription. This has fostered a better understanding of orthoses in general and biomechanical principles as well as wider applications. The authors believe, however, that a better understanding of orthoses in children can be gained by reviewing them as they relate to specific diagnoses. This chapter is not an exhaustive representation of children's orthoses but rather a brief review of some of the more common orthoses in wide usage, their applications, and some biomechanical issues and questions as they relate to developmental dysplasia of the hip (DDH), Legg-Calvé-Perthes disease (LCP), torsional deformities, and paraplegia.

A wide variety of reasons exist for the application of orthoses in children. Much of the beginning of the discipline of orthoses arose from fracture care, and this remains one of the common reasons for an orthotic prescription. The prevention and correction of deformities are among the most prevalent indications for the use of an orthosis. Examples include DDH, LCP, tibia vara, cerebral palsy with joint contractures, and rotational deformities of the lower extremity. The efficacy of orthoses in the correction of many deformities is not universally accepted.[35] Some believe that the soft tissues of the foot, ankle, and knee absorb such a degree of any angular or derotational force applied to the lower extremity that the remaining force on the bone is negligible.[39] Orthoses are also used to stabilize or maintain joints in a functional range of motion, thus augmenting use, stability, and mobility.

In the treatment of specific disease entities, orthoses in children have gained their widest and most universal acceptance in the management of diseases of the hip (specifically the spectrum of DDH and hip dysplasia) and to a slightly lesser extent in the treatment of LCP. There is also widespread use of orthoses in the treatment of lower extremity rotational deformities; however, universal acceptance of their success is lacking. Orthotic applications are also common and well accepted for the maintenance of limb and joint alignment, prevention of contractures, and assistance with mobilization in cerebral palsy, myelodysplasia, and progressive neuromuscular disorders such as Duchenne muscular dystrophy.

HIP DYSPLASIA AND DEVELOPMENTAL DISLOCATION OF THE HIP

DDH is a spectrum of conditions ranging from hip dysplasia, subluxation, and reducible dislocation to fixed nonreducible dislocation. These diagnoses are based on findings on physical examination, radiographic measurements, and dynamic ultrasonography. Congenital hip disease can occur alone, or it can be a part of a syndrome such as arthrogryposis, which changes the prognosis and has an impact on the success of treatment.

Four orthoses are commonly used in the treatment of DDH (DDH encompasses the aforementioned spectrum of hip disease for the purposes of this writing): the Pavlik harness, the Ilfeld orthosis, the Von Rosen splint, and the Frejka pillow. The goal of any orthotic for DDH should be to obtain and maintain a congruous reduction of the involved hip(s).

Pavlik harness

Pavlik introduced this harness in 1945. In 1957, he published his results for the treatment of nearly 1912 hips. His original harness was fabricated with leather. Since that time, the harness has achieved widespread

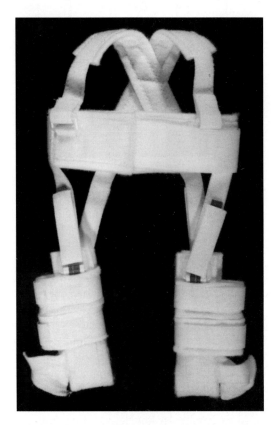

Fig. 34.1. Pavlik harness. Front view.

use and acceptance, and numerous commercially constructed versions have become available.

The harness is used in the dysplastic, subluxated, or dislocated hip in infants up to 12 months but has had higher success rates at younger ages. The Pavlik harness consists of a chest strap positioned at the nipple line, with halter straps that should cross in the back to prevent slipping (Fig. 34.1). The anterior/flexor straps should be at the anterior axillary line; if more medial, they produce an adduction force (Fig. 34.2, A).[28] The posterior straps should overlie the scapula, and the leg straps should not impinge in the popliteal fossa (Fig. 34.2, B). A retaining strap just inferior to the popliteal fossa, however, is necessary to prevent the medial flexion straps from subluxating laterally, creating an adduction force. The anterior strap should be tightened to maintain the hips at 90 to 110 degrees flexion. The posterior straps should be tight enough to prevent adduction, variously reported as allowing 5 to 8 cm between the knees or 20 to 30 degrees of abduction but allowing further abduction freely.[20,28]

Once the child has been placed in the harness, a radiograph should be obtained to ensure that reduction has been obtained. If it has not, this radiograph serves for future comparison. Many hips not immediately reduced reduce with time in an appropriately placed harness, as slow molding of obstructions (capsule, lim-

bus, pulvinar) take place. Also, adductor contracture may make reduction impossible. If after 2 weeks no reduction or adductor stretching has been obtained, an adductor tenotomy may be indicated. It is not advisable to continue Pavlik treatment alone, if reduction cannot be obtained by 3 weeks with or without adductor tenotomy.[11,20] Long-term harness treatment in an irreducible hip may permanently erode the posterior acetabular rim.

Once reduction has been confirmed, a weekly physical examination allows the clinician to ascertain the stability of the hips, adjust for growth of the child, maintain rapport, and ensure parental education in the use of the orthosis. Periodic radiographs (every 4 to 6 weeks) are recommended to document maintenance of reduction. The length of treatment varies according to the age of the patient, the time required to achieve stability of reduction, radiographic evidence of improvement in dysplasia via the acetabular index, and the presenting diagnosis. There are no currently available tables or values for length of treatment. A previous rule of thumb was that treatment was carried out full-time for a period equal to the age of the patient at presentation, followed by a weaning period.[11,20] (Dislocated hips require longer treatment than dysplastic hips.) It is now recommended that treatment be full-time until stability is obtained, then continued for 6 weeks before beginning a weaning period (Fig. 34.3).[14]

The Pavlik harness is inexpensive, relatively simple to use for the health professional, and possesses a reasonable success rate. In his series of 1912 hips of which 632 were dislocated, Pavlik reported successful reduction in 531 (a success rate of 84%). Other authors have cited success rates of 83% to 92%.[3,10,11,28,29,33,38]

Much interest has been placed on the reasons for failure of the Pavlik treatment. Factors that have been found to be significantly associated with failure include age greater than 7 weeks at initiation of treatment, bilateral dislocations, magnitude of displacement, and absence of Ortolani's sign (an irreducible dislocation).[3,14,43] Parental noncompliance, lack of physician familiarity with the harness, and poor construction of the harness have also been cited as contributing factors to failure.[24,28] Degree of femoral anteversion is another possible cause for failure.

Avascular necrosis (AVN) of the femoral head is the worst and most significant complication associated with Pavlik harness treatment. It was this complication (seen in 60% to 70% of patients treated with the Lorenz method) that motivated Pavlik to invent his harness. One cause of AVN is believed to be forced abduction, which causes compression of the superolateral retinacular vessels on the acetabular margin. The extent of AVN is variable,[5,16] but the outcome is universally worse than those hips that are not involved. AVN rates

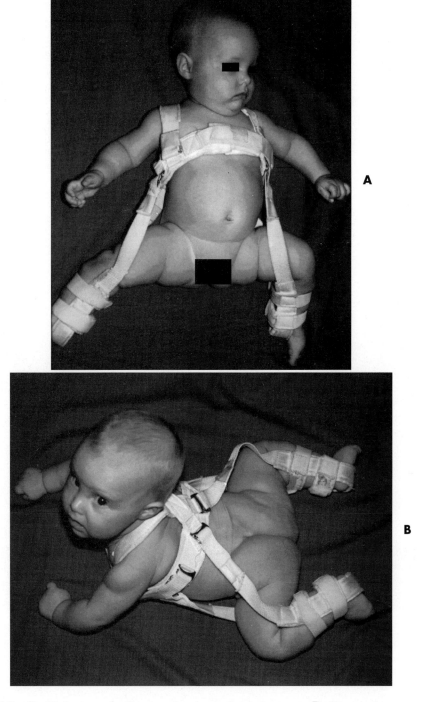

Fig. 34.2. Pavlik harness. **A,** Correct placement of anterior straps. **B,** Correct placement of posterior straps.

are reported as 0 to 16%. Pavlik reported no AVN in the 531 hips in his study that reduced spontaneously but a rate of 18% in dislocated hips that failed harness treatment and were treated by closed reduction/casting.

Ramsey and colleagues[33] reported a 0% rate of AVN and described the "safe zone." Risk factors associated with the development of AVN include the magnitude of the displacement of dislocation, using the Tonnis or other grading system.[10,14,38] Also, age at the time of treatment is cited as a factor, with an increased incidence and a greater degree of head involvement affecting younger children.[16]

Other complications reported less frequently in-

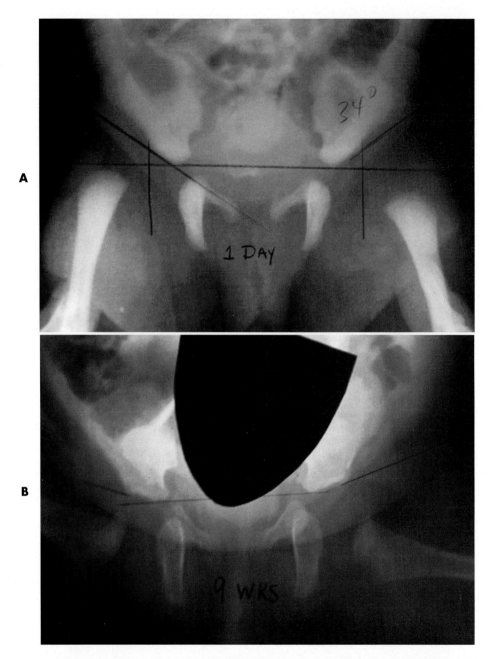

Fig. 34.3. **A,** Radiograph showing bilateral hip dislocation at 1 day of age before beginning treatment with the Pavlik harness. Note that the femoral metaphysis lies lateral to the vertical line of Perkins drawn through the lateral acetabular margin. **B,** Radiograph of pelvis of the same child in (**A**) at 9 weeks of age. Note that the femur is well directed deeply into the acetabulum and that the acetabular index has remodeled into the normal range.

clude inferior obturator dislocation,[34] transient femoral nerve palsy (Fig. 34.4),[28] noncompliance,[24] and residual or late-presenting dysplasia after successful harness treatment.[41] Despite these complications, the Pavlik harness is a relatively safe, effective method of treating most cases of DDH. It is simple, once the physician understands its proper applications and biomechanical principles. The parents must be educated and continually counseled. To them, the treatment is

neither simplistic nor noninvasive, and it adds significant stress to their lives.[24] The success rate and indications may change with time, as more is learned about those patients who fail primary treatment with the harness.

Ilfeld orthosis

The Ilfeld orthosis is primarily an abduction orthosis used in the spectrum of DDH. It promotes flexion to

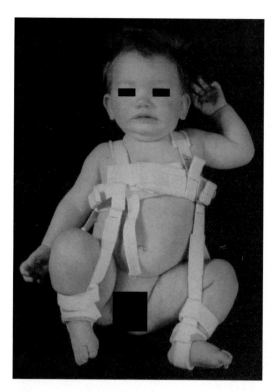

Fig. 34.4. Pavlik harness. Incorrectly applied harness. The hip is hyperflexed because of tightening of the anterior straps. This position can lead to femoral nerve palsy. The hip should be positioned at 90 degrees of flexion, but more flexion is neither necessary nor desirable.

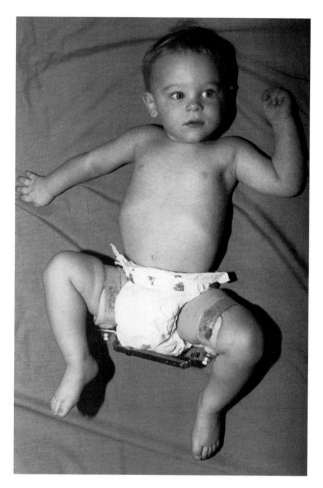

Fig. 34.5. Ilfeld orthosis.

some degree.[16] It differs markedly from the Pavlik harness in that it is a passive device and does not promote motion of the hip joint. Structurally, it is fabricated with two thigh cuffs and an adjustable metal crossbar that allows variation of abduction. Suspension is through a waist strap (Fig. 34.5).[20]

Use of the Ilfeld orthosis for the treatment of hip dysplasia and congenital dislocations is limited by its passive nature. The orthosis, however, is an effective postoperative or postcast treatment to aid in maintaining abduction. It also functions well after Pavlik harness treatment in older and larger children and as a night splint to maintain abduction for a portion of the 24-hour cycle. It is not as popular as the Pavlik harness for the primary treatment of DDH.

Von Rosen orthosis

In 1962, Von Rosen[44] reported his use of a special splint in the treatment of 39 cases of congenital hip dislocations (CDH). He reported only three failures and alluded to the presence of postnatal effects of maternal estrogens on CDH.

The Von Rosen orthosis, similar to the Ilfeld orthosis, is a passive motion restraint, being adjustable in both abduction and flexion. It was originally fabricated from malleable aluminum with a plastic covering (Fig.

34.6). Today the orthosis is made of malleable plastic with three sets of flaps for the shoulders, waist, and thighs. Straps for security of fixation have also been added. Although the Von Rosen orthosis has not found significant use in North America, it is still prevalent in parts of the Scandinavian orthopedic community.

Two articles from Norway and Helsinki compared the results of treatment of CDH with the Von Rosen orthosis versus the Frejka pillow.[13,15] The authors reported better success rates with the Von Rosen orthosis and only one case of AVN. A 19% incidence of skin pressure problems related to wearing the Von Rosen orthosis, however, was noted.

Frejka pillow

Although the Frejka pillow is still used, it is primarily mentioned here for historic interest. Use of the Frejka pillow is nearly anecdotal in most parts of North America. An analogous treatment, double and triple diapering, is still prevalent among primary care providers worldwide.

Frejka was one of Pavlik's professors. Both physicians were concerned that previous methods of CDH

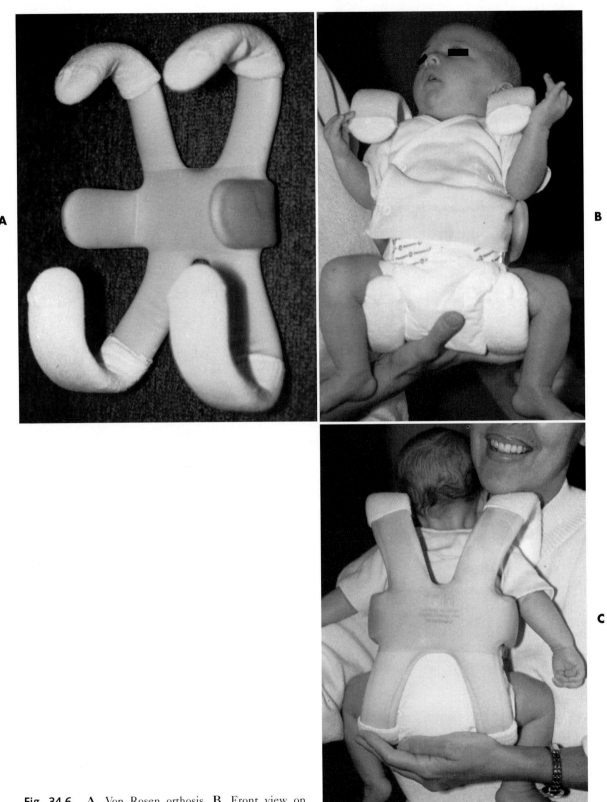

Fig. 34.6. **A,** Von Rosen orthosis. **B,** Front view on patient. **C,** Back view on patient.

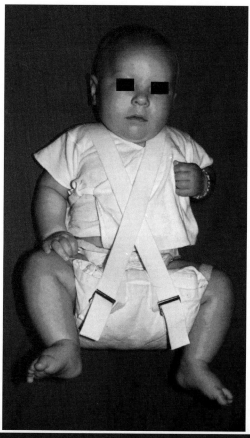

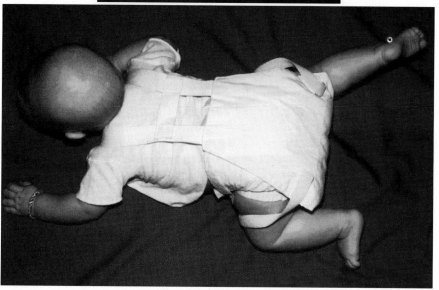

Fig. 34.7. Frejka pillow. **A,** Anterior view. **B,** Posterior view.

treatment had unacceptably high rates of AVN. In 1947, Frejka created the pillow after experiencing some success with abduction treatment. It was noted, however, that a child could overcome the soft pillow and was not reliably maintained in abduction. This also helped to stimulate Pavlik to invent his harness.[29] Another notable drawback was that the Frejka pillow did not provide enough flexion to orient properly the proximal femur toward the triradiate cartilage.[20] The Frejka pillow is constructed as a $9 \times 9 \times \frac{3}{4}$ inch foam pillow, restrained in a cloth harness with securing ties (Fig. 34.7).

LEGG-CALVÉ-PERTHES DISEASE

The natural history of LCP is moderately better understood today than it was when the primary treatment modality of bed rest was first proposed. Long-term outcome studies by Stulberg and colleagues and Mose and coworkers have shown the most significant factors in outcome prediction are age of the patient at disease onset, extent of femoral head involvement, femoral head sphericity, and congruence of the femoral head and acetabulum at skeletal maturity. Early treatment consisted of long-term bed rest while healing occurred. From this treatment, it was noted that slightly better results were obtained when the hip was rested in an abduction brace rather than in traction.[19] Femoral head containment, although not new, evolved as a lone concept that could be influenced by the physician. Methods of containment then came to the forefront and included orthotics, proximal femoral surgery, and acetabular surgery. Containment was shown to influence the outcome positively, but no significant difference in the method of achieving containment was noted.[18] In the late 1960s and early 1970s, a number of orthoses were introduced to contain the femoral head.[7,12,30,31,39]

The Harrison-Turner and Tachdjian orthoses (Fig. 34.8) were designed for abduction with unloading of the hip.[12,39] With the introduction of abduction and internal rotation plasters, Petrie and Bitenc[30] helped to define the principal of ambulatory containment. Orthoses for ambulatory containment were then introduced in Atlanta, Toronto, and Newington. Those designed in Toronto and Newington had similar biomechanical principles; they were designed to hold the hips in 45 degrees of abduction and to provide some internal rotation (usually approximately 20 degrees) while allowing ambulation. Containment achieved by the Scottish Rite orthosis relies on 45 degrees of fixed abduction, with hip flexion to contain the anterolateral portion of the femoral head.

Orthotic application to an irritable hip with decreased range of motion is unwise and does not provide the containment desired.[32] In the face of persistent synovitis, the involved hip adducts, and the uninvolved hip abducts more to compensate. No increase in head coverage or containment is achieved.[32] Thus, in the hip with active synovitis, a period of rest and traction to improve range of motion before orthotic application is recommended. Adductor tenotomy and application of Petrie casts until resolution of the synovitis is a technique used by some physicians, particularly in the child who is incapable of complying with bed rest instructions.

Toronto orthosis

The Toronto orthosis was introduced in 1969 as an ambulatory containment treatment.[4] It consists of thigh

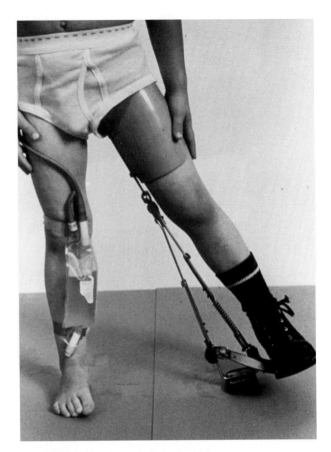

Fig. 34.8. Tachdjian orthosis. The brace provides unilateral abduction. The urine bag on this patient is coincidental because of renal disease and not related to the Perthes disease.

cuffs connected to a triangular frame, which, in turn, attaches to angled foot blocks through a universal joint (Fig. 34.9). This orthosis maintains the feet at 45 degrees to the floor (internally rotated) and the hips in 45 degrees of abduction. It also permits knee motion. This orthosis is custom-fitted to the patient. It is more cumbersome than the Atlanta brace but less so than the Newington orthosis. Crutches are recommended for stability and can be used together in front or split.[20] Rab et al[32] studied femoral head containment in different orthoses and also calculated a "containment index" which reflects the "percentage of the femoral head covered during some part of the gait cycle." They noted two patterns of increased coverage of the femoral head with the Toronto brace, dependent on the patient's gait preference for knees extended or flexed. Increased anterolateral coverage was noted with the knees extended, and increased posterior coverage was noted with the knees flexed. Even in the light of increased head coverage, however, the containment index did not change significantly from a normal hip. The study included only four hips evaluated in Toronto braces.

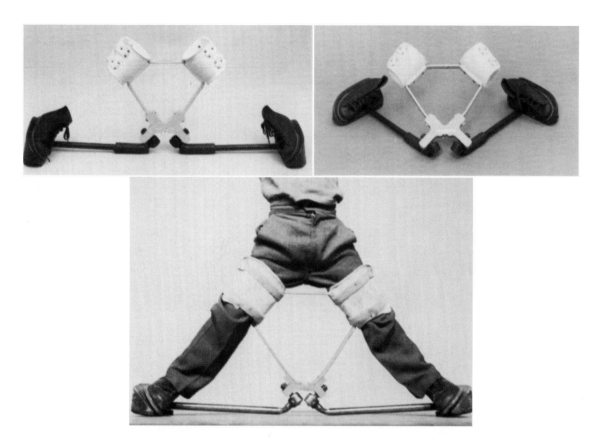

Fig. 34.9. Toronto orthosis.

Newington orthosis

Curtis and associates, published the results of treatment of 19 hips with the Newington orthosis in 1972, noting nearly equal results to treatment with abduction in recumbency. The orthosis itself is cumbersome. It is prefabricated in kit form; it consists of an aluminum frame with nonmobile knee shells (approximately 10 degrees of flexion) and attachable foot plates. It is designed to hold the patient in the same biomechanical position as the Toronto orthosis (45 degrees of hip abduction with internal rotation) (Fig. 34.10). Crutches are required for stability.

Both the Newington and the Toronto orthoses are restricting and have poor cosmesis. They have a significant impact on the clothing and dressing capabilities of the patient. It may be sensible to consider alternatives of a less psychologically intrusive nature but with equal efficacy. This may include surgical options as well as other orthoses.[31,42]

Atlanta orthosis

The Atlanta Scottish Rite orthosis was originally described by Purvis and colleagues[31] in 1971. It consists of two thigh cuffs, with closures attached laterally through hinges to a waist suspension and interconnected by a telescoping rod with universal joints at each end (Fig. 34.11, A). When compared to its counterparts used for the treatment of LCP, it is the least restrictive and easiest to wear. For these reasons, it is the most popular orthosis for LCP. This orthosis is also frequently used for the continued ambulatory treatment of DDH. No crutches are needed, and many activities (bicycling, roller skating, running) are easily performed while in the orthosis (see Fig. 34.11, B).

The Atlanta brace can be modified by removal of the crossbar. This makes it even lighter and less socially intrusive. This modification is called the "cowboy brace" for obvious reasons (Fig. 34.12, A) The orthosis allows free motion of the knees, ankles, and feet. It maintains abduction but does not control internal rotation. The brace has also been used to treat hip dysplasia in children too big for the Pavlik harness (see Fig. 34.12, B and C). As with any orthosis, standing anteroposterior pelvis x-rays should be obtained to document the degree of abduction obtained in the involved hip. In Rab's biomechanical studies, the Atlanta brace increased posterior coverage mostly and lateral coverage by an arc of 20 degrees. Perhaps more notable is that the Atlanta brace was the only one tested that increased the containment index significantly from 64% to 75%.[32]

Two studies, both retrospective and without internal control groups, have compared orthotic treatment using the Atlanta Scottish Rite brace to no treatment and noncontainment treatment.[22,25] Both studies included only small numbers of patients (31 and 34), and those with Caterall stage III/IV disease. The results of the

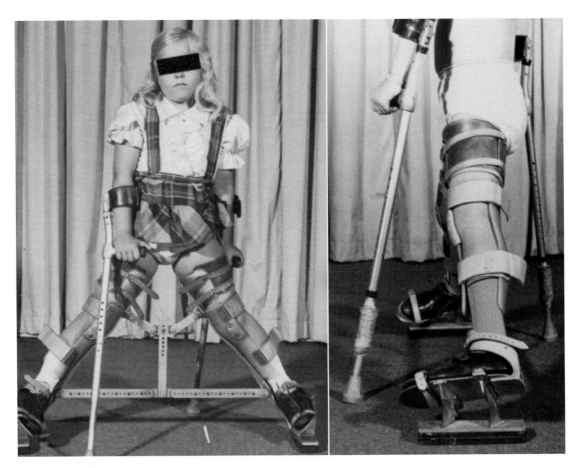

Fig. 34.10.   Newington orthosis.

containment treatment group were then compared to other previous studies, and the authors duly cite their reservations for doing the comparison of results in this fashion. In both series, however, patients treated with orthotic containment had poorer results than expected, with a significantly greater percentage of patients having class III and IV results and a poor outcome using the Mose grading system, as accepted by the Pediatric Orthopaedic Society. A true prospective clinical trial to compare treatment modalities in Perthes disease is still remarkably absent, and orthotic containment, now in question, may not positively affect outcome, as previously thought.

Summary

Indications and length of brace treatment are beyond the scope of this chapter. The natural history of hips in younger children (<8 years) with limited involvement of their femoral heads (Salter Thompson A, or Caterall Group I and II) is so good that it is difficult to show any significant benefit from treatment of any kind in this group. For older children and for those with greater head involvement (>8 years, Salter Thompson B, Caterall Group III and IV), the natural history is not

as good, and a combination of the two usually leads to a loss of femoral head sphericity with skeletal maturity. It is for these patients that ambulatory containment with orthoses or surgery is believed to affect the outcome.[7,8,31] As previously noted, some literature has placed orthotic containment in question as to its ability to affect the natural history of LCP favorably.[22,25] Containment as a general principle has achieved widespread acceptance. There are physicians, however, who do not believe that containment is the true reason behind altered natural histories. Some believe that the improved outcome in surgically treated groups is a result of more rapid healing and resolution of the vascular insult in LCP, secondary to the surgical trauma itself.

No orthosis contains the entire femoral head because the femoral head surface area is greater than that of the acetabulum. Therefore, to maximize femoral head containment requires joint motion in the optimal position to promote coverage and congruency. All of the orthoses mentioned function in this manner. The principal benefit from orthotic application in LCP may be the control of synovitis, which would promote greater range of motion and biomechanically positively affects

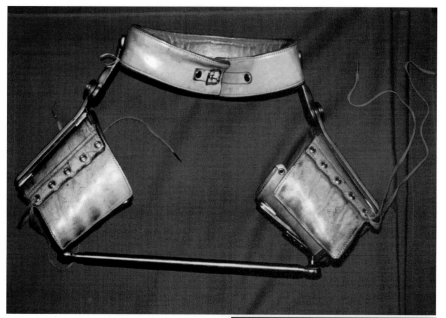

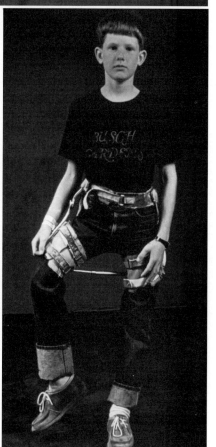

Fig. 34.11. A, Atlanta orthosis. B, The mobility possible with the Atlanta orthosis. Note that in this position the patient has adducted the left hip to neutral.

containment. Bracing should be discontinued when radiographic evidence of the reossification phase is noted.

It is obvious that there is no panacea for the patient with LCP. Many patients have a good outcome with no treatment, and some patients have a poor outcome no matter what is done. Orthoses offer a nonsurgical ambulatory containment option. They also serve to reduce the synovitis associated with LCP and thus make the disease symptomatically more tolerable.

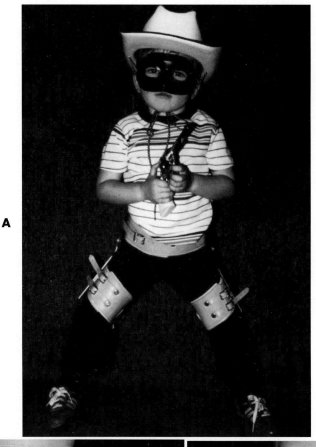

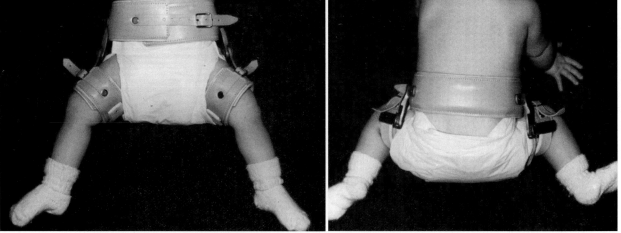

Fig. 34.12. **A,** Denver modification of the Atlanta orthosis, termed the *cowboy brace.* The crossbar is not used, which makes the brace less cumbersome. **B** and **C,** Cowboy brace demonstrating its use for hip dysplasia in a child too large for the Pavlik harness.

TORSIONAL DEFORMITIES

The use of orthoses for the treatment of rotational deformities in children is controversial. The two most common diagnoses that are considered for bracing are internal tibial torsion and excess femoral anteversion. Staheli and colleagues[35–37] have performed a number of studies of rotational profiles and the surgical management of these deformities in older children. They noted a broad normal range in the infant and young child and made no attempt to establish a magnitude of rotation that would indicate brace treatment.

There are no prospective, randomized clinical studies that show a clear benefit to brace treatment of rotational deformities. There is significant spontaneous correction of both tibial rotations and femoral version.[35]

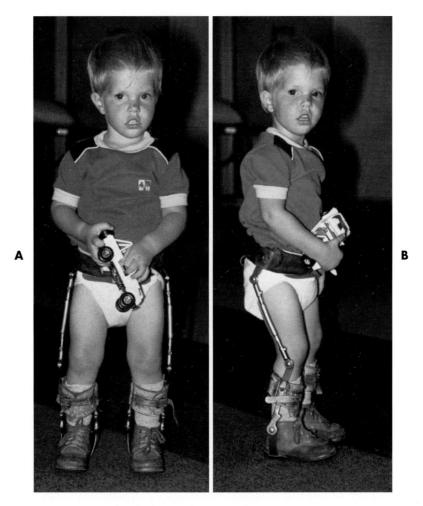

Fig. 34.13. Torsional shaft orthosis. **A,** Front view. **B,** Side view. The "twister cables" have been used for intoeing gait because of femoral anteversion.

Additionally, opponents to brace correction of rotational deformities state that the forces actually imparted to the bone are extremely small after dissipation through soft tissues and joints.[39] If one is going to brace for rotational deformities, however, it should be initiated at a young age when the child tolerates wearing the orthosis, and it is more convenient for the parent to apply. It is also safer when the child is still confined to a crib to minimize the fall risk of a child getting out of bed with the feet or lower extremities tethered together.

Denis Browne orthosis

This is the most commonly prescribed orthosis for the treatment of lower extremity rotational discrepancies. It is a single bendable metal bar to which adjustable foot plates are attached. The patient's feet can be positioned at any rotation desired, and the bar can be bent to correct or accommodate for varus and valgus at

the hind foot or knees. Again, this orthosis is best tolerated as a nighttime brace in the young child.

Torsional shaft orthosis

This orthosis is commonly known as the *twister* or *twister cables*. It consists of a foot stirrup connected via an adjustable spring to a pelvic band (Fig. 34.13). The tension (hence, torsion force) imposed by the spring can be adjusted. There is controversy about the amount of force that actually is transmitted to the bone. This orthosis is not commonly used.

Twister cables are effective in improving the foot progression angles during use only. A role of this orthosis may be in the rotational deformity in a child with flaccid paralysis (spina bifida) until the child is at an age when surgical intervention may be beneficial.

Staheli[35] believes that use of the twister for correction of femoral version is ineffective and that those

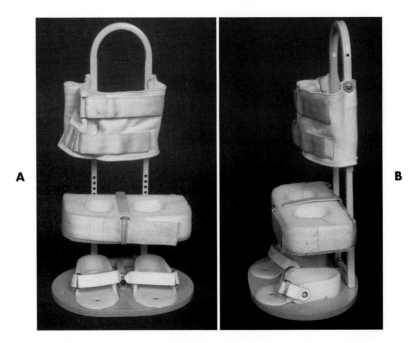

Fig. 34.14.   Standing frame orthosis. **A,** Anterior view. **B,** Lateral view.

patients with marked anteversion require surgical management.

PARAPLEGIA

The use of orthoses in paraplegic children is ubiquitous. Also, in no other area is the impact of bracing so dramatic. In myelodysplasia, depending on the level of involvement, standing and walking can be nearly equal to that of neurologically normal children or with some form of orthosis.

The benefits of erect posture and independent ambulation are myriad. Physiologically the forces of gravity may result in improved pulmonary function and pulmonary toilet, improved bladder emptying, and increased bone mass. Functionally, orthoses free the upper extremities for use and allow independent mobilization. The emotional and motivational benefits for this patient population are significant and should not be underestimated. Almost all myelodysplasic children are candidates for orthoses and can achieve independent ambulation for at least a short period of time. Children have an abundant amount of energy that is not usually seen in adults; therefore, many children who walk independently with orthoses do not maintain that level of function into adulthood. Eventually, they may become wheelchair ambulators only.

The use of orthoses for the management of myelodysplasia is covered in another chapter. Therefore, only a few of the more common orthoses used to provide independent standing support and ambulation for this patient group are discussed here.

Standing frame orthosis

The standing frame orthosis (Fig. 34.14) is a commonly available kit that consists of an unhinged upright frame posteriorly, with attached foot plates, knee supports, and a chest abdominal strap. It is designed for independent standing and allows free use of the upper extremities.[21]

A-frame orthosis

This orthosis, similar to the standing frame, supports the patient in an erect posture. In addition, it also has a pommel that provides for abduction of the hips and can support some of the patient's weight. The A-frame is indicated in the slightly older child, 18 months to 4 years of age.[21] With the A-frame, the hip positions of abduction and internal/external rotation can be controlled.[20] This is advantageous in a population that has a high incidence of hip subluxations and dysplasia.

Parapodium

This orthosis provides the patient with the advantage of sitting and standing as well as the independent ability to change between these two positions. Both the standing frame and the parapodium orthoses were designed at the Ontario Crippled Children's Hospital. (Figs. 34.15 and 34.16).[24,25]

The parapodium is indicated for children older than 3 years. It consists of a prefabricated kit with chest

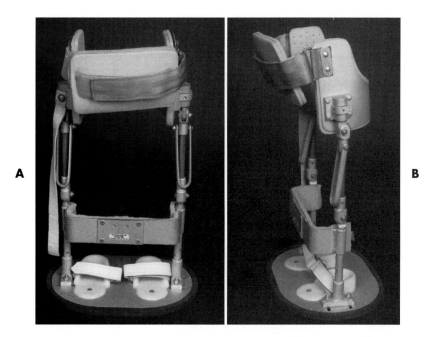

Fig. 34.15. Parapodium. **A,** Anterior view. **B,** Lateral view.

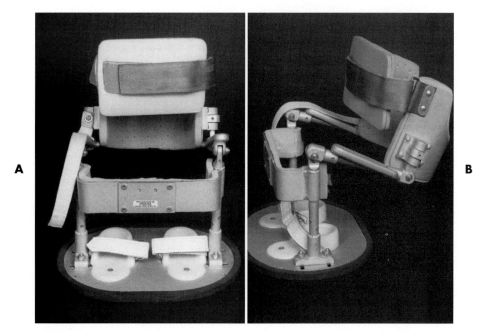

Fig. 34.16. Parapodium. **A,** Anterior view, lowered for seating. **B,** Lateral view, lowered for seating.

abdominal support fixed to a metal lower extremity, which has a knee joint and foot plates attached to a wide metal base. The hip and knee joints unlock with a lever to permit sitting. A four-bar linkage in the hip and a telescoping bar allow patients to roll and ratchet themselves from the sitting to the standing position.[20] Patients old enough to use crutches may also be independently ambulatory in any of these orthoses.

Reciprocating gait orthosis

The reciprocating gait orthosis (RGO) (Fig. 34.17) was originally described by Motloch[27] and has been further modified by Yngve and coworkers.[42] It consists of bilateral KAFOs attached through hinges to a rigid pelvic band with a thoracic extension. A cable system couples hip flexion on one side to hip extension on the contralateral side and thus compensates for the lack of

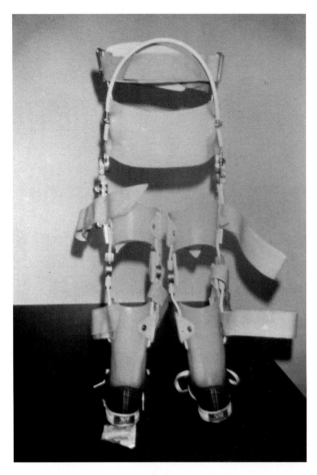

Fig. 34.17. Reciprocating-gait orthosis.

extensor power commonly seen in the patient population.[9] This helps to prevent forward pelvic tilt and lordosis. Assistive devices (crutches or walker) are usually necessary for balance and control.[20]

A study that compared energy expenditure for RGO with swing-through crutch ambulation versus wheelchair ambulation found RGO to be close to wheelchair ambulation in energy requirement.[9] No significant differences were noted in gait velocity with RGO, and all patients achieved community ambulation status with the RGO.[9,23]

REFERENCES

1. American Academy of Orthopaedic Surgeons: Orthopaedic appliances atlas, Vol 1, Ann Arbor, MI, 1952, IW Edwards.
2. American Academy of Orthopaedic Surgeons: Atlas of Orthotics, ed 2, St. Louis, 1985, CV Mosby.
3. Bennett JJ, MacEwen GD: Congenital dislocation of the hip: Recent advances an current problems, Clin Orthop 247:15–21, 1989.
4. Bobechko WP, McLaurin EA, Motloch WM: Toronto orthosis for Legg-Perthes disease, Artif Limbs 12:36–41, 1968.
5. Carey TP, Guidera KG, Ogden JA: Manifestations of ischemic necrosis complicating developmental hip dysplasia, Clin Orthop 281:11–17, 1992.
6. Cooperman DR, Stulberg SD: Ambulatory containment treatment in Perthes disease, Clin Orthop 203:289–300, 1986.
7. Curtis BH, et al: Treatment for Legg-Perthes disease with the Newington ambulation-abduction brace, J Bone Joint Surg 56A: 1135–1146, 1974.
8. Evans IK, Deluca PA, Gage JR: A cooperative study of ambulation-abduction bracing and varus derotation osteotomy in the treatment of severe Legg-Calve-Perthes disease in children over 6 years of age, J Pediatr Orthop 8:676–682, 1988.
9. Flandry F, et al: Functional ambulation in myelodysplasia: The effect of orthotic selection on physical and physiologic performance, J Pediatr Orthop 6:661–665, 1986.
10. Grill F, et al: The Pavlik harness in treatment of congenital dislocating hip: Report on a multicenter study of the European Pediatric Orthopaedic Society, J Pediatr Orthop 8:1–8, 1988.
11. Harris IE, Dickens R, Menelaus MB: Use of the Pavlik harness for hip displacements: When to abandon treatment, Clin Orthop 281:29–33, 1992.
12. Harrison MH, Turner MH, Nicholson FJ: Coxa plana: Results of a new form of splinting, J Bone Joint Surg 51A:1057–1069, 1969.
13. Heikkila E: Comparison of the Frejka pillow and Von Rosen splint in treatment of congenital dislocation of the hip, J Pediatr Orthop 8:20–21, 1988.
14. Herring JA: Conservative treatment of congenital dislocation of the hip in the newborn and infant, Clin Orthop 281:41–47, 1992.
15. Hinderaker T, Rygh M, Uden A: The Von Rosen splint compared with Frejka pillow: A study of 408 neonatally unstable hips, Acta Orthop Scand 63:389–392, 1992.
16. Ilfeld FW: The management of congenital dislocation and dysplasia of the hip by means of a special splint, J Bone Joint Surg 39A:99–104, 1957.
17. Kalamachi A, MacEwen GD: Avascular necrosis following treatment of congenital dislocation of the hip, J Bone Joint Surg 62A:876–888, 1980.
18. Kamhi E, MacEwen GD: Treatment of Legg-Calve-Perthese disease: Prognostic value of Catterall's classification, J Bone Joint Surg 57A:651–654, 1975.
19. Katz JF: Conservative treatment of Legg-Calve-Perthes disease, J Bone Joint Surg 49A:1043–1051, 1967.
20. Kruger LM: In American Academy of Orthopaedic Surgeons: Atlas of Orthoses, St. Louis, 1985, CV Mosby.
21. Letts RM, et al: Mobility aids for the paraplegic child, J Bone Joint Surg 58A:38–41, 1976.
22. Martinez AG, Weinstein SL, Dietz FR: The weight-bearing abduction brace for the treatment of Legg-Perthes disease, J Bone Joint Surg 74A:12–21, 1992.
23. McCall RE, Schmidt WT: Clinical experience with the reciprocal gait orthosis in myelodysplasia, J Pediatr Orthop 6:157–161, 1986.
24. McHale KA, Corbett D: Parental noncompliance with Pavlik harness treatment of infantile hip problems, J Pediatr Orthop 9:649–652, 1989.
25. Meehan PL, Angel D, Nelson JM: The Scottish rite abduction orthosis for the treatment of Legg-Perthes disease: A radiographic analysis, J Bone Joint Surg 74A:2–12, 1992.
26. Menelaus MB: Lessons learned in the management of Legg-Calve-Perthes disease, Clin Orthop 209:41–48, 1986.
27. Motloch W: The parapodium: An orthotic device for neuromuscular disorders, Artif Limbs 15:36–47, 1971.
28. Mubarak S, et al: Pitfalls in the use of the Pavlik harness for treatment of congenital dysplasia, subluxation, and dislocation of the hip, J Bone Joint Surg 63A:1239–1247, 1981.
29. Pavlik A: The functional method of treatment using a harness with stirrups as the primary method of conservative therapy for infants with congenital dislocation of the hip, Clin Orthop 281:4–10, 1992.

30. Petrie JG, Bitenc I: The abduction weight-bearing treatment in Legg-Perthes disease, J Bone Joint Surg 53B:54–62, 1971.

31. Purvis JM, et al: Preliminary experience with the Scottish rite hospital abduction orthosis for Legg-Perthes disease, Clin Orthop 150:49–53, 1980.

32. Rab GT, et al: A technique for determining femoral head containment during gait, J Pediatr Orthop 5:8–12, 1985.

33. Ramsey PL, Lasser S, MacEwen GD: Congenital dislocation of the hip: Use of the Pavlik harness in the child during the first 6 months of life, J Bone Joint Surg 58A:1000–1004, 1976.

34. Rombouts JJ, Kaelin A: Inferior (obturator) dislocation of the hip in neonates: A complication of treatment by the Pavlik harness, J Bone Joint Surg 74B:708–710, 1992.

35. Staheli LT: Rotational problems in children, Instr Course Lect J Bone Joint Surg 75A(6), 1993.

36. Staheli LT, Engel GM: Tibial torsion: A method of assessment and survey of normal children, Clin Orthop 86:183–186, 1972.

37. Staheli LT, Lippert F, Denotter P: Femoral anteversion and physical performance in adolescent and adult life, Clin Orthop 129:213–216, 1977.

38. Suzuki S, Yamamuro T: Avascular necrosis in patients treated with the Pavlik harness for congenital dislocation of the hip, J Bone Joint Surg 72A:1048–1055, 1990.

39. Tachdjian MO, Joueff LD: Trilateral socket hip abduction orthosis for the treatment of Legg-Perthes disease, J Bone Joint Surg 50A:1272, 1968.

40. Tredwell SJ, Davis LA: Prospective study of congenital dislocation of the hip, J Pediatr Orthop 9:386–390, 1989.

41. Tucci JJ, et al: Late acetabular dysplasia following early successful Pavlik harness treatment of congenital dislocation of the hip, J Pediatr Orthop 11:502–505, 1991.

42. Yngve DA, Douglas R, Roberts JM: The reciprocation gait orthosis in myelomeningocele, J Pediatr Orthop 4:304–310, 1984.

43. Viere RG, et al: Use of the Pavlik harness in congenital dislocation of the hip: An analysis of failure of treatment, J Bone Joint Surg 72A:238–244, 1990.

44. Von Rosen S: Diagnosis and treatment of congenital dislocation of the hip joint in the newborn, J Bone Joint Surg 44B(2):284–291, 1962.

Orthoses for the Muscle Disease Patient

John D. Hsu

Patients with generalized, trunk, and extremity muscle weakness may be afflicted with a neuromuscular disorder originating in the motor unit. The manifestation of muscle weakness can be the result of a disease originating in the motor neurone, the peripheral nerve, the neuromuscular junction, or the muscle tissue itself. Weakness in the muscles originating in the muscle tissue is considered to be a *myopathy*. Muscle weakness secondary to a disorder in the motor unit proximal to the muscle is a *neuropathy*. *Muscle disease* can also be referred to as a *motor unit disorder*.[12]

When a patient has muscle weakness, whether it be in the trunk, the proximal portion of the body, or the distal extremities, orthoses may be used for support. Depending on the underlying condition, weakness can be generalized, regional, unilateral, bilateral, or symmetrical. Contractures result from weakness around a joint and occur because the extent of the disorder or rate of deterioration between antagonist or agonist muscle groups may not be the same. They may be influenced by positioning and gravity. Thus, the affected part, for instance, the spine or an extremity, may be constantly pulled into a specific direction without significant resistance. When that occurs over a long period of time, a fixed contracture can develop. Contractures can also result from muscle cell death and fibrosis. Orthoses are designed to support and maintain correction rather than to work against a deforming force. In motor unit disorders, there is no increase in muscle tone. Spasticity is not present in these disorders, and orthoses should not be made to accommodate for this problem.

DIAGNOSIS

The identification of the underlying neuromuscular disorder is an extremely important aspect of the overall planning of treatment and bracing. Many motor unit disorders are associated with a gene defect.[2] Knowl-edge of the family history is important and can frequently help establish the diagnosis. The workup should include information about the onset of weakness, its clinical course and a discussion of progression or stability of the disease process. The areas of weakness also need to be identified and muscle strength recorded by manual muscle testing. Can a pattern be identified: Is the weakness proximal, distal, central, or affecting only a certain area, such as the face, neck muscles, and scapular supporting musculature? Presently, laboratory studies that determine enzyme activity such as the creatine phosphokinase (CPK), reflecting muscle tissue breakdown, are useful to support the clinical impression. CPK is highly elevated with rapidly progressive muscle disorders in which there are significant amounts of breakdown of muscle tissue (e.g., Duchenne pseudohypertrophic muscular dystrophy [DMD]) and not elevated for stable conditions, such as spinal muscular atrophy or congenital myopathies. Blood samples for genetic studies also can give further information as to the nature of the underlying disorder. Other diagnostic tests frequently relied upon include electromyography (EMG) and/or nerve conduction studies (NCV). Muscle biopsy, including histochemical and biochemical studies and dystrophin testing, the presence of which rules out DMD, may give a more definitive answer. Once the diagnosis is established, prognosis and the clinical course the neuromuscular disorder takes can be better understood. This allows for treatment planning to manage the specific patient's immediate or long-term problems and for determining the need for orthotic care.

TEAM APPROACH

Long-term disability with loss of function is associated with most motor unit disorders. Polymyositis with severe generalized muscle weakness can be initially

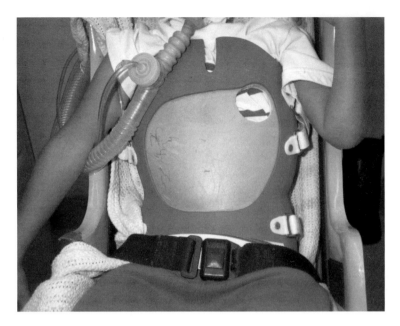

Fig. 35.1.   TLSO for respirator-dependent neuromuscular patient. Note that the main body of the body jacket is made out of fairly stiff material to contain the spine. The anterior aspect is made of softer material, and appropriate cutouts are made to accommodate ventilating and monitoring equipment.

treated with steroids, and improvement in muscle strength and function can be expected with successful treatment leading to control of the acute process. Neuropathies and myopathies require long-term management not only from the medical standpoint but in overall care. A treatment team needs to include *physicians* who have special knowledge of neuromuscular diagnosis and can understand the course of the neuromuscular disorder and disabilities. Expertise in orthopedics, neurology, physical medicine, pulmonary medicine, and pediatrics is needed to manage neuromuscular disorders. *Physical therapists* and *occupational therapists* need to understand the muscle grading and the affected patient's functional abilities together with available self-care aids, mobility devices, and possible environmental adaptives. *Psychologists, liaison nurses, social workers,* and *community workers* support the patient and family's needs, help the school and community understand the disabled child's special problems and concerns, and assist with interfacing with the community and special agencies that provide services to assist the disabled patient. The *certified orthotist,* knowledgeable about support of weakened limbs and trunk, is of utmost importance to the team because of the special experience and training in the construction, fitting, and maintenance of such equipment.

SPINAL ORTHOSES

Spinal deformities are frequently seen in the neuromuscular patient and require support. The orthoses used are generally *containment* devices (Fig. 35.1) and developed in many centers treating neuromuscular patients.[3,7,18,30,32] Frequently, outriggers need to be added to support the head.[26] Principles developed for the use of orthoses in treating the patient with idiopathic scoliosis cannot be directly applied to the patient with neuromuscular scoliosis because this patient has weakness of the supportive musculature of the spine and spinal column collapse.[22]

When spinal orthoses are prescribed, special circumstances may be encountered. Provisions may need to be made for the bracing of:

1. An ambulatory patient.
2. A person with weakened respiratory musculature.
3. A patient with rapid spinal collapse, which requires holding of the spine.

It is important to know the natural history of spinal collapse in the neuromuscular condition being treated.[10,16,18,21] In the ambulatory patient, recognizing the spinal curve pattern and its flexibility becomes important. Encumbering the spine with a corset can interfere with balancing and walking. In a patient with a progressive disease, such as DMD, frequent reassessments of the spine in the seated patient should be done, at least every 6 months. If a spinal curvature is present, it needs to be followed closely, with clinical examinations as frequently as every 3 months. If there is any doubt about the nature and degree of the spinal curvature, an x-ray examination in the sitting position should be made. If the curve progresses, it can become fixed and difficult to correct. Thus, a curve under 35 degrees can be supported by the use of a lightweight body jacket (TLSO), especially in a very slowly progressive condition such as in a spinal muscular atrophy (SMA) or congenital muscular dystrophy (CMD) patient. When the spinal collapse progresses to the degree where sitting becomes difficult and the arms and hands are supporting the trunk, spinal fusion should be made.

Respiratory function tests, including vital capacity, should be measured when the body jacket is used. In patients where respiratory musculature has become weakened to such an extent that respiratory excursion may be even more limited when resistance is applied, large anterior cutouts are used.

It is important to follow the spinal curve clinically and radiographically even though support is used externally through a TLSO or internally via spinal fusion and instrumentation.[6,24,28] In the growing child, posterior spinal fusion can cause arrest of the posterior growth centers resulting in severe lordosis. This presents difficulty in sitting because the head and neck tilt back into extension more and more with increasing age. Modification to the wheelchair or outrigger for support of the head is needed. This lordosis, the result of the "crankshaft phenomenon" needs to be recognized and prevented.

Spinal fusions that are incomplete, too short, or made on growing spines can result in further progression of scoliosis, "falling off", resulting in deformities and bony prominences such as a protuberant rib cage and pain. These present special challenges to the orthotist making special customized supports[5,25] and devices to allow for the maintenance of function and independence.

LOWER EXTREMITY ORTHOSES FOR THE AMBULATORY PATIENT

The use of orthoses in the ambulatory patient is to provide support to the limb at the knee and ankle. The weakened lower extremity with functional muscles can be stabilized at the knee joint or ankle joint using orthotic support. Depending on the strength of the proximal musculature and knee control, long leg (KAFO) or short leg (AFO) orthoses can be selected.[23] Studies of gait disorders and posture changes may assist the clinician and orthotist in recognizing orthotic needs.[11,17,29]

If joint contractures or muscle imbalance is present, surgical release of tightened joint structures is indicated. In the walking child with DMD with fixed knee joint contractures of under 20 degrees, a lateral iliotibial band release to correct the knee to a fully extended position may allow for bracing so that the child can stand either independently in the orthosis or with the help of a standing table.[27,30]

Foot and ankle contractures need to be assessed. In DMD and BMD (Becker muscular dystrophy) we expect an equinovarus deformity,[8,9] but frequently in SMA the feet of patients tend to evert.[20] Fixed contractures may need to be surgically released.[14] Dynamic deformities can be corrected by tendon releases or transfers.[8,13,19,23] When there is sufficient ankle motion to allow for a plantigrade foot, orthoses can help support the weakened joint.

Knee-ankle-foot orthosis

For a neuromuscular patient to continue standing and walking with weakened quadriceps muscles, a long leg brace (KAFO) can be prescribed (Fig. 35.2). KAFOs cannot be successfully used if there is hip flexion contracture of more than 35 degrees. Knee flexion contractures need to be corrected to as close to neutral as possible by serial casting or surgical releases to allow for the knee to be locked into extension by the brace. Ankle and foot deformities also need to be addressed, if necessary, surgically. Special locks need to be incorporated into the orthoses such that a patient with weakened upper extremity musculature and hand function can lock and release the lock from an extended position.

KAFOs for the growing child present a special challenge to the orthotist. Adjustments to growth need to be constantly made by changing the size of the plastic components, the length of the supporting bars, and the position of the knee and ankle joints. The child needs to be seen whenever there is tightness in the brace. Because many children "sit" on the proximal edge their KAFOs, this requires reexamination on a periodic basis because of growth. For good results, this brace almost needs to fit perfectly. Aluminum and steel components can be lengthened easily, but carbon fiber composite upright components that become short need to be replaced by longer ones.

Because of the muscle weakness caused by the inherent disorder and with no need to control abnormal muscle pull or abnormal muscle forces owing to spasticity, lower extremity braces should be made as lightweight as possible.[1] Their function is to support rather than to correct for deforming forces or to hold forcefully.

Ankle-foot orthosis

When ankle dorsiflexors are weak or insufficient, an AFO can be used to support the foot and ankle and stable base, whereas the maintenance of the upright posture and mobility in such a patient is due to normal proximal musculature and good quadriceps strength. AFOs can allow for the limb to continue to function, to prevent the formation of a fixed equinus contracture at the ankle and to support the foot for walking in the ambulatory patient. In the nonambulatory or wheelchair-dependent person, AFOs are used as positioning

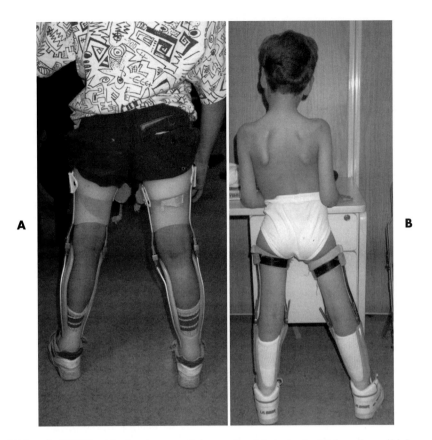

Fig. 35.2. **A,** KAFO with aluminum uprights and molded plastic thigh and pretibial components. **B,** KAFO incorporating lightweight carbon fiber composite supports.

devices to keep the foot and ankle supported so that wheelchair foot rests can be used and tiredness is prevented.[14]

The most appropriate AFO for the neuromuscular patient should be made out of the most lightweight materials possible. Today, polypropylene is used and can be ultra-lightweight by carbon fiber reenforcement and ventilated through cutouts. Such an orthosis can be fitted inside a shoe and is preferable to the standard double upright brace connected by a joint to the shoe (Fig. 35.3).

Muscle imbalance needs to be periodically reassessed when an AFO is used. If there is active muscle pull into varus or valgus, callosities or skin breakdown can form at the bottom of the foot or at the orthosis-skin interphase and along trim lines. This is especially important for the patient who may also have a sensory impairment in addition to the muscle weakness, such as the patient with Charcot-Marie-Tooth disease. Rebalancing the foot either surgically or by using dynamic devices, including hinging the orthoses at the ankle in the correct plane, can give some pressure relief. Ambulatory AFOs may support the leg sufficiently to allow for short distance walking.

UPPER EXTREMITY ORTHOSES

Orthoses for the upper extremity are to support and to prevent contractures (Fig. 35.4). They are seldom used to control positioning of a limb or to prevent excessive forces or movement. A knowledge of the available and remaining muscles functioning through manual muscle testing and functional assessment is of utmost importance before a prescription for an orthosis can be considered. Contractures may be present and acceptable as long as function can be improved. Surgical releases are seldom necessary except for extreme conditions where a clenched fist or hand prevents use of the fingers or make the remaining musculature pull so inefficiently that they are nonfunctional.[15] For example, in the case of a severely contracted DMD hand, where hygiene and finger movement have been severely compromised, release of finger flexors through a sublimus to profundus transfer (STP) operation may be indicated.[33] In the daytime, the released fist can clench over a knob for control of wheelchair movement.

There is controversy with regards to the use of orthoses for the wrist and hand of a patient with PIP and DIP joint contractures due to intrinsic and extrinsic

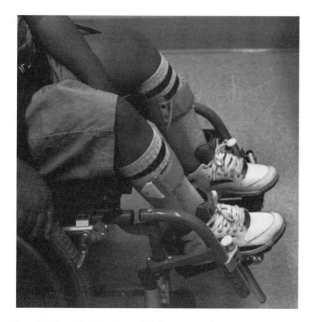

Fig. 35.3. Positioning AFOs used by a wheelchair-dependent DMD patient.

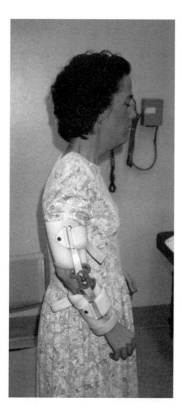

Fig. 35.4. Adjustable elbow splint used after casting for elbow contracture.

weakness. These contractures should be minimized by a preventive program of splinting and stretching. Static splinting is useful to maintain range. Dynamic splinting is rarely used by neuromuscular patients with hand weakness and contractures because they can readily

compensate with substitute motions and activities rather than accept an encumbering and possibly unsightly device.

Mobile arm supports

Function of a patient with proximal weakness can be improved when fitted with a mobile arm support (MAS). With this device, the hands and fingers can be positioned for function. The author has used a MAS successfully in DMD patients during a time when the progressive proximal weakness prevents the hands and fingers to be used for tabletop activities, thus positioning them for continued use. With further weakness, however, finger function becomes more limited. Scoliosis may impact on the position of the arm as spinal curve allows the patient to lean toward the concave side. This could allow the elbow to be propped at table edge. Thus, a unilateral MAS can be useful in this instance. With spinal fusion, however, this advantage can be lost. Persons prescribing and using MAS should understand the limitations of this piece of equipment and the need for appropriate training and frequent initial adjustments to the equipment.[4,31]

ACKNOWLEDGMENTS

The author expresses his appreciation to Ms. Leslie Sakioka for typing the manuscript.

REFERENCES

1. Barnett SL, Bagley AM, Skinner HB: Ankle weight effect on gait: Orthotic implications, Orthopedics 16:1127–1131, 1993.
2. Bruns GAP: Assigning genes to chromosomes: Family studies, somatic cell hybridization, chromosome sorting, in situ hybridization, translocations. In Rowland LP, et al, editors: Molecular genetics of brain, nerve, and muscle, New York, 1989, Oxford University Press.
3. Carlson JM, Winter R: The "Gillette" sitting support orthosis, Orthot Prosthet, 32:35–45, 1978.
4. Chyatte SB, Long C II, Vignos PJ Jr: Balanced forearm orthosis in muscular dystrophy, Arch phys med 46:633–636, 1965.
5. Drennan JC, Renshaw TS, Curtis BH: The thoracic suspension orthosis, Clin Orthop Rel Res 139:33–39, 1979.
6. Galasko CSB, Delaney C, Morris P: Spinal stabilization in Duchenne muscular dystrophy, J Bone Joint Surg 74B:210–214, 1992.
7. Gibson DA, Wilkins KE: The management of spinal deformities in Duchenne muscular dystrophy: A new concept of spinal bracing, Clin Orthop Rel Res 108:41–51, 1975.
8. Hsu JD: Orthopaedic care for children and adolescents with Charcot-Marie-Tooth disease. In Lovelace RE, Shapiro HK, editor: Charcot-Marie-Tooth disorders: Pathophysiology, molecular genetics, and therapy, New York, 1990, Wiley-Liss.
9. Hsu JD: Management of foot deformity in Duchenne's pseudo-hypertrophic muscular dystrophy, Orthop Clin North Am 7:979–984, 1976.
10. Hsu JD: The natural history of spine curvature in the nonambulatory Duchenne muscular dystrophy patient, Spine 8:771–775, 1983.
11. Hsu JD, Furumasu J: Gait and posture changes in the Duchenne muscular dystrophy child, Clin Orthop Rel Res 288:122–125, 1993.

12. Hsu JD, Gilgoff IS: Muscular dystrophy and neurogenic atrophy. In Nickel VL, Botte MJ, editors: Orthopaedic rehabilitation, ed 2. New York, 1992, Churchill Livingstone.

13. Hsu JD, Hoffer MM: Posterior tibial tendon transfer anteriorly through the interosseous membrane: A modification of the technique, Clin Orthop Rel Res 202–204, 1978.

14. Hsu JD, Jackson R: Treatment of symptomatic foot and ankle deformities in the nonambulatory neuromuscular patient, Foot Ankle 5:238–244, 1985.

15. Hsu JD, Taylor D: Upper extremity deformities in Duchenne muscular dystrophy patients. In Fredricks S, Brody GS, editors: Symposium on the neurologic aspects of plastic surgery, St. Louis, 1978, CV Mosby.

16. Lord J, et al: Scoliosis associated with Duchenne muscular dystrophy, Arch Phys Med Rehabil 71:13–17, 1990.

17. Melkonian GJ, et al: Dynamic gait electromyography study in Duchenne muscular dystrophy (DMD) patients, Foot Ankle 1:78–83, 1980.

18. Merlini L, et al: Scoliosis in spinal muscular atrophy: Natural history and management, Dev Med Child Neurol 31:501–508, 1989.

19. Miller GM, et al: Posterior tibial tendon transfer: A review of the literature and analysis of 74 procedures, J Pediatr Ortho 2:363–370, 1982.

20. Moosa A, Dubowitz V: Spinal muscular atrophy in childhood, Arch Dis Child 48:386–388, 1973.

21. Rideau Y, et al: The treatment of scoliosis in Duchenne muscular dystrophy, Muscle Nerve 7:281–286, 1984.

22. Robin GC, Brief LP: Scoliosis in childhood muscular dystrophy, J Bone Joint Surg 53A:466–476, 1971.

23. Rochelle J, Bowen JR, Ray S: Pediatric foot deformities in progressive neuromuscular disease, Contemp Orthop 8:41–50, 1984.

24. Seeger BR, Sutherland ADA, Clark MS: Orthotic management of scoliosis in Duchenne muscular dystrophy, Arch Phys Med Rehabil 65:83–86, 1984.

25. Siegel IM, Silverman O, Silverman M: The Chicago insert: An approach to wheelchair seating for the maintenance of spinal posture in Duchenne muscular dystrophy, Orthot Prosthet 35:27–29, 1981.

26. Silverstein F, Siebens AA: Head-control-system for severely paralyzed patient, Arch Phys Med Rehabil 64:604–605, 1983.

27. Spencer GE Jr: Orthopaedic considerations in the management of muscular dystrophy, Curr Pract Orthop Surg 5:279–293, 1973.

28. Sussman MD: Treatment of scoliosis in Duchenne muscular dystrophy, Dev Med Child Neurol 27:522–531, 1985.

29. Sutherland DH: Gait disorders in childhood and adolescence, Baltimore, 1984, Williams & Wilkins.

30. Vignos PJ, Jr, Spencer GE Jr, Archibald KC: Management of progressive muscular dystrophy of childhood, JAMA 184:89–96, 1963.

31. Yasuda YL, Bowman K, Hsu JD: Mobile arm supports: Criteria for successful use in muscle disease patients, Arch Phys Med Rehabil 47:253–256, 1986.

32. Young A, et al: A new spinal brace for use in Duchenne muscular dystrophy, Dev Med Child Neurol 26:808–813, 1984.

33. Yu W, Schweigel JF: Flexor digitorum sublimis to profundus tendon transfer for flexion deformities of the hand and wrist in spastic paralysis, J Bone Joint Surg 55B:664, 1973.

Cerebral Palsy

John R. Fisk
Terry J. Supan

Cerebral palsy is a disorder of movement and posture (a motor disability) resulting from a nonprogressive central nervous system insult.[3] Although this is a classic definition, it does not go far enough in helping the reader understand the full breadth of the disorder dealt with in this chapter. The orthotic needs of these individuals are affected by the age of the child; severity of the disorder; presence or absence of deformities in the child; and expectations of the care providers, be they health professionals, parents, family, or institutions.

The disorder may stem either from an insult to a normally developing brain or from a central nervous system that developed in an anomalous fashion from an early stage.[4] The important consideration is that although the abnormality is nonprogressive, with growth of the child the brain is developing. Consequently, there may be an evolving neurological picture. Some believe that this can be influenced positively, whereas others believe the evidence for this is lacking.[8,23] In any event, the needs at any given time may differ. Those needs are influenced by the level of central nervous system involvement, by its stage of development, by the size and/or strength of the patient, and by the presence or absence of deformities.

The insult that has occurred to the developing brain has frequently been blamed on birth trauma. Although this does happen, the definition of cerebral palsy encompasses prenatal events as well as postnatal events. Some set the limit arbitrarily at 2 years, although there is motor plasticity up to 6 to 8 years, and there is a significant development in cognitive function up until 16 to 18 years. The point that needs to be made is that a child who sustains an insult to the brain from an encephalitis or an automobile accident has the same needs therapeutically as the child born prematurely with a periventricular hemorrhage. Etiologic studies suggest that anywhere from 33% to 65% of cerebral palsy cases are related to perinatal events, whereas

cerebral palsy acquired postnatally is consistently quoted around 10%.[21,32]

William John Little first linked cerebral palsy to a difficult birth.[1] In a lecture to the London Obstetrics Society in 1862, he demonstrated an early understanding of etiologic factors and of the consequences of poor management undoubtedly present in his day. Osler (1888) is given credit for the term *cerebral palsy*. Freud, in his classic text *Infantile Cerebral Palsy* (1897), emphasized the existence of associated problems such as mental retardation, epilepsy, and visual problems.[1]

Treatment and research activities have varied widely in years past as a result of disagreements over definitions and classifications. Treatment ranged from inhibiting motion with braces to facilitating it with various stimulating techniques.[51] A classification was developed by the American Academy of Cerebral Palsy[29] in 1956. The system is a clinical one based on the physiology of the motor dysfunction and the number of limbs involved. It offers an orderly approach to the description of the patient's motor involvement but provides little insight into the severity, cause, or pathology of the problem. Gage[14] submits that a more complete description of the patient's condition should include (1) functional capacity, (2) associated problems, and (3) causative and/or risk factors.

The broad nature of the definition of cerebral palsy can mislead because it is imprecise and poorly understood. The breadth of the definition is, however, helpful as well. Third-party payers understand poorly some of the nomenclature involved in classifying cerebral palsy and are more willing to provide coverage when the global definition is used. The health care deliverer, however, when using the term in its broadest sense, must not lose sight of the individual needs of a client.

The importance of understanding the scope and definition of cerebral palsy and the possible causative factors and associated conditions is obvious to any clinician faced with the responsibility of explaining to a

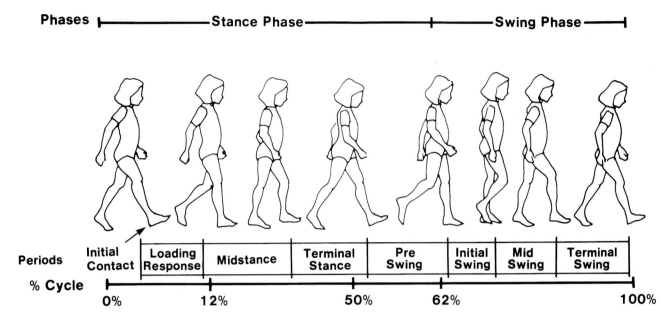

Fig. 36.1.   Illustrated gait periods as defined by Perry. These terms are best used to describe the gait of persons with cerebral palsy. *(From Thomas SS, Supan TJ: A comparison of current biomechanical terms,* J Prosthet Orthot *2:107–114, 1990.)*

parent how it is that their child has that diagnosis. All of those involved in the treatment of individuals with cerebral palsy need to be cognizant of the level of understanding and concern expressed by the families.

UNDERSTANDING GAIT

The role of orthoses in the care and treatment of individuals with cerebral palsy is no different than that for any other condition: to protect a part, to prevent deformity, and to improve function. With this population, there is a limited need for protection and a questionable ability to prevent deformity. Both of these concerns are discussed under specific prescriptions. The primary goal in cerebral palsy is to help the individual walk better.

Perry[33] defined the requisites of normal gait to include stability in stance, the means for progression, and energy conservation. Gage[14] expanded these to five requisites: (1) stability in stance, (2) clearance in swing, (3) preposition of the foot in terminal swing, (4) adequate step length, and (5) energy conservation. When not present, these requisites may be facilitated by therapy, the use of orthoses, and/or by surgery. The reader is referred to Gage's text, *Gait Analysis in Cerebral Palsy,*[14] for an excellent discussion of the role and importance of a motion analysis evaluation of each individual being considered for surgery or orthotic prescription. Even if a laboratory is not available, the added insight gained from the experience of oth-

ers[7,24,37,41,46,47] who use such a facility warrants a familiarity with the material presented by Gage.

Figure 36.1 illustrates the terminology now in common use for describing the stages and dynamics of the gait cycle. There are two phases: stance phase, which makes up typically 60% of a cycle, and swing phase, which makes up the remaining 40%. Current terminology differs slightly from that used in the field of prosthetics. Instead of heel strike, *initial contact* is used as the first event in the cycle because many individuals with cerebral palsy do not initially contact the floor with their heel. *Loading response* replaces foot flat as that transitional period when the weight shifts from double support to single limb weight bearing. *Midstance* remains the same, whereas *terminal stance* replaces heel-off as the beginning of double support. *Preswing* is the period when the weight is transferred to the other limb. Prosthetically, this is indicated as push-off. Normal gait, however, does not exhibit any push-off until the individual's speed starts to accelerate. *Swing phase* is divided into three areas: initial swing or, prosthetically, acceleration; midswing; and terminal swing, which has been known as deceleration.[48]

Frequent mention is made of the three rockers of gait[34] because it is these portions of the foot and ankle dynamics that clinicians commonly seek to influence with orthoses. The first rocker is from initial contact to foot flat and generally involves an external plantar flexion moment. The second rocker is from foot flat to heel-off and is generally a dorsiflexion moment. During this period of the cycle, the tibia passes forward over the ankle mortise and is controlled by an eccentric contraction of the gastroc/soleus muscle. The third rocker is from heel-off until toe-off. Here there is actually a plantar flexion motion that occurs at the ankle and a dorsiflexion motion at the metatarsophalangeal joints. The kinetics during the first and second rockers are of deceleration. With the third rocker, there is generally the acceleration of push-off. The three rockers constitute but a small portion of all of the kinetics and kinematics involved in the gait cycle. They are, however, important considerations when determining proper orthotic prescriptions. Elsewhere in this text, Perry has presented an excellent discussion of the sequences of muscle activity that occur in normal gait (see Chapter 4). An understanding of these is basic to an appreciation for the abnormal sequences seen in a child with cerebral palsy.

Fish and Nielsen[13] described not only the pathologic gaits in both swing and stance phase, but also they described what has been become known as *pathomechanical gait*. Fish and Nielsen[13] define pathomechanics as "the branch of physical science that deals with the static and dynamic forces and their abnormal effect on the human body affected by neurological, muscular, or skeletal disorders." In an external rotational deformity (ERD), the femur is externally rotated, the knee tends to hyperextend, the tibia is externally rotated, the calcaneus goes into a varus position, the forefoot moves medially, and the foot becomes supinated. In an internal rotational deformity (IRD), the opposite is true, in that the femur is internally rotated, the knee tends to be flexed and move into a valgus position, the tibia is internally rotated, the heel goes into a valgus position; the forefoot is abducted, and the midfoot is pronated.

There are marked differences between hemiplegic, diplegic, and quadriplegic gait. More lower limb internal rotation and upper extremity involvement is present with the later two than hemiplegic gait. Spastic hemiplegia has been subdivided by Gage[14] into four different types. Type I patients show equinus during swing phase, and initial contact is with the foot flat or with the toe. There is no first rocker, second rocker begins with initial contact, and there are no limitations to dorsiflexion. The knee is in increased flexion at terminal swing, initial contact, and loading response. The hips have persistent flexion during swing phase, and there is increased lordosis.

Type II spastic hemiplegia has plantar flexion during swing and stance phase. There are contractures of the calf muscles. The second rocker is arrested prematurely. There is hyperextension of the hip and knee in stance phase.

Ankle motion is similar in type II and type III spastic hemiplegia, exhibiting an ERD.[13] The knee is similar with the exception of a limitation to knee flexion in

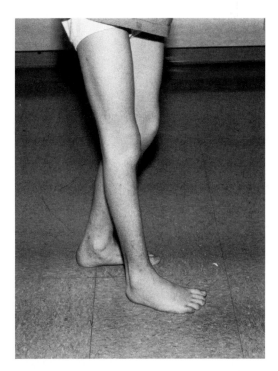

Fig. 36.2. Typical midstance posture of a child with spastic hemiplegic cerebral palsy (type III).

swing phase because of a cospasticity of the hamstrings and the rectus femoris muscles. Therefore, the individual with type III is vaulting like someone who wears a locked knee-ankle-foot orthosis (KAFO) (Fig. 36.2). There is also a hyperextension of the hip in stance and swing causing an increased lordosis.

In type IV spastic hemiplegia, the involvement of the ankle and knee is identical to that of the type III. Differences exist in the hip and the pelvis. There are flexion and adduction contractures at the hip and increased lordosis at terminal swing.

Diplegic and quadriplegic gait patterns are similar to each other. The difference between the two is the intensity of the involvement of the upper extremities so that if the lesser involved quadriplegic is able to ambulate, his or her gait pattern is similar to that of the diplegic (Fig. 36.3). The diplegic exhibits a classical IRD as indicated by Fish and Nielsen.[13] There is usually valgus in the hindfoot, a pronated midfoot, and an abducted forefoot, resulting in stance phase instability. The individual walks with a toe-to-toe or toe-to-heel gait, and the foot is in equinus during swing phase and stance phase. There may be external rotation between the knee and the ankle. Furthermore, the knees are in flexion throughout stance phase with a reduction of the flexion/extension range during swing. Restricted knee extension at terminal stance and terminal swing produces a shortened stride length. Flexion, adduction, and internal rotation are all present at the hips. Stance phase instability is present with exces-

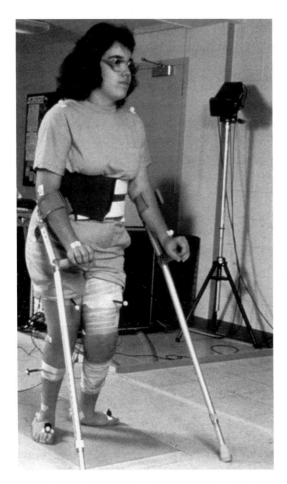

Fig. 36.3. This child with spastic diplegia walks with an internal rotational deformity. Note the classic knee flexed posture with the tarsal bones internally rotating on the calcaneous and pronation of the midfoot.

sive pelvic drop during swing phase. These individuals have a difficult time getting clearance between their legs because of the internal rotation in the hips and the external rotation of the feet.

After a patient's gait pattern has been evaluated, orthotic recommendations are made based on the biomechanical ability of a given device to improve the gait. Design changes (Fig. 36.4) have greatly improved the ability of orthoses to have a positive impact, and as new components become available, orthotic design will continue to alter prescription recommendations.

TYPES OF ORTHOSES

Foot orthoses

The goal of the University of California at Berkley Laboratory (UCBL) foot orthosis is to stabilize the subtalar joint without restricting ankle motion.[9] Foot motion may also be controlled depending on the pliability of the foot and how distal the trim line is. Trim

lines may vary widely. Some practitioners bring the sides to a supramalleolar level and call it a SMO. The important consideration is that there must be good hind foot correction and control to be able to maintain proper alignment through the remainder of the foot. Except in the very young, too much pressure under the navicular area causes only discomfort and skin irritation.

Ankle-foot orthoses

The premade ankle-foot orthosis (AFO) is used primarily for swing phase control. It provides dorsiflexion assist and reduces foot slap. Occasionally a premade device can aid in evaluating the orthotic impact on an individual before prescribing a custom-made orthosis. Seldom are they of adequate fit to be used for extended periods of time.

The custom-made solid AFO can be made in different styles.[16] Specific motions can be controlled around the foot depending on how the orthosis is designed (Fig. 36.5). It increases stability of both the ankle and the subtalar joint and affects knee control as a result of the alignment of the tibia. A hyperextended knee secondary to a plantar flexed foot can be positively influenced by preventing the offending plantar flexion.[7,38] As with the UCBL, hind foot control is key to effecting proper posturing in the remainder of the foot. This AFO provides dorsiflexion assist during swing phase.

The custom-made dorsiflexion assist orthosis is trimmed more posterior to the malleoli than the solid ankle AFO. This allows more flexibility and has less effect on the knee during third rocker. It provides limited stability at the ankle but does not control subtalar motion unless it is specifically designed with a varus/valgus control trim. Historically the metal spring-loaded dorsiflexion assist AFO was used to aid with clearance in swing phase. It is still seen in instances where physiology and biomechanics have been overlooked. The stretch reflex, pathologic in the individual with cerebral palsy, is only worsened by the addition of a spring under extreme tension. Plantar flexion inhibition is the function that is desirable, not augmented dorsiflexion.

The spiral orthosis[26] and the thermoplastic elastomer[45] orthosis function differently than the standard polypropylene orthoses by allowing a more gradual plantar flexion. The first is designed to absorb and use the torques that are in normal walking. It has limited stability at the ankle and the subtalar joint. The second provides a dorsiflexion assist and allows a limited plantar flexion resistance because of the elastomer material. These functions are inherent to their materials and design.

The custom-made articulated orthosis has undergone the most changes in recent years.[2,25,50] Modifica-

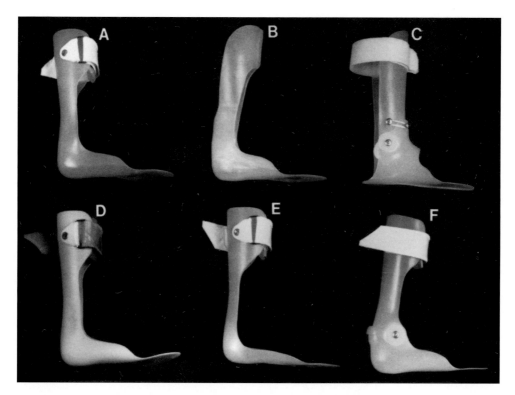

Fig. 36.4. Thermoplastic AFOs. **A,** Solid ankle. **B,** Floor reaction. **C,** Articulated floor reaction. **D,** Thermoplastic elastomer. **E,** Dorsiflexion assist. **F,** Articulated.

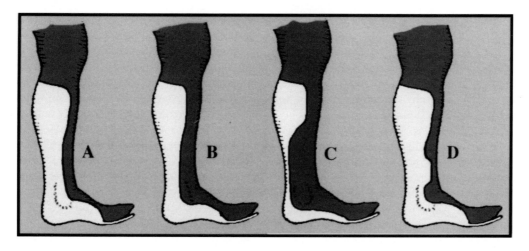

Fig. 36.5. Four possible trim lines for a custom-made AFO. *Trim A* provides the greatest amount of ankle stability, whereas *Trim C* provides more flexibility at the ankle. *Trim D* illustrates the biomechanical three-point force system to provide control of ankle inversion in spastic hemiparesis.

tions have allowed the Certified Orthotist to concentrate on preventing unwanted ankle motion while allowing more normal kinematics. Improved gait is beneficial in the child with cerebral palsy during development stages because the orthosis interferes less with neuromuscular pattern formation. This orthosis can be designed to stabilize the subtalar joint, while preventing unwanted ankle motion; it may assist in preferable

ankle motions; and it gives limited control of knee motion. All of these functions are the result of the way that the orthosis is designed and the type of modifications that are made.

The articulated AFO can be set up to range from a free to a rigid ankle. This type of versatility can allow one device to function as clinical needs vary from a postsurgical state to complete convalescence.[40] There

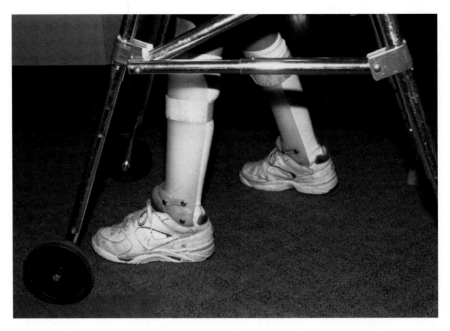

Fig. 36.6.   The articulated floor reaction AFO allows planar flexion during loading response (first rocker) of the left leg while helping to maintain knee extension during midstance and terminal stance of the contralateral limb (second rocker).

can be excellent subtalar control while still allowing free ankle motion. With an adjustable posterior stop, the orthotist can better evaluate and maintain the desired knee posture during stance phase by controlling the effect of the orthosis on the second rocker. Finally a dorsiflexion assist spring can be incorporated into the design. Care must be taken, as alluded to earlier, not to introduce an unwanted spastic response to a potential stretch caused by the spring.

The articulated AFO best takes into consideration control of unwanted dynamics in the rockers of the foot and ankle while facilitating the desirable rockers. With a 90-degree plantar flexion stop, there is swing phase control and prepositioning for stance. During stance, there is subtalar control for stability and facilitated second rocker motion. A flexible toe plate allows forefoot dorsiflexion of the third rocker, whereas limitation in the articulation prevents excessive plantar flexion in early swing. The net effect is a smoother rollover.

Floor reaction ankle-foot orthoses

Two types of floor reaction orthoses, solid and articulated, are frequently used. Originally designed to provide the amount of force needed to prevent unwanted motion and be able to provide more stability to the knee for a patient having postpolio paralysis,[39] the floor reaction orthosis has been modified over the years.[18] The idea behind this orthosis is that while it stabilizes ankle and subtalar motion, it minimizes knee flexion because of the floor reaction forces onto the knee, and it may provide dorsiflexion assist.

The custom-made articulated floor reaction orthosis (Fig. 36.6) is a more recent example of the orthosis trying to better facilitate normal motion.[14] The concept is to minimize orthotic involvement at the first and third rockers while assisting a knee extension moment at second rocker. This orthosis stabilizes the ankle and subtalar joint, allows first rocker plantar flexion, and prevents second rocker dorsiflexion so that the tibia cannot progress anteriorly over the top of the talus. The result is to prevent knee flexion in stance. Free dorsiflexion of the toes at third rocker is dependent on how the orthosis is trimmed in the metatarsal area. Rubber bands may be added for dorsiflexion assist. These bands add control of first rocker and slow plantar flexion in the minimally involved client during loading response.

By understanding normal gait and the pathologic patterns of cerebral palsy, custom-made orthoses for ambulation can be used to their best biomechanical advantage. Gage's five requisites must be kept in mind when performing a patient evaluation:

1. Is there instability during stance?
2. Is there insufficient foot clearance during swing?
3. Is there a problem with prepositioning of the foot at the end of swing?
4. Is there a difference in the stride length, or is it inadequate?
5. Is there increased energy consumption?

If the answer to any of these questions is yes, then the goal of any orthotic or surgical intervention should be to create a more efficient gait.

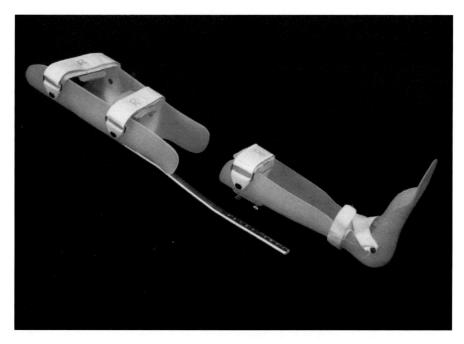

Fig. 36.7. Modular thermoplastic KAFO with removable posterior metal bar allowing disassembly and reassembly of AFO and thigh sections. The assembled orthosis is used at night to hold the knees in extension.

Positioning devices

KAFOs and even those incorporating the hip have been used in the past and continue to be used by some clinicians today. They have little or no role to play with the care and treatment of the ambulatory client. They may be useful for positioning and the prevention of deformities in the nonambulatory child (Fig. 36.7).

Night splinting to prevent knee flexion or hip adduction contractures does have intuitive attractiveness. Some clinicians use night splints extensively, whereas others question their contribution. Conventional hip abduction orthoses (Fig. 36.8) are helpful after surgical procedures done to regain hip stability.[6] Whether they can prevent hip instability in the face of hip flexion or adductor spasticity is debatable. Night splinting for the prevention of equinus contractures in the spastic is also controversial.

All lower extremity orthoses have a time-limited effectiveness in children with cerebral palsy. Skeletal growth, of course, alters the fit of a particular device but may not change the specific prescription. Growth of muscle and body mass may, however, change what is effective for a particular client. Not only does body weight increase but also muscle strength. There may come a time when a particular orthosis cannot perform its desired function because it cannot control those forces on which it was designed to have an effect. At this point, surgical intervention is generally indicated.

The question may also be raised whether surgery is sometimes indicated to allow an orthosis-free existence. Spastic muscle does not elongate as readily as normal tone muscle during the growth of long bones. As a consequence, orthoses may be more important during the adolescent growth spurt just when there is an increasing desire on the part of the teenager to be without them. To hope to be orthosis-free during this phase of development may be discouraging, but to aim for an orthosis-free existence after the cessation of growth is optimistic. At that time, the recurrence of deformity is less likely; however, there must be sufficient control present to effect a smooth function.

Along with the many design alterations (articulated versus nonarticulated, spiral versus conventional, location of trim lines, and choice of materials) AFOs have been designed to have tone-reducing capabilities. They have been a natural outgrowth of inhibitive casting.[11,17,20,42,43,49] Modifications of the trim lines and the footplates are examples of these modifications. The principles behind tone inhibition (Fig. 36.9) are to increase the pressure along the metatarsal arch and the peroneal arch, provide relief under the metatarsal heads, provide a dorsiflexion moment to the toes, provide control of the proximal portion of the calcaneus in the areas medial and lateral to the Achilles' tendon, provide relief on the plantar surface of the calcaneus, and provide support in the sustentacular tali area of the calcaneus.[22,40] As with the casting, controversy exists about their effectiveness. There are many arti-

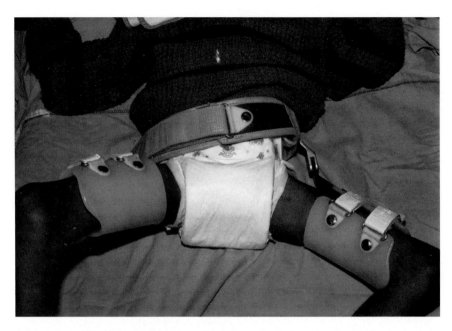

Fig. 36.8. A modified Scottish Rite hip orthosis is used to help maintain the hips in an abducted position after surgery. Polyethylene cuffs are used with the older-style clevis joints. These joints are easier to bend if the abduction angle needs to be changed.

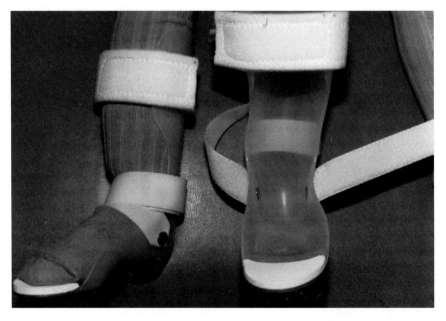

Fig. 36.9. AFO with tone inhibitive modification in the interior plantar surface. Pressure is applied to the metatarsal arch, the sustentacular tali, peroneal arch, and toes with relief under the metatarsal heads and calcaneous. The crepe toe ramp can be moved distally as the child grows.

cles[12,19,31,45,53] in the literature claiming far-reaching benefits from tone-reducing orthoses. Some claim short-term alterations in tone; others suggest that there may be a lasting change in primitive reflexes. Unfortunately, none of these studies are controlled or randomized. Most are single observer reports. Another problem with interpreting reports in the literature about reducing orthoses is the inconsistency in the material used, the basic designs, the trim lines, and the areas of relief. Evidence is still lacking for the role of so-called tone-reducing orthoses.[5]

Spinal and upper extremity orthoses

The reader is referred to the discussion of spinal orthoses in Section Three and orthoses for the upper extremity in Section Four.

CONCLUSION

It has often been said that the care and treatment of the disabled child needs to be by a team approach, and this is certainly the case with the orthotic management of children with cerebral palsy.[10,27,36] The prescription needs to be the consensus of a careful evaluation by physician, therapist, and orthotist. In addition, the expectations of the child, the family, and the child's educators must be addressed. The setting best suited to this type of an approach is a clinic environment where all can be in attendance. When this is impossible, all need to be consulted. Only then are the needs of the child optimally served.

REFERENCES

1. Accardo PJ: William John Little and cerebral palsy in the nineteenth century, J Hist Med Allied Sci 44:56–71, 1989.
2. Banziger E, Hewitt C, Ford RL: Dynamic dorsiflexion assist polypropylene ankle foot orthosis, J Assoc Child Prosthet Orthot Clin 26:65–68, 1991.
3. Bax M: Terminology and classification on cerebral palsy, Dev Med Child Neurol 6:295–297, 1964.
4. Blasco PA: In Sussman MD, editor: The diplegic child, Rosemont, IL, 1992, American Academy of Orthopaedic Surgery.
5. Bleck EE: Current concepts: Management of the lower extremities in children who have cerebral palsy, J Bone Joint Surg 72A:140–144, 1990.
6. Boyd R, Drake C: Effectiveness of the hip abduction and spinal orthosis for postural management in a group of non ambulant bilateral cerebral palsy children, Newsletter ISPO, Summer:26–27, 1993 (abstract).
7. Butler PB, Thompson N, Major RE: Improvement in walking performance of children with cerebral palsy: Preliminary results, Dev Med Child Neurol 34:567–576, 1992.
8. Campbell SK: Efficacy of physical therapy in improving postural control in cerebral palsy, Pediat Phys Ther 2:135–140, 1990.
9. Carlson MJ, Berglund G: An effective orthotic design for controlling the unstable subtalar joint, Orthot Prosthet 33:39, 1979.
10. Diamond M: Rehabilitation strategies for the child with cerebral palsy, Pediatr Ann 15:230–236, 1986.
11. Duncan WR: Foot reflexes and the use of the "inhibitive cast," Foot Ankle 4:145–148, 1983.
12. Embrey DG, Yates L, Mott DH: Effects of neuro-developmental treatment and orthoses on knee flexion during gait: A single-subject design, Phys Ther 70:626–637, 1990.
13. Fish DJ, Nielsen JP: Clinical assessment of human gait, J Prosthet Orthot 5:39–48, 1993.
14. Gage J: Gait analysis in cerebral palsy, London, 1991, MacKeith Press.
15. Gans BM, Erickson G, Simons D: Below-knee orthosis: A wrap-around design for ankle-foot control, Arch Phys Med Rehabil 60:78–80, 1979.
16. Glancy J, Lindseth RE: The polypropylene solid-ankle orthosis, Orthot Prosthet 26:14–26, 1972.
17. Hanson CJ, Jones LJ: Gait abnormalities and inhibitive casts in cerebral palsy, J Am Podiat Med Assoc 79:53–59, 1989.
18. Harrington ED, Lin RS, Gage JR: Use of the anterior floor reaction orthosis in patients with cerebral palsy, Orthot Prosthet 37:34–42, 1983.
19. Harris SR, Riffle EK: Effects of inhibitive ankle-foot orthoses on standing balance in a child with cerebral palsy: A single-subject design, Phys Ther 66:663–667, 1986.
20. Hinderer KA, et al: Effects of "tone-reducing" vs. standard plaster-casts on gait improvement of children with cerebral palsy, Dev Med Child Neurol 30:370–377, 1988.
21. Holm MVA: The causes of cerebral palsy: A contemporary perspective, JAMA 247:1473–1477, 1982.
22. Hylton NM: Postural and functional impact of dynamic AFOs and FOs in a pediatric population, J Prosthet Orthot 2:40–53, 1989.
23. Kanda T, et al: Early physiotherapy in the treatment of spastic diplegia, Dev Med Child Neurol 26:438–444, 1984.
24. Khodadadeh S, Patrick JH: Force plate studies of cerebral palsy hemiplegic patients, J Hum Move Stud 15:273–278, 1988.
25. Knutson LM, Clark DE: Orthotic devices for ambulation in children with cerebral palsy and myelomeningocele, Phys Ther 71:947–960, 1991.
26. Lehneis HR: Plastic spiral foot-ankle orthoses, Orthot Prosthet 28:3–13, 1974.
27. Mcdonald KC, Valmassy RL: Cerebral Palsy: A literature review, J Am Podiatr Med Assoc 77:471–483, 1987.
28. Middleton EA, Hurley GRB, Mcilwain JS: The role of rigid and hinged polypropylene ankle-foot-orthoses in the management of cerebral palsy: A case study, Prosthet Orthot Int 12:129–135, 1988.
29. Minear WL: A classification of cerebral palsy, Pediatrics 18:841, 1956.
30. Mossberg KA, Linton KA, Friske K: Ankle-foot orthoses: Effect on energy expenditure of gait in spastic diplegic children, Arch Phys Med Rehabil 71:490–494, 1990.
31. Mueller K, et al: Effect of a tone-inhibiting dynamic ankle-foot orthosis on the foot loading pattern of a hemiplegic adult: A preliminary study, J Prosthet Orthot 4:86–92, 1992.
32. Paneth N, Kiely J: The frequency of cerebral palsy: A review of population studies in industrialized nations since 1950. In Stanley F, Alberman E, editors: The epidemiology of the cerebral palsies:clinics in developmental medicine. Oxford, 1984, Blackwell Scientific.
33. Perry J: Normal and pathologic gait In Bunch W H, editor: Atlas of orthotics, ed 2, St. Louis: 1985, CV Mosby.
34. Perry J: Kinesiology of lower extremity bracing, Clin Orthop Rel Res 102:20–31, 1974.
35. Powell MM, Silva PD, Grindeland T: Effects of two types of ankle-foot orthoses on the gait of children with spastic diplegia, Dev Med Child Neurol 31(suppl): 8–9, 1989, (abstract).
36. Rogers JP, Vanderbilt SH: Coordinated treatment in cerebral palsy—where are we today? J Prosthet Orthot 2:68–81, 1989.
37. Rose SA, Ounpuu S, Deluca PA: Strategies for the assessment of pediatric gait in the clinical setting, Phys Ther 71:961–980, 1991.
38. Rosenthal RK, et al: A fixed-ankle below-the-knee orthosis for the management of genu recurvatum in spastic cerebral palsy, J Bone Joint Surg 57A:545–547, 1975.
39. Saltiel J: A one-piece laminated knee licking short leg brace, Orthot Prosthet 23:68–75, 1969.
40. Shamp JK: Neurophysiologic orthotic designs in the treatment of central nervous system disorders, J Prosthet Orthot 2:14–32, 1989.
41. Simon SR, et al: A multi-institution prospective study of ambulatory patients with spastic diplegia: Part 1, Dev Med Child Neurol 31(suppl):9, 1989.

42. Sussman MD: Casting as an adjunct to neurodevelopmental therapy for cerebral palsy, Dev Med Child Neurol 25:804–805, 1983.

43. Sussman MD, Cusick B: Preliminary report: The role of short-leg tone-reducing casts as an adjunct to physical therapy of patients with cerebral palsy, John Hopkins Med J 145:112–114, 1979.

44. Sutton R: Thermoplastic elastomer (TPE): The TPE ankle-foot orthosis and the TPE biomechanical-foot orthosis, J Prosthet Orthot 2:164–172, 1990.

45. Taylor CL, Harris SR: Effects of ankle-foot orthoses on functional motor performance in a child with spastic diplegia, Am J Occup Ther 40: 492–494, 1986.

46. Thomas SS, et al: Quantitative assessment of AFOs for children with cerebral palsy, Dev Med Child Neurol 31(suppl)7, 1989 (abstract).

47. Thomas SS, et al: Preliminary report on the effect of gait analysis on the clinical decision making process for children with cerebral palsy, Orthop Trans 16:10, 1992 (abstract).

48. Thomas SS, Supan TJ: A comparison of current biomechanical terms, J Prosthet Orthot 2:107–114, 1990.

49. Watt J, et al: A prospective study of inhibitive casting as an adjunct to physiotherapy for cerebral-palsied children, Dev Med Child Neurol 28:480–488, 1986.

50. Weber D: Use of the hinged AFO for children with spastic cerebral palsy and midfoot instability, J Assoc Child Prosthet Orthot Clin 25:61–65, 1991.

51. Weiss H, Bets HB: Method of rehabilitation in children with neuromuscular disorders, Pediatr Clin North Am 14:1009, 1967.

52. Winters TF, Gage JR, Hicks R: Gait patterns in spastic hemiplegia in children and young adults, J Bone Joint Surg 69A:437–441, 1987.

53. Zachazewski JE, Eberle ED, Jefferies M: Effect of tone-inhibiting casts and orthoses on gait: A case report, Phys Ther 62:453–455, 1982.

Bracing in Myelomeningocele

Mary Williams Clark

Most individuals born with myelomeningocele need the help of orthoses to stand and walk because of the lower limb paralysis resultant from their basic developmental anatomic spinal defect. Braces stabilize joints with inadequate muscle control; prevent progression of deformity (and, in certain instances, correct deformity); provide weight bearing on the lower limbs for both physiological and psychological benefits; and, for most of these individuals, facilitate active mobility.

There is now a plethora of available orthoses for these people, and the choice of a device for a particular patient is made more difficult by the need to make that device appropriate for both motor and developmental levels. The basic principles of alignment, stability, and range of joint motion combined with considerations of developmental, motor, and cognitive function must be applied to varied patient situations. Differences in patients' physical and lifestyle situations produce many permutations of appropriateness and choice. The changing economic climate of medical practice ensures that clinicians must also know and take into consideration the financial coverage arrangements of the patient. There are no current inclusive cost-benefit studies of these devices, and decisions are often tailored to local experience and expertise, without regard to (or even knowledge of) cost.

In this chapter, the words *orthosis* and *brace* are used synonymously. The use of spinal braces for myelomeningocele patients is covered in Chapters 8 and 14. Similarly, upper limb orthoses are applicable only in a few situations, and specific devices for myelomeningocele are not necessary. Therefore, this review is confined to orthoses of the lower limbs.

Bracing for those with myelomeningocele is usually not corrective but supportive; that is, most of the braces to be described cannot correct malalignment that is not passively correctable. Some flexion contractures at hip or knee, usually less than 25 degrees, can be accommo-

dated by knowledgeable orthotists, as can mild varus or valgus at the knee. (Most *apparent* varus/valgus seen at the knee during ambulation in these patients, however, on closer assessment is found to be hip rotation combined with some knee flexion.)

The effects of developmental stage and body size mean that a particular brace may be appropriate for a particular patient at one time but not earlier or later. This variability of need may also occur because many of these patients have changing effective motor levels due to the effects of tethered spinal cords or syringomyelia or hydromyelia, with progressive weakness and/or spasticity. These problems must be recognized and addressed by a knowledgeable neurosurgeon before orthoses are prescribed.

Clinicians in this field have different philosophies of bracing, influenced by their experience. Two of the broad approaches are opposite in intent and can be called *brace high, move lower as possible* versus *brace low, move higher as necessary*. Both are effective as long as follow-up is careful so that overburdening and understabilization are both altered as they become evident.

What follows is a descriptive list of available orthoses used for this population, beginning with those for the foot and working upward. Options at lower levels (e.g., AFOs) are all component options for higher-level braces as well (e.g., as part of hip-knee-ankle-foot orthoses [HKAFOs]). A Bibliography of published studies of orthoses for those with myelomeningocele follows at the end of the chapter.

FOOT ORTHOSES

Foot orthoses for sacral motor levels are not necessary in young children (preadolescent), but as foot deformities develop, secondary to weak or absent intrinsics or other muscle imbalance and increasing body

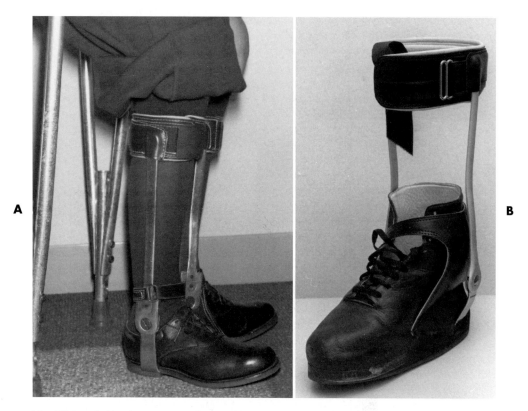

Fig. 37.1.   **A,** Double-upright AFO with medial leather T-strap, attached to steel-shank shoe.
B, Double-upright AFO with custom-molded shoe, steel-shank, and medial T-strap.

size, some improvement of pressure distribution can be provided by *custom-molded insoles*. In the author's experience, rigid orthoses are poor choices for this population because the plantar insensitivity predisposes to ulcers. The insoles may be semirigid, soft, or a combination of materials such as Plastazote, PPT, and Poron. These may be layered in various combinations, usually with the softer-durometer material (pink Plastazote or Poron) next to the foot because these durometers are closest to that of the fat pads of the foot or of the skin itself and with firmer material below to improve durability. These must be replaced at least every six months, frequently as often as every 2 or 3 months, when they bottom-out and no longer provide cushioning. These may replace the existing insoles in regular shoes, or, if necessary, shoes with toe boxes of extra depth can be ordered; these are now available in sneaker styles. The effectiveness of the insoles and the contours can be measured by the absence of thick localized callus on the feet and the absence of skin breakdown.

Congenital or neurogenic foot deformity, such as clubfoot, vertical talus, or calcaneus foot, may have been surgically corrected but with residual deformity and must also be accommodated by a pressure-distribution system of insole and shoe. In those few situations where the families have not allowed surgical correction, similar but more extensive combinations of accommodative orthoses and shoes must be designed.

ANKLE-FOOT ORTHOSES (AFOs)

S2 innervation or lower is rare in myelomeningocele patients, and therefore most of them have weak or absent gastrocnemius-soleus complex muscles. This allows their tibias unrestricted forward motion during mid-stance and late stance phases of gait, without the deceleration provided by the triceps surae. The ankle joints of these patients are usually without significant protective sensation; therefore at risk of Charcot's degenerative changes or physeal fractures over time. The gait pattern without ankle support is a crouch gait with maximum passive ankle dorsiflexion, knee flexion, and significant reliance on quadriceps strength. Therefore, the need for AFOs is almost universal among these people, whatever their additional bracing needs. The term *AFO* refers to any orthosis that controls the foot and ankle. The most commonly used at this time are molded plastic inshoe braces, but those with single or double metal uprights are also still used, particularly by some older members of this population.

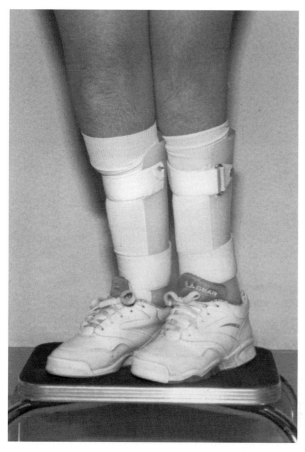

Fig. 37.2. Molded AFO in high-temperature thermoplastic (copolymer), with hook-loop straps, through D-rings.

Metal AFOs

Single or double uprights ("bars") are attached to a steel-shank shoe, with a leather or plastic cuff proximally (Fig. 37.1, *A*). A dorsiflexion stop is needed for protection of ankle joint and of the physes in the skeletally immature. Ankle joint options include adjustable springs or locks in dorsiflexion or plantar flexion. Leather T-straps are often added at the ankle to attempt control of varus/valgus (Fig. 37.1, *B*). *Advantages* include fewer skin problems, especially in warm weather; shoes usually leather "orthopedic" shoes and conform well to foot deformities; shoes may be custom-molded and extra-depth as needed; and shoes are paid for as part of the orthosis. *Disadvantages* include limited control of foot and ankle joints may allow progressive deformity and/or fracture and Charcot's changes. Metal AFOs are heavier than plastic braces and shoe style choice is limited.

Plastic AFOs

Plastic AFOs are molded in-shoe orthoses of thermoplastic material (Fig. 37.2). They may be material molding at low temperature (150 to 180° F) or high temperature (325 to 400° F).

- *Low-temperature materials,* such as Aquaplast and Kaysplint (polycaprolactone), can be molded directly onto the patient over stockinette or socks for same-day delivery. These are useful for infants and children up to age 4 or 5 years or about 45 lb; they last 2 to 4 months for temporary/trial use in older children. *Advantages* are immediate delivery and lower cost. *Disadvantages* are greater thickness than many other materials and lower durability. Also, these materials can be used only for young or small children.
- *High-temperature materials,* such as polypropylene, polyethelene, and copolymer (a combination of the two), are the current standard. They require a cast of the limb to be braced, which is used to produce a poured plaster positive over which the brace is fabricated. *Advantages* are that these materials can be modified for relief and weight-bearing areas on the plaster positive and the orthosis can be vacuum-formed for accurate fit. These materials are durable and can be molded quite thin. *Disadvantages* are that it usually takes several weeks to delivery and more expensive material and labor time are involved.

Solid ankle (nonarticulating) AFOs

Posterior shell with anterior calf strap is currently the "standard" molded AFO (MAFO) in use. The AFO is molded in 2 to 5 degrees of dorsiflexion to improve rollover from heel strike to foot flat during gait, if worn alone. Straps are usually hook-and-loop tape, and fit best and most snugly if used with a D-ring. Those intended for wear at night (e.g., postoperatively) may have a strap over the ankle and/or toes also. Posterolateral trim lines can vary to tailor the flexibility at the ankle. The footplate may be trimmed behind the metatarsal heads or more distally.

Articulating AFOs

Articulating AFOs feature the addition of plastic or metal ankle hinges, medial and lateral; they can be made with motion stops, to limit motion in dorsiflexion, and/or plantar flexion. Posterior straps, inelastic or elastic, may be added, running midline posteriorly as a dorsiflexion stop. The combination of both elastic and inelastic straps provides a good substitute for an absent quadriceps muscle, with the elastic simulating eccentric contraction, controlling forward progress of the tibia over the foot; the inelastic strap provides the ultimate stop, the allowable dorsiflexion range fixed by the length of the strap. (These straps tend to stretch over time, and the degree of dorsiflexion must be periodically inspected.) As mentioned previously, people with no active triceps surae require a dorsiflexion stop to protect their ankle.

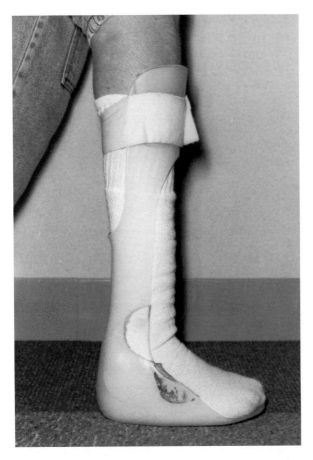

Fig. 37.3. Floor-reaction AFO, standard solid-ankle design.

Floor-reaction AFOs

Glancy and Lindseth described a molded AFO with an extended anterior shell, intended for midlumbar motor level patients. The design includes a rigid ankle, and floor-reaction force is thereby transmitted to the knee and becomes an extension vector. This can reinforce quadriceps that are becoming insufficient to extend a loaded knee against body weight. Lindseth also posits that pressure against the innervated area of skin just anterior and distal to the knee joint, which exists in the usual L4 sensory dermatome, provides proprioceptive feedback, which may also reinforce quadriceps contraction.

Options include:

1. *Single-unit FRAFO* (Fig. 37.3). *Advantages*—closely fitting, easy to fabricate, and the lightest weight of this design; may have dense foam lining, fabricated in same process and bonded to the outer plastic. *Disadvantages*—donned by inserting the foot and leg through the opening below the proximal anterior shell, from rear; may require rotation of the foot, which is difficult for some clients to do independently (and most difficult for a clinic physician to assist with);

outgrown rapidly during growth spurt and difficult to relieve or adjust to extend wear.

2. *Extendable FRAFO*—proximal section separates and overlaps medially and laterally; can be extended lengthwise to improve fit after growth in height, allowing longer period of fit.

3. *Rear-Entry FRAFO*—anterior shell extends entire way to proximal trimline and includes foot circumferentially. Easier to don than single-unit; stronger.

KNEE-ANKLE-FOOT ORTHOSES (KAFOs)

A patient with a strong L3 or L4 level has no active hip extensors (other than medial hamstrings at L4). As height increases, with increased upper body weight also, quadriceps may be insufficient to support the knee adequately in stance, especially with fatigue. Patients with relatively weak (some L3) or absent (L2) quadriceps need positive knee control; others may need medial-lateral knee joint control. These patients need KAFOs. If they have full passive hip range of motion, specifically hip extension, patients with even higher levels (L1) can walk without orthotic hip control. KAFOs consist of AFOs with attached metal uprights and thigh cuffs (Fig. 37.4). Design and fabrication options are as follows:

1. Uprights—*single* (in lightweight patients; usually placed lateral) or *double;* may be steel, aluminum, titanium, or carbon fiber composite.

2. Hinges and locks.

   (a) Drop lock—traditional and safe (stable); may be on lateral upright only or on lateral and medial; need to be moved by hand—difficult for some small and/or young hands (see Fig. 37.7, *B*).

   (b) Posterior offset hinges—place axis of rotation behind knee axis, allowing weight bearing in mild flexion to produce stability (extension moment in front of axis) without a lock; somewhat less wear on clothing than drop locks (see Fig. 37.4, *A*).

   (c) Bail lock—half-ring extending posteriorly; can be passively unlocked by pressing against chair etc. to allow flexion; locks automatically on extension.

   (d) Plastic hinges—single-axis joints through overlapping plastic thigh and calf cuff extensions; useful for lightweight patients only.

3. Cuffs

   (a) Plastic—lightweight; easier to keep clean; can be heat molded to modify fit. Usually posterior (Fig. 37.4, *A*); can be anterior for sitting ease or rotational control (Fig. 37.4, *B* and *C*).

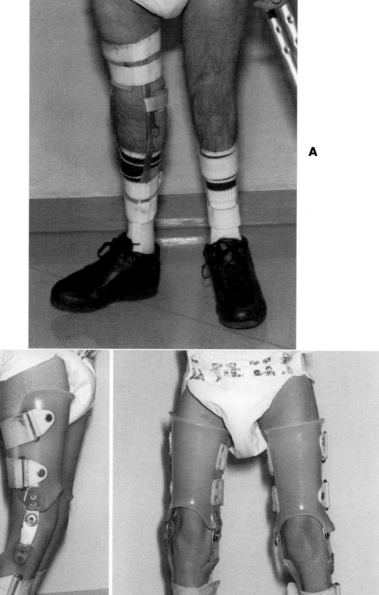

Fig. 37.4. **A,** KAFO with in-shoe molded AFO, thermoplastic posterior (traditional) thigh cuff, and posterior offset knee hinge. (This patient converted happily from double-upright to in-shoe orthoses at age 34.) **B** and **C,** KAFOs with nontraditional anterior thigh cuffs.

(b) Leather—more forgiving for skin; stain easily; heavier.

KAFOs may use in-shoe or attached-to-shoe AFOs; many older patients have successfully and happily made the transition from attached "orthopedic" shoes to molded in-shoe AFOs and more shoe variety (see Fig. 37.4, *A*); many others happily continue to wear attached shoes (see Fig. 37.1, *A*).

HIP-KNEE-ANKLE-FOOT ORTHOSES (HKAFOs)

Rotational control

Patients with motor levels at upper lumbar or thoracic levels usually require some orthotic hip control for stability; those with lower levels may need some rotational control. Young patients of all levels may benefit from total support for their initial upright experiences (see Standing Frames below), those with more active muscle distally weaning out to lower braces. Technically, rotational-control orthoses are termed *HKAFOs* even though they do not control the knees. There are two types in use: twister cables and rotation straps.

1. *Twister cables* have a pelvic band with attached cables of twisted spring steel with torque to produce internal or (usually) external rotation by attaching to the shoes or AFOs. These were used in the past for femoral anteversion. *Disadvantages* are weight and clothing wear (Fig. 37.5).
2. *Rotation straps* are elastic and attach to a fabric pelvic band and to buckles on AFOs or to an eyelet attachment to shoestrings; they can be wrapped around the thigh and leg to produce internal or external rotation. *Disadvantages* are frequent need for replacement for stretching and occasional skin problems (Fig. 37.6).

Traditional HKAFOs

Traditional HKAFOs include pelvic band attached to the uprights, hip hinges, knee hinges, and a form of AFO. Hip and knee hinges may have drop locks if needed (Fig. 37.7). They may also include a larger molded pelvic girdle or thoracic support. The hip control eliminates the trunklurch necessitated by weak hip abductors and controls limb rotation. Gait in these is usually swing through (or for younger or weaker patients, "drag to") with walker or crutches; some patients take advantage of "play" in the system and accomplish reciprocal foot-after-foot gait in these. Some design options have improved the ability to reciprocate in HKAFOs:

1. *Thrust-bearing hip joints*—Hinges that contain cylindrical bearings allow hinging in the face of lateral thrust, without binding; they can be made

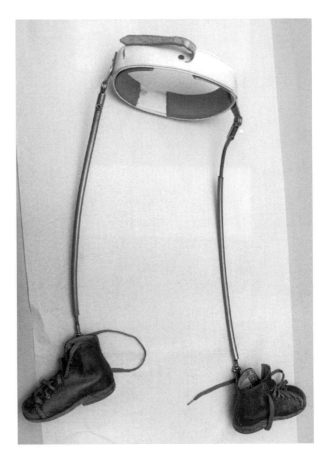

Fig. 37.5.   Twister cables, with molded pelvic band.

with a drop-lock or a specific range of motion, customized by grinding an arc on the base plate behind the hinge (Fig. 37.8). Materials and other options are as for KAFOs.

2. *Hip guidance orthoses*—These are a form of HKAFO with a rigid body brace; low-friction hip joints with flexion, and extension stops, holding limbs somewhat abducted; optional thigh cuffs; and platforms for feet in shoes (rather than in-shoe AFOs). These orthoses are used with a walker or crutches (Fig. 37.9).

Reciprocating gait orthoses (RGOs)

The category of HKAFOs now includes RGOs, braces designed to enable an easier foot-after-foot gait. These braces appeal to families who define (consciously or unconsciously) "walking" as putting one foot ahead of the other. Clinics that use them for selected (thoracic and upper lumbar motor level) patients note ability to achieve independent mobility at a younger age (e.g., 20 to 24 months) with less apparent energy expenditure than seen with traditional HKAFOs and swing-through gait. *Disadvantages* are expense, difficulty with independent catheterization

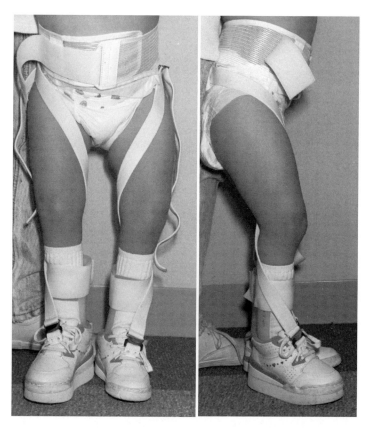

Fig. 37.6. Elastic rotation straps, with fabric pelvic girdle and buckle attachments to shoes; here wrapped for external rotation.

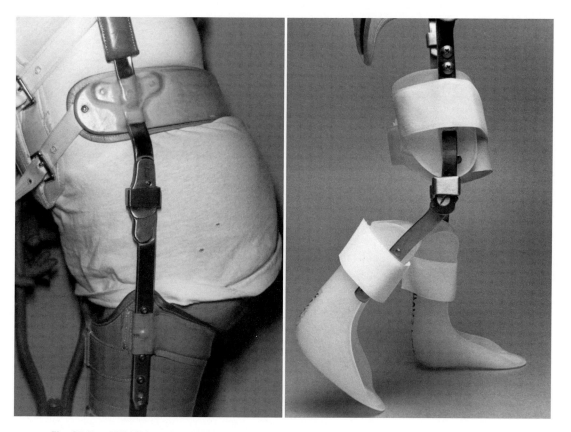

Fig. 37.7. HKAFOs, with single uprights, molded AFOs, drop locks at hips and knees, molded pelvic band, and extended lateral uprights for attachment of fabric anterior thoracic support.

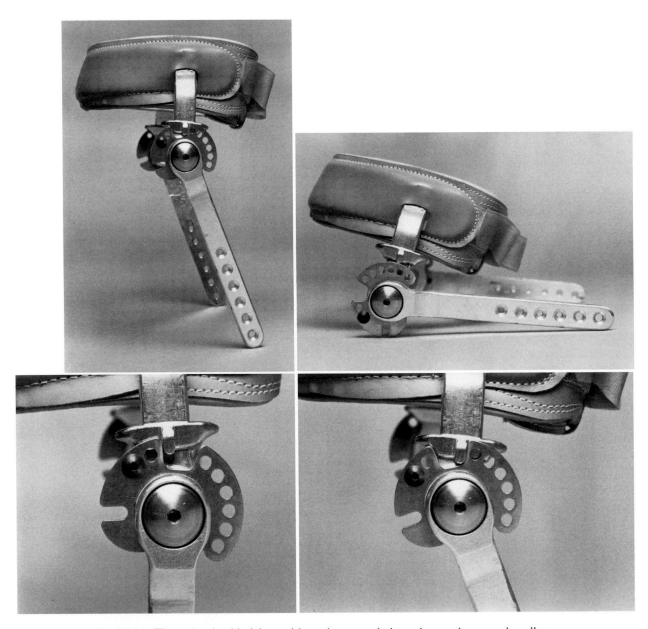

Fig. 37.8.   Thrust-bearing hip joints, with motion-control plates that can be ground to allow a range of flexion and extension (here 0 to 20 degrees of flexion). The hinge itself has cylindrical bearings, arranged radially, to allow motion without binding under lateral stress.

but the cable plate has its own arc of motion, which allows an active flexor (in an L1 or lower patient) to advance one leg, and the pull is transmitted by the cable to extend the other hip. The leg may also be advanced by momentum, as provided by trunk muscles to the pelvis, or by passive extension of the trunk over the hip on the opposite side, providing passive assisted flexion.

2. *Horizontal cable RGO*—Designed by Motloch, this eliminates the arching cables, uses a different hip joint, but provides essentially the same effect without the awkwardness of cables over or under clothing; this RGO is less heavy than the isocentric RGO.

3. *Isocentric RGO*—Another attempt to avoid the space and dressing problems of the original cable system, this provides a centrally pivoting posterior bar on the pelvic band, which attaches to hip joints at each end. It is a significantly heavier brace than the other RGOs.

Frame-type orthoses

Another form of HKAFO is the frame-type orthosis, usually mounted on a base plate, which allows hands-free, crutchless standing and may allow mobility by swiveling.

1. *Standing frame*—These are usually for children ages 10 months to 2 years: rectangular or oval base and a frame posteriorly, against which the patient can be supported by pelvic and thoracic straps; may have a padded knee bar anteriorly and foot-plates to accept and stabilize shoes (Fig. 37.11).

2. *Parapodium*—This was originally designed at Ontario Crippled Children's Centre, Toronto; rounded oval base plate with tubular uprights, knee and thoracic supports; hip and knee locks controlled by rotating handles at hips allow sitting in the frame (Fig. 37.12, *C*); a later version has a fixed anterior extension assist, an upright on the base that allows a *pull-to-stand* motion (Fig. 37.12).

3. *Rochester parapodium*—A team at the University of Rochester Medical Center, Rochester, New York, developed modifications to the parapodium as follows: separate locking mechanisms for hips and knees (allowing more controlled descent to sitting and activities to be done with knees locked and hips flexed—sitting, bending down, lock releases operating flat (not into rotation) by one hand (freeing a hand for balance or support in going from stand to sit and requiring less lateral space), and flat side bars (providing more rigidity).

4. *ORLAU swivel walker*—This was originally developed at the Orthotic Research and Locomotor

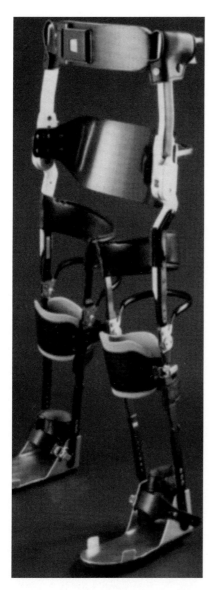

Fig. 37.9. Hip guidance orthosis (HGO) designed at the Orthotic Research and Locomotor Assessment Unit (ORLAU), Robert Jones and Agnes Hunt Hospital, Oswestry, England. Limbs are abducted slightly, hip joints are low friction, and foot pieces are platforms to accept shoes.

(also a problem with other HKAFOs), and some clothing problems. They have been shown in one study to allow faster walking speed, but large and/or controlled studies have not yet been done.

Options available are:

1. *LSU RGO*—Motloch developed the original RGO design while at Ontario Crippled Children's Centre, Toronto. With Motloch's permission, Douglas, at Louisiana State University, modified the original design (Fig. 37.10). The arching cables attach to the outside plate of double hip joints; the hip hinge joint can be locked, preventing forward flexion at the hips,

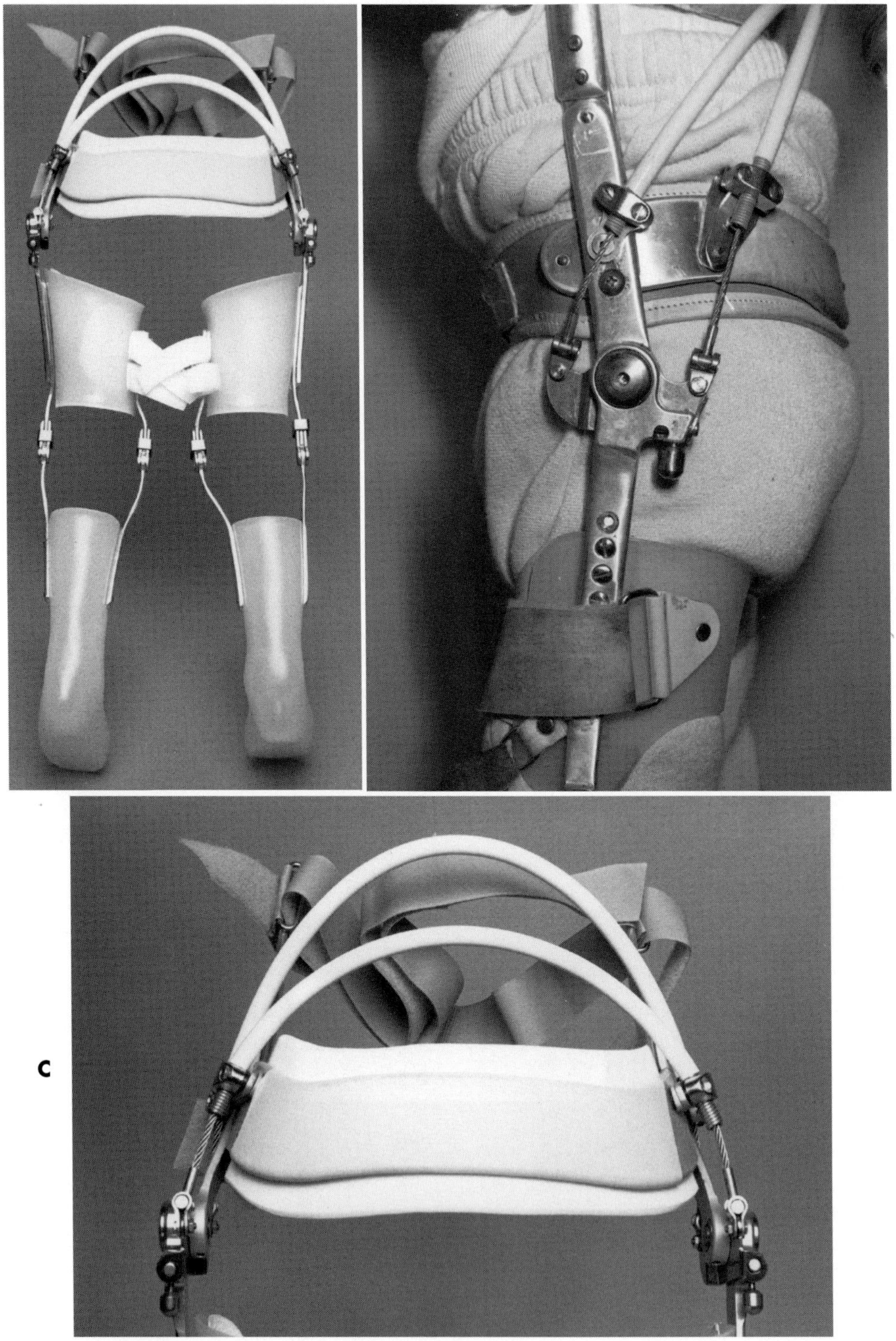

Fig. 37.10. LSU reciprocating gait orthosis (RGO) designed at Ontario Crippled Children's Centre, Toronto, and modified at Louisiana State University, New Orleans. Posterior view (**A**) shows double cables in low-friction housing, attaching to latch plates at hips (**B**); hip lock (inferior and posterior [**B** and **C**]) prevents forward flexion at hips, and force exerted at one hip (e.g., active hip flexion or passive hip extension by thoracic extension) is transmitted to the other by the cables, so that flexion of one hip produces extension force at the other.

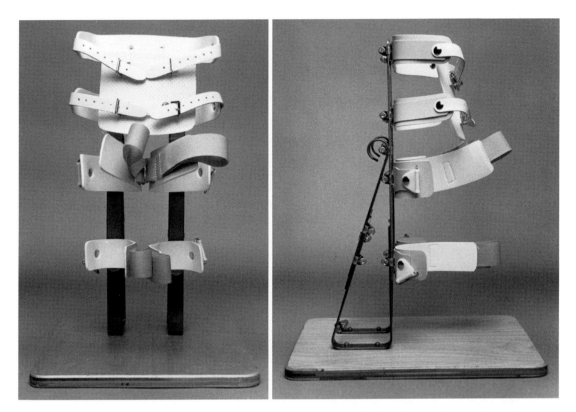

Fig. 37.11. Standing frame, anterior and side views; this version is stable; another version with smaller oval base plate, posterior A-frame, and molded footplates (into which shoes can fit) can allow early swivel walking with training.

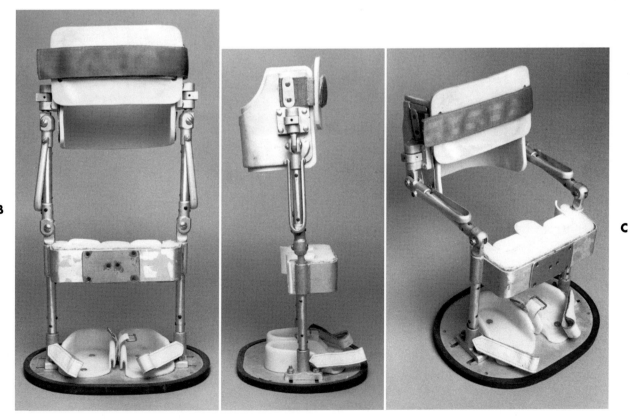

A,B

C

Fig. 37.12. Parapodium designed at Ontario Crippled Children's Centre, Toronto. Anterior standing view (**A**) shows anterior knee bar and thoracic pad, with locking handles lateral, in locked position (hip and knee joints transversely oriented). **B**, Lateral view of same. **C**, Frame in seated position, handles anterior, which has rotated the lateral tubes and joints 90 degrees.

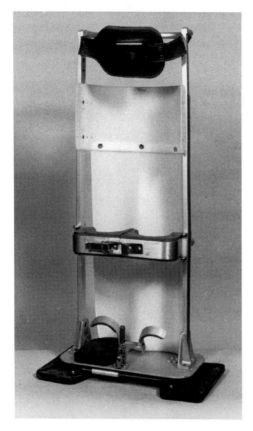

Fig. 37.13. Swivel walker, ORLAU version, with base plates upon which the frame pivots when the other side is unloaded by lateral weight shift.

Assessment Unit, Oswestry, England, for adult paraplegics; similar to a parapodium but without hip or knee joints and with the base mounted on a pair of swivel footplates. Weight shifting laterally allows the patient and brace to swivel automatically forward on the weight-bearing limb; this requires less energy for advancement than (and is a different motion from) swiveling by upper trunk and limb rotation, which advance the parapodiums. The parapodiums and swivel walker are usually used without crutches but may provide swing-through gait with crutches when desired (Fig. 37.13).

BIBLIOGRAPHY

Asher M, Olson J: Factors affecting the ambulatory status of patients with spina bifida cystica, J Bone Joint Surg 65A:350–356, 1983.

Beaty JH, Canale ST: Current concepts review: Orthopaedic aspects of myelomeningocele, J Bone Joint Surg 72A:626–630, 1990.

Bick EM: Classics of orthopaedics, Philadelphia, 1976, JB Lippincott.

Charney EB, Melchionni JB, Smith DR: Community ambulation by children with myelomeningocele and high-level paralysis, J Pediatr Orthop 11:579–582, 1991.

Douglas R, et al: The Louisiana State University reciprocating gait orthosis, Orthopedics 6:834–839, 1983.

Findley, Agre: Ambulation in the adolescent with spina bifida: II. Oxygen cost of mobility, Arch Phys Med Rehabil 69:855–861, 1988.

Flandry F, et al: Functional ambulation in myelodysplasia: The effects of orthotic selection on physical and physiologic performance, J Pediatr Orthop 6:661–665, 1986.

Gram MC: The parapodium, Woodridge IL, 1991, MM Therapeutics.

Glancy J, Lindseth RE: The polypropylene solid-ankle orthosis, Orthot Prosthet 26:14–26, 1972.

Lindseth RE, Glancy J: Polypropylene lower-extremity braces for paraplegia due to myelomeningocele, J Bone Joint Surg 56A:556–563, 1974.

Hoffer MM, et al: Functional ambulation in patients with myelomeningocele, J Bone Joint Surg 55A:137–148, 1973.

Hullin MG, Robb JE, Loudon LR: Ankle-foot orthosis function in low-level myelomeningocele, J Pediatr Orthop 12:518–521, 1992.

Korpela RA, Siirtola TO, Koivikko MJ: The cost of assistive devices for children with mobility limitation, Pediatrics 90:597–602, 1992.

Mazur JM, et al: Orthopaedic management of high-level spina bifida: Early walking compared with early use of a wheelchair, J Bone Joint Surg 71A:56–61, 1989.

Mazur JM, et al: Swing-through vs. reciprocating gait patterns in patients with thoracic-level spina bifida, 3 Kinder chir. 45 (suppl 1):23–25, 1990.

McCall RE, Schmidt WT: Clinical experience with the reciprocating gait orthosis in myelodysplasia, J Pediatr Orthrop 6:157–161, 1986.

Motloch W: The parapodium: An orthotic device for neuromuscular disorders, Artif Limbs 15:37–47, 1971.

Rang M: Anthology of orthopaedics, New York, 1977, Churchill Livingstone.

Rose GK, Sankarankutty M, Stallard J: A clinical review of the orthotic treatment of myelomeningocele patients, J Bone Joint Surg 65B:242–246, 1983.

Rose J, et al: Energy cost of walking in normal children and those with cerebral palsy, J Pediatr Orthop 9:276–279, 1989.

Rose J, et al: The energy expenditure index: A method to quantitate and compare walking energy expenditure, J Pediatr Orthrop 11:571–578, 1991.

Yngve DA, Douglas R, Roberts JM: The reciprocating gait orthosis in myelomeningocele, J Pediatr Orthop 4:304–310, 1984.

ASSISTIVE DEVICES

INTRODUCTION
Bertram Goldberg

In the *Atlas of Orthotics,* Second Edition, Norris C. Carroll,[1] in his introductory paragraph to "Wheelchairs and Mobility Aids," aptly started with a quote from Nichols: "Mobility is the foundation upon which the skills of daily living are built." The pertinence and continued relevance of this quote are well brought out in this section, which discusses the assistive devices so necessary for the continued mobility and enjoyment of patients with diseases or traumatic conditions of the central nervous and musculoskeletal systems.

From the most basic devices such as canes and crutches to the more complex such as sip-and-puff wheelchairs, all are unique in their function and can and should be specifically prescribed to the patient according to his or her needs. Each patient must be individually evaluated regarding age, disease or post-traumatic deficit, and economic or social needs in or-der to provide the most efficient and cost-effective system to permit that patient to continue to exist and, more than that, function at the highest level, both physically and cognitively, in an increasingly complex society.

The authors in this section have accomplished their task of providing the reader with the most up-to-date data on these devices, not only from the technical aspects but also from the aspects of how the patient and the device, after having been properly prescribed, should interact. By keeping up to date with this information, both the patient care provider and patient will find satisfaction in the final result.

REFERENCES
1. Carroll NC: Atlas of orthotics, ed 2, St. Louis, 1985, CV Mosby.
2. Nichols PJR: Prescription of wheelchairs. In Murdoch G, editor: The advance in orthotics, London, 1976, Edward Arnold Publishers.

Canes, Crutches, and Walkers

Bertram Goldberg
Maurice LeBlanc
Joan Edelstein

The use of assistive devices for ambulation dates back to antiquity. It would seem obvious that early man, when hindered by injury or disease, would have come up with some sort of support to enable him to get about, or else early death would have been the result, either from starvation or predators. The earliest known evidence of the use of a supportive device dates to ancient Egypt; a carving on the entrance portal of Hirkouf's tomb about the time of the Sixth Dynasty, 2830 B.C., depicts a figure leaning on a crutch-like staff. (Fig. 38.1).[15,35] From that time on, the crutch remained a simple "T" design until the use of the saw around 1800 made it possible to split the staff, spread the two halves, and insert a cross-piece for the hand.

Today, new developments in materials and design, guided by further knowledge of man and his diseases, have led to a myriad of cane, crutch, and walker designs that, when properly prescribed, enable a person to continue to function in society at the maximum level possible (Figs. 38.2 and 38.3).[29,51] To these have been added various types of tips to permit safer, more comfortable ambulation, such as metal tips or spikes, which can be retractable, to use in the winter (Fig. 38.4), or the energy-storing crutch tip (Fig. 38.5), which purports to provide a bit more spring during lift-off, not dissimilar in concept to the new family of prosthetic dynamic response feet.[51] Another design is that of the ISY Walking Crutch Attachment permitting somewhat smoother rollover during gait (Fig. 38.6).

Assistive devices serve one or more functions for a given user:
- Broaden the base of support.
- Improve balance and stability.
- Reduce load on one lower limb.
- Assist propulsion.
- Transmit sensory cues through the hand(s).
- Notify passersby that the user requires special con-

siderations, such as additional time when crossing streets or a seat on the bus or train.
- Enable the individual with paralysis to maneuver in places inaccessible to a wheelchair and to obtain the physiological benefits of upright posture.[1,12,36,96]

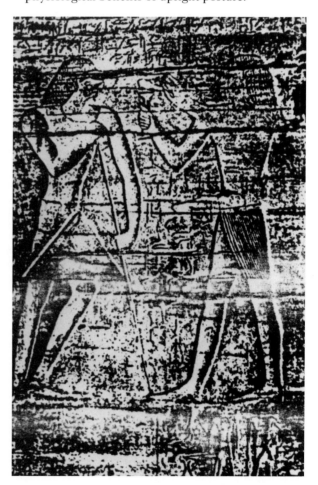

Fig. 38.1. Tomb of Hirkouf in the Isle of Elephantine, Egypt, Sixth Dynasty (2830 B.C.). *(From Epstein S: Art, history and the crutch, Ann Med Hist 9:304, 1937.)*

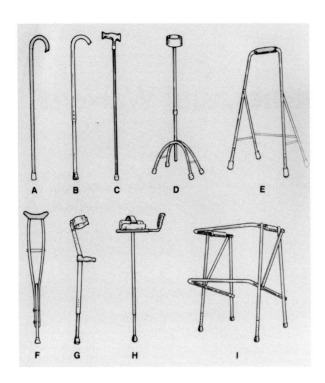

Fig. 38.2. **A,** C-handle or crook-top cane. **B,** Adjustable aluminum cane. **C,** Functional grip cane. **D,** Adjustable wide-base quad cane. **E,** Hemi-walker. **F,** Adjustable wooden axillary crutch. **G,** Adjustable aluminum Lofstrand crutch. **H,** Forearm support or platform support. **I,** Walker or walkerette. *(From DeLisa DA, editor: Rehabilitation medicine: Principles and Practice, ed 2, Philadelphia, 1993, JB Lippincott.)*

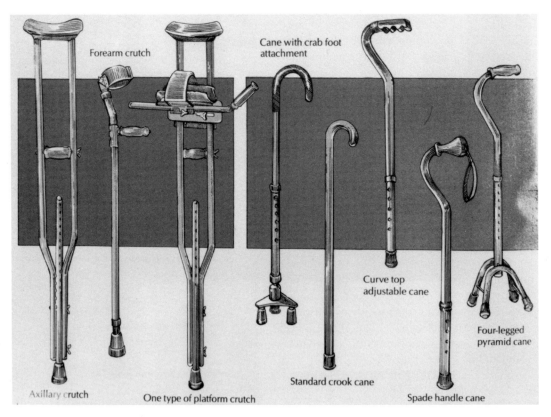

Fig. 38.3. Commonly used crutches and canes. *(From Joyce BM, Kirby RL: Canes, crutches and walkers, Am Fam Pract 43:535, 1991.)*

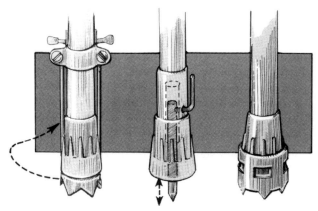

Retractable metal tip   Retractable metal spike   Removable mace tip

Fig. 38.4. Various tips to winterize ambulation aids. *(From Joyce BM, Kirby RL: Canes, crutches and walkers, Am Fam Pract 43:535, 1991.)*

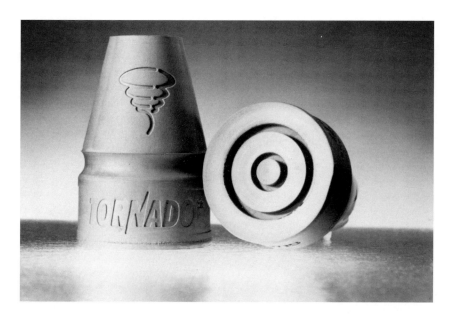

Fig. 38.5. Energy-storing crutch tip. *(Courtesy of Guardian Products, Inc., Simi Valley, CA.)*

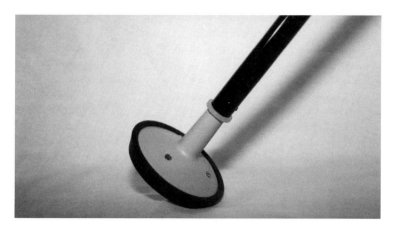

Fig. 38.6. ISY walking crutch attachment. *(Courtesy of Blooming Company, Hong Kong.)*

CANES

Canes, made of either wood or adjustable aluminum (Fig. 38.7), are the simplest of the assistive devices and for that reason tend to be forgotten in the total care of patient's whose need for such a device may not be apparent early on in their care, such as in the patient with early degenerative arthritis/synovitis of the hip or knee. In fact, all too often the patient, when offered the use of a cane will refuse, thinking that it is a sign of disability or senility. Blount, in his classic treatise of 1956, *Don't Throw Away the Cane,* demonstrated how important its use is.[15]

Cane design consists of the standard crook handle, enabling the person to hang it over the forearm or the back of a chair; the spade handle cane, making grip more comfortable; and the curve top cane, combining grip comfort with a more physiologic position of the tip relative to the grip handle (see Figs. 38.2 and 38.3). The Klik telescopic cane, developed in Canada, lengthens from a compact size of 22½ inch (57.2 cm) to a maximum size of 39¾ inch (101 cm), thus making transport more convenient (Fig. 38.8).

By adding a widened base to the tip of the cane, the total base of support can be increased, thus increasing stability during gait (Fig. 38.9).[51] Milczarek and colleagues[66] have stated, however, that in the hemiparetic individual, the four-footed cane offers no advantage over a standard cane.

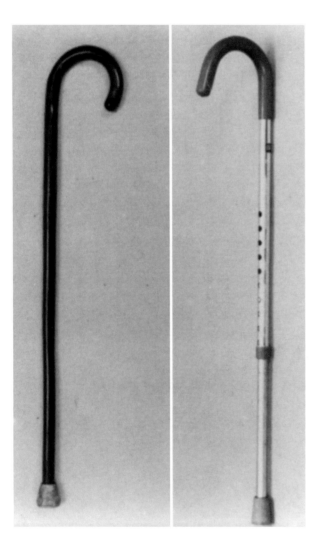

Fig. 38.7. Wooden cane and adjustable aluminum cane. *(From Atlas of orthotics, ed 2, St. Louis.) 1985, CV Mosby.*

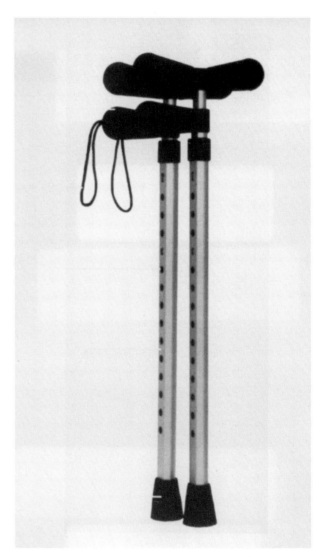

Fig. 38.8. KLICK telescopic cane. *(Courtesy of KLICK Product Sales Corp., Lynn, MA.)*

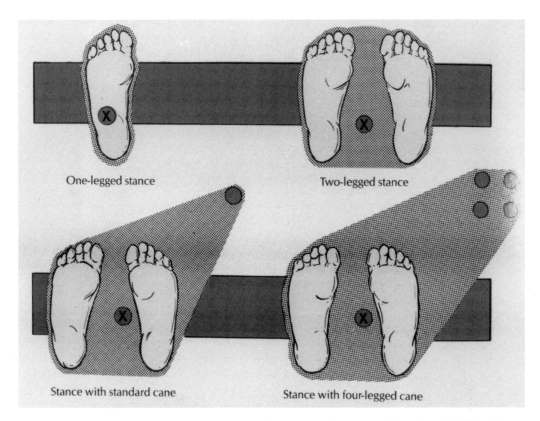

Fig. 38.9.   Stability can be increased by enlarging the base of support. *(From Joyce BM, Kirby RL: Canes, crutches and walkers, Am Fam Pract 43:535, 1991.)*

CRUTCHES

Crutches are of three major types (see Figs. 38.2 and 38.3):[51]
- Axillary or underarm crutches
- Forearm or Lofstrand crutches
- Platform crutches

Axillary crutches are adjustable for both hand height and overall length. They have classically been made of wood (Fig. 38.10). The newer models are made of aluminum and have a ball-detent adjustment, which permits fitting time to be reduced to seconds, and a quick-adjust hand system (Fig. 38.11).

Forearm or Lofstrand crutches are also made of aluminum and are adjustable in length and cuff position (Fig. 38.12).

Platform crutches provide a trough to permit forearm weight bearing for those patients whose upper limb cannot bear the full force of weight transmission (Fig. 38.13). Even though crutches permit up to 80% weight bearing of the body, they also require a significant increase in energy expenditure. This is due mostly to the vertical rise of the body to clear the ground during swing-to or swing-through gait.[56,86,94]

Complications are not uncommon with the use of crutches and must be watched for, especially in the patient whose ability to communicate is impaired. These problems can occur in the region of the hand, arm, shoulder, or axillary area.[56] Injury to the ulnar or median nerves can occur and adaptations have been made in crutch grips, such as in the hand piece of the Right Grip forearm crutch, to prevent this from taking place (Fig. 38.14). Other complications are axillary artery thrombosis and compression of the radial nerve.[4,18,87]

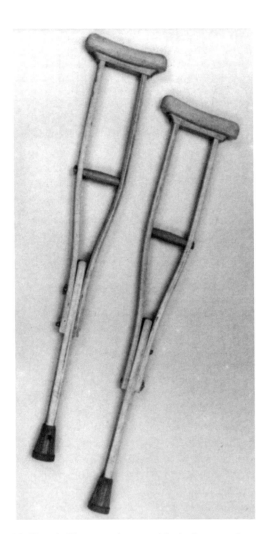

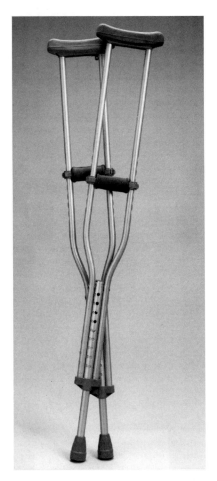

Fig. 38.10. Axillary crutches provide the best trunk support and can transfer up to 80% of body weight. *(From Atlas of orthotics, ed 2, St. Louis, 1985, CV Mosby.)*

Fig. 38.11. Red Dot crutches with a quick-adjust hand adjustment to assist in rapid fitting. *(Courtesy of Guardian Products, Inc., Simi Valley, CA.)*

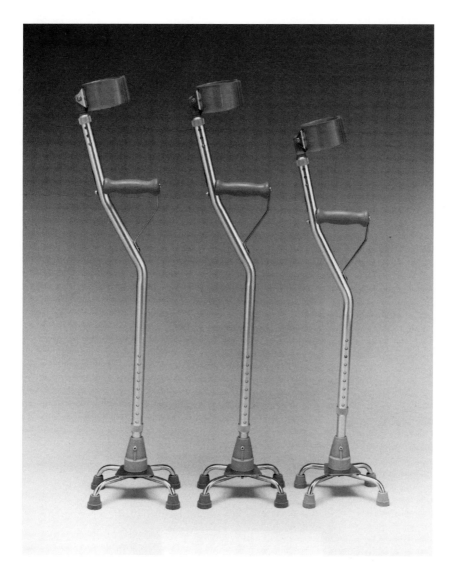

Fig. 38.12.   Gaiter-Aid crutch. Pivoting quad base provides solid footing, and the cuff helps in forearm positioning. *(Courtesy of Guardian Products, Inc., Simi Valley, CA.)*

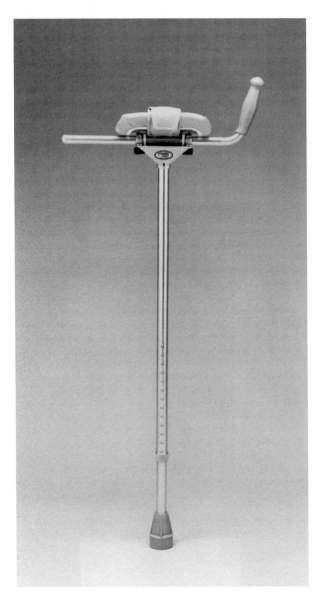

Fig. 38.13. Platform crutch for forearm support. *(Courtesy of Guardian Products, Inc., Simi Valley, CA.)*

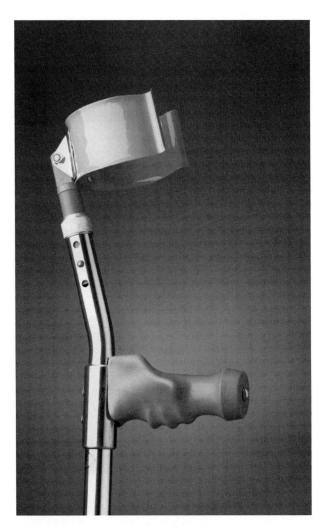

Fig. 38.14. The Right Grip forearm crutch distributes weight bearing to the hypothenar muscles and thus away from the carpal tunnel area. *(Courtesy of Guardian Products, Inc., Simi Valley, CA.)*

WALKERS

Walkers, as crutches, come in a variety of types (see Fig. 38.2; Fig. 38.15):[51]
- Standard
- Folding
- Reciprocating
- Rolling
- Platform

The standard walker, made of aluminum, consists of the four-post base and adjustable limbs to permit proper positioning for the patient. The folding, rolling, and platform walkers are variations on this basic design to enable the individual to get about more comfortably with the least amount of energy expended as possible. The Red Dot walker with swivel wheels and rear glide brakes is an excellent example of how this can be accomplished (Fig. 38.16). The Strider family of walkers conforms to the needs of both the adult and the pediatric populations with adjustable wheels and handles (Fig. 38.17). For the geriatric population, the Gemstone rolling walker, which comes in three basic designs, enables the individual to ambulate with the appropriate amount of support and to become more independent in society, with its built-in seat and basket (Fig. 38.18).

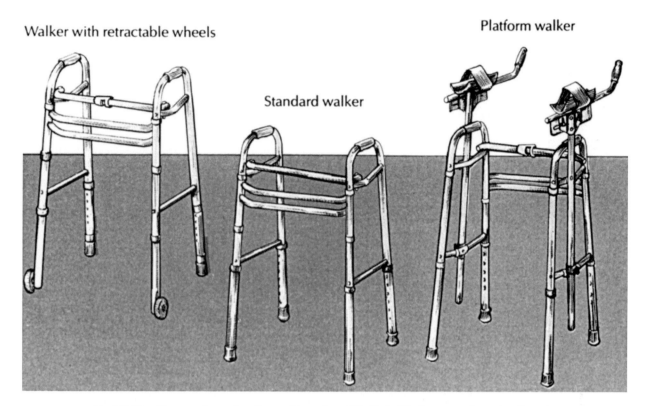

Fig. 38.15. Commonly used walkers. *(From Joyce BM, Kirby RL: Canes, crutches and walkers, Am Fam Pract 43:535, 1991.)*

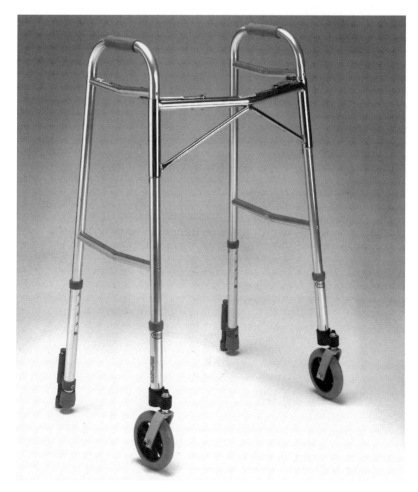

Fig. 38.16. Red Dot walker with 5-inch swivel wheels and rear glide brakes, which are in contact with the ground only when weight is applied. *(Courtesy of Guardian Products, Inc., Simi Valley, CA.)*

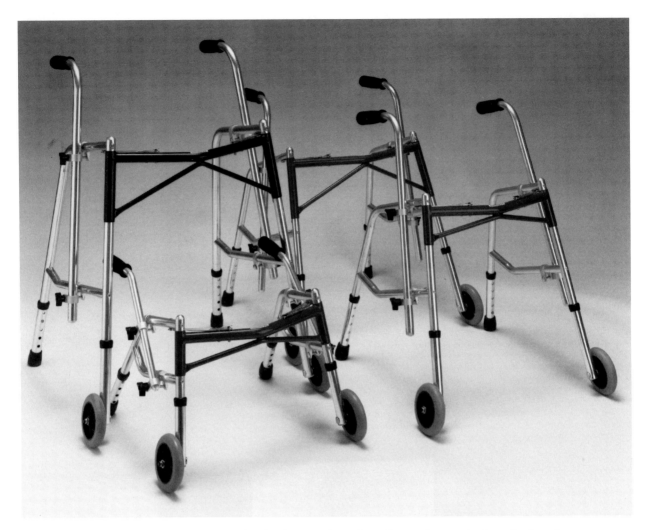

Fig. 38.17. The Strider family of walkers conform the walker to the user in that wheels and handles can be adjusted for postural requirements. *(Courtesy of Guardian Products, Inc., Simi Valley, CA.)*

Adaptations, as necessary, can be added to any particular walker, such as for the child with cerebral palsy, in which a hip guard can be built on to permit a more stable upright position (Fig. 38.19). Aquaplast can be used to make a walker handle more conforming so as to prevent some of the complications in the hand mentioned earlier with crutch usage (Fig. 38.20).[103]

Reciprocating walkers, such as the ORLAU VCG swivel walker (Fig. 38.21), are prescribed for the child with more severe neuromuscular disease to permit maintenance of an upright posture and ambulation, albeit with a significant amount of energy expenditure.[97]

MEASUREMENT GUIDELINES FOR ASSISTIVE DEVICES

Having decided on the type of device the patient needs, the practitioner must ensure that it is fitted properly. This should be a combined approach involving not only the practitioner and patient but the medical equipment supplier.[69] Ross[85] has shown, in a study of 86 women and 58 men, 61 to 80 years of age, that this integrated approach provides a significant improvement in function and reduction in falls.

Correct height of the assistive device and proper positioning of the handle or cuff enable the user to walk with the least effort and the greatest comfort. Measure-

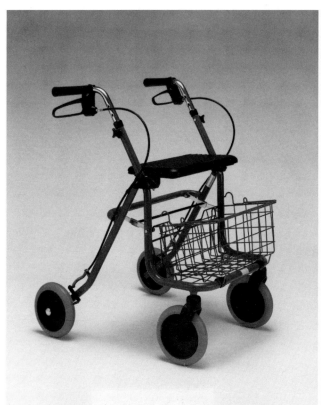

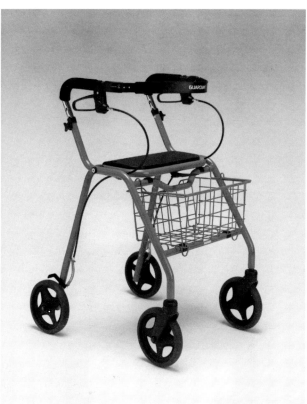

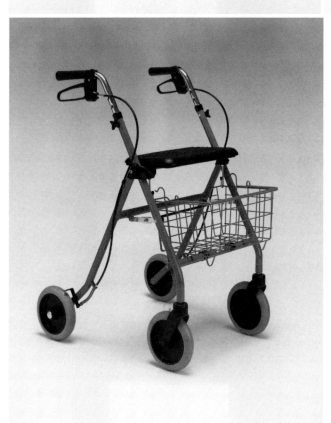

Fig. 38.18. Gemstone rolling walker with hand-activated brakes, seats, and baskets. *(Courtesy of Guardian Products, Inc., Simi Valley, CA.)*

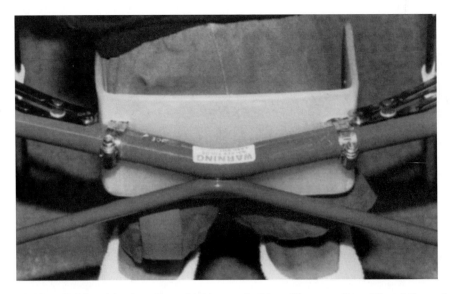

Fig. 38.19. Child position in walker with hip guard. *(From Thompson-Rangel T, et al: Customized walker adaptions for a child with cerebral palsy, JACPOC 27:97, 1992.)*

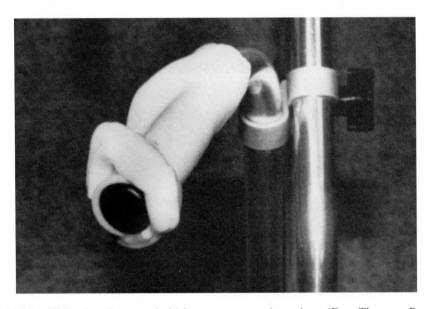

Fig. 38.20. Walker handle covered with low-temperature Aquaplast. *(From Thompson-Rangel T, et al: Customized walker with adaptions for a child with cerebral palsy, JACPOC 27:97, 1992.)*

ment is strongly influenced by the type of gait pattern used and the shoe heel height.

Improper cane measurement may be related to increased risks of falls among the elderly, as mentioned previously.[88] Misfitted canes generally are too long, causing the user to lean forward; too short a cane imposes undue stress on the lumbosacral region. Crutches that are too short compel the user to lean forward, whereas those that are too long force the

shoulders up and risk compression of the radial nerve[18,63,81,87] or suprascapular nerve.[93] Even when crutches are adjusted properly but used incorrectly, some patients experience redness, pain, and abrasion of the lateral chest; tenderness over the medial aspect of the arm; cramping of the triceps; bruising of the medial epicondyle; shoulder pain; and ulnar neuropathy.[22] Individuals with severely limited walking ability are more apt to use walkers, as compared with other assis-

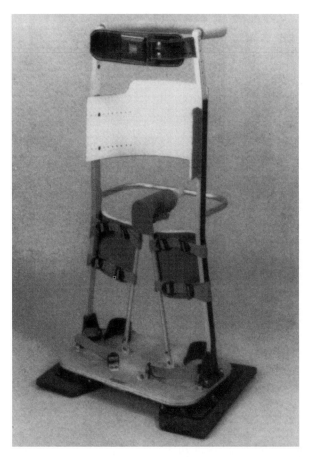

Fig. 38.21. ORLAU VCG swivel walker. *(From Stallard J, et al: The ORLAU VCG swivel walker for muscular dystrophy patients, Prosthet Orthot Int 16:46, 1992.)*

tive devices. Although walkers provide considerable stability, they do not eliminate the risk of falling.[19]

The methods suggested include the total height of the device with accessories, such as rubber tip, hand cushion, and axillary pad in place. Unless specified, the individual should be wearing the type of shoes that will be worn when using the device. The procedures are guidelines that may need to be altered to suit a given patient, with particular consideration paid to the individual's body proportions and motor power.

Cane

With the cane held perpendicular to the floor, the highest point of the cane should be level with the greater trochanter[63] or the wrist crease.[26,55,67]

Walker

Most patients prefer having the walker adjusted so that the handle lies at the ulnar styloid when the individual stands erect with the elbow flexed 15 degrees.[44]

Forearm crutch

The patient should stand with the crutch hand piece adjusted to provide 15 to 30 degrees of elbow flexion; more elbow flexion is required for gait patterns that require the user to lift both feet from the floor simultaneously. The crutch should contact the floor 5 to 10 cm lateral and 15 cm anterior to the foot. The cuff should lie on the proximal third of the forearm, approximately 2.5 to 4 cm below the olecranon process.[63,90]

Triceps crutch

The upper cuff should contact the proximal third of the arm, approximately 5 cm below the anterior fold of the axilla. The lower cuff should lie 1 to 4 cm below the olecranon process to avoid bony contact, yet provide adequate stability to the arm.[63]

Axillary crutch

The crutch should extend from the lateral chest to a point slightly in front and to the side of the foot. Hand piece placement should enable the patient to have a 30-degree resting elbow flexion angle.[83] Less flexion is suitable for the individual who walks by alternating foot steps. Ideally, one should measure each crutch with the patient standing in a secure environment, such as the parallel bars. Axillary crutches should extend from a point approximately 4 to 5 cm (2 finger breadths) below the axilla to a point on the floor 5 cm lateral and 15 cm anterior to the foot or to a point 15 to 20 cm directly lateral to the foot.[77] Alternative methods to determine crutch height are to subtract 40 cm from the patient's height[11,73] or make the crutch equal 77% of the subject's height.[9]

In the supine position, the crutch should extend from the anterior axillary fold to a point 10 to 15 cm lateral to the anatomic heel.[27,54,77] In the sitting position, the patient can abduct both arms to shoulder level and extend the elbows. Crutch length is the distance from the tip of the middle finger to the tip of the olecranon process of the opposite arm.[70]

The hand piece should provide 15 to 30 degrees of elbow flexion.[77] An easy way of determining hand piece placement is to position the hand piece so that its distance from the bottom of the axillary piece equals the distance from the patient's olecranon to outstretched thumb.[70] If the crutch has a forearm platform, it should be angled so that the patient has maximum comfort and control of the crutch; ordinarily the forearm rests on the platform at a 90-degree angle to the upper arm. Measuring may be facilitated with the use of special devices[2,16,102] or variations on the techniques described.[25,101]

GAIT PATTERNS

The way one uses assistive devices can be described by indicating the sequence of foot movement.[8,14,20,21,28,46,61,62,71,74,95,109] Selection of gait pattern(s) depends on the patient's ability to move the feet reciprocally, tolerate full load on each leg, push the body off the floor by pressing on the hands, and maintain balance. A crowded environment or a slippery or sloping floor also affect the choice of gait pattern.

Alternating (reciprocal) gait pattern

Most individuals move reciprocally, one foot at a time, alternating with the walking aid. Alternating gaits are relatively stable and less stressful on the cardiovascular system and the upper limbs, but movement is rather slow.

Four-point gait.   Using two canes or crutches, the patient advances the right aid, then the left foot, then the left aid, followed by the right foot.

Two-point gait.   With two aids, the patient advances the right aid and the left foot, followed by the left aid and the right foot.

Three-point gait.   With two aids, usually crutches, the patient advances both aids together with the affected foot, then advances the unaffected foot. The three-point gait reduces load on the affected leg.

Cane gait.   The cane is usually held on the side opposite the affected leg. The patient advances the cane and the affected foot, then moves the unaffected foot.

Walker gait.   The patient advances the walker. The standard walker should be placed so that all four tips touch the floor simultaneously; walkers with two or four wheels should be wheeled forward slightly. Then the patient steps forward with one foot, following with the other foot.

Swinging (simultaneous) gait patterns

These patterns require use of a pair of axillary or forearm crutches rhythmically to eliminate load from both feet by forceful shoulder depression and elbow extension.

Drag-to gait.   Both crutches are advanced, either individually or together, followed by dragging both feet on the floor to an imaginary line just behind the crutches.

Swing-to gait.   Both crutches are advanced individually or together, followed by swinging the feet slightly off the floor to an imaginary line just behind the crutches.

Swing-through gait.   Both crutches are advanced together, followed by swinging the feet beyond the line of the crutches.[20,86] The swing-through gait is the fastest mode of crutch ambulation but requires the most floor space. The patient must be able to support the trunk and lower limbs for a period of time long enough to allow the legs to swing from behind to in front of the crutches. In addition, the patient must have confident balance when the posteriorly placed crutches are out of sight.

KINETIC AND KINEMATIC CONSIDERATIONS

The duration and amount of force that patients apply to an assistive device vary considerably.[10,53,68] Most individuals keep the cane on the floor during stance phase on the disabled limb, particularly those with a fractured pelvis or arthritis of the knee. In contrast, a person with paralysis agitans contacts the floor with the cane just before stance on the more disabled limb, using the cane in a manner similar to that of individuals with visual impairment. Those with hemiparesis lift the cane only during the double-support phase of gait.

A force transducer in the device can register the applied load.[17,23,33,34,41,65,68,75,84,91,92] Some investigators used a force plate to register loads on the cane or crutch.[98,107] Individuals with bone and joint disabilities apply significantly more force to the cane than do those with neuropathies. A single cane can support approximately a quarter of body weight, whereas a forearm crutch can bear almost half of one's weight.[50] When greater weight relief is required, the patient needs a pair of canes or crutches.

A cane reduces force throughout the hip, particularly when the cane is held in the contralateral hand,[15,17,33,34] which reduces abductor muscle pull and decreases the moment arm between the center of gravity and the femoral head, thereby lessening the force transmitted through the affected leg substantially. Some individuals prefer to hold the cane in the ipsilateral hand, using the device as a splint to reduce foot contact force.[12] Some patients insist on using the cane in the dominant hand, regardless of the side of pathology.

Kinematic studies of patient with hemiparesis confirmed that a cane held on the uninvolved side reduced mediolateral and anteroposterior sway, regardless of whether a standard or a four-footed cane was used.[66]

With a four-wheeled walker, elderly individuals were able to walk somewhat faster and negotiate sidewalk cracks more easily than with the conventional walker, which has no wheels.[31,32] Less attention is needed to maneuver a rolling walker as compared with a standard model.[108] Wheeled walkers, however, are more difficult to maneuver on carpets[52] and, being relatively bulky, are more difficult to put in the car. Children with cerebral palsy did not exhibit significant differences in step dimension, cadence, or velocity when walking with a wheeled walker (Rollator) with vertical handles as compared with one with horizontal handles.[59] Nondisabled children using a standard forward walker and then a two-wheeled posterior walker had a longer stride time with the posterior control walker and greater anterior trunk lean with the standard forward walker.[42] Similar results were obtained with a four-wheeled posterior walker.[57] Disabled children had more upright posture and faster gait with a posterior walker as compared with an anterior walker.[43,58,60]

Using forearm crutches to perform the three-point gait, subjects sustained an average vertical force to the unimpaired leg of 1.32 times body weight, 16% higher than during normal walking.[98] Patients with tibial fractures exhibited higher medially than anteroposteriorly directed force.[75] With axillary crutches and the same gait pattern, subjects applied 44% of body weight to the arms.[41]

Investigations of disabled and nondisabled subjects using the swing-through gait indicate that the vertical excursion of the shoulders is greater than that of the hip and that, lacking the normal shock-absorbing function of the lower limbs, the person who uses crutches absorbs the shock of ground contact with the crutch tips and the upper limbs.[94] Because the shoulder girdle has limited capacity to absorb shock, the swinging gaits impose high loads on the lower limbs[75,80]; conventional crutches do not absorb shock adequately.[78] In addition, children may lack the necessary arm adductor strength to anchor the axillary piece of the crutch against the chest.[65] The swing-through gait pattern with axillary crutches imposed dynamic loads at the hands from 1.14 to 3.36 times body weight and horizontal loads at the chest of 3% to 11% of body weight.[98]

PHYSIOLOGIC FACTORS

Ambulating with assistive devices imposes physiologic stresses on the client, as indicated by heart rate and energy expenditure higher than resting values.

Heart rate

Clients who use forearm crutches to relieve one lower limb of all weight have a significantly higher heart rate,[45] as do elderly women using a walker.[6] Among various designs of underarm crutches, the triceps version is associated with less increase in heart rate than the Sure-Gait and Ortho Crutches. Nondisabled adults using axillary crutches to perform the three-point gait had significantly higher heart rates than in normal walking; an average subject with a pulse rate limit of 130 beats per minute sustained equal stress whether crutch walking at 60 m/minute or running at 134 m/minute.[79] Heart rate increase and oxygen consump-

tion were less with axillary crutches than with a standard or wheeled walker for nondisabled subjects performing the three-point gait.[48] Healthy subjects who received preambulatory training with arm ergometry or free weights and push-ups did not differ in heart rate from subjects who practiced the three-point gait with axillary crutches; all subjects displayed elevated heart rate.[13]

Energy expenditure

Energy demand based on oxygen utilization may be expressed as rate (i.e., consumption per time) or cost (i.e., consumption per distance). The three-point gait performed by patients with lower-limb disorders required oxygen uptake as much as a third greater than for normal walking and a heart rate of more than 50% higher.[5,24,38,49,82,104] Consequently, elderly patients using a cane or crutches reduced walking velocity to maintain tolerable energy expenditure.[76,105] Energy demand is particularly high with the swing-through gait because of muscular demands in the upper limbs to lift the trunk and legs to initiate body-swing phase and then provide stability while the patient swings through the line of the crutches.[86] Walking speed affects metabolic cost, with patients using more energy when crutch walking at faster velocities[64,106] except when required to walk so slowly that rhythm was disturbed.[39]

Crutch design appears to have little effect on energy expenditure. Nondisabled subjects using Ortho axillary crutches to perform the three-point gait initially used less oxygen and had lower heart rates than with standard axillary crutches; differences, however, disappeared after they walked an average of 11.5 minutes.[47] Oxygen consumption and heart rate among nondisabled young adults was not affected by the type of crutch, axillary or forearm, that they used.[24,30,37,64] Most investigators found that the use of axillary crutches with a curved bottom (Sure-Gait) did not decrease the physiologic stress of crutch walking among nondisabled adults[3,72,100] and among orthopedic patients.[7] The curved bottom was associated with a 9% lower oxygen uptake; efficiency was attributed to the reduced height of vertical displacement.[40] The triceps crutch seems to exact a slightly lower metabolic cost, followed by the forearm crutch and the axillary crutch when used for the swing-through gait.[89,99]

SUMMARY

The development of new materials along with a better understanding of a particular patient's needs, goals, and future potential, relative to his or her particular disease process, have enabled the health care team to prescribe more effectively and efficiently the appropriate assistive device for the patient. By adhering to the aforementioned principles and working closely as a team, we should all benefit, especially, and most importantly, the patient.

REFERENCES

1. Allison BJ: Current uses of mobility aids, Clin Orthop 148:62–69, 1980.
2. Ang EJ, et al: Biofeedback device for patients on axillary crutches, Arch Phys Med Rehabil 70:644–646, 1989.
3. Annesley AI, et al: Energy expenditure of ambulation using the Sure-Gait crutch and the standard axillary crutch, Phys Ther 70:18–23, 1990.
4. Ball NA, et al: Radial nerve palsy: A complication of walker usage, Arch Phys Med Rehabil 70:236, 1989.
5. Bard G, Ralston HJ: Measurement of energy expenditure during ambulation, with special reference to evaluation of assistive devices, Arch Phys Med Rehabil 40:415–420, 1959.
6. Baruch IM, Mossberg KA: Heart-rate response of elderly women to non-weight-bearing ambulation with a walker, Phys Ther 63:1782–1787, 1983.
7. Basford JR, Rhetta HL, Schleusner MP: Clinical evaluation of the rocker bottom crutch, Orthopaedics 13:457–460, 1990.
8. Basmajian JV: Crutch and cane exercises and use. In Basmajian JV, Wolf SL, editors: Therapeutic exercise, ed 5, Baltimore, 1990, Williams & Wilkins.
9. Bauer DM, et al: A comparative analysis of several crutch-length-estimation techniques, Phys Ther 71:294–300, 1991.
10. Baxter ML, Allington RO, Koepke GH: Weight distribution variables in the use of crutches and canes, Phys Ther 49:360–365, 1969.
11. Beckwith JM: Analysis of methods of teaching axillary crutch measurement, Phys Ther 45:1060–1065, 1965.
12. Bennett L, et al: Locomotion assistance through cane impulse, Bull Prosthet Res 10:38–47, 1970.
13. Bhambani YN, Clarkson HM, Gomes PS: Axillary crutch walking: Effects of three training programs, Arch Phys Med Rehabil 71:484–489, 1990.
14. Blodgett MI: The art of crutch walking, Occup Ther Rehabil 25:27–32, 1946.
15. Blount WP: Don't throw away the cane, J Bone Joint Surg 18-A:695, 1956.
16. Bosanny JJ, Molitor Z: A measuring crutch to assist in rapid crutch fitting, Phys Ther 47:123–124, 1967.
17. Brand RA, Crowninshield RD: The effect of cane use on hip contact force, Clin Orthop 147:181–184, 1980.
18. Brooks AL, Fowler SB: Axillary artery thrombosis after prolonged use of crutches, J Bone Joint Surg 46:863–864, 1964.
19. Charron P: Epidemiology of walker-related accidents in the United States, Arch Phys Med Rehabil 1974:1240, 1993 (Abstract).
20. Childs TF: An analysis of swing-through crutch gait, Phys Ther 44:804–807, 1964.
21. Cicenia EF, Hoberman M: Crutches and crutch management, Am J Phys Med 36:359–384, 1957.
22. Clarkson H, Bhambhani Y: Complications of using axillary crutches and a three point non-weight bearing gait, Phys Ther 68:451, 1988 (Abstract).
23. Cochran GV, Gand R, Blossom B: Force measurement device for canes and crutches, Arch Phys Med Rehabil 54:43–46, 1973.
24. Cordrey IJ, Ford AB, Ferrer MT: Energy expenditure in assisted ambulation, J Chronic Dis 7:228–233, 1958.
25. Davenport J: Improved method for fitting crutches and canes, Phys Ther Rev 40:591, 1960.
26. Dean E, Ross J: Relationships among cane fitting, function, and falls, Phys Ther 73:494–504, 1993.
27. Deaver GG: What every physician should know about the teaching of crutch walking, JAMA 142:470–472, 1950.
28. Deaver GG, Brown ME: The challenge of crutches: I, II, III, IV, V, VI. Arch Phys Med 1945; 26:397–405, 515–523, 573–583, 747–758, 1945; 27:141–157, 683–703, 1946.
29. DeLisa, JA, editor: Rehabilitation medicine: Principles and practice, ed 2, Philadelphia, 1993, JB Lippincott.
30. Dounis E, et al: A comparison of efficiency of three types of crutches using oxygen consumption, Rheumatol Rehabil 19:252–255, 1980.
31. Eblen C, Koeneman J: A multidimensional evaluation of a four-wheeled walker. Assist Tech 3:32–37, 1991.
32. Eblen C, Koeneman JB: A longitudinal evaluation of a four-wheeled walker: Effects of experience. Top Geriatr Rehabil 8:65–72, 1993.
33. Edwards BG: Contralateral and ipsilateral cane usage by patients with total knee or hip replacement. Arch Phys Med Rehabil 67:734–740, 1986.
34. Ely DD, Smidt GL: Effect of cane on variables of gait for patients with hip disorders, Phys Ther 57:507–512, 1977.
35. Epstein S: Art, history and the crutch, Ann Med Hist 9:304, 1937.
36. Farmer LW: Mobility devices, Bull Prosthet Res 10:47–118, 1978.
37. Fisher SV, Patterson RP: Energy cost of ambulation with crutches, Arch Phys Med Rehabil 62:250–256, 1981.
38. Ganguli S, et al: Biomechanical approach to the functional assessment of the use of crutches for ambulation. Ergonomics 17:365–374, 1974.
39. Ghosh AK, et al: Metabolic cost of walking at different speeds with axillary crutches. Ergonomics 23:571–577, 1980.
40. Gillespie FC, et al: A physiologic assessment of the rolling crutch, Ergonomics 26:341–347, 1983.
41. Goh JC, Toh SL, Bose K: Biomechanical study on axillary crutches during single leg swing through gait, Prosthet Orthot Int 10:89–95, 1986.
42. Gorski L, et al: 3-dimensional kinematic analysis of effects of walker design on normal children's gait, Phys Ther 71:S58, 1991 (Abstract).
43. Greiner BM, Czerniecki JM, Deitz JC: Gait parameters of children with spastic diplegia: A comparison of effects of posterior and anterior walkers, Arch Phys Med Rehabil 74:381–385, 1993.
44. Hall J, Clarke AK, Harrison R: Guidelines for prescription of walking frames, Physiotherapy 76:118–120, 1990.
45. Hall J, et al: Heart rate evaluation of axillary and elbow crutches, J Med Eng Tech 15:232–238, 1991.
46. Harris DM: Crutch balancing. Phys Ther Rev 30:424–429, 1950.
47. Hinton CA, Cullen KE: Energy expenditure during ambulation with Ortho crutches and axillary crutches, Phys Ther 62:813–819, 1982.
48. Holder CG, Haskvitz EM, Weltman A: The effects of assistive devices on the oxygen cost, cardiovascular stress, and perception of nonweight-bearing ambulation, J Orthop Sports Phys Ther 18:537–541, 1993.
49. Imms FJ, MacDonald IC, Prestige SP: Energy expenditure during walking in patients recovering from fractures of the leg, Scand J Rehabil Med 8:1–9, 1976.
50. Jebsen RH: Use and abuse of ambulation aids, JAMA 199:5–10, 1967.
51. Joyce BM, Kirby RL: Canes, crutches and walkers, Am Fam Pract 43:535, 1991.
52. Karpman RR: Problems and pitfalls with assistive devices, Top Geriatr Rehabil 8:1–5, 1992.
53. Klenerman L, Jutton WC: A quantitative investigation of the forces applied to walking sticks and crutches, Rheumatol Rehabil 12:152–158, 1973.

54. Knocke I: Crutch walking, Am J Nurs 61:70–73, 1961.
55. Kumar R: Methods to estimate the proper length of a cane, Arch Phys Med Rehabil 74:1235, 1993 (Abstract).
56. LeBlanc MA, et al: A quantitative comparison of four experimental axillary crutches, J Prosthet Orthot 5:20, 1993.
57. Levangie PK, et al: The effects of the standard rolling walker and two posterior rolling walkers on gait variables of normal children, Phys Occup Ther Pediatr 9:19–31, 1989.
58. Levangie PK, et al: The effects of posterior rolling walkers vs. the standard rolling walker on gait characteristics of children with spastic cerebral palsy, Phys Occup Ther Pediatr 9:1–17, 1989.
59. Levangie PK, et al: Effects of altering handle position of a rolling walker on gait in children with cerebral palsy, Phys Ther 69:130–134, 1989.
60. Logan L, Byers-Kinkley K, Ciccone C: Anterior vs. posterior walkers: A gait analysis study, Dev Med Child Neurol 32:1044–1048, 1990.
61. Lovett RW: The tripod method of walking with crutches, JAMA 74:1306–1308, 1920.
62. Lowman EW, Rusk HA: Self-help devices: Crutch prescriptions: Gaits, Postgrad Med 31:392–394, 1962.
63. Lowman EW, Rusk HA: Self-help devices: Crutch prescriptions: Measurement, Postgrad Med 31:303–305, 1962.
64. McBeath AA, Bahrke M, Balke B: Efficiency of assisted ambulation determined by oxygen consumption measurement, J Bone Joint Surg 56:994–1000, 1974.
65. McGill SM, Dainty DA: Computer analysis of energy transfers in children walking with crutches, Arch Phys Med Rehabil 65:115–120, 1984.
66. Milczarek JJ, et al: Standard and four-footed canes, their effect on the standing balance of patients with hemiparesis, Arch Phys Med Rehabil 74:281–285, 1993.
67. Mulley GP: Walking sticks, BMJ 296:475–476, 1988.
68. Murray MP, Seireg AH, Scholz RC: A survey of the time, magnitude and orientation of forces applied to walking sticks by disabled men, Am J Phys Med 48:1–13, 1969.
69. Nabizadeh SA: Technical considerations in the selection and performance of walkers, J Burn Care Rehabil 14:182, 1992.
70. Najdeski P: Crutch measurement from the sitting position, Phys Ther 57:826–827, 1977.
71. Nelson D: Crutch walking, Am J Nurs 39:1088–1093, 1939.
72. Nielsen DH, et al: Energy cost, exercise intensity, and gait efficiency of standard versus rocker-bottom axillary crutch walking, Phys Ther 70:487–493, 1990.
73. Olmstead L: Crutch walking, Am J Nurs 45:28–35, 1945.
74. Olsson EC, Smidt GL: Assistive devices. In Smidt GL, editor: Gait in rehabilitation, New York, 1990, Churchill Livingstone.
75. Opila KA, Nicol AC, Paul JP: Forces and impulses during aided gait, Arch Phys Med Rehabil 68:715–722, 1987.
76. Pagliarulo MA, Waters R, Hislop HJ: Energy cost of walking of below-knee amputees having no vascular disease, Phys Ther 59:538–542; 1979.
77. Palmer ML, Toms JE: Manual for functional training, ed 3, Philadelphia, 1992, FA Davis.
78. Parziale JR, Daniels JD: The mechanical performance of ambulation using spring-loaded axillary crutches: A preliminary report, Am J Phys Med 68:193–195, 1989.
79. Patterson RP, Fisher SV: Cardiovascular stress of crutch walking, Arch Phys Med Rehabil 62:257–260, 1981.
80. Peacock B: A myographic and photographic study of walking with crutches, Physiotherapy 52:264–268, 1966.
81. Platt H: Occlusion of the axillary artery due to pressure by a crutch, Arch Surg 20:314–316, 1930.
82. Pugh LGCE: The oxygen intake and energy cost of walking before and after unilateral hip replacements with some observations on the use of crutches, J Bone Joint Surg 55B:742–745, 1973.
83. Reisman M, et al: Elbow moments and forces at the hands during swing through axillary crutch gait, Phys Ther 65:601–605, 1985.
84. Robinson HS: Cane for measurement and recording of stress, Arch Phys Med Rehabil 43:570–573, 1962.
85. Ross DE: Relationships among cane fitting, function, and falls, Phys Ther 73:494, 1993.
86. Rovic JS, Childress DS: Pendular model of paraplegic swing-through crutch ambulation, J Rehabil Res Dev 25:1–16, 1988.
87. Rudin LN, Levine L: Bilateral compression of radial nerve (crutch paralysis), Phys Ther Rev 31:229, 1951.
88. Sainsbury R, Mulley GP: Walking sticks used by the elderly, BMJ 284:1751, 1982.
89. Sankarankutty M, Stallard J, Rose GK: The relative efficiency of "swing-through" gait on axillary, elbow and Canadian crutches compared to normal walking, J Biomed Eng 1:55–57, 1979.
90. Schmitz TJ: Gait training with assistive devices. In O'Sullivan SB, Schmitz TJ, editors: Physical rehabilitation: Assessment and treatment, ed 3, Philadelphia, 1994, FA Davis.
91. Seidel GK, Soutas-Little RW: The intelligent walker: A potential aid for hip fracture patient rehabilitation, Arch Phys Med Rehabil 72:1159, 1991 (Abstract).
92. Seireg AH, Murray MP, Scholz RC: Method for recording the time, magnitude and orientation of forces applied to walking sticks, Am J Phys Med 47:307–314, 1968.
93. Shabes D, Scheiber M: Suprascapular neuropathy related to the use of crutches, Am J Phys Med 65:298–299, 1986.
94. Shoup TE, et al: Biomechanics of crutch ambulation, 7:11, 1974.
95. Smidt GL: Crutch attachment for special cases, Phys Ther 44:112, 1964.
96. Sowell TT: The role of canes, Inter-Clinic Information Bull 17:9–17, 1981.
97. Stallard J, et al: The ORLAU VCG swivel walker for muscular dystrophy patients, Prosthet Orthot Int 16:46, 1992.
98. Stallard J, et al: One leg swing through gait using two crutches: An analysis of the ground reaction forces and gait phases, Acta Orthop Scand 51:71–77, 1980.
99. Stallard J, Sankarankutty M, Rose GK: A comparison of axillary, elbow and Canadian crutches, Rheumatol Rehabil 17:237–239, 1978.
100. Stevenson CA, et al: Assessment of ambulation using Sure-Gait and standard axillary crutches, Phys Ther 71:S28, 1991 (Abstract).
101. Stuart L: Method of measurement for walking appliances, Can J Occup Ther 32:87–88, 1965.
102. Tagawa TT: Adjustable measuring crutch, Phys Ther 43:113–114, 1963.
103. Thompson-Rangel T, et al: Customized walker adaptions for a child with cerebral palsy, JACPOC 27:97, 1992.
104. Waters RL, Campbell J, Perry J: Energy cost of three-point crutch ambulation in fracture patients, J Orthop Trauma 1:170–173, 1987.
105. Waters R, Turburn L, Mulroy S: Energy expenditure in elderly patients using assistive devices, Top Geriatr Rehabil 8:12–19, 1992.
106. Wells RP: Kinematics and energy variations of swing-through crutch gait, J Biomech 12:579–585, 1979.
107. Wilson JF, Gilbert JA: Dynamic body forces on axillary crutch walkers during swing-through gait, Am J Phys Med 61:85–92, 1982.
108. Wright DI, Kemp TI: The dual-task methodology and assessing the attentional demands of ambulation with walking devices, Phys Ther 72:306–315, 1992.
109. Wright WG: Crutch-walking as an art, Am J Surg 1:372–374, 1926.

Positioning and Wheeled Mobility for Children and Adults with Disabilities

Jan Furumasu
Gail Gilinsky
Betti J. Krapfl

The number of Americans with disabilities continues to grow. In 1990, there were 1.4 million people in the United States who used wheelchairs; one tenth of whom were children.[22] There are more people with severe disabilities who are surviving and reentering the work force or educational system. In the past, the opportunity to integrate into society was hampered by severe deformities, pressure sores, limited functional abilities, and lack of equipment technology. New advances in technology have made a difference in controlling deformities, preventing pressure sores, and expanding each individual's potential in life.

For children and adults with a disability, mobility bases and seating systems have made social, educational, and vocational participation a reality. The mobility system provides support needed for an upright, symmetrical posture and prevents or delays spine and pelvic deformities. Better anatomical alignment of the pelvis and trunk may enhance physiological functions such as swallowing, cardiopulmonary function, and improved upper extremity control.[2,4,18,27,29,30,34] Positioning can influence tone and reflexes, thereby improving upper extremity use and access to technologies, such as power wheelchair controls, communication devices, or computers.[39] The mobility system should be user friendly for the person in the wheelchair and the caregiver. It should also be visually appealing so that the person is seen and not the system. It needs to be comfortable, provide pressure relief, and prevent pressure sores. This system should strive to be as dynamic as possible to allow changes in a child's physical and cognitive growth as well as the changes the adult user may experience. The best selection is achieved through an evaluation process involving a team of professionals knowledgeable in the person's medical needs and a resource person who is familiar with commercially available products so that the appropriate medical equipment can be prescribed.

Understanding the basic principles and concepts rather than a specific brand or model of wheelchair or seating system is important in the functional outcome. The eclectic approach, using the most appropriate parts from different manufacturers instead of limiting the prescription of equipment to a single company, is often the best to provide the exact system that the user needs in the most cost-effective manner. The user, family, and caregivers play key roles and must be interviewed extensively about environmental and functional needs. From these needs, specific positioning and mobility goals are determined by the therapists, the user, or family. The end result is the recommendation of a useful and functional system (Fig. 39.1). Simultaneously, positioning needs are assessed along with mobility needs. This chapter discusses the assessment, principles of positioning, and manual and power mobility bases for the adult and pediatric populations.

IDEAL SEATED ALIGNMENT

Understanding normal alignment is essential in problem solving difficult positioning needs. In the ideal seated position, the pelvis is relatively neutral, and the trunk is upright with the hips at approximately 90 degrees and at slight hip abduction and neutral rotation.[23] The knees should be flexed to approximately 90 degrees depending on the amount of muscle tone present and its influence on balance and control. The dorsiflexed foot allows weight bearing for stability, decreases excessive tone, and prevents equinus deformities. Finally, an upright, symmetrically balanced trunk over a stable pelvis facilitates upper extremity reach. The pelvis influences the alignment of the thoracic and cervical spine and therefore the head position (Fig. 39.2).[8]

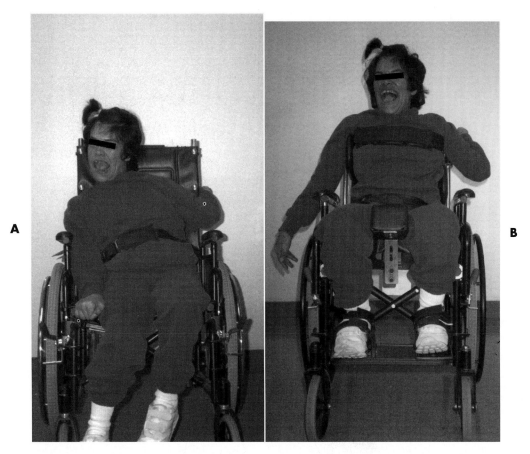

Fig. 39.1. **A,** Young woman before evaluation of seating system. **B,** Same woman with seating system that provides support and alignment, increasing functional abilities.

SEATING AND MOBILITY SYSTEM CONSIDERATIONS

A seating and mobility system evaluation should address all aspects of a person's medical and personal lifestyle issues. The following categories should be assessed thoroughly.

Medical history

Pertinent history is collected that has an impact on mobility or positioning needs. Is the condition progressive rather than stable? Is mechanical ventilation or future surgical intervention, such as spinal fusion, muscle releases, or amputations, possible or likely in the future?

Tone

Is the muscle tone low or hypotonic rather than high or hypertonic? How does tone affect positioning and functional ability?

Reflex influenced posturing

Is the posturing obligatory or nonobligatory, a functional or nonfunctional reflex posturing? For example, the child with opisthotonic posturing demonstrates extension of the trunk and head or asymmetric tonic neck reflex posturing causing rotation of the head, trunk, and pelvis. This reflex posturing may be used functionally to extend the upper extremity to drive a power wheelchair or to point to a communication device. Persons with athetosis or dyskinetic-type movement disorders use reflex posturing for stability to use their extremities functionally.

Skin sensation and integrity

Sensation needs to be evaluated carefully. Is it intact, absent, or impaired? Information about previous history of pressure areas, scar tissue, and surgical repairs is needed. This information, along with problem solving any current reddened areas, is needed for a successful cushion prescription. Specific cushion evaluation is addressed in detail in the section on pressure relief.

Motor control and strength

Is motor control dyskinetic, such as athetosis, or patterned in synergies? Are deformities or posturing a result of muscle paralysis, weakness, or imbalance?

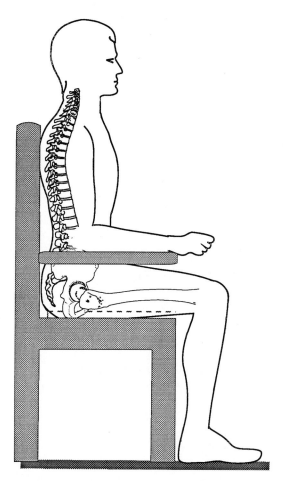

Fig. 39.2. Ideal seated alignment.

Range of motion

Are deformities of the pelvis, hip, trunk, and extremities fixed or flexible?

Functional abilities and goals

How are activities of daily living, transfers, and lifestyle accomplished? Observation of actual activities is critical for the problem-solving approach for seating and mobility.

Cognitive status and behavioral issues

Does the person have cognitive or behavioral issues, such as the inability to attend, reasoning that is concrete versus abstract, or destructive-type behavior, that influence the prescription of equipment, especially in regards to safety features?

Visual and perceptual ability

What visual or perceptual deficits are present? Positioning affects visual field for those individuals who cannot separate head movement from eye movement; visual field cuts can be well compensated for by head posturing or trunk movement. Compro-

mises in support are necessary to assure maximal function.

Environmental accessibility

How will the person access his environment? All environments need consideration, whether it is within the home, school, or work. For example, as part of academic goals, the need to integrate lap-tray or communication devices with the seating system may be present.

Transportation

Is the driver or passenger safe and independent in regards to wheelchair lockdowns, wheelchair seat height, and breakdown of system for loading into a car, and does the mobility base fit on van lifts?

Ancillary equipment needs

Has all equipment necessary for daily living, such as ventilator trays, communication devices, or lap trays, been considered as part of the overall mobility base?

Other considerations

Aging or overuse syndromes. Aging or overuse syndrome affect positioning and the need for added supports. For example, pain and fatigue in the upper back and neck of an adult with polio may be relieved by adding a head support.

Cosmesis. Cosmesis is an important factor in overall compliance with seating intervention and reflects the person's personal identity.

Finances. At a time when technology is at its peak with more functional equipment, cost containment, and reimbursement have become a real constraint. When writing wheelchair prescriptions, the clinician must be conscientious about costs.

Caregivers. Caregivers included in the initial interview provide insights important in ensuring successful prescriptions and follow-through after the delivery. Any equipment provided must be easily managed and maintained by the caregiver.

Changes in height and weight. Height and weight changes, particularly in the child and the hospitalized person with a new injury, may greatly influence what the clinician orders now and as it relates to growth factors in the future.

SEATING ASSESSMENT

After the medical history and functional and environmental assessment have been completed, hands-on evaluation of the physical problems begins. Preferably this evaluation is done both in the supine position and in the sitting position. Three main areas of the hands-on

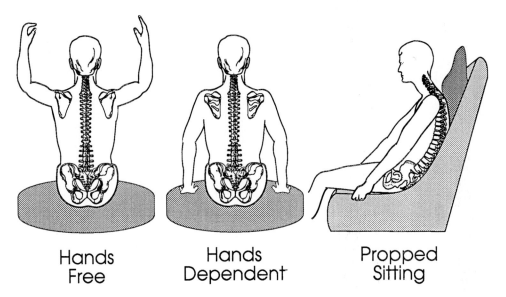

Hands
Free

Hands
Dependent

Propped
Sitting

Fig. 39.3. Classification of sitting ability has been grouped according to the amount of trunk control present and the amount of support needed in a seating system.

evaluation include the person's ability to sit, patterns of deformities in the sitting position, and whether these deformities are fixed or flexible.

Classification and description of sitter

The degree of independent sitting is one important factor in determining the type of seating system and mobility base that are needed. Hoffer[17] classifies a persons' ability to sit according to the amount of trunk control present. His grouping has been modified to include generalizations as to the type of seating and mobility bases that are needed (Fig. 39.3).

Hand-free sitters are individuals who can sit independently for long periods of time without use of their hands for support. They have good trunk balance and the ability to weight shift. In general, they need a simple seating system designed primarily for pelvic stability, comfort, and mobility. An example of a hand-free sitter is a person with a T_{12} paraplegia.

Hand-dependent sitters are persons who require either one or both hands for support. In general, their trunk control and balance are poor and spine deformity is common. Trunk supports are needed to allow hand use for functional activities. Providing a more stable base of support may change a hand-dependent sitter, such as a person with a weak trunk and scoliosis, to a hand-free sitter.

Propped sitters are the people who, because of severe physical involvement or structural deformity, are unable to sit without total body support. Trunk and head control are usually poor. Positioning of the trunk, head, and all four extremities is needed, such as for the child who has cerebral palsy with total body involvement.

Pattern of deformity or alignment

There are three common patterns of postural malalignment:

- *Symmetrically slouched*
- *Lordotic* posture
- *Asymmetrical* posture

Table 39.1 describes possible causes and equipment solutions for these postural alignment problems. It should be noted that the position of the pelvis influences the alignment of the trunk and therefore the shoulders, upper extremities, and head. The *symmetrically slouched* position begins with a posterior pelvic tilt. The most common cause of a posterior pelvic tilt in persons who have cerebral palsy is hypertonicity in the hamstring muscles.[23] The *lordotic* posture, often the position of balance for persons with proximal muscle weakness, begins with an anterior pelvic tilt. This alignment allows trunk movement to increase upper extremity reach, which is limited by proximal weakness.[11] The *asymmetrical* or windswept posture, one hip adducted and internally rotated with the opposite hip abducted and externally rotated, is seen in combination with pelvic rotation, a dislocated hip, pelvic obliquity, and scoliosis of the spine.[23]

Severity of deformity (fixed versus flexible)

Rang and colleagues[32] have categorized severity of deformity according to three stages: flexible or preventable deformities, deformities amendable to surgical correction that need to be maintained, and deformities that are fixed and not surgically correctable. This information is important in deciding the type of seating components needed. For example, many flexible de-

Table 39.1.   Causes and equipment for patterns of deformities

PROBLEM	CAUSE	EQUIPMENT SOLUTIONS
Slouched posture		
Posterior pelvic tilt	Sling upholstery	Three-point control: solid seat, firm back, and pelvic/hip seat belt
		Rigid anterior pelvic support: subasis bar, knee blocks
	Inappropriate seat depth	Measure from PSIS to popliteal, include fixed kyphosis
Hip/knee extension	Extensor tone (hip and knee)	Antithrust seat
	Hip extension contracture:	Wedge seat cushion
	Unilateral	Increase hip angle >90 degrees
	Bilateral	Increase knee angle >90 degrees (foot placement behind knee)
Thoracic kyphosis	Trunk weakness/paralysis	Unilateral split seat or leg trough, to maintain trunk upright
	Fixed deformity	Recline back
		Lower back height
Shoulder protraction	Spasticity	Firm back
	Weakness/scapular	Appropriate back height
		Accommodate with molded back
		Shoulder straps pulling up and back
		Rigid shoulder
Forward head posture	Weakness	Occipital support with capital extension
	Spasticity	Head band (stationary or dynamic) attached to head rest
	Reflex posturing if too reclined	Recline back or tilt back to seat angle
Rotational/oblique posture		
Pelvic obliquity/pelvic rotation	Sling seat	Firm seat
	Scoliosis	Lateral hip guides
	Hip dislocation	Flexible: build up under low side
	Asymmetrical hip ROM	Fixed: build up under high side, relieve pressure under low side
		Custom-molded seat
		Off-set cut-out in cushion
		Accommodate seat depth for leg length discrepancy
		Anterior pelvic belt
		Two-piece subasis bar
Hip problems	Sling seat	Firm seat with medial thigh support
Hip adducted—internal rotation	Adductor tone	Lateral thigh cuffs
Hip abduction—external rotation	Hypotonia	Lateral thigh/knee stabilizers
	Fixed deformity	
Windswept hips	Pelvic rotation	Three-point control: hip guides, medial, and lateral thigh support
Adducted thigh with abducted thigh	Dislocated hip	
	Scoliosis	Custom-molded seat
Thoracic scoliosis	Pelvic obliquity and rotation	Three-point control: pelvic/trunk supports
Flexible	Weakness	
	Spasticity	Rotational deformity: curved supports
Fixed	Asymmetric tone/muscle strength	Custom-molded back or system to accommodate to rib hump deformity
Asymetrical head posture	Scoliosis	Appropriate support of pelvis, trunk, and shoulder girdle
	Fluctuating tone	
	Reflex posturing	Three-point control: head and neck support. Extension of occipital support to mastoid process or over the ear to the temple for lateral control
	Weakness	
	Visual compensation	
		Stationary or dynamic headband

Continued.

Table 39.1.   Causes and equipment for patterns of deformities—cont'd

PROBLEM	CAUSE	EQUIPMENT SOLUTIONS
Lordotic posture		
Anterior pelvic tilt	Muscle imbalance	Placement of belt across ASIS
Hip flexion	Abdominal weakness	Wedge seat/cushion to accommodate if
Thoracic lordosis	Contractures	fixed
		Tilt in space manual or power frame,
		adjustable seat angle
		Anterior chest support: molded chest
		plate, wide Velcro strap
Retracted shoulders	Spasticity	Appropriate pelvic/trunk positioning
	Posturing for trunk weakness	with sternal support
		Shoulder wedges
Extended head posture	Spasticity	Neck ring
	Weakness	Occipital support

formities can be supported by adjustable, commercially available positioning components, whereas fixed deformities may need more customized solutions.[32]

BIOMECHANICAL PRINCIPLES OF SEATING

The following biomechanical principles should be considered when prescribing a person's seating and mobility system.

The pelvis is the key!

The influence of pelvic stability on alignment and function cannot be overemphasized. As stated earlier, stabilizing the pelvis improves trunk balance, head control, and upper extremity control. Each body part influences alignment and function of the part above and below. The three main points of control are support beneath the pelvis, capturing the ischial tuberosities in the seat cushion to prevent a posterior tilt; posterior support such as lumbosacral back support; and anterior support such as that provided by a hip belt.

Seating components that improve pelvic position. Positioning the flexible pelvis begins at the pelvis itself; however, positioning the fixed pelvic and trunk deformity begins with the head because a level visual field is the priority. Support beneath the pelvis begins with providing support of soft tissues and relieving pressure of the ischial tuberosities. (Pressure-relieving cushions are discussed in the section on incorporating pressure relief into seating systems.) Maintaining an upright pelvis by preventing the ischial tuberosities from sliding forward is the purpose of the *antithrust* seat. The ischial tuberosities are captured in a dish of softer foam blocked from moving forward by a denser foam under the thighs (Fig. 39.4).

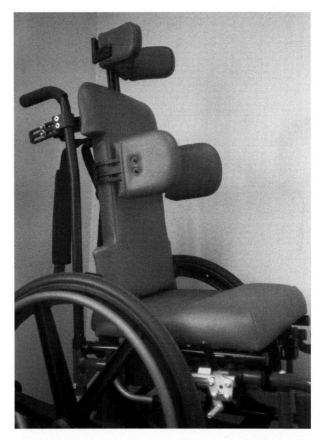

Fig. 39.4.   Antithrust seat prevents ischial tuberosities from sliding forward and maintains pelvic positioning.

Pelvic rotation must also be evaluated with depth of the seat. A longer sitting surface under the thigh of the forward anterior-superior iliac spine (ASIS) is needed for adequate support. Likewise, the depth should be cut back on the side of the backwardly rotated pelvis to prevent the pelvis from being pulled into posterior tilt (Fig. 39.5).

ASYMMETRICAL LEG-LENGTH

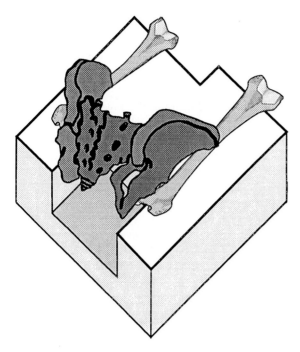

Fig. 39.5. Accommodation of seat depth because of leg length discrepancy, pelvic rotation, or hip dislocation.

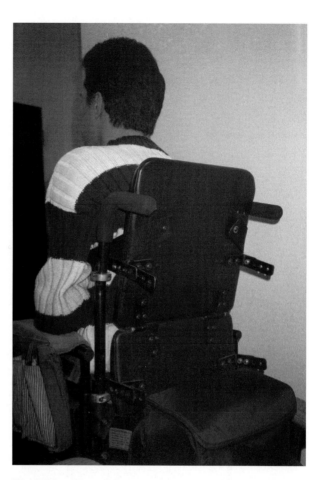

Fig. 39.6. Biangular back consists of support of the pelvis separate from the trunk.

Posterior support of the pelvis begins with a solid back or upholstery, either of which may need adjustable lumbosacral support. Providing support of the pelvis separate from the upper torso in a seating system has been a clinical challenge. Sacral support has been fabricated into a number of different designs. A "biangular back" consists of two components. The lower component supports the pelvis upright and the upper component adjusts separately to align the trunk (Fig. 39.6).

Anterior support, usually a crucially placed seat belt, is used to provide the third point of stability for the pelvis. The angle of pull, between 45 and 90 degrees, from the seat rail depends on the position of the pelvis and the amount of support needed.

Firm versus flexible supports

Firm supports hold posture better than flexible supports. For example, a sling seat upholstery does not provide as much pelvic support as a rigid seat.

Three points of control

To control deformities, opposing forces are applied around the joint center. Controlling forces should be as far away from the joint as possible; for example, to support a scoliosis, off-set trunk and pelvic pads are needed (Fig. 39.7).

Increase surface area contact to disperse pressure

To optimize pressure distribution, the contact surface area should be increased to disperse the pressures over a larger area of contact. For example, a seat cushion with a long seat depth is used to distribute sitting pressures from the pelvis to the thighs.[3]

Accommodation versus correction of deformity

Fixed deformities as well as functional posturing need to be accommodated. To accommodate a fixed pelvic obliquity with the right side down, the cushion must be built up on the left and relieved under the right to distribute the weight-bearing pressures as evenly as possible. If functional compromises are needed, accommodation is needed as well—for example, the child who must turn his head because of a visual field deficit. His posturing should be accommodated, not corrected, if it is his way of visually compensating. In this case and others where reflex posturing is used functionally, compromises in positioning are needed.

Positioning for function

There are a number of reported studies on functional activities and how they relate to seating.[18,19,26,27] Clearly, positioning greatly influences upper extremity function.[29]

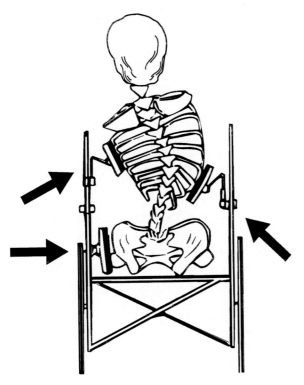

Fig. 39.7.   Three points of control for scoliosis.

Position in space.   Position in space can affect a person's trunk balance and control. In a more upright position, the trunk movement forward and laterally can be balanced with minimal muscle activity. This is especially important for people with proximal weakness, such as children and adults with spinal muscular atrophy. If reclined, they would not be able to reach forward and use the distal strength in their hands (Fig. 39.8). Similarly, children with cerebral palsy have less extensor muscle activity in their paraspinals when the back is positioned upright rather than at a 15- or 30-degree recline. With the trunk reclined, upper extremity and head control in this population is affected by the tonic labyrinthine reflex.[28] Nonetheless, for those with poor trunk or head control, the back needs to be slightly reclined to assist with support. Positioning for persons with quadriplegia is critical for mouthstick activities as well as for mobile arm support (MAS) use. To provide the best mechanical advantage for MAS use, a nearly upright trunk position is needed (Fig. 39.9).[42]

Circumferential support may also be provided by a thoracolumbosacral orthosis (TLSO) in the pediatric population for those at risk for spinal deformity. This support allows them to sit more upright and maximize the use of their head and neck or weak shoulder girdle. Similarly, adults with quadriplegia also may benefit from circumferential support from using thoracolumbar corsets.

Seat-to-back angle.   Seat-to-back angle is important in maintaining the pelvic position. Muscle tone and range of motion are assessed simultaneously to deter-

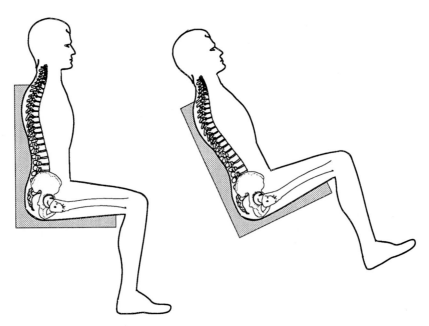

Fig. 39.8.   *Left:* The trunk is upright with hip and knee angle flexed to 90 degrees. *Right:* Fixed tilt in space with the trunk reclined and a fixed hip and knee angle.

mine seat-to-back angle, specifically for those persons whose motor control is patterned. Hip flexion range of motion should be carefully checked for asymmetry. At least 90 degrees of hip flexion is ideal. If there is less than 90 degrees in one hip, an asymmetrical seat or cushion is needed.

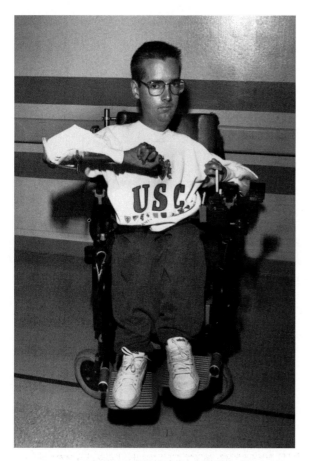

Fig. 39.9. Young man with spinal muscular atrophy (SMA) sits upright for mobile arm support (MAS) use.

The amount of extensor tone should be assessed as the hips are being flexed; this determines the amount of hip flexion needed in the seating system. Hypertonicity in the hamstrings can pull the pelvis into a posterior tilt causing the hips to slide down and forward. Stabilizing the pelvis and flexing the hips and knees more than 90 degrees may decrease the influence of extensor tone. The popliteal angle determines foot placement to eliminate the pull of tight hamstring muscles (Fig. 39.10).[23] Preventing hip adduction also assists in decreasing extensor tone and needs to be maintained with the hips flexed.

Another alternative for maintaining pelvic and hip positioning is through a fixed seat-to-back angle in the reclined or *tilted* position. If the person cannot tolerate an upright position and must be reclined, the seat-to-back angle can remain fixed. This can be accomplished in two ways. The seat and back can be statically mounted in a tilted position on the wheelchair frame, or the wheelchair frame itself can be tilted back dynamically. Usually the tilted position is needed because trunk and head control are poor; however, this position compromises upper extremity function and may limit visual field (Fig. 39.11).

SIMULATION

To choose or predict accurately the functional effect of the system, a trial of the system is needed. Attempting to evaluate the effect of support while manually holding the person is difficult. Simulation is a method of assessing the person in a mock-up chair before the final product is ordered. This simulation process can be accomplished in an evaluation wheelchair or in a commercially available simulator chair. With simulation, tone fluctuations can be observed by varying positions

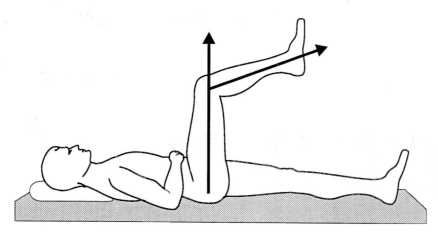

Fig. 39.10. Evaluation of popliteal angle to determine hamstring tightness with 90 degrees of hip flexion.

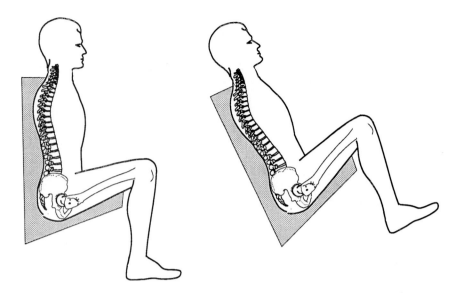

Fig. 39.11. Hip and knee flexion greater than 90 degrees to decrease extensor tone. Trunk upright on the left and position tilted for trunk recline on the right.

Table 39.2. Components of a seating system

Solid seat	Planar, contoured, antithrust, seat cushion incorporated into the surface
Solid back	Planar, contoured, biangular, molded surface interfaced to accommodate deformities
Medial thigh stabilizer (abductor, pommel)	Used to maintain thigh abduction or prevent adduction
Knee blocks	To prevent sliding out of a seat and allow repositioning by the user
Trunk supports	Straight for lateral stability and curved swing away for better support of rotational or kyphotic deformities
	Three-point control, trunk and pelvis for scoliosis
Shoulder retractors	Straps pulling up from trunk supports and anchoring midline behind the back. Rigid shoulder retractors needed for upper trunk stability to improve head control and not affect upper extremity function
Head supports	Neck ring to maintain head midline and support below occiput to prevent stimulation of the tonic labyrinthine reflex, which causes head extension with pressure under the occiput in the cerebral palsy patient
	Lateral head control asymmetric for asymmetric tonic neck reflex posturing
	Occipital support of capital extension
Foot rests	Placement important in overall positioning. Solid footboard with leather straps or shoe holders

in space and adding or changing pelvic or trunk supports. The effect of changing asymmetric posturing on functional ability can be addressed. Simulation of the supports needed begins at the pelvis, hip, and trunk and proceeds to the extremities. This anatomical systematic approach is followed to reevaluate the effect on the person's overall posture and control before proceeding onto the next body segment in hopes of preventing "overseating." Table 39.2 describes various types of seating components that aid in the simulation process and eventually the final system.

Measurements during the simulation process are taken supine and in the sitting position. To ensure accurate fit for seating and mobility systems, the following planar measurements are needed for both sides of the body (Fig. 39.12):

- Hip to top of head (A)
- Hip to top of shoulder (B)
- Seat depth (C)
- Leg length—knee to heel (D)
- Chest depth and width (E,F)
- Hip width (trochanter to trochanter) (G)
- Hip to underarm—left and right (HL) (HR)

TYPES OF POSITIONING SYSTEMS

The severity of the deformity or deforming forces influences the type of seating system. Flexible deformities can usually be held prophylactically with modular planar systems. These systems with multiple flat or slightly curved components are adjustable and can be

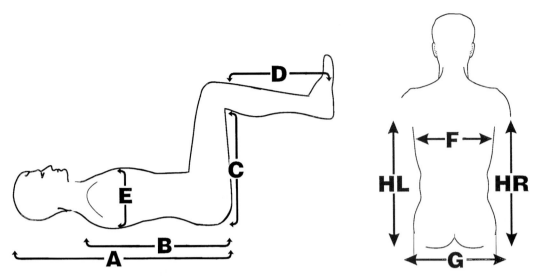

Fig. 39.12. Planar measurements needed for modular seating systems.

interchanged between manufacturers. Severe fixed deformities usually need to be accommodated in custom-molded systems. Both types of systems have evolved from orthotic principles and fabrication techniques.

Planar systems

Planar systems are flat (as opposed to contoured) such as a solid seat and back, and allow the user the freedom to move (Fig. 39.13). These systems are composed of many positioning components, which are interchangeable and provide rigid postural support. They can be easily adjusted as the person grows or changes. Many components from different manufacturers can be used together to create the best overall system.

Simple contoured systems

These are commercially available systems that provide basic generic contoured support of the pelvis and trunk. They offer increased contact of the body to distribute pressures more evenly as compared to the planar systems. Therefore, they provide more stability and perhaps less freedom of movement for those that would benefit, such as individuals with athetoid cerebral palsy (Fig. 39.14).

Custom-molded systems

Custom-molded systems are commonly used for the population with fixed deformities that need to be accommodated. With these systems, intimate contact of body contours distributes pressures evenly over surface areas—to provide control while providing pressure relief. This is especially important for those individuals with severe fixed deformities who may not

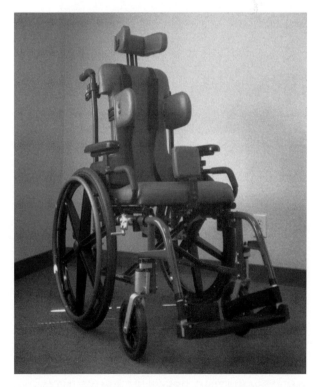

Fig. 39.13. Planar seating system with modular components.

tolerate weight bearing on planar or generically contoured surfaces and are at risk for skin breakdown. There are two basic techniques to create custom-molded systems (Fig. 39.15).

Negative cast mold. A negative plaster mold of a client is taken directly or by using a simulator. This model, or its digitized contours, may be sent to the manufacturer for fabrication. Once the contoured sys-

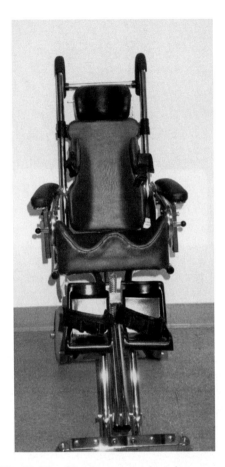

Fig. 39.14. Simple contoured seating system.

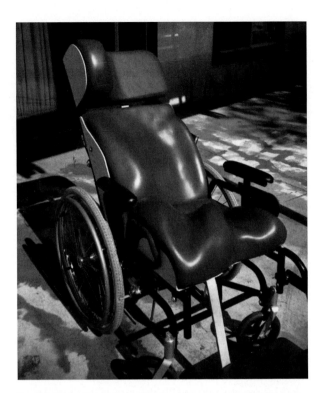

Fig. 39.15. Custom-molded seating system with negative cast mold seat and a direct mold back.

tem is received it is fitted to the individual. If changes or adjustments are needed, the molded system may need to be redone.

Direct mold. The individual's own wheelchair frame is used. Two chemicals are mixed with a catalyst to create foam. This foam expands and molds around the body contours as the person is held in place. Positioning the person correctly at the time of foaming is critical and can be difficult and sometimes hard to control. This process, however, can be done in one session. Adjustments or remolding can be done in one session. This technique is commonly called *foam in place.*[15]

INCORPORATING PRESSURE RELIEF INTO SEATING SURFACES

Cushions

All seating systems should address pressure relief according to the needs of that individual. Pressure can be defined as the perpendicular force divided by the area over which it acts. Forces acting parallel to the skin are called shear stresses.[9] Sitting surfaces must provide skin protection from excessive buildup of pressure under the pelvic bones and from shearing forces. The qualities of the sitting surface are influenced by the presence or absence of protective sensation, the prominence of bony areas, and the ability or inability to shift one's body weight.[10]

There are three bony areas that are at particular risk for tissue breakdown from pressure or shear. They are the ischial tuberosities, the sacral/coccygeal area, and the greater trochanters.[31] Any bony prominence, however, can be susceptible to breakdown, especially if it is subject to the shearing movement of body tissue against the bony prominence.[21] Body heat and moisture collection can also cause skin maceration.[36] Pressures exceeding normal capillary pressure can lead to tissue necrosis.[33] There are several types of cushions that assist with pressure relief: foam, gel, and air.

Foam. Various types of foam are available in a variety of thicknesses and densities. For example, a medium 3 lb foam (1 cubic foot weighs 3 lb) distributes sitting pressures by contouring to the pelvis.[38] This may be most appropriate for the geriatric population or individuals with sensation who have the ability to weight shift independently. Higher-density foam, 4 or 5 lb, compresses less, lasts longer, and may be appropriate for people with spinal cord injury and others with decreased sensation. Specific cut-outs for pressure relief under bony prominences can be made in the foam to redistribute sitting pressures to soft tissues (Figs. 39.16 and 39.17). Pliable closed cell foams can be used

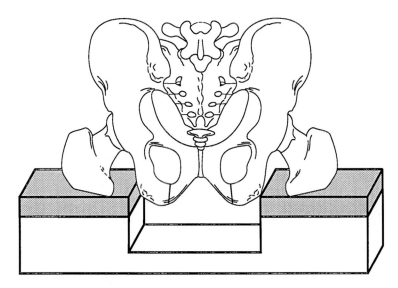

Fig. 39.16.   Ischial tuberosities suspended in a cut-out in a foam cushion.

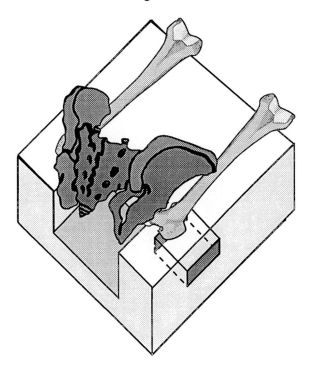

Fig. 39.17.   Trochanter suspended in cut-out in foam cushion for pressure relief.

as a buffer over cut-outs to prevent edge pressure and shearing. As a rule, foam cushions are lighter weight and economical but tend to deteriorate, needing frequent replacement. Foam is also a poor conductor; thus it insulates body heat and may result in dampness, which contributes to skin breakdown.

Gel.   A second type of cushion easily distributes sitting pressures by immersion of bony prominences in a gel-like substance or fluid. The fluid surrounds or conforms to the shape of a person's buttocks. When a person moves or does a weight shift, shearing that might

occur tends to be reduced by the gel material. Some manufacturers incorporate this fluid on top of a contoured base; others pocket it within contoured foam. Both methods provide excellent positioning of the pelvis. Although gel fluid cushions weigh more than foam or air, they usually provide good skin protection against pressure, shear forces, and heat buildup (Fig. 39.18).

Air.   A third type of cushion uses air to distribute sitting pressures and protect the skin. Some manufacturers use a single bladder or compartment that is inflated; others use multiple air cells from 2 to 4 inches in height and many different compartments. These can be customized to any configuration to relieve specific pressure areas or correct deformities while still supporting the pelvis. Air cushions are lightweight and durable and provide excellent skin protection against pressure and shear forces. Air pressure must be maintained, however, and air flotation can decrease a person's stability and balance. Because the bony prominences are surrounded by air, heat dissipates easily (Fig. 39.19).

All cushions need to be evaluated beneath the person to determine whether the bony areas are coming in contact with the bottom of the cushion base or wheelchair seat, commonly known as bottoming-out. If so, then reevaluation and modification of the cushion are needed. All postural deformities of the pelvis and hips need to be addressed with the cushion itself. Evaluation of whether the deformity is fixed or flexible determines if the modifications need to accommodate or correct. Pelvic obliquity, if flexible, can be reduced by using an insert, increasing the amount of air pressure, or using a higher-density foam on the low side of the pelvis. If the obliquity is fixed, the insert, the increase in air pressure, or the denser foam must be under the high side of the obliquity to accommodate the fixed pelvic deformity and redistribute sitting pressures.

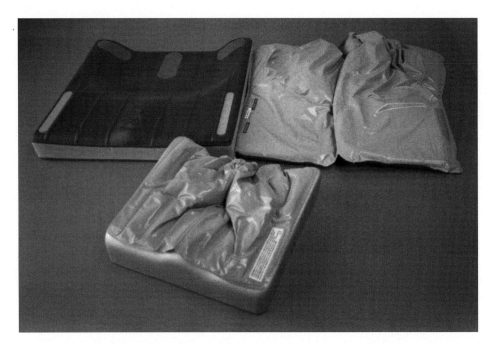

Fig. 39.18.   Jay cushion with contoured base and gel interface.

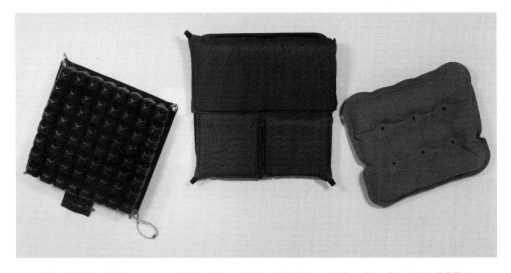

Fig. 39.19.   Three types of air cushions: Roho, Varilite, and Bye-Bye Decubiti (BBD).

Recline systems

In addition to pressure-relieving cushions, a mechanical method for pressure relief is needed for those unable to weight shift. Two of these methods are discussed: *back recline* or *tilt in space*. Both can be accomplished either manually by the caretaker or by a power system that can be controlled independently by the user.

Back recline.   A full back recline system redistributes sitting pressures from the buttocks to the back by opening the hip angle (Fig. 39.20). Because this method of recline can contribute to shearing forces, manufacturers have incorporated different designs to reduce the amount of movement between the person and the back, thereby decreasing the amount of shear. If a person is not positioned correctly, shearing can contribute to skin breakdown, and it can cause the body to slide down, changing the orientation of drive mechanisms and displacing positioning devices. Advantages of the back recline, however, include discreet weight shifts and the ability to maintain hip extension range as well as the orientation of lap-trays. Back recline can also allow for easier access for bladder catheterization.

Tilt in space.   If the orientation of the seat-to-back angle must be maintained for positioning, such

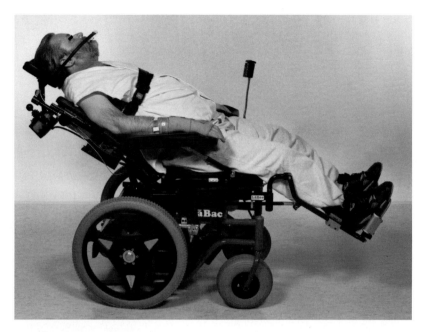

Fig. 39.20.   C4 quadriplegic weight shifting in power recline wheelchair.

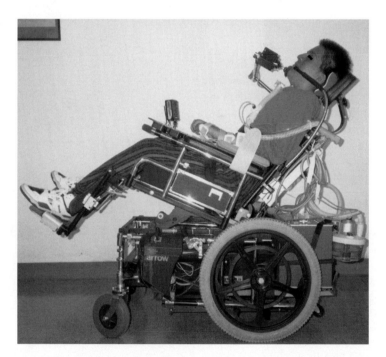

Fig. 39.21.   Power wheelchair with a tilt in space recline system.

as with contoured systems, a fixed tilt in space recline may be preferred (Fig. 39.21). These tilt in space systems accommodate hip flexion contractures. They eliminate shear and maintain orientation of drive controls. Severe total body extensor patterning or spasticity is more effectively controlled with a fixed positioning system than with the back recline systems described previously. A combination back and tilt recline system is shown in Figure 39.22.

MOBILITY SYSTEMS

When prescribing a wheelchair, the following questions should be asked: What situations warrant the use of a wheelchair? Is the person no longer able to ambulate? Will the person be a part-time user? Is the chair required for longer distances because of low endurance? Will it be the person's primary means of mobility? Will the person be in the chair for most of the day, every day? The answers to these questions determine the technology to be used for each individual. The same technology that revolutionized such sports as skiing, bicycling, and tennis was later applied to wheelchair manufacturing. Before 1980, manual wheelchairs were heavy and difficult to maneuver. New technology and engineering now provide wheelchairs that weighed half what their predecessors did. People learn to maneuver these chairs over indoor and outdoor terrains with greater success. For example, C5 spinal cord–injured individuals were formerly not considered candidates for a manual chair. Many of these individuals can propel a lightweight wheelchair with quad pegs or vertical projections on the wheel rims. As a result, they experienced greater levels of functional independence. In addition, the lighter-weight wheelchairs were easier to manage for caregivers.

The 1990s brought yet another revolution in technology to the manual wheelchair industry. While aluminum and titanium had been standard lightweight materials, composite plastic materials were introduced to the wheelchair arena. They still are being evaluated. The advantages are that they are light, rigid, and strong. So far, the overwhelming opinion of wheelchair users is positive. They express some common benefits, such as the smooth, quiet ride of the wheelchair and lack of vibration through the user's joints. Even more than the lightweight metal chairs, the composite chairs seem to offer greater shock absorption so that fatigue is not as much of a problem. This is an important advantage, especially in an aging population. It is anticipated that composite technologic advances will be incorporated into more equipment in the future.

MANUAL WHEELCHAIRS

Frame types

There are two major frame types: folding and rigid. The *folding* frame (Fig. 39.23) is usually constructed of two cross braces, which give a more forgiving ride as the frame *flexes*, thus absorbing the shock. Because

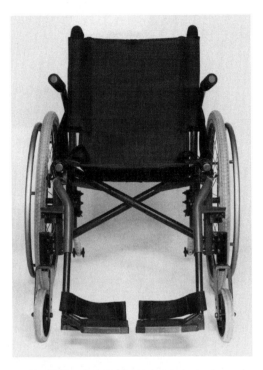

Fig. 39.23. Folding wheelchair (cross braces).

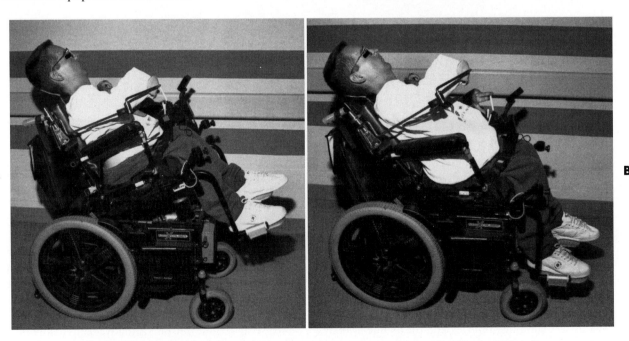

Fig. 39.22. Combination tilt in space and back recline power system. **A,** Tilted position. **B,** Recline position with open hip angle.

of the frame construction, the chair is heavier. It folds easily into a more compact unit and can be stored in the back seat of a small car or in the trunk. The user could fold the chair and, using leverage, roll it into the car. The rear wheels do not have to be removed.

The *rigid* chair gives a more responsive ride; is easier to push for an active wheelchair user, such as a spinal cord–injured person; and is lighter (Fig. 39.24). Because it has fewer parts, it responds as one unit. It does, however, give a rougher ride without as much shock absorption. The back folds forward onto the seat (Fig. 39.25). The rear wheels must be removed to load it into a car (Fig. 39.26).

Weight types

Ultra-lightweight chairs can be either folding or rigid; are made of aluminum, titanium, or composite materials; and presently weigh approximately 22 lb. These are excellent wheelchairs for the active, athletic paraplegic who is involved in many sporting activities.

Lightweight chairs can also be either folding or rigid; are made of aluminum, steel, or composite materials; and weigh about 30 lb. These chairs tend to be more for everyday, all-purpose use than the ultra light chairs. These have become the most popular wheelchairs for a large variety of individuals, ranging from children with cerebral palsy to adults with a neurologic deficit.

Standard chairs are folding only, usually made of steel, and weigh about 40 lb. These wheelchairs are durable, less expensive, and generally used indoors by the less active person.

All the aforementioned categories are available with a folding frame. In addition, there are reclining, folding wheelchairs as well as a variety of strollers for pediatric clients. The rigid chair is limited to the ultralight and lightweight categories but also includes a tilt in space chair (Fig. 39.27).

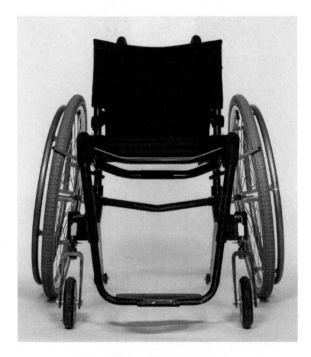

Fig. 39.24.   Rigid wheelchair.

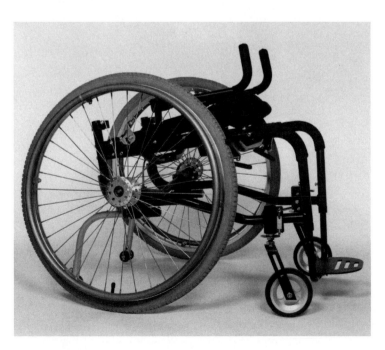

Fig. 39.25.   Rigid wheelchair with back folded forward.

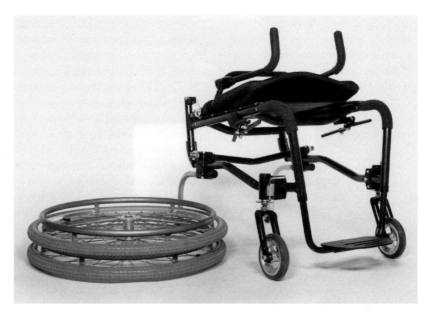

Fig. 39.26.   Rigid wheelchair—rear wheels off for loading into a car.

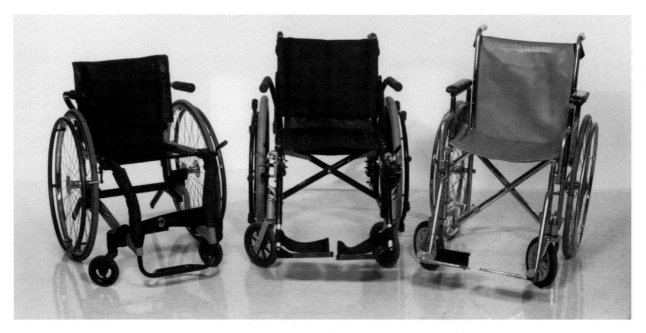

Fig. 39.27.   Ultralight, lightweight, and standard wheelchairs.

WHEELCHAIR PARTS AND ACCESSORIES

Wheels

Rear.   There are two common types: *mag* and *spoke* (Fig. 39.28). *Mag* wheels have a plastic hub and spokes, weigh more, but are low maintenance. *Spoke* wheels are the same as bicycle wheels and are much more efficient. The tires can be pneumatic (air filled) or hard rubber. A pneumatic tire gives a smoother ride, especially on outdoor, rough terrain. They are subject to flats, however. Being stranded with a flat tire can be extremely frustrating.

Solid rubber tires give a much rougher ride but are maintenance-free—no flats. Both air and solid tires are available in treaded or smooth patterns. Tread gives more friction and bite on outdoor terrain, such as gravel, sand, or ice. On carpet, however, it requires more energy expenditure. Smooth tires are more appropriate on indoor terrain. They usually are not efficient for active outdoor use.

The size of rear tires varies from 20 to 26 inches in diameter for manual wheelchairs. The industry standard is 24 inches. Power chairs have 10- to 20-inch diameter tires available. Choosing a specific size of

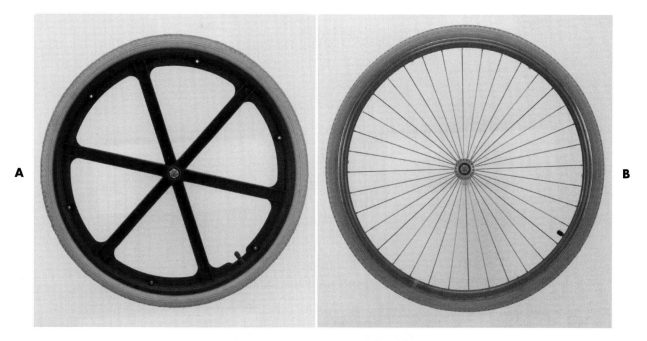

Fig. 39.28. **A,** Rear mag wheels. **B,** Rear spoke wheels.

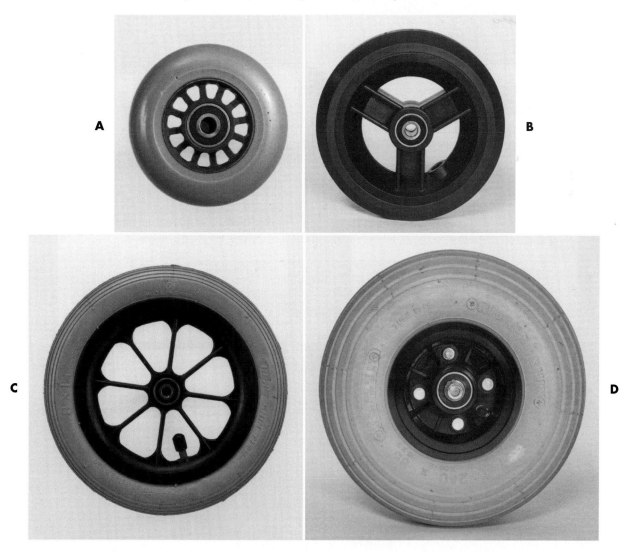

Fig. 39.29.   Front caster wheels. **A,** 3-inch manual polyurethane. **B,** 5-inch manual polyurethane. **C,** 8-inch manual pneumatic. **D,** 10-inch power pneumatic.

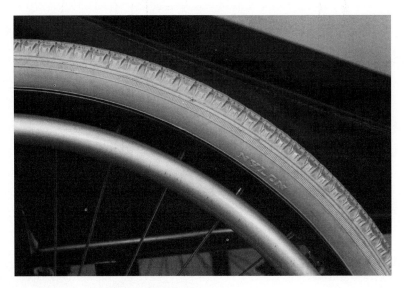

Fig. 39.30. Standard hand rims.

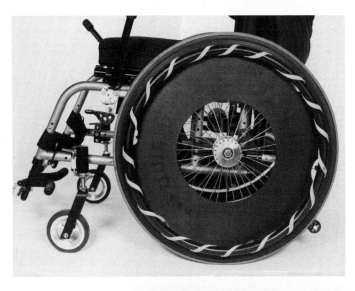

Fig. 39.31. Wrapped hand rims with surgical tubing to provide greater friction.

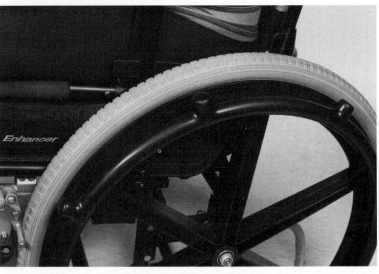

Fig. 39.32. Quad pegs—nubbies.

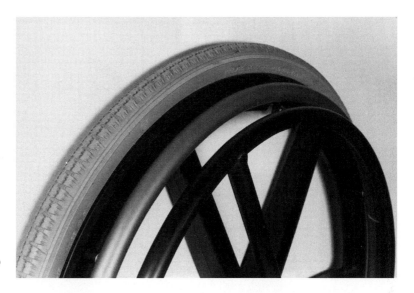

Fig. 39.33.   One-arm drive wheelchair; two rims on one side.

wheel or tire depends on the terrain at home, work, or school. In making the decision on the size of tires, the clinician must consider if the person will be functioning primarily indoors with carpet on smooth floors or outdoors on rough terrain.

Front (caster).   Lifestyle and terrain also affect the choices for front tires. All the aforementioned parameters such as smooth, tread, pneumatic, and hard rubber exist for casters as well. Common sizes are 3, 5, 6, and 8 inch diameter. The types for manual chairs are pneumatic and molded polyurethane. Power chair sizes are 8 to 10 inches diameter, in the same types (Fig. 39.29). The larger the caster, the more difficult turning quickly and maneuvering is, but the overall ride is smoother. The most effective setup for a manual wheelchair for general, overall indoor and outdoor terrain is 24-inch spoked rear wheels and treaded pneumatic tires and 6-inch polyurethane front casters.

Hand rims (manual wheelchairs)

Each rear wheel comprises a tire and a hand rim. *Standard* hand rims are metal (aluminum or steel) (Fig. 39.30). *Friction wrapped* or *plastic-coated* rims are also available. These cover the metal hand rim and provide grip or friction for the person who has limited hand function (Fig. 39.31). Some people with normal hand function, however, also prefer the coated rims to avoid extremely cold or hot metal rims.

Quad pegs or *projections* are metal knobs on the rims that are covered with rubber. They can be full-size or nubbies (Fig. 39.32) and provide leverage against which to push. People with limited or absent hand function may benefit by using quad pegs. The number of pegs varies from 8 to 12; they are equally spaced around the rim.

One arm drive wheelchairs usually have two rims located on one wheel (Fig. 39.33). These rims are available in metal or plastic coated. This manual wheelchair system can be used by the individual who has only one functional upper extremity. Both rims are used to go forward and backward; one rim is used to turn right and the other left.

Wheel locks

Rear.   *High mount—push or pull to lock*—(Fig. 39.34, *A*) are preferred by most people because they are conveniently accessible. People with limited hand function require the high mount location if brake extensions are used.

Low mount—scissors or push/pull to lock—(see Fig. 39.34, *B*) are used by people who are active and have normal reach. The low mount location is out of the way for wheelchair skills and prevents individuals from hitting the thumbs or hands on the locks during rapid wheelchair propulsion.

Caster locks.   The purpose of these wheel locks is to control the front tire, provide a more stable wheelchair, and prevent the front wheels from pivoting during transfers or functional activities. The lock is usually a swivel mechanism (Fig. 39.35).

Brake extensions.   These give leverage and access to wheel locks and allow persons with limited upper extremity function to reach them easier (Fig. 39.36).

Hill climbers/grade aids.   These allow the individual who has weak upper extremities or poor hand control to push or roll up a hill with greater ease (Fig. 39.37). While he reaches back with his arms to take another stroke, the hill climber holds the rear wheels, preventing the wheelchair from rolling or slipping backward.

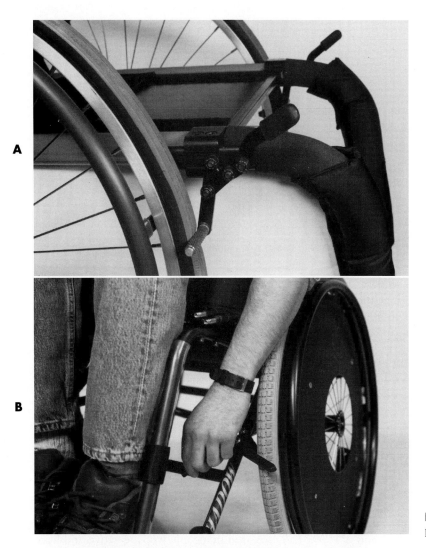

Fig. 39.34. **A,** Wheel locks—high mount push/pull. **B,** Low mount scissor or push/pull.

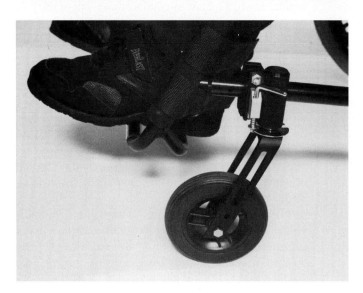

Fig. 39.35. Caster locks.

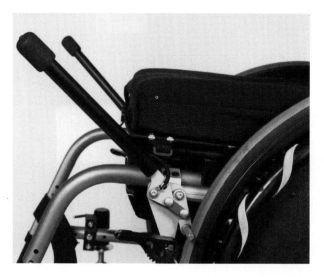

Fig. 39.36.   Brake extensions.

Anti-tippers

These are small extra wheels or bars at the rear of the wheelchair, which, when correctly positioned, keep the wheelchair from tipping over backward (Fig. 39.38). Safety is the primary concern. They can be flipped up for practicing "wheelies" and/or going up/down curbs.

Axles (manual wheelchairs)

Non-removable.   These axles are used for the person who has a folding wheelchair and does not need to remove the wheels quickly.

Quick-release.   These axles provide easy access for wheelchair maintenance or repair of flat tires. Quick-release axles are required on rigid wheelchairs if the person is a driver and plans to load the chair into the car independently.

Amputee axle.   A plate may be added to the rear of the axle to move the center of gravity back, providing an

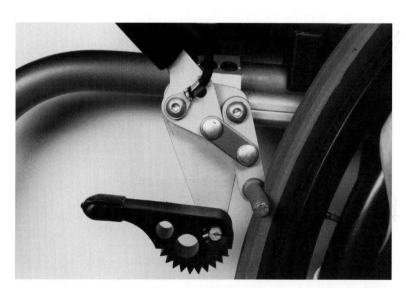

Fig. 39.37.   Hill climbers/grade aids attached to lower aspect of wheel lock.

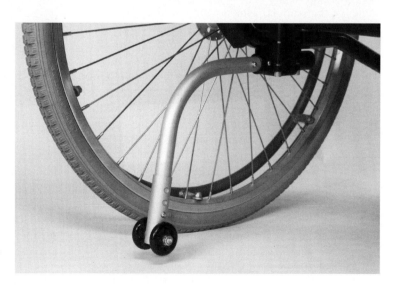

Fig. 39.38.   Anti-tippers mounted at rear of wheelchair.

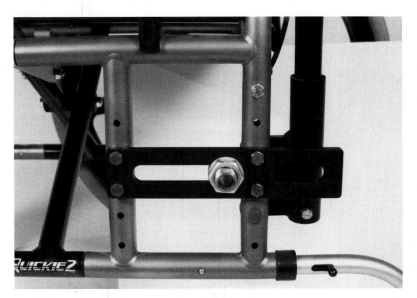

Fig. 39.39.   Amputee axle plate shown parallel to seat rail and lower frame rail.

increase in stability by counterbalancing the loss of weight on the front of the chair (Fig. 39.39) from lower limb amputation.

Back frame of wheelchair

Back heights.   There are various ranges available, depending on the manufacturer or type of wheelchair, for example, ultralight, lightweight, manual, or power. Back heights range from 8 to 20 inches in standard sizes. These can be adjusted up or down. Examples of specific ranges available are 8 to 12 inches, 12 to 16 inches, 16 to 20 inches, or custom heights. Lower-priced wheelchairs have fewer options and usually have a fixed back height. Back heights for recliner or tilt-in-space systems may extend up to 25 inches.

In choosing a back height, the person's level of activity should be considered. If the person is active and will be pushing the wheelchair independently and performing independent activities of daily living (ADL), the ideal back height is 1 to 2 inches below the inferior angles of the scapula. This height gives back support yet does not interfere with function or allow rubbing or catching of the scapula on the top edge of the back.

Another consideration is for the less active person who will not be propelling the wheelchair independently and needs a higher back height for better trunk support and control. In this case, the ideal height would be 1 to 2 inches above the inferior angle of the scapula. This also prevents any rubbing, potential skin problem, or discomfort on the inferior angle.

Seat-to-back angle.   In the ultralight, lightweight, standard, manual, and power wheelchairs, the seat-to-back angle can be varied from true perpendicular by 0 to 10 degrees. Although 0 degrees might suffice for most people, some might need to recline 3 to 8 degrees for balance and function.

Seat-to-back angle in a recliner back is a dynamic system that can vary from 0 to 180 degrees. A tilt

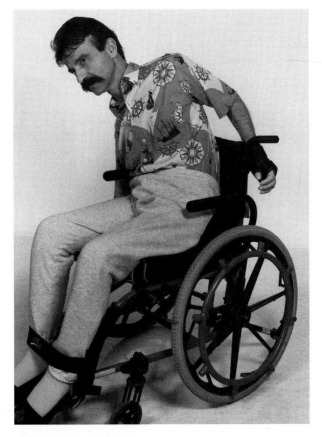

Fig. 39.40.   Individual using push handle for weight shift.

wheelchair can recline as a unit from 0 to 50 degrees; however, the seat-to-back angle remains at static, usually between 70 and 90 degrees.

Push handles.   These are optional on ultralight wheelchairs and standard on lightweight, standard, and recliner wheelchairs. The advantages of push handles are that they offer the active person the opportunity to "hook" an arm for independent weight shifts (Fig. 39.40) and facilitate moving around or repositioning

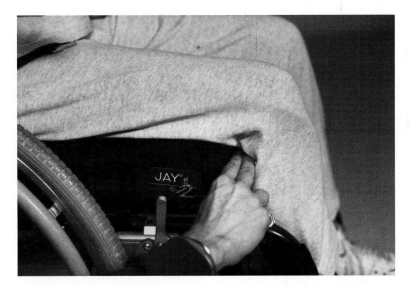

Fig. 39.41.   Seat depth—ideally 1 to 2 fingers' space behind knees.

oneself in the wheelchair. In addition, wheelchair handling, by an attendant, whether indoors or outdoors on uneven terrain, curbs, or stairs is far easier and safer with push handles.

Seat

Seat depth.   Seat depth is crucial in maintaining hip and pelvic positioning. If the seat is too long or too short, the pelvis may tilt. Adequate seat depth prevents the pelvis from sliding forward into a posterior tilt (Fig. 39.41). It is important in the pediatric population to address growth adjustment in the most cost-effective and timely manner, by providing adjustable hardware and growth-expandable seating systems and wheelchair frames. For example, the seat depth is ordered long, and the back support hardware moved forward or reversed as the child grows. Seat depth varies:
- *8 to 16 inches*—Pediatrics
- *14 to 18 inches*—Ultralight, lightweight, standard
- *19 to 22 inches or deeper*—Custom frame construction or by seating system or the cushion

Seat width.   Seat width is vital in preserving lateral stability in both seat and back. It is important to have as narrow a seat width as possible, while still allowing approximately 0.5 to 1 inch on each side of the hips (Fig. 39.42). This prevents rubbing on tires, clothing, side guards, or arm rest parts. The ability to maneuver through narrow doorways is enhanced. It also allows the active person to propel the manual wheelchair in the most efficient manner without having to abduct the upper extremities (Fig. 39.43). Seat width sizes are:
- *8 to 16 inches*—Pediatrics
- *12 to 20 inches*—Adults
- *20 to 36 inches*—Custom, heavy-duty construction

The wheelchair and cushion must be fitted *to the person's* measurements, not vice versa. Too often, a tall

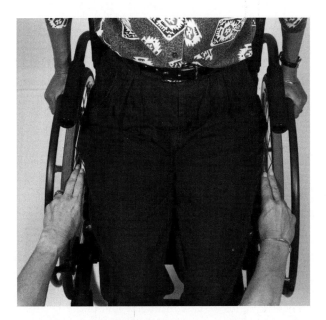

Fig. 39.42.   Seat width—½ to 1 inch on each side of hips.

person with long legs is fitted to a wheelchair because it occupies less space and allows him or her to function in smaller confines within the environment. Regardless of architectural barriers, if the wheelchair is not fitted to the individual's specific dimensions, the consequences could be severe: major skin sores, permanent postural contractures, and decreased level of independence.

Head rests

Head rests are most often used with recline and tilt in space wheelchairs. They can be used to support weak neck musculature, correct or support deformities, or provide a resting surface in a reclining position. There

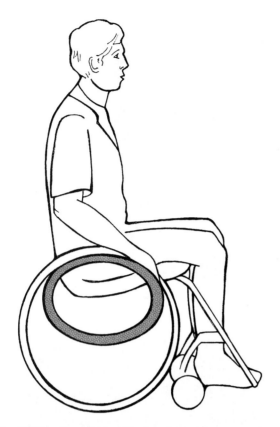

Fig. 39.43.   Seat width—Ideal push or stroke on rear tires or rims.

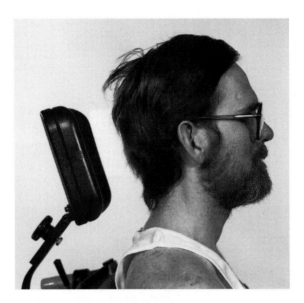

Fig. 39.44.   Simple head rest.

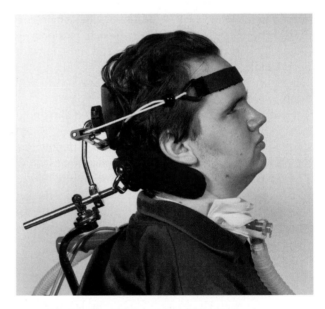

Fig. 39.45.   Three-piece adjustable head rest.

are a wide variety of commercially made head rests ranging from simple pads to custom, adjustable three-piece models (Figs. 39.44 and 39.45).

In choosing a head rest, a person's neck strength influences the complexity of the head rest design. For example, a spinal cord–injured individual with normal neck musculature requires only a simple pad to rest on while in the recline position. While in the upright position, the head rest should not be touching or interfering with head movement. Conversely, a child with cerebral palsy and severe spasticity, causing asymmetric posturing, requires a more complex, customized model to control the head and neck.

Arm rests

Arm rests not only assist in proper postural alignment when elbows are rested on them, but also they provide an important function for several methods of weight shifts.

Tubular swing away. These have limited height adjustments and are very light. They are available on lightweight and ultralight wheelchairs (Fig. 39.46).

Desk. These are desk height and are cut away to allow an easy approach to desks, tables, and other furniture. They usually are heavier and fully adjustable (Fig. 39.47). The design, weight, and adjustability vary with each manufacturer.

Sliding/low profile. Sliding or low-profile arms are used on manual or power recline systems. When a person requires support for the upper extremities in both the upright and the reclined position, these are ideal because they move in conjunction with the back as it reclines (Fig. 39.48).

Arm troughs. These can be added to either type of arm rest (Fig. 39.49). They are designed to support a person's forearm, usually at 90 degrees at the elbow. For a person with no upper extremity musculature, arm troughs provide stabilization and support of the glenohumeral joint as well as assisting with upper body balance.

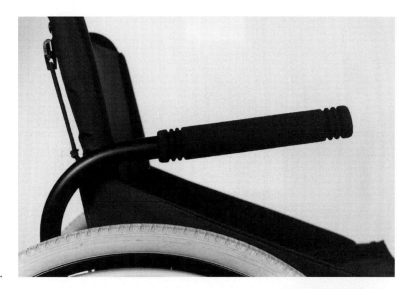

Fig. 39.46. Tubular arm rests.

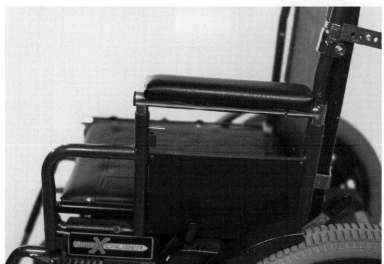

Fig. 39.47. Desk arm rests.

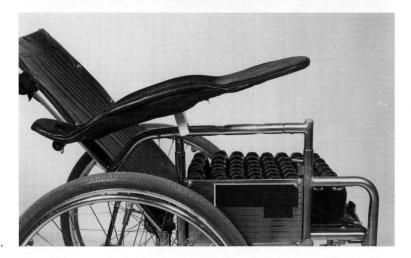

Fig. 39.48. Sliding arm rests.

Foot rests

Foot rests are an integral component of a wheelchair and are available in many different designs. Common options for footrests include:

1. *Rigid "cage"*—built into the frame (Fig. 39.50)

2. *Swing-away* (Fig. 39.51)
3. *Elevating*

Rigid. On a rigid chair, the foot rest, front-end or cage, is generally built into the frame. Some manufacturers, however, offer the option of removable

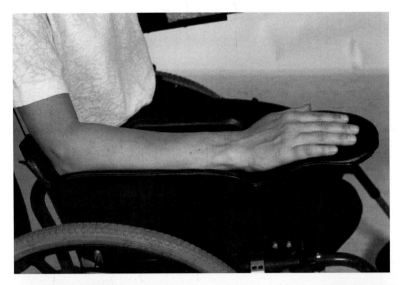

Fig. 39.49.   Arm trough.

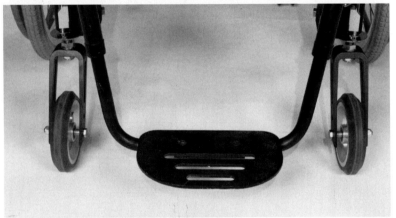

Fig. 39.50.   Rigid wheelchair "cage" foot rests.

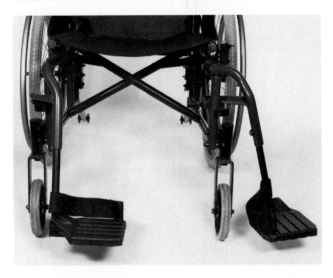

Fig. 39.51.   Removable, swing-away foot rests.

swing-away foot rests. This combines the best of a rigid, one-piece lightweight wheelchair with removable swing-aways for easy access to a tub, shower, or furniture. It does add weight to the chair. Without this option, the rigid wheelchair usually has a tighter turning radius because the rigid foot rest/leg rest assembly does not add overall length to the wheelchair (Fig. 39.52). Additionally, there are fewer parts to interfere with transfers or wheelchair mobility.

Swing-away.   In the past several years, manufacturers have heeded the recommendations from many wheelchair users and caregivers about having a smaller

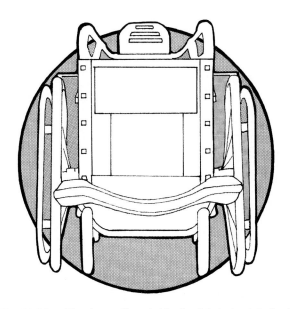

Fig. 39.52. Turning radius: rigid wheelchair (aerial view).

front end. Previously, the foot rests were at a 60-degree angle and took up so much space that it required wider hallways and a larger turning radius in homes, schools, and offices. By changing the angle to, at first, 70 degrees and now 80 degrees, the front end is far more compact, which enhances function (Fig. 39.53).

The primary advantage of swing-away foot rests is ease of access to a bed, tub, car, or furniture for transfers. This feature allows the independent person to be closer to the object to which he is transferring, thus increasing safety. It also provides better access for the attendant or caregiver who is assisting with a transfer. The ability to swing the foot rests out of the way allows the attendant better, safer, more secure foot placement when doing stand pivot or front approach transfers.

If the person's most independent method of wheelchair propulsion is with one or both feet, swing away foot rests are essential. Otherwise, the feet become tangled in the foot rests while trying to propel (Fig. 39.54).

Elevating leg rests. Elevating leg rests are removable on standard manual reclining wheelchairs and lightweights. They are appropriately used on reclining wheelchairs but are unusual on manual lightweights. Power recliner system prescriptions almost always include elevating leg rests. The other option is nonelevating leg rests, appropriate if a person does not have a problem with edema in the lower extremities or history of hypotension. This keeps the already large power wheelchair from taking up so much space when the client is reclined in a weight shift or resting (Fig. 39.55). This feature is especially appealing at school, work, or out in the community. Elevating leg rests can interfere with transfers due to the gooseneck portion.

Foot plates. There are numerous foot plates available from a variety of manufacturers; however, they fall into two general categories: one piece or two pieces. Some are tubular metal, often covered with foam; others are composite materials (Fig. 39.56).

A patient's foot size, body frame, level of activity, and amount of spasticity all influence what type foot plate is chosen. Foot support can be vital in preserving ideal postural alignment.

HOW TO WRITE A WHEELCHAIR PRESCRIPTION

Ideally a wheelchair prescription should be written by a clinician who is well versed in what equipment is available and what the needs of the patient are. Keeping current on state-of-the-art technology and changes, options, and accessories is difficult. Figures 39.57 and 39.58 illustrate an organized method of writing a wheelchair prescription for a manual or power wheelchair.

POWERED WHEELCHAIRS

In the past, powered wheelchairs had not been readily prescribed because it was believed they would promote dependency. It has become apparent, however, that powered mobility can enhance rather than impede one's abilities. A powered wheelchair should be considered for a person who is unable to propel a manual wheelchair functionally and efficiently in his home, vocational and/or avocational environment. Factors that may interfere with efficient manual wheelchair propulsion include decreased upper extremity strength, coordination, and/or range of motion. Poor muscle strength, diminished endurance, decreased cardiopulmonary function, or pain may interfere as well. Aging that results in degenerative damage to shoulders from overuse also may cause a manual wheelchair user to consider a power wheelchair for joint protection and conservation. Energy-efficient mobility during daily activities is important for participation in educational, vocational, and social activities. Therefore, a person's lifestyle must be closely examined to determine the need for power mobility. In other words, the person's physical status, functional necessity, and environment must be considered.

Though powered wheelchairs may enhance a user's personal mobility, environmental accessibility may be adversely affected. It is virtually impossible for a powered wheelchair user to negotiate curbs or stairs independently. Power wheelchairs weigh 200 lb or more

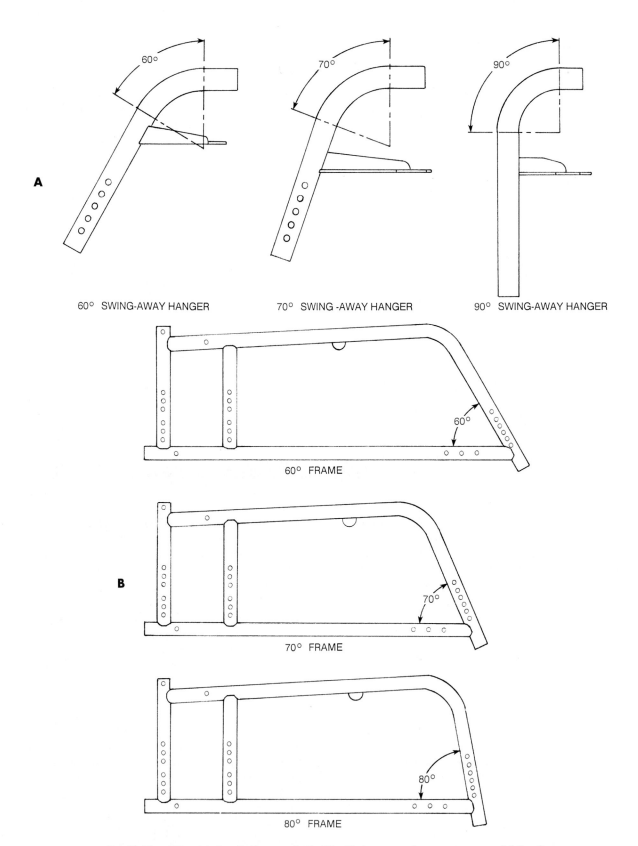

Fig. 39.53. Wheelchairs. **A,** Front end: 60-, 70-, 90-degree angle measurements; folding frame. **B,** Front end: 60-, 70-, 80-degree angle measurements; rigid frame.

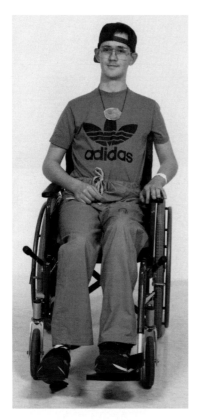

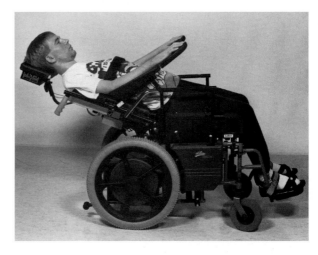

Fig. 39.55. Reclining wheelchair with nonelevating leg rests.

Fig. 39.54. Person propelling wheelchair with one foot; foot rest swing away.

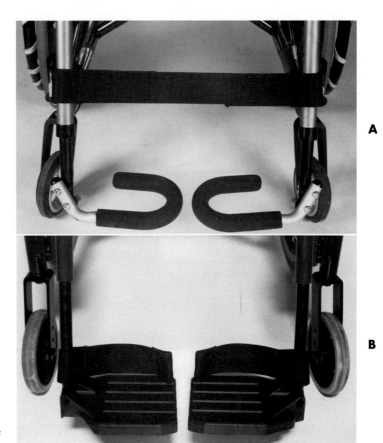

Fig. 39.56. **A,** Tubular footplates. **B,** Composite footplates.

PATIENT EQUIPMENT PRESCRIPTION

Date _____ Unit # _____ Estimated Date of Discharge _____

Patient Name

Address

Name _____ Therapist _____

Reason for Need _____ Physician _____

Wheelchair Make _____ Model # _____

FRAME & ACCESSORIES	WHEELS, CASTORS, ACCESSORIES	FOOTRESTS & ACCESSORIES
❏ Folding	❏ Rear Wheels ❏ 20 ❏ 22 ❏ 24 ❏ 26	❏ Front End Angle
❏ Rigid	❏ Wheel Rim Type	❏ Swing-Away Detachable Footrests
❏ Frame Size	❏ Rear Tire Type	Extension Length
		Other
❏ Frame Color	❏ Hub Type	❏ Elevating Legrests
❏ Upholstery Color	❏ Quick Release Axles	Type
ARMS & ACCESSORIES	❏ Standard ❏ Quad Release	❏ Troughs
❏ Armrests (describe)	❏ Extras	❏ Flip up Footrests
	❏ No More Flats	Type
❏ Block Type Armrests	❏ Air Tight	❏ Cage
❏ Arm Troughs ❏ R ❏ L	❏ Thorn Resistant Tubes	❏ Large Footplates
Type	❏ Other	❏ Heel Loops
Model #	❏ Spokes	
Size ❏ S ❏ M ❏ L	❏ Spoke Guards	❏ Toe Strap
❏ Reclining Armrest Assembly	❏ Mag Style Spokes	❏ Leg Strap
❏ Power Drive Control ❏ R ❏ L	❏ Camber	❏ Single
Type	❏ None ❏ Standard	❏ "H" or Double
	❏ Other	**MISCELLANEOUS ACCESSORIES**
BACK OF CHAIR - ACCESSORIES	❏ Hand Rims	❏ Crutch Holder ❏ R ❏ L
❏ Back Type	❏ Standard	❏ Detachable Back Pack
Model #	❏ Plastic Coated Gray/Black	Type
	❏ Quad Pegs	❏ Front End Roller Bar
❏ Back Height	Make	❏ Anti Tip Bars
Adjustable Range	❏ Nubbies 8 10 12	❏ Batteries and Charger
❏ Save Upholstery	❏ Vertical 8 10 12	Type
❏ Push Handles	❏ Oblique 8 10 12	❏ Under Seat Pouch
❏ Degree of Bend	❏ Inches Between Wheel Rim and Hand Rim	❏ Wet Weather Guards
❏ Folding Back	❏ Standard ❏ Other	Type
❏ Safety Belt ❏ Velcro ❏ Buckle	❏ Extra: ❏ Wheel ❏ Tire ❏ Tube ❏ Caster	❏ Tool Kit
❏ Location	❏ Casters ❏ Diameter ❏ Width	❏ Impact Guards
❏ Length R	❏ Rim Type ❏ Aluminum ❏ Composite	Type
❏ Length L	❏ Caster Tire Type	❏ Touch up Paint
	❏ Hard Rubber	❏ Other
❏ Location	❏ Urethane	
❏ Length R	❏ Semi Pneumatic	
❏ Length L	❏ Pneumatic	
	❏ Other	**CUSHIONS & ACCESSORIES**
❏ Head Rest	❏ Air Tight ❏ Airless Insert	❏ Cushion Type
	❏ Stem Bolt Length	Size
❏ Lateral Trunk Supports	❏ Caster Form Length	
Type	❏ Caster Locks	❏ Solid Insert
Size	❏ Wheel Locks	
SEAT OF CHAIR	❏ Mount Location ❏ High ❏ Low	❏ Cushion Cover Type
❏ Seat Type	❏ Toggle ❏ Push ❏ Pull	
❏ Seat Width	❏ Scissors	Size
❏ Seat Height	❏ Brake Extensions	❏ Other
❏ Seat Depth	Length	
	❏ Hill Climbers	

VENDOR (S) ❏ BID _____

PRE-DELIVERY ADJUSTMENTS _____

DELIVERY INSTRUCTIONS _____

TOTAL COST
$

ATTENDING PHYSICIAN SIGNATURE

2022 (REV 1/94)   WHITE - RECORD   CANARY - VENDOR   PINK - FILE   GOLD - THERAPIST

Fig. 39.57. Wheelchair prescription—manual wheelchair.

and do not fit into a standard car. Therefore, a van, modified with a ramp, lift, wheelchair tie down, and various other adaptions, is required for safe transportation.

When prescribing powered mobility, the following questions should be asked:

1. Does the user have sufficient and consistent motor function, cognitive ability, and judgment to access the drive control mechanism? In the pediatric population, does the child display cognitive developmental readiness?

2. What are the functional needs; will the system be used for the household or community?

3. What are the seating and positioning needs?

4. Are there accessibility or transportation issues that need to be considered?

5. What other technologies need to interface with the wheelchair controller, for example, environmental control unit, computer, or communication device?

6. Will transfers be affected such as independent standing, sliding board?

Types

Powered scooters. A powered scooter is appropriate for a person who has adequate trunk and lower

PATIENT EQUIPMENT PRESCRIPTION • OCCUPATIONAL THERAPY

Date _____ Unit # _____ Estimated Date of Discharge _____
Patient Name _____ Therapist _____
Name _____
Address _____
Reason for Need _____ Physician _____

WHEELCHAIR BASE	WHEELCHAIR DIMENSIONS	LEGRESTS
❑ Make ❑ Model	❑ Seat width " ❑ Depth "	❑ Elevating ❑ non elevating ❑ pad gooseneck
RECLINER TYPE	❑ Wedge	❑ Trough ❑ Pad Type
Make	❑ Custom flr. to seat ht "	Legrest angle
❑ LoShear ❑ Adjustable sliding back	❑ Back height "	❑ Foot plates ❑ 6" ❑ 9"
❑ Tilt ❑ Tilt/Recline	❑ Scapular cutout	❑ Adj. angle ❑ plastic coated
❑ Other	dimensions	❑ Ankle Strap ❑ Toe Strap Type
RECLINER SWITCHES	❑ Gibbus cutout/size	❑ Heel loops ❑ Double ❑ Kydex
❑ Pneumatic ❑ Tape Switches	❑ Extra foam for lumbar size	**WHEELS**
❑ Toggle Extended toggle	❑ Deliver unupholstered	❑ Rear wheel
Placement	❑ 90° vertical cams (LaBac)	Std. base ❑ flat-free ❑ pneum ❑ thorn res.
❑ Other	❑ Other	Pwrbase ❑ flat-free ❑ pneum
DRIVE CONTROLS		❑ Casters
❑ Pneumatic ❑ Chin		Std. base ❑ semi pneum ❑ pneum
Placement ❑ Rt ❑ Lt	**TRUNK SUPPORTS**	Size
❑ Type gooseneck	❑ Type	Pwrbase ❑ flat-free ❑ pneum
❑ Extra mouthpieces #	Size ❑ Rt ❑ Lt	Size
❑ Drive display ❑ Rt ❑ Lt	Custom	**BELTS**
❑ off armrest ❑ gooseneck ht "	**HEADREST**	❑ Velcro ❑ Buckle ❑ D-ring ❑ Quadloops
❑ Mounted on w/c back	❑ Standard	❑ 45° hip ❑ chest
❑ Hand Drive	❑ Ottobock Type	❑ Attach ❑ Do not attach
Placement ❑ Rt ❑ Lt	❑ 3 piece adjustable Type	❑ Other
❑ Retractable bracket Type	❑ Custom	❑ Length
❑ Control pieces	❑ Other	**MISCELLANEOUS**
❑ t-bar ❑ u-bar ❑ ball	**ARMRESTS**	❑ Utility bag ❑ back ❑ side
❑ Extended toggle	❑ Standard adj. desk style ❑ Rt ❑ Lt	❑ Lapboard · ❑ extra brackets
Other	❑ Sliding adj. desk style ❑ Rt ❑ Lt	❑ Standard ❑ Custom
❑ Head Control	❑ Low Profile ❑ Rt ❑ Lt	❑ Ventilator tray Vent Type
Make	❑ Flat arm pads ❑ Rt ❑ Lt	❑ Vent battery and charger ❑ Vent Cable
❑ Remote adjustment box	Make	❑ Batteries ❑ new ❑ demo ❑ dry ❑ wet
❑ Attendant drive	Size/Length	❑ Gel cell
EMERGENCY OFF SWITCH	❑ Arm Troughs ❑ Rt ❑ Lt	☒ Battery charger and tester
❑ Leaf switch ❑ Tape switch	Make	☒ Instruction manual
❑ Dufco sensitouch (only on dufco system)	Size/Length	☒ Prep. and assembly
❑ Other	❑ Straps	❑ Emergency supply and repair kit
Placement ❑ Rt ❑ Lt	❑ Custom	❑ Ship w/c
		❑ Upholstery color
		❑ Frame color ❑ Accessories

COMMENTS: _____

DELIVERY INSTRUCTIONS:
VENDOR (S) ❑ BID _____   TOTAL COST $ _____

_____ Physicians Signature

3033 (Rev 2/94)   WHITE - Medical Records   CANARY - Vendor   PINK - File   GOLDEN - Therapist

Fig. 39.58. Wheelchair prescription—power wheelchair.

extremity control for balance and upper extremity control to maneuver the steering device, also known as the tiller assembly (Fig. 39.59). There is usually a lever on either side of the tiller that is operated by the thumb in a grasping motion. One hand makes the scooter move forward and the other reverse. Many scooter users have the ability to ambulate part-time but need more efficient mobility for the community. Users must be able to transfer independently and shift their weight to counterbalance moving turns. The units can be disassembled for the car but not typically by the user. They are front or rear wheel driven and are available in three-wheeled or four-wheeled models. The four-wheeled models tend to be more stable.

Power add-on units. A modular system that makes it possible for the user to disassemble a power system is referred to as a power add-on unit (Fig. 39.60). Adding a power system to a manual wheelchair is an economical alternative to having both a manual and a power wheelchair. Although the individual power components can be taken off the frame of the chair, they are heavy and can be difficult to manage by the user or the caregiver. Smaller batteries are used both for portability and to fit into the front aspect of the frame. The chair, therefore, has a decreased driving range per battery charge. Wet weather can cause slipping of the drive system on the tires, limiting the use of these chairs in inclement weather or on varied terrain.

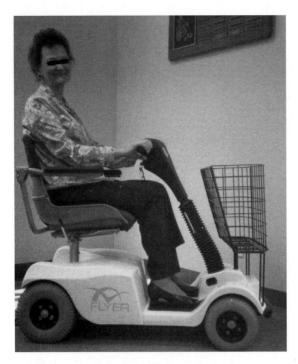

Fig. 39.59.   Scooter.

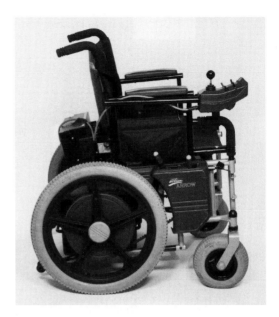

Fig. 39.61.   Standard belt driven wheelchair.

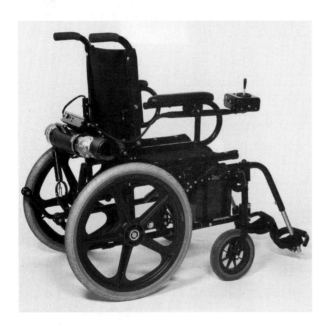

Fig. 39.60.   Power add-on unit.

Thus, the overall performance of add-on systems is limited. These systems are often used for the individual who has minimal funds for a power wheelchair and confines mobility to short distance and smooth terrain. It is also appropriate for the person who does not have a van to transport a power chair.

Standard belt driven.   A standard belt driven wheelchair has two belts connecting the right and left motors to each rear wheel (Fig. 39.61). Each motor works independently of the other. When engaged by the clutch assembly, the belts are tightened between the motor and the rear wheel, which engages the drive system. The seating is incorporated into the frame of the wheelchair; therefore, if there is a need for a greater seat width, the overall width of the chair is increased. This can affect a user's accessibility to his or her environment. The conventional frame does allow for variability in floor-to-seat height, can accommodate a ventilator between the cross frame, and is compatible with public transportation. The rear wheels are usually 20 inches diameter, and the front casters are 8 inches.

Direct drive or power base.   On a direct drive system, the rear wheel is attached directly to the motor unit, which consists of the motor and gear box. There is no pulley or belt system, thus allowing more efficient use of power. These systems are often said to handle rough or uneven terrain better than the conventional chairs. They can give the user a slightly rougher ride, however, and may be more difficult to maneuver indoors in tight quarters because of the large front casters. The front casters tend to be about 10 inches and the rear wheels no larger than 12 inches.

The ease of freewheeling when the clutches are disengaged varies greatly between manufacturers. Freewheeling is important to consider for the user who may need assistance by another to maneuver the wheelchair in a van or align it by a bed for transfers. The ease of freewheeling is important if it malfunctions or has low batteries.

Front wheel drive.   Front wheel drive chairs are direct drive systems similar to the powerbase units; however, the motors are attached to the front wheels

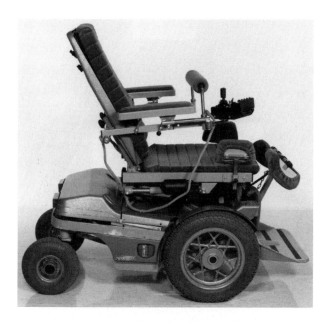

Fig. 39.62.   Frontwheel drive wheelchair.

rather than the rear wheels (Fig. 39.62). With these systems, the front wheels are larger than the rear. This allows for a shorter turning radius and the ability to maneuver over most curbs, something that the other systems may not be able to manage. Because the drive wheels are in the front, the leg rests cannot be detached, and transfers over the wheel may be difficult.

Drive inputs

A person's physical and cognitive abilities determine the type of controller or input method that is needed to operate the wheelchair. Different manufacturers have several varieties of power wheelchairs, which may or may not be compatible with specialty controls. A specialty control is used when a person is unable to operate the standard joystick control by hand or if there is a need to interface multiple technologies through the drive control, such as computers, environmental control units, or communication devices. To access these additional devices, one can simply use a single input control. By using a series of commands through a single input device, the user can move from a wheelchair drive mode to the mode that would access, for example, the communication device. There is usually a standby mode that is a temporary off position or waiting position, to ready the system for the command the user will give. Specialty controls can include systems such as pneumatic (sip and puff), head controls, or chin drive. These usually increase the cost of the wheelchair. Drive control input can be *microswitch* or a *proportional* operation.

Microswitch.   Microswitches allow wheelchair input by simply activating switches in either on or off positions. If a user has motor control of four switches, each switch controls a direction (i.e., forward, reverse, left, and right). There are options for three-switch or one-switch scanning methods available as well. However, these latter options are less efficient. Scanning is a very slow and tedious process.

There are two types of microswitch controls: *latch* or *momentary*. Latched input is similar in concept to a car's cruise control. The activation of a switch engages the wheelchair until another command is given. For example, by moving the joystick forward and then letting go, the wheelchair moves forward. The wheelchair stops when the opposite command is given by pulling the joystick in the reverse direction and letting go. Latched input is much more abstract and requires quick response time, memory, and the ability to give two different commands. Latch is most commonly used with pneumatic (sip and puff) systems, which are described later.

Whenever any type of latched system is used, a safety off switch must always be included. This is a secondary way to stop the wheelchair in case of an emergency, such as the user losing the straw in a sip and puff system or a chin control inching itself out of reach. Safety switches can be such things as a tape switch on a head rest, a leaf switch placed at the chin or shoulder, a fiberoptic switch, or a touch sensor that requires contact to the skin and is activated when that contact is broken. Any single microswitch placed in a reliable position can act as a safety switch. This safety switch may also serve a dual purpose as a mode select switch.

Momentary microswitch controls are designed so the wheelchair responds only when the control is being activated. This allows the chair to go only one speed, no matter how long the control is engaged or how far the joystick is displaced. For example, the chair moves in a forward direction as long as the user is pushing the joystick forward. When the command is no longer given by letting go of the joystick, the wheelchair stops.

Proportional.   The most commonly used hand drive systems are proportional. In other words, the speed of the chair is determined proportionally by the displacement of the joystick from the neutral position. The movement of the wheelchair is also relative to the direction the joystick is placed. The joystick always returns to the neutral position when not engaged and the wheelchair comes to a stop. Proportional systems can also be used as a chin drive but can be fatiguing for one's neck when driving long distances because of the constant need to control the joystick. Proportional hand drive or chin drive systems seem to be the easiest systems for most people to learn conceptually. It is a specific cause-and-effect method (i.e., if you push the joystick forward, the wheelchair goes forward; the

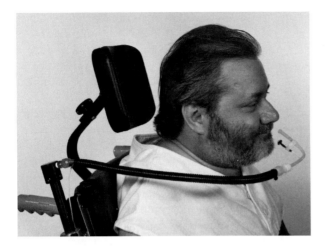

Fig. 39.63.   Pneumatic control (sip and puff).

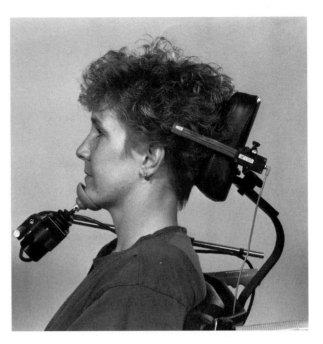

Fig. 39.64.   Chin drive control.

further you push the joystick, the faster the wheelchair will go; if you move the joystick to the left, the wheelchair goes left; and so on).

Drive controls mechanism

Standard joystick control. Standard joystick control is best used with someone who has some upper extremity muscle control and is typically a proportional drive system. Those who drive with their arm or hand must be strong enough with or without adaptive aids, such as mobile arm supports or deltoid aids, to place their hand on and off the joystick, and to bring it to the neutral position to start and stop the wheelchair safely. The same is true for wherever the joystick control box is placed, whether it be mouth, chin, or foot access. Endurance is also a consideration for long distances. Spasticity or movement disorders such as ataxia may interfere with safe control. Many manufacturers have incorporated a tremor dampening that delays the response of the joystick to protect against unintentional motion. A joystick control comes standard on all power wheelchairs and is the simplest and most reliable of systems.

Pneumatic/sip-and-puff. Sip-and-puff or pneumatic controls are ideal for those individuals who have no available motor power to manage a joystick and can cognitively learn the commands (Fig. 39.63). A typical user is a person with a high cervical (C1-4) spinal cord injury. The pneumatic switch is a microswitch activated by the pressure formed in one's mouth rather than actually moving air. Therefore, a person on a ventilator or with little vital capacity can manage this system as long as he or she can achieve good lip closure creating a vacuum on the drive straw. The sip-and-puff system requires little endurance, because it operates similar to cruise control in a car. Because it is a latched system, it allows the user to talk while operating the chair. The

gooseneck and straws for the systems have become quite small, making them more cosmetically acceptable. Using a sip-and-puff system over uneven terrain allows greater control than a chin drive because the tube can be held in the mouth. Two different methods of changing speed are available, depending on the type of controller. One system requires a single puff for each new speed up to five speeds; the second requires one long puff to ramp up to the speed that is desired. The turns are usually set in momentary input. Therefore, a softer sip or puff than the command for forward or reverse is given and maintained until the turn is completed.

Chin drive. Chin or mouth drive is appropriate for individuals with no use of their extremities but who have fair to good use of their neck musculature (Fig. 39.64). Chin drive systems can be accomplished either by positioning the proportional joysticks used for hand drive at the chin or mouth or by using specialty controls, with either latched or momentary input. As discussed earlier, although a proportional system is easier to learn, it may require more neck endurance for driving long distances. A latched system, on the other hand, may require less neck range of motion but more cognition and quicker responses to give both a drive and stop command. Mounting of a chin drive system must be stable to ensure accurate control by the user and to avoid being jarred loose after continued use. A variety of devices on the end of the joystick can be used, such as cups, balls, and extensions, to operate the joystick mechanism.

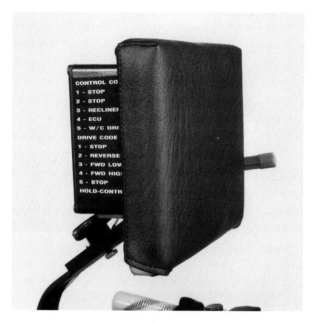

Fig. 39.65. Peachtree Head Control System.

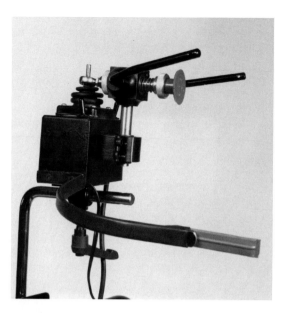

Fig. 39.66. Proportional/RIM head control.

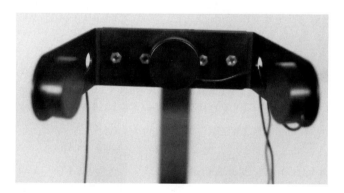

Fig. 39.67. Microswitch.

Head controls. Head controls are another alternative to using a standard joystick. There are three types of head controls: (1) sensor or magnetic fields, which are interrupted by head motion (Fig. 39.65); (2) proportional/RIM (Rehabilitation Institute of Montreal) (Fig. 39.66); or (3) microswitch control (Fig. 39.67).

Systems that are controlled by magnetic fields are by far the most cosmetic type of specialty control. There are no switches, brackets, or controls in or near the user's face. One simply activates the switch within the head rest to change modes (i.e., drive, recline, forward, reverse), then by flexing the head forward, the wheelchair moves forward. The further one moves the head forward, the faster the wheelchair goes—thus, this is a proportional input. To turn, the head is laterally flexed in the direction of the turn. To stop the chair, the switch in the head rest is activated by hitting it or bringing the head back to zero or center.

The RIM system requires a joystick placed behind one's head, which is either incorporated into a head rest or with a special pad and side levers. Alternate switches such as leaf switches are required to change modes or to reverse the function of the joystick. The chair is activated by pushing the head back on the pad or head rest. To change the direction of the wheelchair from forward to reverse, the alternate switch must be activated.

A latched microswitch system can also be used for head control systems. The switch on each side of the head rest controls turns, and the switch behind the head moves the chair forward. An alternate switch changes the forward switch to a reverse mode. With this system, turns cannot be combined with a forward or reverse motion, making it a more tedious drive system.

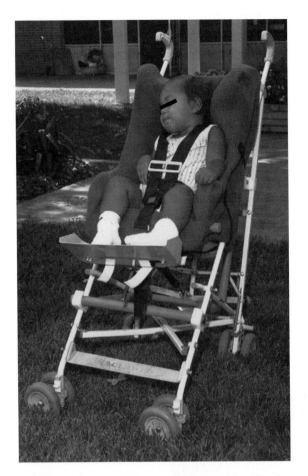

Fig. 39.68. Car seat–type seating insert on a stroller base.

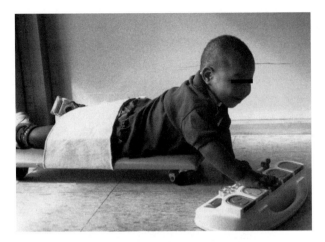

Fig. 39.69. Prone scooter for independent floor mobility.

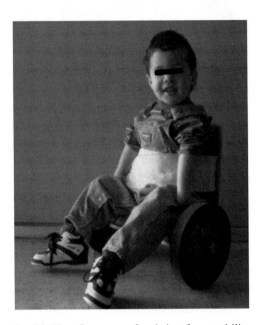

Fig. 39.70. Caster cart for sitting floor mobility.

Performance adjustments

Many powered wheelchairs have a variety of adjustments that determine how the wheelchair functions and allow use of a variety of input methods, depending on the sophistication of the electronics. Some of the performance adjustments include speed, acceleration, and braking. The speed setting determines the maximum speed attainable in the high and low settings of the chair. Acceleration determines how quickly the wheelchair achieves the maximum speed, and braking determines how quickly or smoothly the chair comes to a stop. Torque, sensitivity, short throw, and dampening can also be found on some systems. The torque or power of the wheelchair can be increased to accommodate heavier loads or hilly terrain. The sensitivity setting affects the response of the joystick. If a person is unable to move the joystick its maximum distance because of weakness or decreased range of motion, short throw can be adjusted to decrease the distance the joystick needs to travel to achieve the highest speed. Depending on the manufacturer, the short throw can be adjusted in separate quadrants or in percentages of joystick travel distance. Dampening is an adjustment that decreases the response of the wheelchair to unin-

tentional joystick motion. This is particularly helpful for someone who has severe spasticity or ataxia, such as in cerebral palsy.

Different manufacturers' systems make it possible for the user to program the wheelchair drive inputs to be momentary, proportional, or latched. This is especially useful in the clinical setting, allowing one clinician to evaluate many individuals' needs. It is also helpful and cost-effective for the individual who has changing needs.

Another option available on many systems allows for environmental control access through the drive inputs on the wheelchair. This makes it possible for the user to operate such things as computer systems, power recline systems, controls for televisions, radios, and communication devices through one switch. It is extremely

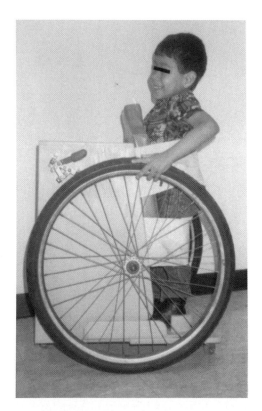

Fig. 39.71. Standing mobility frame.

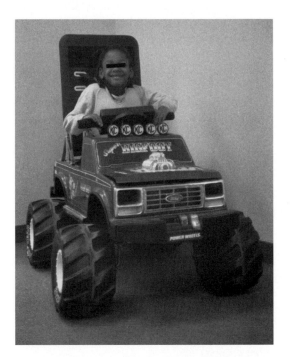

Fig. 39.72. Power toy car—hand operated.

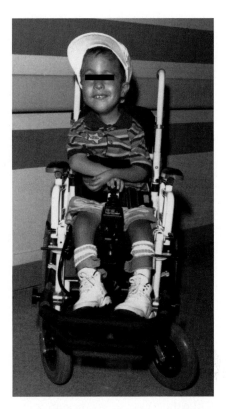

Fig. 39.73. Three-year-old boy with arthrogryposis using a center mount joystick for independent powered mobility at school.

important to ensure compatibility of the electronic interface for each of these systems. This has opened many avenues for independent living and vocational success and has made schooling more of a reality for many individuals. When interfacing all of these systems, however, one must be aware that if the wheelchair controller fails, the ability to control the rest of the environment may fail as well.

The technology that has enabled the fine-tuning and adaptability of wheelchair performance has provided many options that can allow people with disabilities more independence in mobility. Clearly the many options in technology described here dictate the need for thorough evaluations before ordering powered mobility.

Safety features

In the past few years, manufacturers of powered wheelchairs have made many improvements in safety features. Most manufacturers now have electromagnetic braking in the drive motors that locks the motor when the drive controls are not activated. This is an excellent safety feature, especially on hills, on ramps, and in vehicles.

On many systems, if the wheelchair on/off switch is turned on while the user is activating the drive input switch, for example, if the joystick is in the forward position, the power does not come on. There is a delay of several seconds after the joystick returns to neutral before the power returns. This eliminates any accidental start ups when turning on the wheelchair.

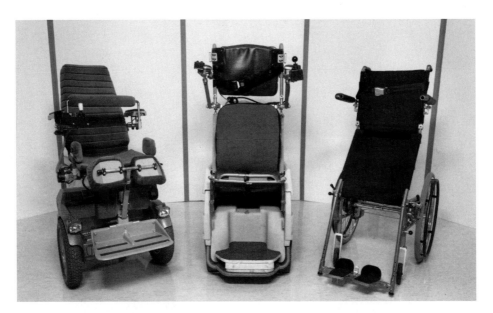

Fig. 39.74.   Variety of specialty wheelchairs.

Another feature that protects against accidental start ups is the standby mode on some specialty control systems. Depending on how the controller is programmed, the drive system always goes to a standby or waiting mode after several seconds. For instance, if the user is driving the chair and stops, after a programmed 10 seconds, the chair resets to standby. The first command given to the wheelchair determines the mode, such as drive, recline, or environmental controls. The second command performs the actual function, such as driving the chair.

Also, the power wheelchairs of the past fluctuated greatly in speed on hills and ramps. With newly available technology, the electronics built into the wheelchair can sense whether it is going up or down hills and then adjust accordingly without the user having to move the joystick to compensate.

Batteries

Batteries are a crucial part of maintaining a power wheelchair. Most power chairs operate with two 12-V acid-filled or gel cell batteries. Although acid-filled batteries require more care and maintenance, they generally hold a charge longer than gel cell batteries. If a user travels frequently on airplanes, gel cell batteries may be a better choice because most airlines accept only dry batteries that cannot accidentally spill battery acid.

Battery access for care and maintenance is a consideration as well. There are several power wheelchairs that allow access to the batteries only when the person is not sitting in the wheelchair. This can limit the times when the wheelchair can be serviced. Unless the user has a second wheelchair, this may necessitate bed rest simply to have batteries changed or serviced.

MOBILITY EQUIPMENT FOR PEDIATRICS

Developmental assessment of mobility impairment begins at birth. There have been many studies done on the importance of independent mobility on the development of spatial cognition and as a facilitator of psychological growth. A number of studies have found that the inability to move has a significant negative impact on development. In children with disabilities, lack of independent movement may cause further delays in cognitive and psychosocial development because the effects of immobility are cumulative and are important at each stage of development. Therefore, mobility is assessed at an early age, and limited mobility because of physical impairments should be augmented (Figs. 39.68 to 39.73).

SPECIALTY WHEELCHAIR SYSTEMS

There are a variety of special systems that allow standing in both power and manual versions as well as seats that raise and lower. These are usually prescribed in rare cases for individuals who may require specific vocational or medical needs (Fig. 39.74).

CONCLUSION

Whether addressing seating or positioning needs, ordering a new wheelchair, or a combination of the above, several factors need to be emphasized. Wheelchair and positioning equipment design is still evolving and ever-changing. While new technology is constantly being developed, conversely, funding sources are committing fewer dollars to pay for such systems. This can certainly create havoc and frustration within a clinical team whose primary goal is to assess and order what is best for the client. It definitely provides an opportunity for increased creativity, all the more reason to involve a team of knowledgeable professionals and a resource person familiar with commercially available products or with the ability to custom-fabricate products.

Understanding basic principles and concepts of seating and positioning and wheelchair fitting is vital. Assessing and ordering the appropriate equipment with clients is mandatory. Educating clients and their families is the long-term goal: a challenge indeed.

ACKNOWLEDGMENTS

The authors gratefully acknowledge the contributions of Lydia Cabico in the preparation of the illustrations and Antje Hunt, Clinical Manager of the Seating Center, Rancho Los Amigos Medical Center, and Linda Bowen, Julie Wolff, RPT, Kelly Root, RPT, and Craig Hospital Staff for reviewing the text.

REFERENCES

1. Anderson GBJ, et al: The influence of back rest incline and lumbar support on lumbar lordosis, Spine, 4:52, 1979.
2. Bergen AF, Colangelo C: Positioning the client with CNS deficits: The wheelchair and other adapted equipment, Valhalla, NY, 1985, Valhalla Publications.
3. Cooper D: Biomechanics in postural control, Proc Seating the Disabled, Vancouver, 1990.
4. Crenshaw RP, Vistnes LM: A decade of pressure sore research: 1977–1987, J Rehabil Res Dev 26:63–74, 1989.
5. Dilger NJ, Ling W: The influence of inclined wedge sitting on infant postural kyphosis, Proc Seating the Disabled, Memphis, 1987.
6. Drummond D, Breed AL, Narechania R: Relationship of spine deformity and pelvic obliquity on sitting pressure distributions and decubitus ulceration, J Pediatr Orthop 5:396–402, 1985.
7. Dolan P, Adams MA, Hutton WC: Commonly adopted postures and their effect on the lumbar spine, Spine 13:197–201, 1988.
8. Engstrom B: Seating for function: Angles, pitch and facilitation, Proceedings of 7th International Seating Symposium, Memphis, 1991.
9. Ferguson-Pell MW: Seat cushion selection, J Rehabil Res Dev 2(suppl):49, 1990.
10. Ferguson-Pell MW, et al: Pressure sore prevention for the wheelchair bound spinal injury patient, Paraplegia 18:42–51, 1980.
11. Furumasu J, et al: Functional activities in spinal muscular atrophy patients after spinal fusion, Spine 14:771–775, 1989.
12. Garber SL, Krouskop TA: Wheelchair cushion modification and its effect on pressure, Arch Phys Med Rehabil 65:579–583, 1984.
13. Gilsdorp P, et al: Sitting forces and wheelchair mechanics, J Rehabil Res Dev 27:239–246, 1990.
14. Greenfield J: Personal communication, LARIE, Rancho Los Amigos Medical Center, 1993.
15. Hobson D: MPI and foam in place seating systems, Proc International Seating Symposium, Vancouver, 1983.
16. Hobson DA, Nwaobi O: The relationship between posture and ischial pressure for the high risk population, Proc. of the 8th Annual RESNA, Memphis, 1985.
17. Hoffer MM: Basic considerations and classifications of cerebral palsy, in American Academy of Orthopedic Surgeons: Instructional Course Lectures, Vol 25, St. Louis, 1976, CV Mosby.
18. Hulme JB, et al: Behavioral and postural changes observed with use of adaptive seating in clients with multiple handicaps, Phys Ther 67:1060, 1987.
19. Hundertmark LH: Evaluating the adult with cerebral palsy for specialized adaptive seating, Phys Ther 65:209–212, 1985.
20. Krouskop TA, et al: Inflation pressure effect on performance of air filled wheelchair cushions, Arch Phys Med Rehabil 67:126, 1986.
21. Krouskop TA, et al: The effectiveness of preventive management in reducing the occurrence of pressure sores, J Rehabil Res Dev 20:74–83, 1983.
22. Letts RM: Principles of seating the disabled, Boca Raton, FL, 1991, CRC Press.
23. Letts M, et al: The windblown hip syndrome in total body cerebral palsy, J Pediatr Orthop 4:55, 1984.
24. Medhat MA, Trautman P: In Redford J, editor: Orthotics etcetera, ed 3, Baltimore, 1986, Williams & Wilkins.
25. Miedaner J: The effects of sitting positions on trunk extension for children with motor impairment, Pediatr Phys Ther 2:11–14, 1990.
26. Myhr U, Wendlt L: Improvement of functional sitting position for children with cerebral palsy, Dev Med Child Neurol 33:246–250, 1991.
27. National Center for Health Statistics: 1977 National Health Survey, Vital and Health Statistics, Series 10, No. 135.
28. Nwaobi OM: Effects of body orientation in space on tonic muscle activity of patients with cerebral palsy, Dev Med Child Neurol 28:41–44, 1986.
29. Nwaobi OM: Seating orientations and upper extremity function in children with cerebral palsy, Phys Ther 67:1209–1212, 1987.
30. Nwaobi OM, Smith P: Effects of adaptive seating on pulmonary function in children with cerebral palsy, Dev Med Child Neurol 28:251–354, 1986.
31. Peterson M, Adkins H: Measurement and redistribution of excessive pressures duing wheelchair sitting, Phys Ther 62:990–994, 1982.
32. Rang M, et al: Seating for children with cerebral palsy, J Pediatr Orthop 1:279, 1981.
33. Rogers JE: Tissue trauma group, Annual Report of Progress, 1973.
34. Seeger BR, Caudrey DJ, O'Mara NA: Hand function in cerebral palsy: The effect of hip flexion angle, Dev Med Child Neurol 26:601–606, 1984.
35. Seikman A: The anti thrust cushion—a twelve year retrospective review, 6th Int Seating Symposium, 1990.
36. Seymour RJ, Lacefield WE: Wheelchair cushion effect on pressure and skin temperature, Arch Phys Med Rehabil 66:103–108, 1985.
37. Shields RK, Cook TM: Effect of seat angle and lumbar support on seated buttock pressure, Phys Ther 68:1682, 1988.
38. Sprigle S, Chung KC, Brubaker CE: Factors affecting seat contour characteristics, J Rehab Res Dev 27:127–134, 1990.
39. Taylor S: Evaluating the client with physical disabilities for wheelchair seating, Am J Occup Ther 41:711–716, 1987.
40. Tredwell S: Overview of seating conditions, 2nd Int Seating Symposium, Vancouver, 1986.
41. Yamashita T, Letts M: Use of the soft Boston orthosis in seating, 6th Int Seating Symposium, Vancouver, 1990.
42. Yasuda Y, Bowman K, Hsu JD: Mobile arm supports: Criteria for successful use in muscle disease patients, Arch Phys Med Rehabil 67:253, 1986.

Assistive Devices for Recreation

Sam Andrews

During the rehabilitation process, the person with newly acquired disabilities goes through a difficult period of psychological and physiologic readjustment. Through recreation and leisure planning, independence and quality of lifestyle can be restored regardless of the disability. Therapeutic recreation can help to ease the traumatic adjustment process. The overall goal of therapeutic recreation is to assist and encourage each person to reach his or her fullest potential no matter how limited his or her abilities may be.

With those who have experienced physical impairment, this goal is accomplished by introducing new activities in which they can successfully participate or by reintroducing activities they enjoyed before injury. It should be demonstrated to the individuals and their families that they are still capable of participating in the entire spectrum of recreational activity, using a few appropriate modifications. One focus of therapeutic recreation intervention is to promote self-acceptance and confidence by helping individuals develop skills and talents to compensate realistically for the disability. Success is an essential part of the implemented program. A patient's involvement in recreation must provide a measure of success with a minimum of frustration. Enjoyment, fun, and accomplishment are obvious rewards for participating in recreation. The following applies to individuals incurring any form of disability regardless of severity. Often, severe disability is addressed. The reader is encouraged to understand the adaptation, and the intervention process requirement may be less complex if the severity is reduced from some of the examples noted. Peterson and Gunn's *Therapeutic Recreation Program Design—Principles and Procedures*[7] is the cornerstone reference for service delivery. Coyle et al[2] cite the many benefits of therapeutic recreation service.

EVALUATION

Early evaluation of the patient is essential to obtain important information not only about the patient's leisure background but also that of friends and family. Typically the therapeutic recreation specialist makes early acquaintance with the patient and family, stating the purpose of that type of intervention and, when the appropriate time comes, what therapeutic recreation entails. It is generally believed that a patient with a relatively new injury and the family are understandably preoccupied with the severity of the medical situation and not receptive to much more than words of optimism and encouragement. This applies regardless of the severity.

Additional information can be obtained from the family at appropriate times. They are often willing at least to discuss the leisure and sports activities the patient enjoyed before injury.

Functional information should be gathered through FIM[10] (Functional Independence Measure developed at State University of New York at Buffalo) or FAM[9] (Functional Assessment Measure developed at Santa Clara Valley Medical Center, San Jose, Calif.) protocols in a coordinated effort with other treating disciplines. The LCM[4] (Leisure Competence Measure, developed at Parkwood Hospital and Oklahoma State University) should also be used to focus on leisure concerns. The LCM assesses leisure skills, attitudes, and preferences. These items in conjunction with FIM and FAM can give clear information on patient status and, more importantly, an indication of what should be addressed in a collaborative and cooperative interdisciplinary approach to an effective, efficient treatment program. It must be understood that any measurement should be used as just that, and the ultimate focus must be on effective outcome well beyond discharge. Assessment modalities have been compiled in a three-volume series entitled *Assessment Tools for Recreational Therapy.*[1] The authors present a vast array of assessment processes that can be of value in therapeutic recreation intervention.

ACTIVE INTERVENTION

As soon as the patient has become medically stable and settled into the routine of daily therapies, the time is typically appropriate for the therapeutic recreation specialist to begin working in earnest to implement leisure assessment modalities. Long-term (discharge and postdischarge) and short-term (main amount of time of patient's initial stay) goals can be established. Again, collaboration with other disciplines is imperative to implement fast and efficient use of staff. Almost invariably the physician, nurses, and other therapists and counselors are able to provide information to assist the therapeutic recreation specialist in determining the proper timing and intensity of therapeutic recreation intervention.

During the time of the assessment, it is important to review with the patient and family the exact role of therapeutic recreation so that realistic expectations of the recreation staff are formulated. Recreation has such broad and general meaning to people of varied backgrounds that it cannot be assumed patients and family will automatically understand the role therapeutic recreation staff intend to play.

Early intervention with the patient is frequently and effectively enhanced by strong, active physician support. Further, initiating activity in conjunction with other therapy activities and/or appropriate nursing functions also greatly enhances the relationship between therapeutic recreation specialist and patient and family. Examples are as follows: (1) coordinating with the physical therapists using a basketball to work on strength and endurance, along with eye-hand coordination, while exploring basketball and its required adaptations as a viable sports and recreational pursuit; and (2) nursing staff and therapeutic recreation specialists coordinating sitting tolerance, self-medication protocol, or implementation of meaningful activity designed to reduce unnecessary dependency on nurses.

Therapeutic recreation specialists should be adequately and properly trained, and any process essential to the general safety and comfort of the client should be implemented. Although other staff generally work with the patient when all the specialty support disciplines are more readily available, the therapeutic recreation specialist often works with the patient during times or in locations when or where those services are somewhat reduced or unavailable. This is not to say

that the therapeutic recreation specialist should go beyond what is deemed reasonable by the attending physician, but more to say functions that family are ordinarily expected to perform should also be performed in competent fashion by the therapeutic recreation specialist. This clearly enhances patient availability for therapeutic recreational activities and sessions. It also serves as a positive example, often encouraging family to become proficient in those functions sooner.

The skill training phase of therapeutic recreation intervention is seen to include four general components. Those components are values clarification, communication, use of adaptive techniques, and use of adaptive equipment. Values clarification is an important component because often it provides the high quadriplegic enhanced insight to the types of events and activities most important to him or her. He or she can often learn not only what aspects of his or her life are important but, more importantly, why. A clearer understanding of why certain events, thoughts, and activities are important greatly enhances a perception of needs. When needs are more clearly understood, it obviously becomes easier to identify those needs that must be met. The therapist and the patient can then more easily set out to meet those needs rather than expend unwarranted time and energy trying to duplicate activities in which the patient is engaged before injury. The patient's time and the therapeutic recreation specialist's time together is limited, and it is essential to make the most of it through a process similar to the one just described. This becomes increasingly essential as the average time the patient spends in a the health care facility is steadily decreased.

It is important to review communication skills and the decision-making skills of the patient and family. There is not time to review completely and make major changes in the patient's communication techniques with family and friends, and it is not practical to attempt to make major changes in the family's communication style with the patient. It is important, however, to review with each the value of communicating needs beyond those basic survival needs in such a way that positive outcomes from such discussion are enhanced.

All rehabilitation disciplines should strive to encourage all parties to communicate clearly values and needs, while the same parties remain open about hearing and understanding the values and needs of others. The recreational setting is an excellent medium in which to review and possibly refine such skills. It is a more realistic or practical setting with real issues in value judgment, community interaction, and interpersonal communication among family members and friends that constantly but naturally occur. For example, having the older children assist a hemiplegic parent into the car to go to a movie gives both parties a "hands on"

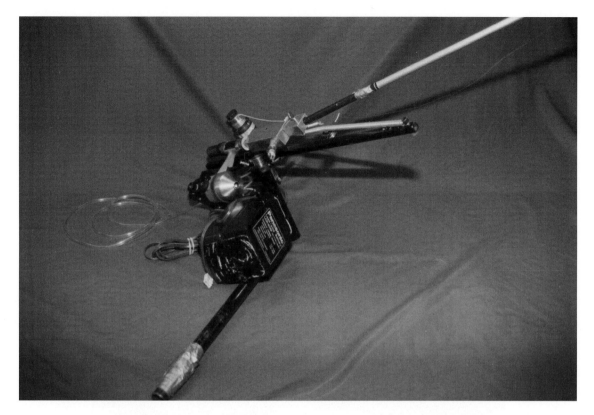

Fig. 40.1. Adaptive fishing device with pneumatic sip-and-puff controls.

experience of the effort involved (which is sometimes less involved than feared).

Clearly sharing needs and desires with others, through assertive behaviors, and realistic expectations of others (meaning family or friends accompanying the patient) are extremely important tools for successful social and leisure encounters, thus helping the individual and family to become less dependent on the health care system in the long run. Therapeutic recreation specialists should dedicate substantial time and effort in communication skill enhancement as well as decision-making training with the patient and family if possible. A shopping trip is an excellent medium to practice effective options for requesting assistance, while the patient is provided the opportunity to exercise self-directed decisions. Dealing with a store clerk, cashier, waiter, and family in a public forum provides the essential components to practice these vital interactions.

Adaptive techniques must be learned to take the place of the typical way functions were performed. For example, the individual may need to learn to throw a ball or draw with the hand and arm opposite the one used before the disability. The use of one hand instead of two to perform a motor task takes effort and innovation to achieve. Adaptive swim strokes to compensate for imposed limitations can be appropriately implemented.

Skills in the use of adaptive equipment, whether it be durable medical equipment or equipment considered to be less medically essential, must be learned. A broad spectrum of equipment, such as a mouth-operated long bow trigger or a bowling ball with a retractable handle in place of the traditional three holes, exists. Another example is a fishing device that casts and reels without requiring the use of hands (Fig. 40.1). The social/recreational experience is greatly enhanced as the individual learns and practices appropriate and effective use. Modification of a pool cue can be done (Fig. 40.2). A weakened trigger finger can be supported by a simple splint apparatus, which is much more desirable than modifying the trigger mechanism of a firearm (Fig. 40.3).

EQUIPMENT AND RESOURCES

The individual with physical disability may or may not use a great deal of adaptive equipment. It is extremely important that the therapeutic recreation specialist work closely with other treating disciplines, early on, so that basic equipment also meets as many recreational needs as possible. Some examples of these considerations are prosthetic devices, such as an arm prosthesis designed to hold pottery tools; enhancing equipment, such as a mechanical device to cock a

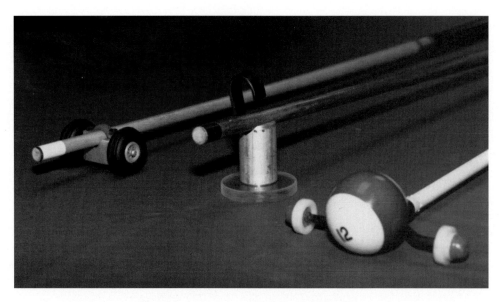

Fig. 40.2.   Simple modifications to pool cues.

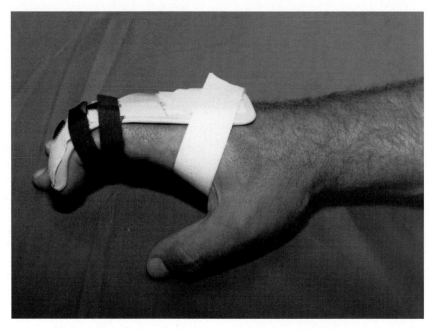

Fig. 40.3.   Moldable plastic trigger finger splint.

crossbow and brackets and wheelchair superstructure allowing for bipod mounts for camera or rifle; appropriate main tires and casters or crutches to properly negotiate anticipated encountered terrain. This can reduce long-range costs to the disabled patient as well as third-party payers. Further, early coordination of customizing equipment can reduce the need for additional specialized equipment, which would represent additional bulk and increase the user's vulnerability to equipment malfunction.

Specialized equipment for recreational activity is often needed. It is important that no equipment should be recommended until a thorough investigation into its practicality has been made. Too often, in their enthusiasm for the patient's success, the staff assist in the aquisition of specialized equipment without enough consideration to such issues as storage, maintenance, and installation away from the rehabilitation setting (e.g., a mechanical adaptation for pinball machine flippers). The danger of the equipment becoming a useless reminder of the disability to the patient must be carefully avoided.

Resource exploration is an essential component to any recommendation the therapeutic recreation specialist might make to the patient. As patient values and needs are explored, immediate consideration for resources to meet those needs and values should be made. Consideration for such things as transportation resources (e.g., accessible bus and taxi availability or personal vehicle), human assistance resources (e.g., service organizations, family, friends, community outdoor and/or recreation personnel), financial resources (understanding the costs of activities and any possible adaptive costs), and accessibility for the highly specialized wheelchair or the prosthetic leg and cane should be given for both the short-term (i.e., during the rehabilitation process) and the long-term (subsequent to discharge). Even under the best of conditions in resource planning for leisure activity after discharge, resources often break down. The therapeutic recreation specialist must be prepared to follow up in some fashion to attempt to assure that planned resources have, in fact, been placed in effect and remain so.

Entities that solely exist to provide resource information are growing in number daily (e.g., *Sports 'n Spokes* magazine, *Disabled Outdoors* magazine, and *Easy Access to National Parks*[8]). The Americans with Disabilities Act (ADA) has, in part, begun to have an effect on the fostering of potential resources in communities across the United States. Organizations (e.g., Flying Wheels, located in Minnesota; local Multiple Sclerosis Society chapters; PVA; Outdoor Buddies, located in Denver, Colorado; Handicapped Scuba Association; National Sports Center For the Disabled, in Winter Park, Colorado; POINT, an outdoor adventure organization located in Dallas, Texas, to name a few) that address assistive needs of individuals with disabilities are rapidly increasing in numbers. Information sharing about these entities is imperative.

PRECAUTIONS

Precautionary considerations for leisure activity should be taught by therapeutic recreation specialists as well as members of other disciplines. Beyond general safety and precautionary considerations for the individual with greater disability, there are three categories of additional consideration that play an important role in the success of leisure pursuits. They are social, mechanical, and environmental.

From a *social* standpoint, certain considerations by the disabled individual truly enhance his or her recreational experience in a number of ways. One example is clear communication by the individual with the disability with other participants of a social situation, beforehand, what physical needs he or she will have during the event and how he or she intends to handle them, rather than asking for assistance continually from those who would not know what is to be asked next. Often, that type of situation can be easily remedied by having an attendant accommodate his or her needs. Another example of a difficult social situation is one in which full consideration for those attending an event is not given, such as the noise adaptive equipment might make during a movie in a theater. Practical remedies might include prearranged seating by theater management in an area of the theater next to an exit with easy entry and exit so that the individual could quietly and quickly be moved outside to a part of the lobby where attending to a personal need would be much less of a spectacle. Advising those seated nearby of unusual sounds or excessive noise or movement should be done as a courtesy so that those who might be disturbed would have the opportunity to move away if they so chose. Remedies to these situations can create a more acceptable and, therefore, more satisfying recreational situation.

The second category concerns *mechanical* considerations. The therapeutic recreation specialist can give a great deal of information on the use of back-up mechanical equipment by demonstrating its use in recreational activities. One example of a simple mechanical adaptation for safety back-up is a connection to the electrical system of a vehicle that allows for auxiliary electricity to operate a ventilator or the mechanical components of the wheelchair, especially suctioning equipment, in the case of power failure. Systems such as this might eliminate the need to carry along extra batteries. Gel cell batteries powering equipment can make air travel much more convenient. Considerations such as this tend to remove some of the factors that may serve as deterrants to leaving the comforts of home to participate in recreational activity.

The third category is *environmental* conditions. The therapeutic recreation specialist should spend educational time with the patient discussing the effect of various environmental conditions. Through close collaboration with the physician and nursing staff, information should be shared on the effects of such conditions as dust, heat, sun, cold, ice, altitude, and, humidity, to name a few. Again the aim of such education is to give the individual the opportunity to enjoy the success of the activity rather than suffer negative consequences of preventable environmentally induced problems.

It is extremely important to identify individual needs when designing individual programs. The individual's interests, values, recreational needs, leisure resources, and capabilities must be taken into consideration so that realistic goals can be set with a high probability of achievement in preparing the patient for effective leisure time use. Use of the various diagnostic and profile assessments published by therapeutic recreation and psychological specialists can be used. A compilation of many of these instruments is available.[1]

ACTIVITIES

Socially an individual with a disability needs to nurture a sense of belonging, of being accepted by society. When a person with a disability is able to accomplish a project or fill a role successfully, he or she then has an opportunity to build his or her self-image.

For practical consideration, examples of extreme situations are noted, understanding that less demanding situations require less drastic adaptation.

Enhancing of one's self-image may be accomplished

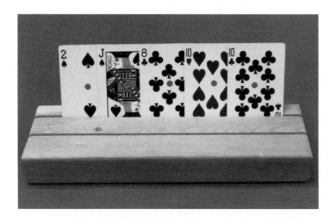

Fig. 40.4.   Adapted card holder and adapted cards.

through such activities as decoupaging with a paint brush in the mouth or becoming a licensed Ham radio operator using a sip-and-puff Morse coder. A device such as the sip-and-puff Morse coder can be designed on the same principle as the sip-and-puff control of the electric wheelchair. All activities that can be accomplished with head, mouth, or chin control should be explored. Even in extreme cases, keeping modifications as simple and practical as possible is important. The rule of thumb is to get by with the least elaborate modification as is necessary. This reduces complexity of the activity and makes repair of modification at a later date easier.

Again in extreme situations, simple table games with magnetic pieces moved by a mouthstick can be used. These games can be played with a friend, family, or a staff member. Card games can be played by cutting holes in the upper middle portion of the cards so that a mouthstick can be inserted to move them. Cards from any type of table game can be arranged in a simply constructed card holder along with the use of a bird beak (a hooklike item held in the mouth) device with which to pick them up and/or move them (Fig. 40.4).

Electronic video games and personal computers can be adapted with a chin control and/or pressure-sensitive switch that allows the disabled individual to operate them independently or with a partner (Fig. 40.5).

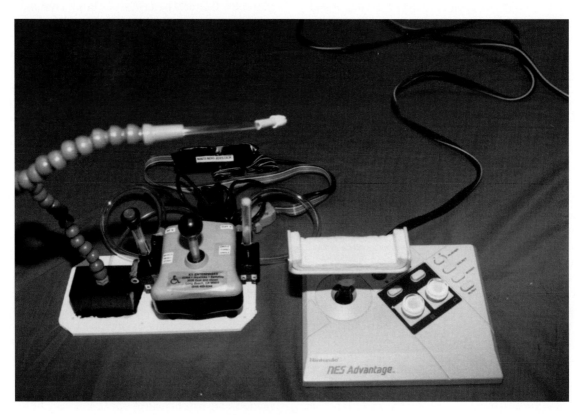

Fig. 40.5.   Adapted video game controls.

Various brands and quality levels of stereo cassette players, compact disk players, and AM/FM receivers have total push button or remote switching and controls allowing for adaptive operation. These units are also configured in such a way that the use of bird beak devices and adaptive storage libraries gives the high quadriplegic the capability to insert or remove disks or cassettes himself or herself.

For fishing, there is an adapted fishing reel that is operated by disengaging the drive belt of an electric or sip and puff wheelchair. More simply commercially produced fishing rod holders can work well for an individual with use of only one hand or arm by placing the holder in a convenient location for maximum use. A more sophisticated adaptive self-casting rod and reel apparatus is pictured. The fisherman can reel in fish by simply operating a switch, thus creating opportunities to fish with casting assistance or fishing off the side or back of an appropriately configured moving boat. More sophisticated and reliable casting and reeling devices are being tested at the time this chapter is being written. A growing amount of adaptive equipment is being designed as microswitch or sip and puff controlled to work off the electrical system of the electric wheelchair opening, many new horizons for the high quadriplegic and, of course, anyone with less severe limitations.

Aquatic activities can also provide an environment for socialization and some independence. Radio-controlled sailing is one type of aquatic activity. The same skills are needed to operate a model sailboat or a full-sized boat. A control is positioned so that the two radio-control joystick levers are within the range of the high quadriplegic's mouth, chin, or mouthstick. These same controls can be used with less modification and more appropriate modification as well. When the boat is in the water, the individual level of disability becomes moot. Family and friends can also participate in this type of activity, and no previous sailing experience is required because the basic skills can be learned quickly. This type of activity also provides an avenue for competition through model yachting clubs across the United States that organize races featuring these radio-controlled boats. In a case such as this, the disability presents no disadvantages or handicaps to competition. Even with mouth controls, a high quadriplegic or double arm amputee can compete on an equal basis with anyone. The same operational principles for the sailboats apply to radio-controlled cars, airplanes, gliders, and power boats (Fig. 40.6). Activities such as these lend themselves to valuable family interaction (especially with youngsters) affording a wide spectrum for activity involvement.

Other aquatic activities to consider are rafting and high-performance sailing. These are extremely high-risk activities and are not generally recommended because much preliminary work must be done to insure appropriate safety conditions. Under exceptional circumstances, however, even the ventilator-dependent quadriplegic might be a candidate for rafting if proper

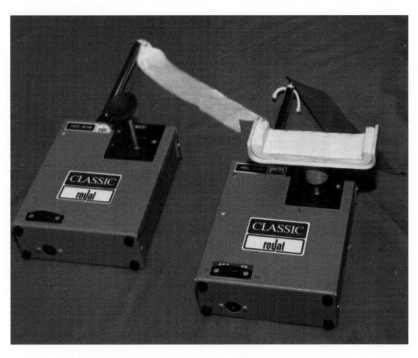

Fig. 40.6. Adapted radio control transmittal boxes.

attention is given to the many safety considerations that can be controlled. Each situation presents its own safety considerations. Some common ones are the recruitment of highly qualified rafting specialists, highly stable rafts, well-studied appropriate waters, ideal weather conditions, spare manual ventilating equipment, and appropriate protection for ventilator equipment (to name just a few).

The physically limited person can exercise mental strategies for tactical maneuvers and be actively involved in operations such as judging weather conditions and other essential variables critical to operation. Again, these are activities in which family and friends can be involved.

Camping is another activity for the individual with a disability. The individual can provide himself or herself the opportunity to be with family or friends away from the typical home or institutional environment. Although the individual may be dependent on others for care, he or she can be responsible for making such decisions as campsite selection, weather-related contingencies, and campsite arrangement. The individual might even participate in hauling firewood by towing it with the electric wheelchair.

In all activities, the physical aspect is only one part. There are also mental, social, and emotional aspects of intervention to be considered. Recreational outings offer a means of testing out self-image in public, and they can be a time for socialization. A successful experience on an outing can encourage a person with disability to try that experience or others similar to it again. Challenging outings can expose the person and family and friends to situations that might be encountered at home. The person can begin to problem solve on his or her own or with others so that these challenges are less threatening later. As families get more opportunity to problem solve, especially with the assistance of staff, the outings subsequent to discharge are less of a burden and more "user friendly," thus enhancing the probability of the individual getting out into the community on a more frequent and likely healthier basis.

Activities once thought impractical, if not impossible, are, in fact, "doable" with appropriate planning and coordination with the members of the other disciplines of the rehabilitation program. Activities of an adventuresome nature include such events as kite flying, ocean cruises, hot air ballooning, and big game hunting. They are highly popular and are becoming less difficult to conduct as experience is gained. Again, it must be emphasized that a great deal of planning, ingenuity, safety consideration, and resource analysis, in all of which the person with the disability should be highly involved, are essential components to short-term and long-term success.

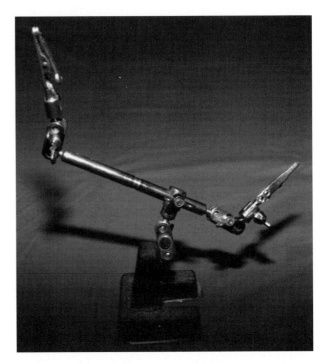

Fig. 40.7.   Standard craft clip vise.

Music and drama also serve as important therapeutic modalities as well as pleasurable activities. Coaching and cheering at athletic events should also be considered as opportunities to allow the person a means for creativity, self-fulfillment, and expression. Creating or participating in skits, dance, talent shows, dramatic productions, athletic events, or other spectator events provides an opportunity to escape the physical confines of the wheelchair. The person may even be able to build up lung capacity and strength while striving to sing or project the voice.

Yet another activity for major consideration is photography. Use of a bi-pod or the camera strap as a stabilizer makes photography or videography quite viable. Great latitude for creativity and self-expression exists. Today's cameras can be purchased with the specific automatic features to meet the individualized need of each person, easily accommodating the person's specific preference. The use of bi-pod or suspension equipment attached to the electric wheelchair, crutch, or walker places the camera in a desirable position for operation by anyone with a disability. Further adaptations of camera controls such as manual focus and light aperture can be made to suit individual desires. The activity can easily be carried on to the darkroom for additional creativity in photo composition.

Literally, most any hand operation can now be adapted by consulting experts in rehabilitation engineering, therapeutic recreation, and adaptation at the noted rehabilitation centers and many community recreation centers. Often over-the-counter materials are most economic and effective. The clip vise shown in Fig. 40.7 is an example of an assistive item that compensates for limited use of hands. Maddox[5] and Nesbitt[6] present a wealth of ideas and information based on practicality and success.

The field of exercise is also available to many through adapted programs. The most noted at the time of the writing of this chapter is "Lisa Erickson's Seated Aerobic Workout."[3] Other more general programs are also available. The Saratoga Cycle and Shadow Cycles are current examples of hand-operated exercise equipment that are commercially available. Figure 40.8 shows an exercise cycle operated by hand. Figure 40.9 shows adaptive hand grips and straps to adapt the hand-operated cycles to individual needs.

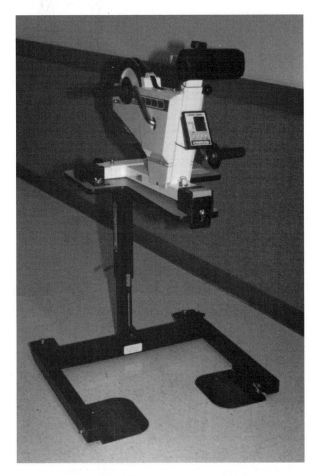

Fig. 40.8.   Exercise cycle on stand.

CONCLUSION

This chapter has discussed experiences that have been demonstrated to be effective in therapeutic recreation intervention. Following a basic format of introduction and assessment, skill training, and resource exploration as previously described, therapeutic recreation intervention provides increased opportunity for the individual to return to a healthy state. The individual and the family should use recreational skills and resources to add strong incentive to live in as healthy and independent condition as possible after all the effort, energy, and resources have been expended to return the individual to typical medical health. Most any activity across the entire recreational spectrum can be adapted. It must be determined whether the activity and its adaptation are meaningful and appropriate.

Once the patient is discharged, follow-up and reevaluation are essential in assuring that appropriate leisure skills are commensurate to the desires and abilities of the individual as conditions in his or her life change. Referral to community resources is a most important transitional step from the health care facility to the community.

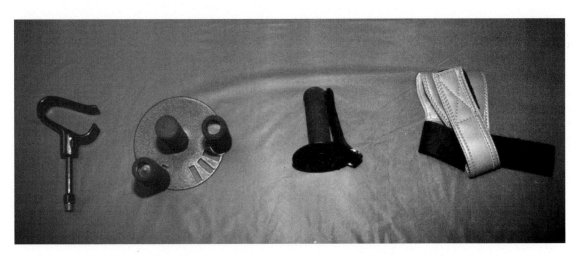

Fig. 40.9.   Assorted modifications to cycle hand grips.

REFERENCES

1. Burlingame J, Blaschko TM: Assessment tools for recreational therapy, Seattle, 1990, Frontier Publishing.
2. Coyle CP, et al, editors: Benefits of therapeutic recreation: A consensus view, Philadelphia, Temple University.
3. Erickson L: Lisa Erickson's seated aerobic workout, Video Tape, Denver, 1993, Aspen Fitness Association.
4. Kloseck, et al: Leisure competence measure, Stillwater, Oklahoma, 1992, Oklahoma State University.
5. Maddox S: Spinal network, Boulder, CO, 1993, Sam Maddox, Publisher.
6. Nesbitt JA, editor: The international directory of recreation-oriented assistive device sources, Marina Del Rey, CA, 1986, Lifeboat Press.
7. Peterson CA, Gunn SL: Therapeutic recreation program design—principles and procedures, Englewood Cliffs, NJ, 1984, Prentice-Hall.
8. Roth W, Tompane M: Easy access to national parks, San Francisco, 1992, Sierra Club Books.
9. Santa Clara Valley Medical Center: Functional assessment measure, San Jose, CA.
10. Uniform Data System for Medical Rehabilitation: Functional independence measure, Buffalo, State University of New York at Buffalo.

Sports Adaptations for the Physically Challenged Athlete

David F. Apple, Jr.
Judy Askins
Ann Cody
Barbara Trader
Grant Peacock

Before 1950, there was not much available in the sporting world for people with disabilities. Largely through the impetus of Sir Ludwig Guttmann at the Stoke Mandeville Hospital outside of London, England, the sports movement for people with disabilities began as the annual wheelchair games. These games took on added significance during the Olympic year when the event became truly international in flavor.

The wheelchair games became the Paralympic Games in 1960 when they were held in Rome, the Olympic host city that year. Since that time, national sports federations have developed around each disabled sport. These federations have held national and international events to promote excellence in the specific sport. In 1988 for the first time, the Paralympic Games were held immediately following the Olympic Games in Seoul, Korea, using the same facilities as the Olympic Games. This scenario was repeated in Barcelona in 1992, and in 1996, the Tenth Paralympia will follow the games in Atlanta by 2 weeks. In the 1996 Paralympic Games, 16 sports will be included, 14 of which are the same as in the Olympic Games.

This chapter lists most of the sports that are available for people with disabilities. Many of them can be competed by athletes with disabilities without special equipment. Others require one or more pieces of adapted devices. Illustrations are provided for many of these.

ARCHERY

Archery can be a competitive or recreational sport. Many different pieces of adapted equipment make it possible for individuals with a variety of disabilities to participate. Archery cuffs and quick release cuffs assist those with limitations in the hands to grip the bow or the arrow and allow them to draw and release the bowstring effectively. Wrist and elbow supports are used by individuals who have arm, wrist, and grasp difficulties. These supports provide additional support and stability to the elbow and wrist of the bow arm.

Trigger releases are another piece of mechanical equipment commonly used by those individuals with upper extremity impairments. These releases assist the archer with the draw and release of the bowstring. Many archers that have upper extremity involvement also use several types of mouthpieces to draw the bowstring with the mouth.

BASKETBALL

This sport requires few adaptations for equipment as well as rules. Participants use sports chairs that are lightweight, have cambered wheels, and have high-pressure tires, enabling them to be maneuvered and make quick turns. Spoke guards are used to protect both the spokes of the wheelchairs and the players' hands (Fig. 41.1).

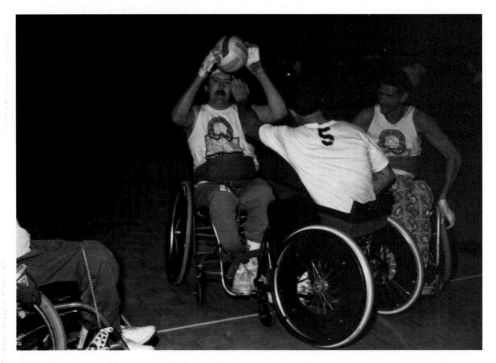

Fig. 41.1.   Basketball. Wheelchairs that can maneuver easily are necessary as well as straps to hold legs in position. For quadriplegics a trunk strap is necessary.

BILLIARDS

Billiards uses several pieces of adapted equipment for individuals with impairments in the upper extremities. Pool cuffs (Fig. 41.2, *A*), which are secured to both the hand and the pool cue, assist with gripping the pool cue. There are two types of pool bridges, both a stationary bridge rest and a mobile bridge, which help support the far end of the pool cue for individuals with balance problems (Fig. 41.2, *B* and *C*).

BOATING/CANOEING/KAYAKING

Boating can be a recreational activity as well as a competitive sport. The area of boating includes a wide variety of possibilities, from canoeing to kayaking to motorboats. Individuals with disabilities can participate in this activity with varying degrees of adapted equipment. In common for most boating activities are cushions or padding for those with sensation deficits. Seating can be customized to provide the appropriate amount of back support and positioning, whether it be in a motorboat seat or on the floor of a kayak. For kayakers, the use of floats or inserts in pant legs is recommended for safety reasons. This helps to prevent the legs from snagging on submerged objects as well as provides buoyancy. Individuals with grasp difficulties can use Ace bandages or

grasping cuffs to hold the paddles effectively. (See also Rowing.)

BOWLING

Bowling is a popular recreational activity that requires minimal modifications to equipment. Bowling balls can be purchased with a spring-loaded handle, used often by those lacking finger dexterity to grip a standard ball (Fig. 41.3). When the ball is released, the handle retracts into the ball, enabling the ball to roll smoothly. Snyder's bowling ball holder ring fits onto the wheelchair, freeing the bowler's hands, allowing the bowler to maneuver the wheelchair. For individuals who do not have the balance or strength to hold a bowling ball, bowling sticks (or a two-pronged ball pusher) can be used. A variety of bowling ramps exist that are used primarily by those unable to bowl free-arm or with the use of a bowling stick. Ramps can easily be made at home or purchased commercially.

CYCLING

The adaptation of cycling for people with disabilities is a natural progression in the development of human-powered vehicles. The innovative elements introduced to adapted bicycles have created opportunities

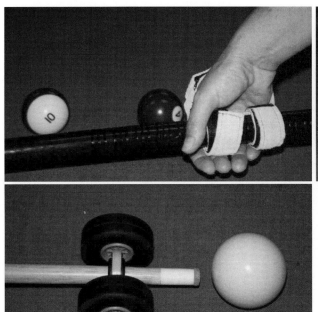

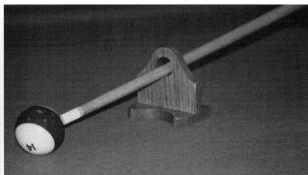

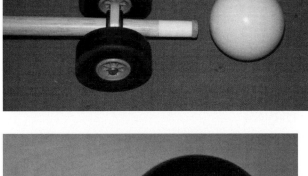

Fig. 41.2. Billiards. **A,** Adaptive device to hold a pool cue. **B** and **C,** Different devices to serve as bridges.

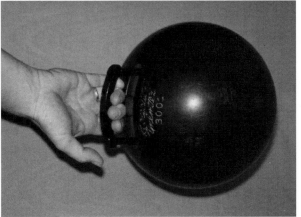

Fig. 41.3. Bowling. Special holding device for the ball.

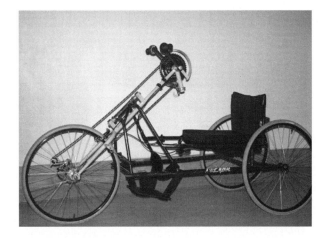

Fig. 41.4. Cycling. Custom triwheeled bike powered by upper extremities.

for people with various disabilities to participate in the sport recreationally and competitively. Cycling is a Paralympic sport for the blind and visually impaired, amputees, and people with cerebral palsy.

The visually impaired use tandem bicycles, amputees customize the bikes to accommodate a prosthesis, and people with cerebral palsy ride custom-built triwheeled bikes. People with spinal cord injuries enjoy recreational and competitive cycling, although it is not a Paralympic event. These bicycles are arm operated with a crank connected to the front fork, which also serves as the steering mechanism. They are typically triwheeled for greater stability with multiple gears and hand brakes (Fig. 41.4).

FENCING

Wheelchair fencing is one of the oldest sports for people with disabilities. Athletes compete in foil, épée, and saber events. Since the first international competition held in 1955 at Stoke Mandeville, England, the rules have been progressively adapted to parallel technical advances in the systems used to stabilize the wheelchair to the piste (platform used in competition).

Fencing is a Paralympic sport for amputees, spinal cord–injured individuals, and persons with cerebral palsy. All competitors must compete from a wheelchair. The adapted equipment used in this sport includes a

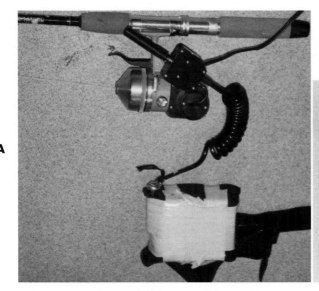

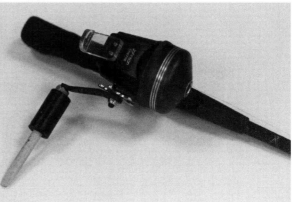

Fig. 41.5.   Fishing. **A,** Electric casting system with a joystick fastened to wheelchair. **B,** Stick attached to reel, which fits into the cuff on the person's hand.

piste and lock down or stabilizing device to secure the athlete's wheelchair to the platform, which allows the athlete freedom of movement in the upper body with a stable seat. There is also a protective cover worn over the athlete's lap to protect lower extremities from incidental contact.

FIELD EVENTS

Field events, part of track and field, are enjoyed by people of all ages and disability groups. There are numerous opportunities recreationally and competitively at regional, national, and international levels. Field events are included in the Paralympic program for athletes with spinal cord injuries, cerebral palsy, amputations, visual impairments, and small stature.

Adapted equipment is used for those individuals who compete from a seated position. Athletes throw implements from their wheelchairs, which are customized for this sport. Most chairs do not have wheels because this is less stable than throwing from a fixed bench seat. The bench is equipped with rails used for seating balance and leverage and is fully padded to protect the athlete's skin. The bench or throwing wheelchair is anchored to the throwing circle by a special device. This device is a strapping system with suction cups that adhere to the medical platform on which the bench sits. Straps are used to secure the bench or wheelchair, and suction cups hold them to the platform. Credit is given to the Paralympic Organizing Committee of Barcelona for developing this innovative system for the 1992 games.

FISHING

Fishing is a recreational and competitive sport that can be accessed by anyone with a physical disability. This is due to the development of adapted equipment to accommodate people with lower and upper extremity impairments.

Rod holders are used to hold a fishing rod to the wheelchair if a person is maneuvering the chair or unable to hold a rod independently.

An *automatic or electric casting system* is used to cast the fishing line automatically with an electric breath or joystick control mounted on the wheelchair. The rod holder is also used in conjunction with this system (Fig. 41.5, *A*).

An *electric reel* operates on the same premise as the electric casting system but is used for reeling in a line or fish. Reeling may also be done manually with modifications to the reel's handle.

Fishing cuffs are used by individuals who have minimal hand function. These cuffs are attached to the person's wrist and hand and have a specially designed strap that holds the fishing rod securely in the person's hand. Individuals with minimal hand function may still be able to cast and reel manually (see Fig. 41.5, *B*).

FITNESS/TRAINING EQUIPMENT

Fitness for people with physical disabilities is important and necessary to obtain a higher quality of life. Manufacturers are recognizing this market by

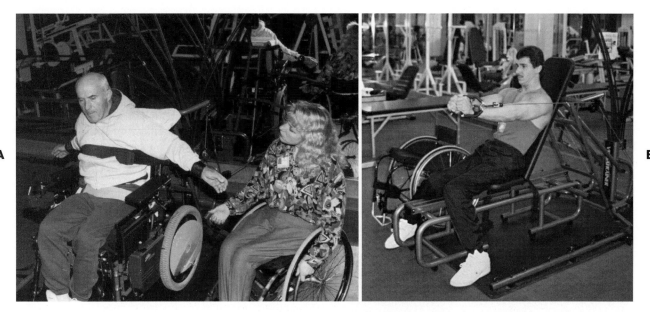

Fig. 41.6. Fitness/training equipment. Many adaptations are available to allow participation by persons with disabilities. **A,** A quadriplegic in a tie down wheelchair using wrist cuffs attached to a pulley weight system. **B,** Stand and bench are easily transferred from a wheelchair using a pulley system for weights.

developing equipment that allows wheelchair access, such as arm ergometers, multistation gyms, and resistance training aids that are arm operated. The manufacturers and specific equipment are too numerous to list; however, a brief description of the major areas is provided.

Arm ergometers provide a stationary aerobic exercise modality for the lower extremity impaired. These come in different designs to accommodate all levels of function. There is a free-standing system that allows a person to arm crank from a wheelchair. Another type sits on a stand, desk, or table top for easy access from a wheelchair. Lastly, there is an ergometer with its own seat, which requires a person to transfer but provides greater stability.

Multistation gyms (weight training) are designed to provide a variety of weight training exercises that can be done from a wheelchair. These gyms are free-standing or wall-mounted units with different resistance settings. They often include wrist or hand cuffs to allow the upper extremity impaired to access each station. There are some units specifically designed for individuals with this type of disability (Fig. 41.6, *A*).

Resistance training aids include wrist or hand cuffs used for grasping equipment (e.g., dumbbells, pulleys, curl bars, ergometer crank handles). These cuffs may be general use grasping cuffs or specifically designed by manufacturers for using their equipment.

Stationary rollers are similar to treadmills or wind trainers for bicycles. The wheelchair is mounted with the rear wheels sitting on top of a drum wide enough to accommodate the chair, and front wheels are secured to the stationary frames. This system is commonly used by athletes who race or others who want to increase their fitness and pushing skills.

GOLF

This sport was once considered inaccessible to people with physical disabilities, but it is quickly gaining in popularity among people with disabilities. The development of adapted equipment for golf has made the sport more accessible. There remains a dispute over whether individuals who golf from carts or wheelchairs should be allowed to gain access to the green because of the delicate turf. It has been suggested that development of adapted equipment that would not damage the green is needed. Adapted equipment available to golfers with disabilities is as follows.

The *adapted golf cart* is designed with a seat that swings out to the side of the cart to allow the golfer to sit or stand over the ball. The seat has a harness that straps the golfer in. This cart provides greater leverage and stability for swinging the club.

There are many *adapted clubs* on the market designed to enhance power, such as the flexible handle clubs. These are excellent for golfers with disabilities. There are also clubs with modified grips and clubs with larger angles for golfers who swing from their wheelchairs (low to the ground) (Fig. 41.7).

The *stand-up wheelchair* is used as an alternative to the adapted cart or standard wheelchair. It is a wheelchair with a mechanical device that puts the person in a standing position. These come in manual and electric models. This allows the disabled golfer to stand and hit the ball while being supported by the standing chair.

HORSEBACK RIDING

Individuals from many disability groups can enjoy horseback riding, not only as a leisure option, but also as a competitive Paralympic sport, beginning in 1996. It also has therapeutic results of increased muscle strength, enhanced balance, and decreased spasticity.

The horse is often mounted by wheelchair users via a ramp that positions the person at the height of an average horse's back. Throughout the instructional phase, one to two spotters walk alongside the horse, balancing the student using a belt with a hand hold on each side. Many students and riders customize their saddles to meet their unique needs—particularly in extra padding to guard against skin sores from pressure as well as shearing (Fig. 41.8). Stirrups can be customized as well and are important for maintaining balance and protecting legs from injury.

HUNTING

Hunting can be pursued by individuals with severe disabilities because of the wide range of innovative equipment available. Mobility in the woods can be managed by all-terrain wheelchairs (wide, nubby tires), all-terrain vehicles such as four-wheelers, or customized vehicles (i.e., golf carts that an electric chair user can roll into, with sip-and-puff controls). Most hunters use camouflage drapes over their vehicles to guard against startling game with shiny chrome reflections.

Gun management depends on the severity of the disability. Trigger pull can be assisted simply by adjusting the trigger but may require a special device. Some hunters use a commercially available trigger mechanism attached to the gun (Fig. 41.9,*A*). Others prefer a custom trigger pull attached to the hand.

For hunters requiring gun support, a gun rest (such as Steady Boy) is available commercially, which may be sufficient. Others use gun rests attached to their ATVs.

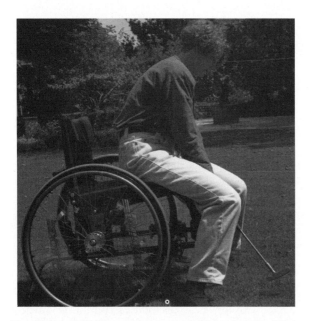

Fig. 41.7.   Golf. Shorter clubs are used from the wheelchair.

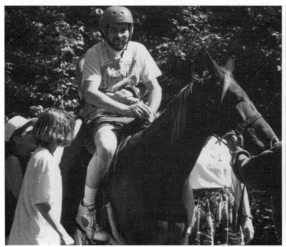
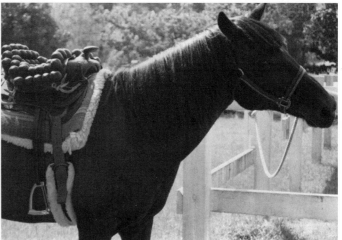

A   B

Fig. 41.8.   Horseback riding. **A,** Chair with strap to hold a paraplegic on the saddle. **B,** Roho cushion attached to saddle for better cushioning.

Many custom-built gun supports support the weight of the barrel and allow for vertical and lateral movement (Fig. 41.9,*B*).

Hunters who are disabled severely have found a sip-and-puff attachment to their rifle to be effective. One commercially available model was designed by a C4 quadriplegic and has been upgraded several times. Once the rifle is mounted properly, this device allows the hunter to position the gun, aim, and fire independently. (See also Shooting.)

ICE HOCKEY

Called *sledge hockey* in Paralympic competition, this sport was developed in Northern Europe and made its debut at the winter Paralympics in Lillihammer, Norway, in 1994. Played primarily by amputees and paraplegics, the rules are virtually the same as traditional ice hockey. It is a fast-paced, aggressive, and exciting sport. The players use sledges, which are lightweight and regulated in design and size. Hockey sticks double as a mobility tool, with a pick at one end to maneuver on the ice, and a hockey stick face on the other end. All players wear face guards on their helmets because of the probability of getting hit by the puck.

MOTOR SOCCER

Designed as a competitive sport, motor soccer is for electric chair users only. A cross between basketball and soccer, it is played on a gym floor and goals are scored by crossing the end line with the ball, by throwing or carrying. It can be highly competitive and aggressive, depending on the players and the sophistication of players strategy. The only additional equipment needed is a guard around the wheelchair foot rests. This serves to protect a player's feet from injury. They are commercially available.

POWERLIFTING

Powerlifting is a Paralympic sport in which all disability groups can participate. Athletes are classified by weight class. The current Paralympic world record is held by U.S. athlete Kim Brownfield at 602 lb.

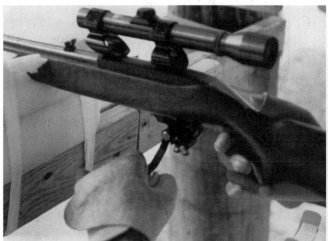

A

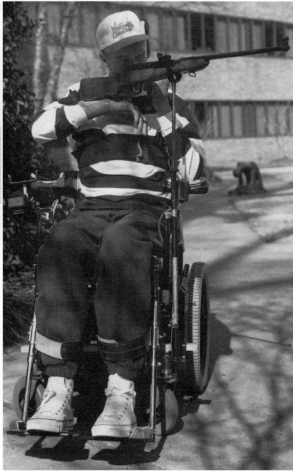

B

Fig. 41.9. Hunting. **A,** Special triggering device. **B,** Gun support for wheelchair.

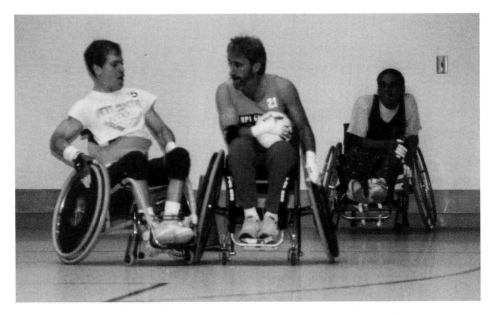

Fig. 41.10. Quad rugby. Sports chair similar to those used in basketball.

The regulation bench used in Paralympic competition is designed for safety and function. The supports for the bar are relatively long and U-shaped, resting on telescoping legs. This allows the athlete to move the bar to the best location without moving his or her body and allows spotters to move the bar up or down to be at the right height above the lifter's chest. The bench is quite wide, and the athlete can be strapped to the bench for safety.

QUAD RUGBY

A highly competitive sport, played mainly in the United States and Canada, quad rugby is for quadriplegics in manual chairs only. A lightweight court chair is used as well as spoke protectors and straps. Strapping is important in maintaining competitor balance as well as good ball control (Fig. 41.10).

This sport is also played on a basketball court. The rules are unique to this sport, and goals are scored by carrying or throwing the ball over the line between the goals, as in motor soccer. Strategy, passing, player positioning, and player speed and mobility determine the success of the team. Four players make up a team.

RACQUETBALL

The adaptation of racquetball for people with disabilities has primarily focused on the wheelchair athlete. The simple adaptation of doorways to courts for wheelchairs and equipment such as grasping cuffs have made the sport totally accessible to people with disabilities. Rules adaptations are limited, including a two bounce rule.

The sport has grown in popularity because of the combined efforts of the American Amateur Racquetball Association (AARA) and the Wheelchair Racquetball–USA member of the Wheelchair Sports USA. This has led to full incorporation of disabled athlete participation into all local, regional, national, and international competition formats. Wheelchair racquetball will be an official demonstration sport in the 1996 Atlanta Paralympic Games.

ROWING

Several modifications can be done to boats to help with potential balance problems for the disabled rower (Fig. 41.11). Seating systems can be adjusted to remain stationary, and a high back can be added for support. Individuals with grasping difficulties can use either Ace bandages or rowing mitts, which also support the wrists as well as securing the hands to the oars. (See also Boating/Canoeing/Kayaking.)

SAILING

The adaptation of sailing for people with disabilities has been extensive. Numerous styles of boats specifically designed to increase access have been developed. Among the more popular boats are trapseat catamarans,

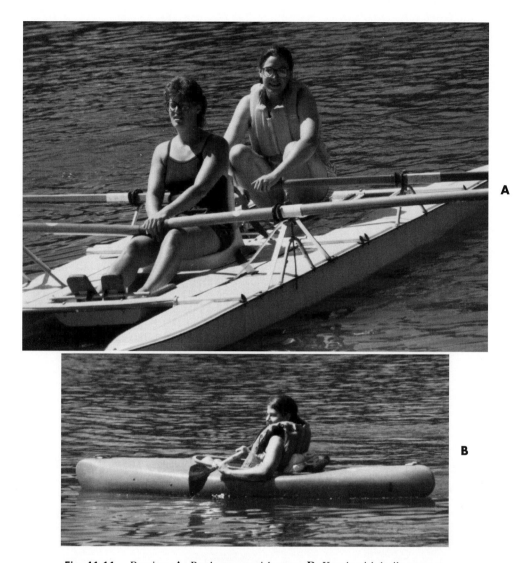

Fig. 41.11. Rowing. **A,** Bucket seat with strap. **B,** Kayak with built-up seat.

trimarans, 2.4 mR, and the International 210. These boats have included single-handed to three- to four-person crews. Adaptations are generally limited to maximize space for mobility in the cockpit of the boat, hand controls, and safety. Events are organized by National Handicapped Sports (NHS) and the U.S. Sailing Committee of Sailors with Special Needs. Sailing has achieved official demonstration sport status in the 1996 Atlanta Paralympic Games.

SHOOTING

Shooting has long been enjoyed by many persons with different disabilities. Events include air rifle and pistol, .22 caliber rifle and pistol, and skeet and trap shooting. Target shooting distances of 10, 25, and 50 m will be used in the 1996 Atlanta Paralympic competition.

The sport is adapted primarily for needed stabilization of the shooter, rifle, or pistol with devices such as tripods, support stands for quadriplegics (Fig. 41.12, *A*), and trigger activators (Fig. 41.12, *B*). The opportunities for competition are developed by Wheelchair Shooting–USA, United States Cerebral Palsy Athletic Association, and National Handicapped Sports, who all are supported by the U.S. Shooting Team/National Rifle Association. (See also Hunting.)

SNOW SKIING

Skiing is by far the most widely enjoyed winter sport activity by all people with disabilities and all age groups. Numerous adaptations and instructional techniques have been developed that allow access to both alpine and Nordic forms of the sport. Included in these are sitski, monoski, outriggers, and bi-skis (Fig. 41.13).

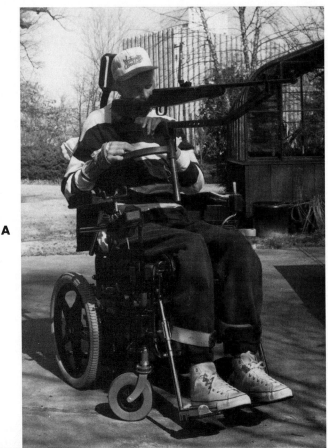

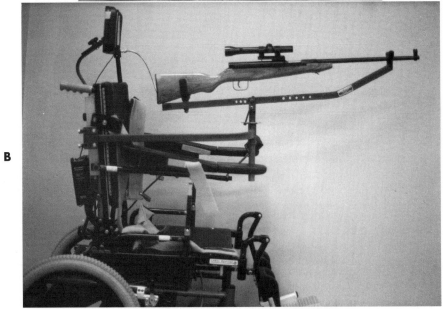

Fig. 41.12.   Shooting. **A,** Gun holder on swivel. **B,** Power chair with gun-holding device and sip-and-puff trigger mechanism.

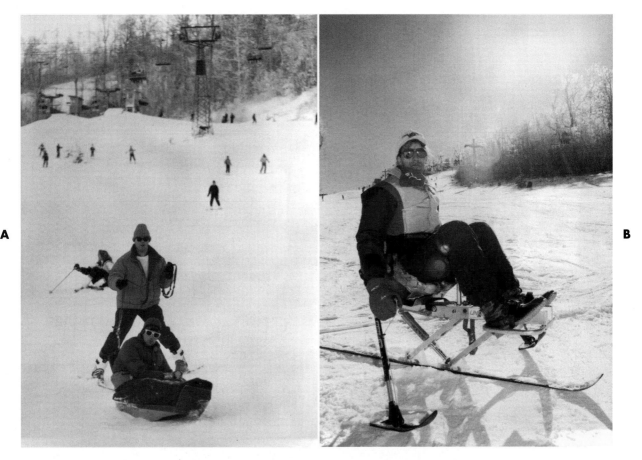

Fig. 41.13.   Skiing. **A,** Bucket ski. **B,** Sit mono ski.

Extensive regional, national, and international event development has taken place through National Handicapped Sports (NHS) and United States Ski Team. Events include downhill, slalom, and cross country with the 1994 Winter Paralympics in Lillihammer, and 1998 Winter Paralympics in Nagano, Japan.

SWIMMING

Swimming is becoming increasingly popular and accessible to people with all disabilities. Access laws and adaptations such as various lifts, ramps, and rails have helped. Devices for flotation (Fig. 41.14) and enhanced propulsion have brought expanded access to fitness, recreational, and competitive swimming opportunities.

Competitive opportunities are available through all National Disabled Sports Programs, which include a full menu of events at distances of 50, 100, 200, 400, and 800 m in all competitive strokes: breast, back, and butterfly. Swimming is a full medal sport in the 1996 Atlanta Paralympics with two competitive systems: one for blind athletes and one for physically disabled athletes.

SCUBA

This sport can often be continued without the use of special requirements, other than needing assistance in and out of a boat or finding a wheelchair-accessible dive site. Selecting equipment for this activity should be done with the assistance of a certified diving instructor and includes some of the following recommendations in reference to physically disabled divers.

For persons with reduced respiratory ability, masks and snorkels should come with a purge valve for easy clearing. Regulators should have an octopus, or additional regulator, for buddy breathing to allow the diver to use his hands for propulsion or for carrying objects.

Buoyancy compensators should have a soft-touch or low-pressure inflator mechanism to avoid the need for oral inflation. Webbed neoprene hand fins are used to increase arm power. Also, diver propulsion vehicles provide an alternative to arm propulsion for divers with lower extremity impairment. Wet suits can be modified for an individual's needs with such items as zippers and Velcro strips, to decrease the difficulty in donning and doffing suits. Fins are recommended for divers with

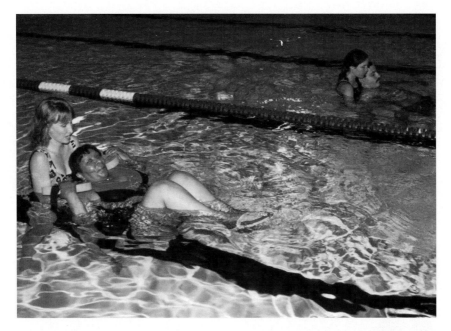

Fig. 41.14.   Swimming. Flotation devices for quadriplegic swimming.

weak or impaired lower extremities. Some individuals also attach small weights to their ankles to prevent them from floating.

TABLE TENNIS

Table tennis, long a popular recreational sports activity, is now a competitive sport and is one of the recognized Paralympic activities. Many sanctioned competitions follow USTTA rules except for international competition. Modifications that allow participation by persons with disabilities are simple to implement and limited. There are few modifications in actual play, and these are centered around the delivery of the serve (Fig. 41.15).

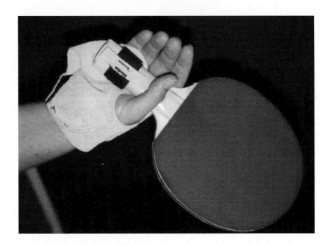

Fig. 41.15.   Table tennis. Adaptive device for paddle.

TEAM HANDBALL

Wheelchair team handball is one of the most exciting sports available to the physically impaired. It is exciting to watch and to play, combining the basic skills of catching, passing, dribbling, and movement into a fast-moving, relatively noncontact sport. It was originally called *wheelchair soccer* and uses nine players per team with two goalies and seven court players. The game is played on a basketball size court requiring two 30-minute halves. The players are allowed 3 seconds in which to decide whether to pass, dribble, or shoot the ball at the goal. Court markings are similar to basketball except there is a goalie's area where no one except the goalies are allowed to enter.

TENNIS

The National Foundation of Wheelchair Tennis was formed in 1976. There has been enormous growth in this sport with many regional and national tournaments held each year. Rule modifications from able-bodied tennis are minimal. The major one is the "two bounce rule," wherein the ball must be returned after bouncing no more than two times compared to once for the able-bodied.

TRACK

Track represents the single largest venue of participation for athletes with disabilities, both in terms of number of events and number of participants. About

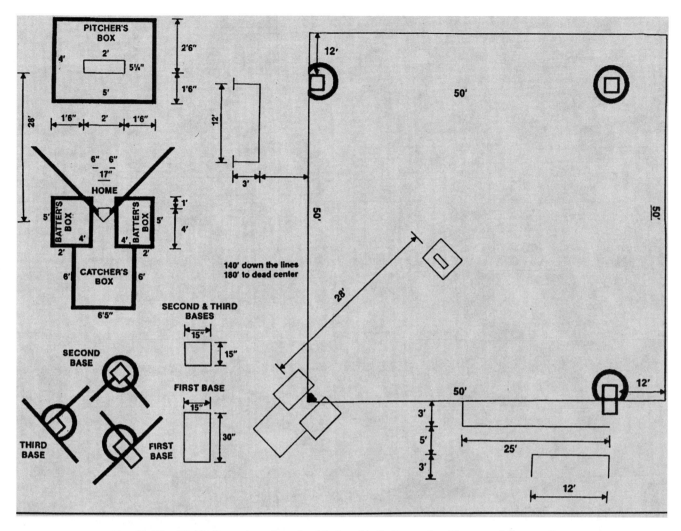

Fig. 41.16. Field dimensions for wheelchair softball diamonds. *(Courtesy of Courage Center [Sports and Recreation for the Disabled].)*

50% of athletes with disabilities are participating in wheelchairs. This has led to a variety of wheelchair designs to meet the specific requirements of each athletic endeavor. Events are as short as 20-m distances, going on up to a marathon for wheelchair athletes. Almost every track and field endeavor that is available to the able-bodied person is available to the person with a disability. Because of the various levels of disability, there are usually multiple places of participation for each single event to allow for the different capabilities within the population of people with disabilities.

WATER SKIING

Water skiing has become popular because of advances in equipment technology and development of instructional techniques that have fostered recreational participation. With the advance in recreational participation, competition has ensued. The development and

awareness of safety precautions and the ever-improving equipment available has made this sport safe and thus much more enjoyable.

WHEELCHAIR SOFTBALL

Softball is a popular sport among the able-bodied and is increasingly popular among people with disabilities, especially those who use wheelchairs for mobility (Fig. 41.16). No matter what the disability, usually there are only minor rule changes necessary to accommodate the disability. In the case of wheelchair softball, the players must participate in a wheelchair, with all chairs having foot rests. The playing field must be a smooth, hard surface. The pitching mound is 28 feet from the plate. A base is a 4 feet in diameter circle. Fielders are penalized for leaving their chairs to catch a ball by awarding two bases to the runner, and throwing errors allow runners to advance an additional base. Rules changes for other disabilities such as for amputations and cerebral palsy are similarly minor.

SUGGESTED READINGS*

Adams RC, Daniel AN, McCubbin JA, Rullman L: Games, sports, and exercises for the physically handicapped, ed 3, Philadelphia, 1982, Lea & Febiger.

Bleck EE, Nagel DA (eds): Physically handicapped children: A medical atlas for teachers, New York, 1975, Grune & Stratton, p. 213.

British Sports Association for the Disabled: Water sports for the disabled, Wakefield, 1983, EP Pub. Ltd.

Christiason MA: Directory of recreational resources for the disabled: A resource handbook, Cerritos, Calif., 1986, Christiason.

Clark MW, Eilert RE (eds): Sports and recreational programs for the child and young adult with physical disability, Chicago, Am. Acad. of Orthopaedic Surgeons, 1983.

Guttmann L: Textbook of sports for the disabled, Aylesbury, 1976, HM & M Publishers.

Kegel B: Physical fitness: Sports and recreation for those with lower limb amputation or impairment, Veterans Adm. J. of Research & Dev., Clinical Supp., No. 1, 1985.

Kelley JD, Frieden L: Go for it: A book on sport and recreation for persons with disabilities, Orlando, Fla., 1989, Harcourt Brace Jovanovich.

Nesbitt JA (ed): The international directory of recreation-oriented assistive device sources, Marina del Rey, Calif., 1986, Lifeboat Press.

Paciorek MJ, Jones JA: Sports and recreation for the disabled: A resource handbook, Indianapolis, Ind., 1989, Benchmark Press.

Rosenberg C: Assistive devices for the handicapped, Atlanta, 1968, Stein Printing Co., p. 73.

Winnick JP (ed): Adapted physical education and sport, Champaign, Ill., 1990, Human Kinetics Books.

*Suggested Readings compiled by Mickey Christiason, M.S., C.T.R.S., Recreational Therapy Supervisor, Rancho Los Amigos Medical Center, Downey, California, and by John D. Hsu, M.D.

Assistive Devices for Driving

Deena Garrison Jones

To many, operating a motor vehicle is a rite of passage. Driving requires responsible action from those operating the vehicle. Therefore, driving is not a right but a privilege that must be earned. Even those with physical and emotional disabilities may be able to learn to operate a motor vehicle safely and efficiently once evaluated and trained with the appropriate techniques and adaptive equipment. Training for persons with disabilities is usually provided by a certified driving instructor or a certified driver rehabilitation specialist (CDRS) who provides driver rehabilitation services (for persons with disabilities) while following and interpreting all applicable federal, state, and local laws and policies. This person may have a background in rehabilitation, education, health, safety, therapy, or a related profession. Many hospitals and private facilities employ driver specialists to instruct their clients in the use of adaptive equipment. The Association of Driver Educators for the Disabled (ADED) is a good place to start to locate driver educators, driver instructors, and/or driver rehabilitation specialists in the United States. ADED is an international group of professionals with a desire to improve the quality of driver rehabilitation for persons with disabilities.

DRIVER'S EVALUATION

When locating a certified driver rehabilitation specialist, one should be sure this professional can and will complete a clinical evaluation before any driver's training. A clinical evaluation should consist of testing the areas of physical, visual, perceptual, and cognitive function. It is important to realize that if one does not feel comfortable evaluating the above-mentioned areas, the client should be referred to an appropriate driving specialist. In most states, these referrals are made by the client's physician.

VISUAL EVALUATION

When looking at the visual system, it is important to note the client's near and distance visual acuity. Testing should be completed with and without the client's corrective lenses. It is also important to evaluate the range of motion of both eyes as well as saccades (rapid eye movement), visual fixation, and visual scanning skills. It should be noted whether the eyes work together or separately of one another. Depth perception (stereopsis) and color perception should also be evaluated during the clinical visual assessment.

PERCEPTUAL EVALUATION

Assessment tools should give the driver specialist an idea of the client's perceptual skills (i.e., spatial relations, figure-ground, visual closure, and visual memory skills).

COGNITIVE EVALUATION

A variety of cognitive tests can be incorporated into the evaluation. Overall, it is important to note deficits in any of the following areas: attention, memory, ability to perform tasks simultaneously, and ability to follow multistep directions.

PHYSICAL EVALUATION

The evaluator must also look at the client's physical status. Are there any hearing limitations? What is the stability of the client when seated? Are there any limitations in neck rotation to the right or to the left? The clinician must look for spasticity of

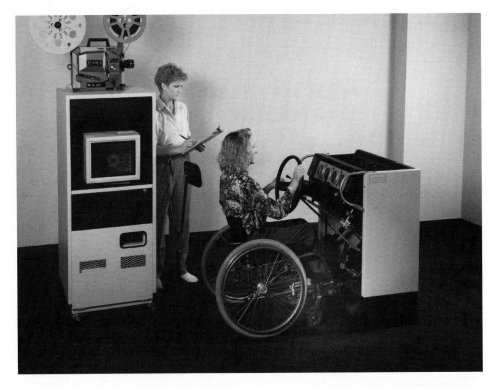

Fig. 42.1. Doron L—300R/A Assessment system. *(Courtesy of Doron Precision Systems, Inc.)*

both upper and lower extremities. Strength and range of motion of the following should also be evaluated: shoulder flexion, shoulder extension, shoulder horizontal movement, elbow and wrist flexion and extension, hip abduction and adduction, knee flexion and extension, and dorsiflexion and plantar flexion of the ankle. The individual's overall endurance and coordination should be assessed. Simple coordination tests such as bringing the index finger to the nose or performing rapid alternating movement (diadochokinesia) can be used. Sensation, position sense, and stimulus localization are important. A seating evaluation may also be needed depending on the individual's trunk stability. This may need to be performed by another specialist such as a physical therapist.

A miscellaneous consideration is finances, not only to pay for the vehicle and vehicle modifications, but also to maintain the vehicle properly. Insurance for the vehicle can be discussed as well as arrangements for transportation to and from driving sessions.

During the evaluation, other issues should also be addressed (i.e. dysreflexia, sensory loss, how to handle the vehicle in an emergency situation, and the need to pull the vehicle to the side of the road to perform pressure releases to maintain good skin integrity).

SIMULATORS/TEST DRIVES

After successful completion of a clinical assessment, the client must be evaluated with appropriate adaptive equipment. The client may be evaluated on a simulator (Fig. 42.1) or through an on-the-road test drive using adaptive equipment. Once the client has been determined to be a candidate for driving with adaptive equipment, training with this equipment should take place in residential, highway, interstate, and city traffic. Parking maneuvers should be practiced and judgment and risk-taking addressed.

EQUIPMENT

It is recommended that persons who are planning to load their own wheelchair purchase a two-door car (a four-door car with a bench-style seat can also be used). Power windows, door locks, and mirrors are also suggested. Vehicles that are to be modified with hand controls must have power brakes, power steering, and an automatic transmission. A seat belt with shoulder harness and side mirrors are also strongly recommended.

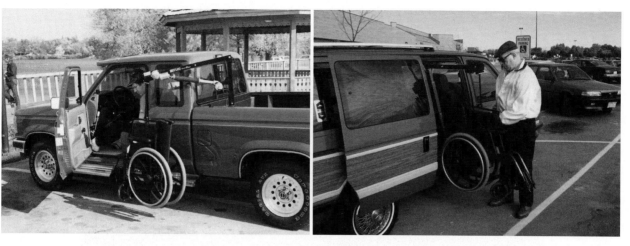

Fig. 42.2. **A,** Pick-up wheelchair loader. **B,** Wheelchair lifter. *(Courtesy of Bruno Independent Living Aids, Inc.)*

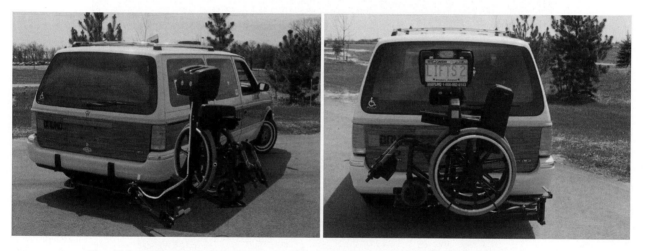

Fig. 42.3. Wheelchair lift—swing away. *(Courtesy of Bruno Independent Living Aids, Inc.)*

WHEELCHAIR LOADERS

For those individuals who are unable to load their own wheelchair, there are four basic types of wheelchair carriers available:

1. *Pickup carrier*—This automatically folds and loads the wheelchair into the back of a pickup truck (Fig. 42.2).
2. *Bumper-dash mounted carrier*—Someone needs to fold and place the wheelchair on the carrier mounted on the rear bumper (Fig. 42.3).
3. *Hitch mounted carrier*—This automatically folds the wheelchair and holds it in place on the back of the vehicle or inside the trunk (Fig. 42.4).
4. *Car-top carrier*—This automatically folds and loads the wheelchair onto the top of the car.

HAND CONTROLS

When operating a vehicle using hand controls, the client should typically steer with the stronger arm. Hand controls can be placed on either the right or left sides and should be adapted with horn and dimmer switch buttons. The hand controls fall into one of three categories:

1. *Right angle (most common)*—These hand controls work by pulling the handle down toward the floor to accelerate and pushing back toward the dash to brake (Fig. 42.5).
2. *Push/pull*—These hand controls work by pulling toward the driver to accelerate and pushing back toward the dash to brake (Fig. 42.6).
3. *Push/twist*—These hand controls work by twist-

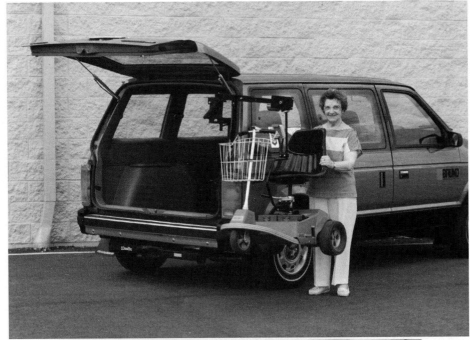

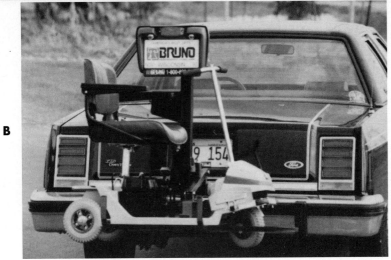

Fig. 42.4. Scooter lift. **A,** Curb-sider. **B,** Out-sider II. *(Courtesy of Bruno Independent Living Aids, Inc.)*

ing the throttle to accelerate (i.e., like a motorcycle throttle) and pushing back toward the dash to brake (Fig. 42.7).

STEERING DEVICE

A person who uses hand controls has only one hand to steer the vehicle and therefore may need a steering device to allow for adequate steering. It is no longer recommended that "expander bars" be installed on vehicles. These expander bars, which are removable and cross the center of the steering wheel, have been known to come off during use and to interfere with the airbag function. The following are types of steering devices (Fig. 42.8):

- Spinner knob
- Amputee ring
- U-grip (used for the loss of finger function, but person has retained wrist motion)
- Tripost spinner knob (used to stabilize the hand and wrist)

DISABILITIES

A list of typically recommended equipment for individuals with specific disabilities is given below.

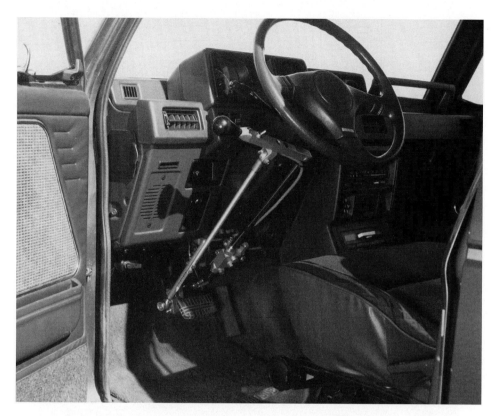

Fig. 42.5. Hand controls—MD 3500. *(Courtesy of Crow River Industries, Inc.)*

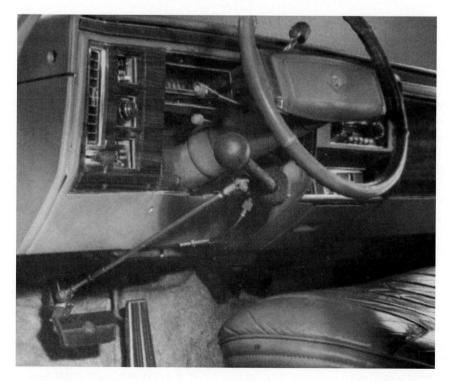

Fig. 42.6. DADC 500 (Throttle-Hand Controls). *(Courtesy of William Perry.)*

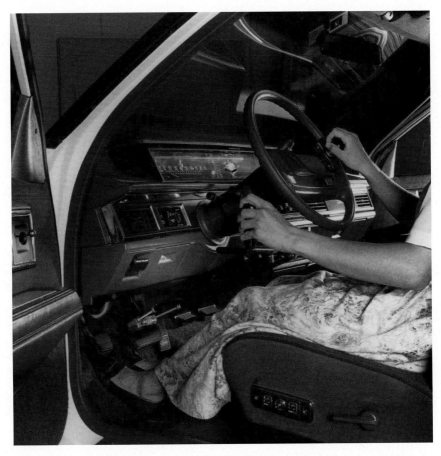

Fig. 42.7. Hand controls—MPD Sure Grip (push/pull hand controls). *(Courtesy of Crow River Industries, Inc.)*

Right hemiplegia
- Left foot accelerator.
- Left spinner knob (usually placed at 8 o'clock position on the steering wheel).
- Automatic transmission.
- May need gear selector extension.
- Hand-operated dimmer switch.

Left hemiplegia
- Regular gas and brake pedals
- Right spinner knob (usually placed at the 4 o'clock position on the steering wheel)
- Automatic transmission
- Right directional signals
- Hand-operated dimmer switch on the right side

Paraplegia
- Hand controls for brake and acceleration with dimmer switch and horn button
- Automatic transmission
- Emergency brake extension
- Possibly a steering knob

Tetraplegia
- Hand control for brake and acceleration with dimmer switch and horn button
- Automatic transmission
- Emergency brake extension
- Shoulder harness/torso support
- Possibly a directional signal adaptor, if necessary
- Steering device (U-grip, spinner knob, tripost)

Some persons with tetraplegia (C5 and above) need to use sensitized equipment or may need to drive from their wheelchair. For more information, please refer to the van information given later.

Bilateral lower extremity/limb amputee
- Hand control for brake and accelerator with dimmer switch and horn button
- Possibly a spinner knob
- Automatic transmission
- Emergency brake extension
- Torso support device
- Directional signal adaptor

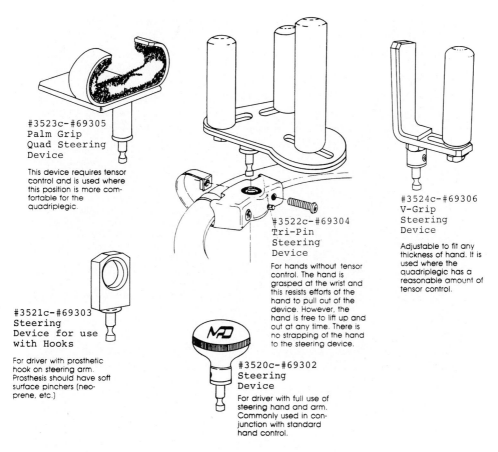

#3523c-#69305
Palm Grip
Quad Steering
Device

This device requires tensor control and is used where this position is more comfortable for the quadriplegic.

#3524c-#69306
V-Grip
Steering
Device

Adjustable to fit any thickness of hand. It is used where the quadriplegic has a reasonable amount of tensor control.

#3522c-#69304
Tri-Pin
Steering
Device

For hands without tensor control. The hand is grasped at the wrist and this resists efforts of the hand to pull out of the device. However, the hand is free to lift up and out at any time. There is no strapping of the hand to the steering device.

#3521c-#69303
Steering
Device for use
with Hooks

For driver with prosthetic hook on steering arm. Prosthesis should have soft surface pinchers (neoprene, etc.)

#3520c-#69302
Steering
Device

For driver with full use of steering hand and arm. Commonly used in conjunction with standard hand control.

Fig. 42.8. MPD Steering Devices. *(Courtesy of Crow River Industries, Inc.)*

Bilateral upper extremity/limb amputee
- One or two rings for steering
- Gear lever extension
- Other right attachments for dash board accessory controls (lights, fans, windows)

Right lower extremity/limb amputee
- Left foot accelerator
- Automatic transmission

Left lower extremity/limb amputee
- Automatic transmission

VAN MODIFICATIONS

When shopping for a full-size van that is to be converted for transportation needs or driving from a wheelchair, it is recommended that the van be ordered as listed here. All of these items can be justified and are usually necessary to accommodate the additional weight of the prescribed equipment and additional drain on the vehicle battery and engine.
- V-8 engine or equivalent
- Long wheel base—138 inches

- Automatic transmission (overdrive optional)
- Power steering and brakes
- Heavy-duty battery (85-A battery with another 500-A cold cranking power)
- 60-A alternator
- Window van with privacy glass (recommended for optimal driving visibility). If interior and windows are customized, specify cargo van with windows in side and rear doors only.
- Side doors. If a rotary lift is chosen, a sliding side door is necessary. Swing doors, however, have fewer mechanical problems when modified for automatic use. They also provide greater room at the door opening.
- Super engine cooling package—includes heavy-duty radiator, transmission cooling
- Tilt steering wheel
- Factory power windows and door locks
- Driver/passenger seats. If the van is to be modified as a wheelchair passenger van and the client will *not* be driving, captain's chairs can be ordered from the factory.

If the client will be driving from his or her wheelchair or transferring to the captain's chair to drive, a vendor should be consulted on the type of captain's chair to

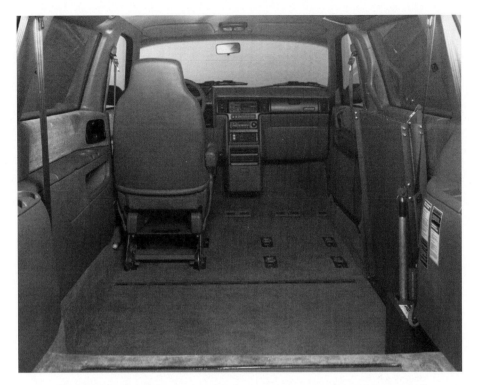

Fig. 42.9.   Braun Entervan (minivan). *(Courtesy of The Braun Corporation.)*

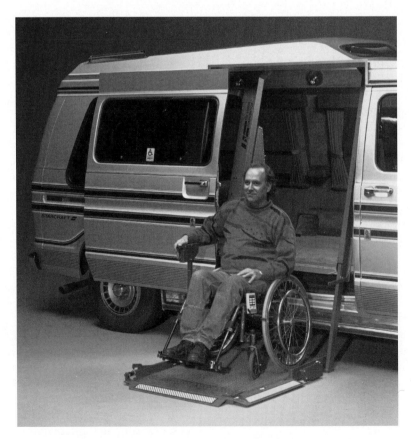

Fig. 42.10.   Wheelchair lift. *(Courtesy of The Braun Corporation.)*

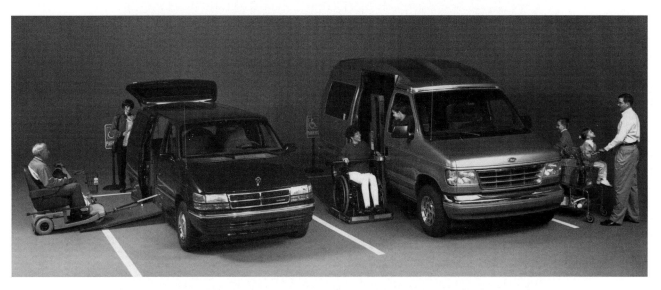

Fig. 42.11. Full-size Ford vans with Braun rotary lift and Entervan. *(Courtesy of The Braun Corporation.)*

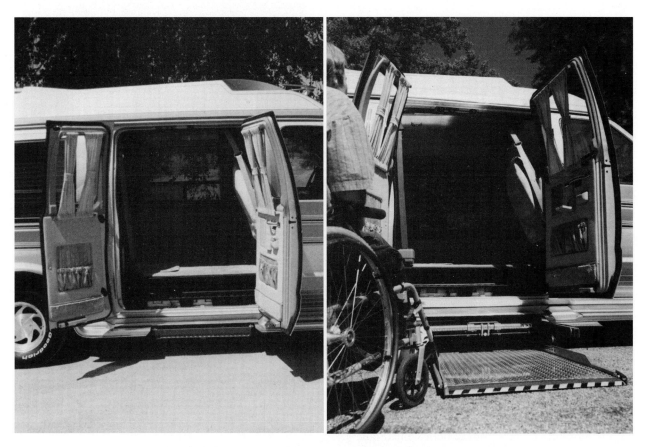

Fig. 42.12. Under car lift. *(Courtesy of Mobile Tech Corporation.)*

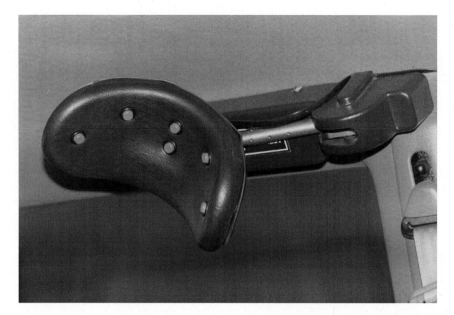

Fig. 42.13. Head mount system (for accessory switches). *(Courtesy of EMC, Inc.)*

order to facilitate adaption of the captain's chair with a power seat base or quick-release casters (Fig. 42.9). This allows for able-bodied individuals also to drive the vehicle.

Interior height of vans

Typically an interior vehicle height at least 2.5 inches taller than the client sits in his or her wheelchair needs to be created. This can be created by completely lowering the floor or raising the roof of the vehicle. When a lowered floor is chosen, it is recommended that the drop floor meets standards that have been set by Safety Automatic Engineering (SAE) and National Mobility Equipment Dealers Association (NMEDA). The drop floor should also be extended up into the driver's area if the person will be driving from his or her power wheelchair. It is typically recommended that the drop floor be undercoated, rust proofed, primed, and painted. Floor lowering is usually attempted only on vans with separate body and chassis designs (such as a Ford van). If a raised roof is added, additional structural supports (i.e., rollbars) are recommended.

Lifts

If the client depends on a wheelchair for mobility and will be using a van, a fully automatic wheelchair lift with automatic door openers/closures, inside/outside mounted controls, and manual back-up system is recommended. There are three basic types of lifts: the platform lift (which comes in both semiautomatic and fully automatic models), the rotary lift, and the under vehicle lift (Fig. 42.10, 42.11, and 42.12). There are advantages and disadvantages to each lift, and this

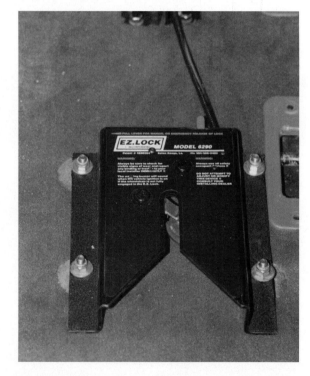

Fig. 42.14. Easy-lock power wheelchair lock down. *(Courtesy of EMC, Inc.)*

should be evaluated depending on the type of vehicle purchased and the type of wheelchair the individual has.

Seat belt system/wheelchair tie-downs

The seat belt system for the driver must also be operated by the client with no assistance and needs

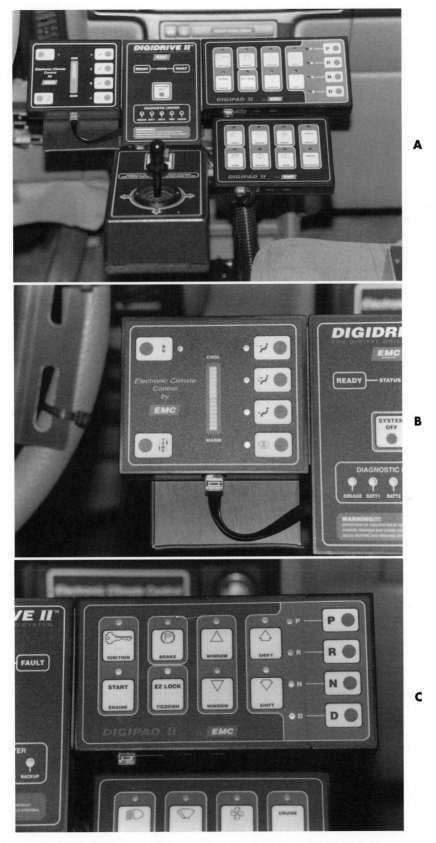

Fig. 42.15.   A, DIGIDRIVE II with accessory console operation. B, Electronic climate control unit. C, DIGIPAD II touchpad console operation. *(Courtesy of EMC, Inc.)*

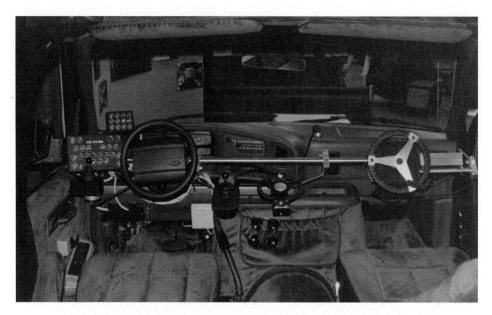

Fig. 42.16. Customized controls. *(Courtesy of As-Tech, Inc.)*

to meet federal motor vehicle safety standards. It is also strongly recommended that a passenger wheelchair restraint system be mounted in the rear of the van. This system must be *forward facing* because side facing is not adequate for safety reasons. The passenger wheelchair restraint must also include lap and shoulder belts separate from the wheelchair. Custom/home-built tie-down systems are not acceptable for safety reasons; commercial tie-downs are available to meet these needs. It is also recommended that the wheelchair tie-down be a four-point tie-down system.

If a person is driving from his or her wheelchair, a power wheelchair lock-down in the driver's area, again with a separate lap and shoulder belt mechanism, must be installed. There are approved crash-tested systems on the market today (Fig. 42.13).

Sensitized equipment

As mentioned earlier, persons with tetraplegia or those with general muscle weaknesses need special adaptations for steering and braking. There are a variety of sensitized steering and braking devices (Figs. 42.14 to 42.16):

- *Reduced/low effort steering*—This adaptation is for those individuals who have limited use of upper extremities. The effort required to steer the vehicle is reduced by approximately 30% to 40%.
- *Zero effort steering*—The effort required to steer the vehicle is reduced by approximately 60% to 70%.
- *Horizontal steering*—The steering wheel sits in a position horizontal to the client's lap, therefore decreasing the need for full range of the upper extremities.

- Joystick—This is similar to the control of a power wheelchair and requires use of only one extremity for steering, braking, and acceleration.

CONCLUSION

It is important to remember that driving is significant for most individuals, especially in today's world. With continual improvement in technology, it is certain that even more driving equipment will be introduced in the future.

RESOURCES

American Automobile Association
1000 999 Dr.
Heathrow, FL 32746-5063

Association of Driver Educators for the Disabled
P.O. Box 49
Edgerton, WI 53534

As-Tech, Inc.
8 Shovel Shop Square
North Easton, MA 02356-1445

The Braun Corporation
1014 S. Monticello
P.O. Box 310
Winamac, IN 46996

Bruno Independent Living Aids, Inc.
1780 Executive Dr.
P.O. Box 84
Oconomowoc, WI 53066

Crow River Industries, Inc.
14800 28th Ave., N.
Minneapolis, MN 55447

DADC (Driving Aids Development Corp.)
9417 Delancey Dr.
Vienna, VA 22180

Doron Precision Systems, Inc.
P.O. Box 400
Binghamton, NY 13902-0400

EMC, Inc.
2001 Wooddale Blvd.
Baton Rouge, LA 70806

Woodrow Wilson Rehabilitation Center
Fishersville, VA 22939

Mobile Tech Corporation
P.O. Box 2326
Hutchinson, KS 67504-2326

National Mobility Equipment Dealers Assoc.
909 E. Skagway Ave.
Tampa, FL 33604

COPYRIGHT HOLDERS AND ADDRESSES

Association of Driver Educators for the Disabled
P.O. Box 49
Edgerton, WI 53534

As-Tech, Inc.
8 Shovel Shop Square
North Easton, MA 02356-1445

The Braun Corporation
1014 S. Monticello
P.O. Box 310
Winamac, IN 46996

Bruno Independent Living Aids, Inc.
1780 Executive Dr.
P.O. Box 84
Oconomowoc, WI 53066

Crow River Industries, Inc.
14800 28th Ave., N.
Minneapolis, MN 55447

DADC (Driving Aids Development Corp.)
9417 Delancey Dr.
Vienna, VA 22180

Doron Precision Systems, Inc.
P.O. Box 400
Binghamton, NY 13902-0400

EMC, Inc.
2001 Wooddale Blvd.
Baton Rouge, LA 70806

Mobile Tech Corporation
P.O. Box 2326
Hutchinson, KS 67504-2326

National Mobility Equipment Dealers Assoc.
909 E. Skagway Ave.
Tampa, FL 33604

Assistive Devices for Daily Living

Y. Lynn Yasuda

From the beginning of time man has relied on tools to accomplish tasks. Many individuals with physical disabilities, however, are not able to use common implements in our environment. Over the centuries, those with impairments, no doubt, have devised ingenious ways to accomplish daily activities. For example, Auguste Renoir, a famous Impressionist painter who had severe rheumatoid arthritis in his later years, found a way to hold his paintbrush despite profound hand deformities. It was not until the mid–twentieth century that assistive devices for those with physical disabilities began to achieve recognition in the literature. Since the 1950s and especially in the last decade, the scope of special tools, better known as assistive devices, has been increasing in the commercial market. This is timely because people are living longer, concurrently increasing the number of people with physical disabilities in the population. Because assistive devices, by nature, should be ergonomically sound, items that were once marketed primarily for those with disabilities are now often found in the general market to allow efficiency for all in daily task performance. An example of this is the use of hook and loop closures (Velcro) on shoes. A few years ago, this was found only on shoes adapted for those with disabilities; now, it can be found on everyday sports shoes and children's shoes for the general public. Assistive devices have enabled those who were dependent on others to now manage in the mainstream of society on their own or with lesser assistance than previously expected.

This chapter presents the range of assistive devices currently available for people with disabilities. Devices described are limited primarily for those with orthopedic disabilities. Devices are categorized into self-care, household management, and community activities. Following description of common problems and device solutions, chacteristics that are often found with good users of assistive devices are given. Resources to assure appropriate device prescription and to obtain assistive devices are then described. Lastly, resources to locate needed devices are provided.

SELF-CARE

Self-feeding

Often, this is the first task a severely involved person is interested in mastering. However, it is a complex task for anyone with significant upper extremity weakness. Before this task is attempted with assistive devices, it is not only important to be able to hold an implement but to assure that the proximal musculature can handle the weight of assistive devices in addition to taking the hand to the mouth. Necessary orthoses for the upper extremities must also be determined before suggesting assistive devices. With appropriate orthoses, assistive device use is enhanced.

Adapted eating utensils come in a variety of forms to accommodate varied needs. *Lightweight utensils with built-up handles* are frequently used by patients with joint pain. With the presence of severe upper extremity weakness, a person using mobile arm supports (MAS) and wrist-hand orthoses (WHOs) to move functionally may require *swivel-handled utensils* to prevent spilling from the spoon in the hand-to-mouth motion (Fig. 43.1). *Knives* with rocker bottoms are useful for those dependent on the use of one hand and for patients with distal pain and weakness. If a patient finds the weight of a cup or glass too heavy to lift, *straw-holders* and *long plastic straws* are useful. A person with limited hand opening or a person with quadriplegia may benefit from the use of a *T-handled mug*, which permits passive hold of the mug between the fingers.

Hygiene/grooming

The tasks of hygiene and grooming all involve bringing the hand to the face or higher or reaching behind the neck and head. Devices used to compensate

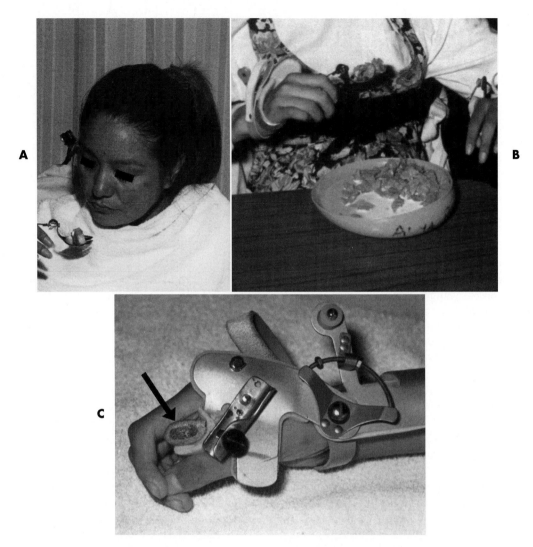

Fig. 43.1.   A, Patient with C5 level cervical spine injury is using a swivel-handled spork (combined spoon and fork), which prevents spilling. It is placed in a pocket attached to her wrist-action WHO. **B,** A dish with a built-up side and a friction pad underneath allows for ease in scooping food. **C,** Side view of wrist-action WHO shows a pocket in which tools, such as a spork, are placed.

for problems in these motions include *comb, brush, shampoo brush, and face sponge with long handles; built-up handled toothbrush, utensil cuff to hold toothbrush, razor,* and/or *make-up* (Fig. 43.2). For the one-handed, resulting from stroke, amputation, or other conditions, a *nail brush holder, nail scissors holder,* and *battery-operated toothbrush* can be helpful.

Dressing

Dressing problems can occur when only lower extremities are involved with hip and/or knee pain and limited motion or if there is upper extremity involvement only. The problems are compounded when both upper extremity and lower extremity disability exist. Fatigue from the effort required with the presence of total body involvement can make this task unrealistic.

With lower-extremity involvement only, the most useful devices are a *dressing stick, sock cone,* and *reacher* (Fig. 43.3). Because of the frequency with which these have been found to be successful, these three items sometimes are commercially packaged together for the postoperative total hip arthroplasty patient, who is asked to restrict hip flexion motion. Other devices useful for the patient unable to reach distal portions of the lower extremities include *long-handled shoe horn, adapted shoes with Velcro closure and looped tabs* (this allows use of a dressing stick to maneuver closure and opening), and/or *elastic shoelaces.* For those with upper body reach problems, *long zipper pulls* and *front-closure*

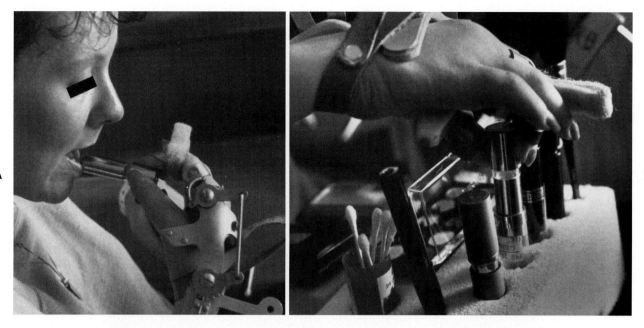

Fig. 43.2. Patient with C6 cervical spine injury is wearing a wrist-driven WHO (**A**) and using an adapted holder for her cosmetics to allow independence in this activity (**B**). The holder is made of high-density foam.

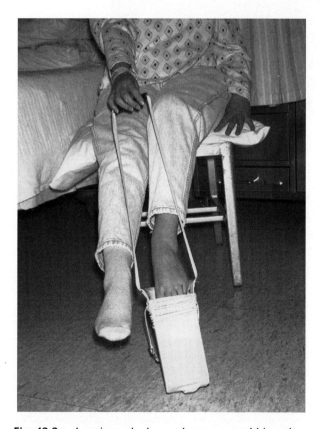

Fig. 43.3. A patient who has undergone a total hip arthroplasty procedure is putting on her socks with a sock aid, secondary to restricted hip flexion postoperatively. Generally a dressing stick and reacher (not seen here) are nearby, which will also help place her pants over her feet while adhering to postoperative hip arthroplasty precautions.

bras as well as the previously mentioned dressing stick can assist. For those with hand weakness, *button hooks, looped zipper pulls, elastic loops in pants, elastic waistbands,* or *Velcro-closure waistbands* are useful. Overall choice of clothing for wearing ease includes garments that are loose-fitting, T-shirts with V-neck openings, elasticized waistbands, front-opening clothing, wrap-around shirts, and garments with few fastenings.

Toileting

Limited reach to the perineum to cleanse one's self can result from limited elbow extension, trunk/hip flexion, limited hand closure, limited wrist flexion, or bilateral upper extremity amputation. Limited mobility (which may prevent timeliness to reach the toilet) can pose a toileting issue. Transferring on and off the toilet is an issue for those with limited hip and knee flexion. Donning and lowering underpants or manipulating other clothing for toileting can also be problematic and has been addressed in the Dressing section.

Commercial devices exist that hold toilet paper or they can be fabricated with wire or plastic. A *bidet* can substitute for cleansing one's self. *Elevated toilet seats* come in a variety of designs as do *grab bars* to assist with transferring on and off the toilet. When limited mobility does not allow timeliness in reaching the toilet, a *male urinal* or a *Freshette* (a funnel that is held covering the perineum and is attached to tubing and a plastic bag) for women can be used while sitting in a wheelchair or sitting to the side of a bed (Fig. 43.4). A bedside *commode chair* can also allow for timeliness problems in the middle of the night.

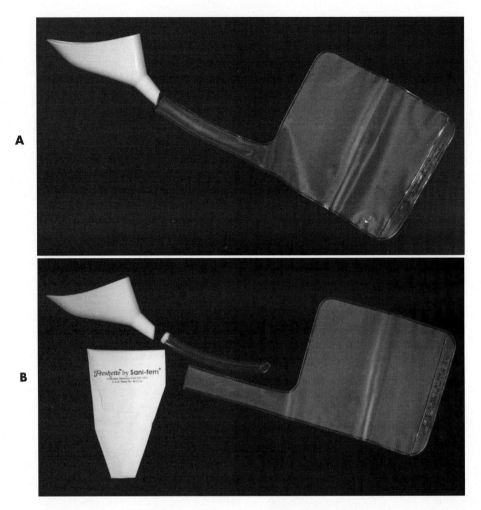

Fig. 43.4.   A, A portable female urinal that can be used while sitting in a wheelchair. The urinal bag can be emptied when convenient. **B,** When not in use, parts can be taken apart and placed in a small envelope for use when traveling.

Bathing

In order to bathe independently, a series of tasks must be accomplished: undress and dress; transfer in and out of bath or shower; maintain sitting or standing balance; manage faucets, soap, and washcloth to reach all parts of body; and dry self. Patients may present with difficulty in any one or more of these tasks. In addition, shampooing hair, which many people perform in the shower, is a task that often is given up because of lack of endurance or strength in using the upper extremities in an overhead position while reaching all parts of the head.

For patients with mobility problems, a vast array of commercially available *bath benches* and *grab bars* exist to assist in transfer. When a bath bench is used, other assistive equipment such as a *long-handled shower hose* is required. This shower hose may need a *remote control attachment* to enable independent operation of the water flow. To wash the lower extremities, a *long-handled sponge* or an *adapted washcloth with strings* may need to be

used (Fig. 43.5). Individuals with hand weakness or pain may need a *mitt, liquid soap pump, soap-on-a-rope,* or *suction soap holder.*

HOUSEHOLD MANAGEMENT

Desk activities

Desk skills (e.g., writing, turning pages, using a phone) require precision handling skills, proximal upper extremity strength to place the hand for function, and neck positioning to view reading materials.

For people who cannot hold writing implements, *commercial pen holders* are available that slip over the finger and thumb. Such devices passively position the fingers and use proximal musculature for writing. Various methods are possible to enlarge the diameter of writing implements to accommodate hand weakness, pain on limited closure, and/or writing with greater comfort and ease. Some pens can be purchased that

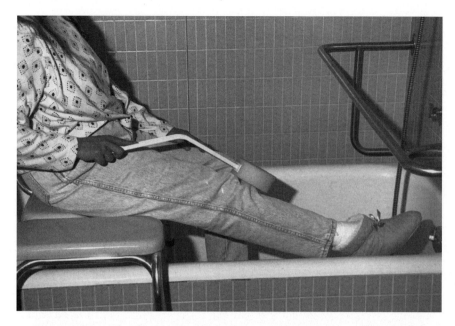

Fig. 43.5. A patient with arthritis with limited lower extremity function sitting on a bath bench and demonstrating how a bent, long-handled sponge can be used to reach lower parts of body while bathing.

have a large circumference. Standard writing devices can be enclosed in various types of *tubing* made specifically for enlarging diameters of gripping surfaces. For those with proximal muscle weakness, a commercially available *gooseneck phone holder with a circuit-breaker attachment* can be used to prevent the need to hold a receiver while using a phone. A commercial *book-holder* can be positioned for those who are dependent on neck motion to turn pages with a mouthstick. *Electrically operated page turners* allow a person to merely push a button to advance a page with a mouthstick or dowel attached to a WHO. Lastly a common device for those who are temporarily immobilized in a fully supine position, such as required postoperatively for cervical spine fusion, or are otherwise unable to look down to a work surface is *prism glasses* (Fig. 43.6). These glasses reflect images at a 90-degree angle, thus allowing the ability to read or work on other lap-top activities when limited neck flexion, trunk flexion, and downward gaze exist.

Safety aids

Falls in the home are a common problem with any elderly person and more so when an orthopedic or neurologic problem exists. A number of assistive devices to prevent falls and other accidents exist to maintain the frail elderly and others with disability in the home.

Light switch adaptations, such as "touch" on-off switches and built-up switches, can be attached to lamps for those with upper extremity weakness. *Environmental control units* are available that can be plugged

into the wall with switches placed in strategic locations in the home. These switches can remotely turn on lights or many electrically operated appliances used in the home. This easy accessibility to lighting and appliances may prevent walking in poorly lit areas where unseen objects could induce tripping and may promote independence in the use of household appliances. Loose floor mats should be replaced with *rubberized scatter mats* to prevent falls. Ideally, it is better to remove all scatter rugs, but this may be against patient preference.

If a patient living alone is totally dependent on ambulatory aids for walking at home and has limited ability to arise from the floor, it is essential that a safety system is installed to call for help, when needed. Fortunately, personal alarm systems are available in many parts of the United States that can be activated with a switch attached around a wrist or neck (Fig. 43.7). Through a phone line, activation of the switch notifies a local hospital that the owner is in trouble.

Meal preparation

Limited standing and walking time secondary to lower extremity pain or weakness may make meal preparation laborious and thus lead to dependency in this task. People in wheelchairs can also find it difficult to prepare meals because the standard kitchen is not easily accessible to them. In addition, any limitations in upper extremity strength or proximal range of motion can make the meal preparation environment inaccessible or use of standard tools difficult.

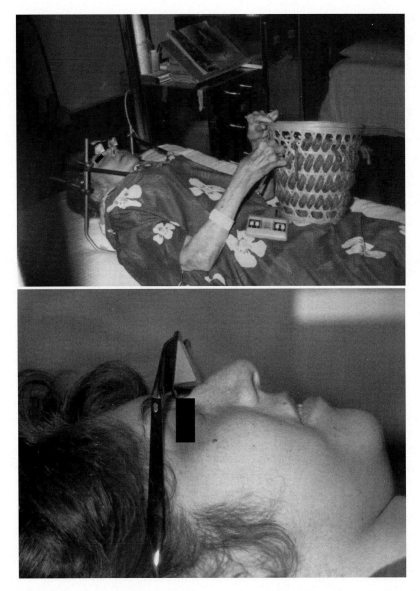

Fig. 43.6. A patient who has undergone a cervical spine fusion requiring the application of a halo apparatus is restricted visually. Prism glasses, which reflect images at a 90-degree angle, allows her to continue working on crafts and other activities at lap level whether in bed or sitting in a wheelchair.

The *Easy Mobile Stand* (Fig. 43.8), which has an adjustable high stool with a bicycle-type seat and wheels, allows a person with limited ambulation or standing time to sit to work at a standard height kitchen counter or travel easily in the kitchen. A *rolling cart* can be used to limit steps in carrying items from place to place. It can often also be used as a momentary replacement for an ambulatory aid. A cane can be suspended from the cart, if needed. For those with upper extremity problems, a large variety of assistive devices are available to compensate for these problems. For weak or painful grip, the *Zim jar opener* allows the use of two hands to hold a jar and easily turn the lid inside a v-shaped serrated surface. A *multipurpose knob turner,* which uses a system of tiny push-buttons that become proportionally depressed according to the size of levered knobs, can be used to turn almost any size knob, using primarily the power of the forearm rotators instead of pinch strength. *Lightweight knives with large handles* that extend perpendicular to the cutting surface have found popular use by those who need to use cylindric grip instead of a form of pinch to prepare foods that require cutting or chopping. Electrically operated tools, such as *food choppers, electric can openers,* and *electric jar openers,* can ease function for those with impaired hands. Additionally the portable *microwave oven* with

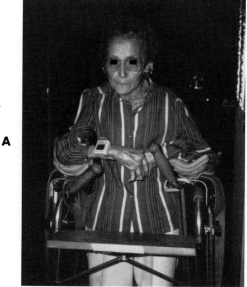

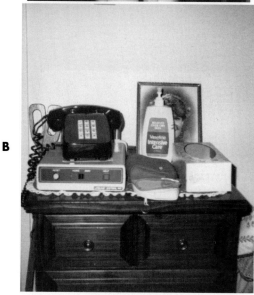

Fig. 43.7. A person with long-standing rheumatoid arthritis requiring full-time use of a walker living alone in an apartment is able, by hitting a button on her wrist attachment (**A**), to be connected immediately to a local hospital via a system (**B**) attached to her phone. If she is not within amplifier distance of the system to be heard, the paramedics are alerted to call on her to find out the problem.

side-opening doors has enabled those with both upper extremity and lower extremity problems to easily access an oven, which can be placed at any height to accommodate wheelchair users or those with ambulatory aids (Fig. 43.9). It also allows for efficiency in cooking by quickly heating foods that can be prepared well in advance and frozen. In addition to assistive devices, cupboards with revolving or pull-out shelves or open shelves without doors increase the available storage space for those with limited reach.

Home maintenance

Heavy homemaking, such as vacuuming, cleaning the bathroom, doing the laundry, and changing bed linens, are often the first activities that may be given up by the person with orthopedic disabilities. These activities require significant strength in the upper extremities. They also require mobility in the lower extremities and spine, as demonstrated by the need to lean over and lift a mattress to change sheets on a bed or to kneel to clean the bathtub.

Items found in selected catalogs or stores available to the general public may be a necessity for those with orthopedic problems to manage heavy home skills. Examples include a *bucket with a dolly or wheels* to prevent the need to carry water needed for mopping floors, *spring-loaded sheet holders* to prevent the need to lift a mattress to replace sheets, *long-handled dustpan* to prevent the need to squat to pick up the dustpan (Fig. 43.10), and *long-handled sponge* to clean the bathtub. Devices mentioned earlier, such as the rolling cart, can be used to transport laundry; the long-handled sponge can be used to clean the bathtub.

Community activities

Community activities, such as shopping, attending school or work, or traveling and staying in hotels, often require use of assistive devices to be able to perform necessary activities in these environments. Some devices used in the home may work in the community with or without modifications.

Doorknobs adapted with long lever arms provide the leverage needed for some with hand weakness to use the power of more proximal musculature to open doors at work (Fig. 43.11). To manage keys at work or school, various types of *keyholders* with long lever arms exist. For wheelchair users or others with limited reach, a *dressing stick or reacher,* mentioned as useful for dressing and other self-care activities, can be invaluable to manage elevator buttons, light switches, or reaching clothing in a closet while staying in a hotel. Compact *fold-up reachers* and *fold-up dressing sticks* are now available to be placed in a purse that can be used for traveling. Another example of a commercially available assistive device is an *adapted shoulder-strap briefcase holder,* which allows those with weak, painful hands and shoulder weakness to suspend the briefcase on a hook located on the side of the body while traveling to a workplace.

Minor or major adaptations may need to be made in the workplace to allow the use of assistive devices (Figs. 43.12 and 43.13). The use of a large electrically operated turntable desk allowed an attorney who was quadriplegic to use assistive devices to practice in an ordinary law office.

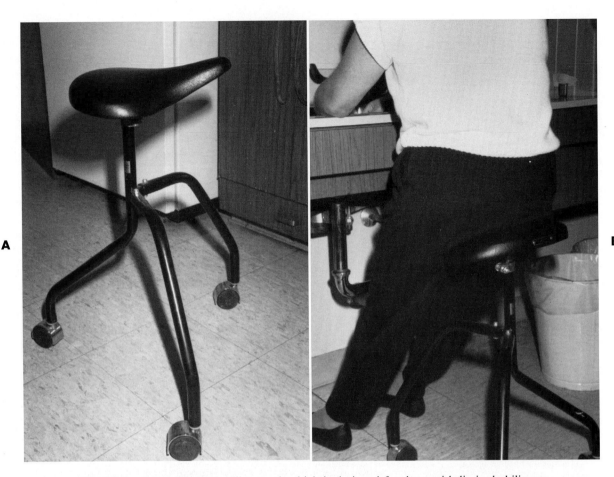

Fig. 43.8. **A,** An elevated rolling stool, which is designed for those with limited ability to ambulate in the home, allows a person to perform upper extremity activities, such as (**B**) washing dishes at a standard height sink, without encountering lower extremity pain or fatigue when ambulation and standing time are limited.

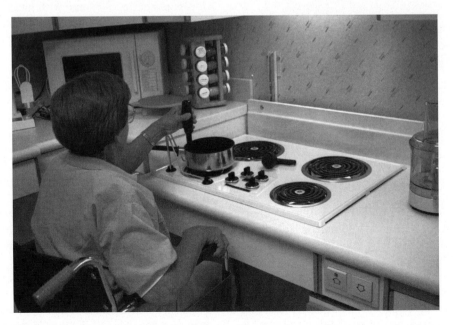

Fig. 43.9. A person in a wheelchair has a lowered stove surface to allow ease in using the stove burners. A suctioned holder prevents the pot from moving while she stirs her food. A microwave oven is also accessible from her wheelchair.

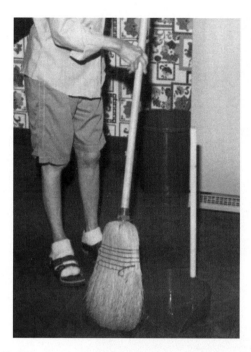

Fig. 43.10. A commercially available long-handled dustpan prevents the need for this person with arthritis and lower extremity limitations to kneel or squat to pick up her dustpan.

CHARACTERISTICS LEADING TO SUCCESSFUL USE OF ASSISTIVE DEVICES

Therapists as well as patients and their families often recognize the possibilities of the use of assistive devices leading to functional independence. However, not all assistive devices that are recommended for, or purchased by, patients are used. In our experience we have found certain patient and environmental characteristics and available resources that encourage successful use of assistive devices.

Patient characteristics

The following four characteristics of patients have been found to enhance the possibilities of patients' use of assistive devices:

Self-initiation. Patients who demonstrate problem-solving behaviors are good candidates to use assistive devices. An example is the patient who laboriously uses a pair of pliers to wind his or her wristwatch when fine prehension is no longer available. These patients show initiation and have functional goals for themselves.

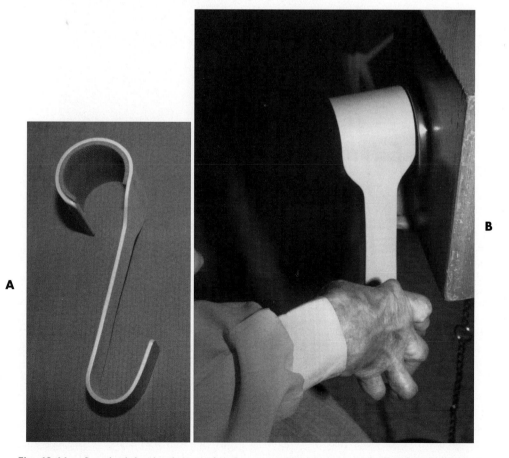

Fig. 43.11. Standard doorknobs can often be managed with the use of a simple, long-levered attachment (**A**) for those with an extremely weak, painful grasp and limited opening (**B**).

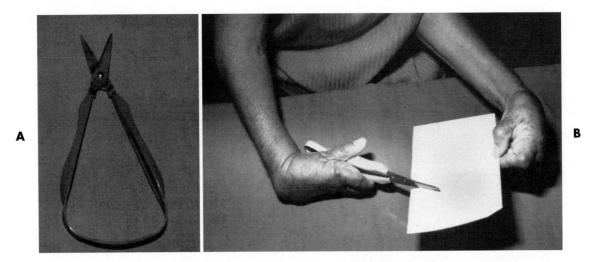

Fig. 43.12. Adapted scissors (**A**) with passive opening through the use of spring wire allows ease in this activity for this person with severe rheumatoid arthritis in her hands (**B**).

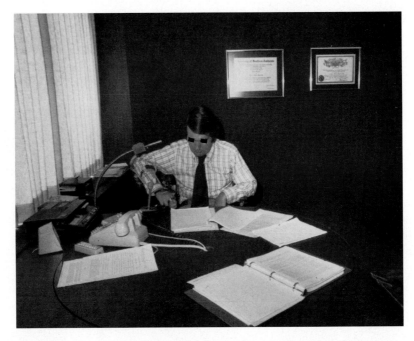

Fig. 43.13. This desk has been adapted for this person with C5 level quadriplegia to continue to work as an attorney. With his right hand in a ratchet-driven WHO and MAS, he is able to trigger the switch attached to a gooseneck on his right-hand side. This will rotate the desk to bring the speaker phone and paperwork within working range of his right upper extremity.

Body image/self-concept. A person who does not like the appearance of his or her body parts, such as "deformed" hands, can find it difficult to use assistive devices in the presence of others because it may represent an extension of poor body image. With low self-concept or self-esteem, which could be combined with depression, the desire for greater independence through the use of assistive devices may not be a priority. This is not to say that assistive devices should not ever be given to this person. Before recommending

devices, the use of rehabilitation team efforts, such as a psychologist and occupational therapist, helping this person find meaning in participating in everyday life despite physical disability may be helpful.

Stage of adjustment to disability. A person who is still mourning the loss of his or her previous skills or who believes that a chronic condition is only temporary may not feel that assistive devices are necessary. Patients in this state may say, "I don't need to struggle to re-learn how to feed myself with devices. When I return to normal, I'll begin doing this activity." Understanding the patient's psychological level of adjustment and helping him to focus on function as he works through various stages of adjustment may allow the patient to feel able to work with assistive devices as a "temporary" solution. He or she may recognize over time that the assistive devices may be for long-term use.

Gadget tolerance.   In the general population, there are those who do and do not have tolerance for learning to work with new devices. If a patient has low tolerance for learning how to use diminished motor abilities to manage assistive devices, it is important to provide the simplest devices for this patient. It also is important to provide training that ends each session with success, even if in small increments. The failure of patients to use assistive devices sometimes falls under this category. Patients in this category may respond with, "I don't use the device because it's so inconvenient to find it when I need it." Overloading patients with multiple pieces of equipment can also be a deterrent to use of these devices. When a single assistive device can perform multiple functions, such as the folding dressing stick, it is more likely to be used.

Environmental characteristics

Social support.   Families who encourage independence, understand the use of assistive devices, and are willing to prepare the environment to allow the patient to use devices aid successful use. The patient's school or workplace personnel can also encourage independence by helping to set up the community environment for activities such as self-feeding. An example is the application of MAS, WHO, and strategic placement of special eating equipment for the person at mealtime.

Architectural barriers.   Architectural barriers in the home or community can prevent the use of assistive devices effectively. For example, high cupboards or cabinets from which a patient in a wheelchair is not able to reach supplies can prevent his ability to perform his job in the community or self-care at home. A narrow bathroom door that does not allow a wheelchair to enter may prevent the ability to toilet or bathe one's self. Solutions, such as room doors that are removed or have *offset hinges*, may increase door width and allow a wheelchair to pass through. Using dresser drawers in the kitchen in place of cupboards or using pull-out cupboard shelves enables the use of low cupboards for someone who cannot squat or bend down.

Patient/family resources to obtain devices

Financial support.   Some assistive devices are covered by third-party payers of health care. If devices are not covered, and many items are not, there needs to be a method to help the family purchase affordable

devices that are effective. Registered occupational therapists (O.T.R.) can often help with this because a range of devices is often found in occupational therapy clinics that the patient may try. When families cannot afford to purchase devices, outside resources may need to be found, such as local churches. If the assistive device does not need to be ordered from a medical supply catalog, but can be found in local department or grocery stores, it generally will cost less.

Construction of devices.   If there is no resource to purchase commercial devices, there may be community resources to build devices. For example, some hospitals have maintenance departments that may make lap trays for wheelchairs or walkers. A local Boy Scout troop may make wooden reachers. Occupational therapy departments often have patterns for assistive devices, which volunteers can use to construct items. There may be a retired engineer who can help construct mechanical devices, such as an adapted laundry or shopping cart to attach to the wheelchair.

RESOURCES TO ASSURE APPROPRIATE PRESCRIPTION OF ASSISTIVE DEVICES

Simple, single device need

When there is need for a simple, single device, such as a crutch-holder to prevent crutches from falling to the floor when not in use, an extensive evaluation is not indicated. Having the patient purchase directly from manufacturers or distributors may be sufficient.

Complex device need or complex patient problems

If a patient has complex or multiple needs, such as room modification and adaptations to manage work tools, an occupational therapy evaluation is indicated. A biopsychosocial approach to identifying the problem and working on a solution is necessary. This can often be done through the occupational therapy evaluation process, which evaluates functional problems in light of musculoskeletal and psychosocial issues.

RESOURCES TO LOCATE ASSISTIVE DEVICES

With the proliferation of commercially available assistive devices for daily living activities, it is important that the best device to suit the patient be chosen. There are several means to locate a preferred device for a patient.

Computerized data bank

At this time, there is one exceptional data bank that stores information about assistive devices. *Hyperable-*

data is a software package that categorizes assistive devices by function (e.g., bookholders). It provides the health professional or consumer with a list of available commercial products and addresses. If purchasing the software package is not economical, *information brokers* can be contacted in various places throughout the United States. They look up Hyperabledata resources for the caller.

Publications

Ideally, it would be useful to collect all manufacturer catalogs of assistive devices. However, this still does not provide pertinent information about advantages and disadvantages of products. Professional journals may evaluate some devices. Research articles regarding assistive devices also can occasionally be found in various journals. There are ongoing publications for people with disabilities that may provide product evaluation or description (e.g., Accent on Living, Paraplegia). Lastly, there are books that describe assistive devices. One that was produced in 1988 by the Arthritis Foundation includes a wide array of devices, categorized by function, that are particularly useful for people with arthritis (*Guide to Independent Living for People with Arthritis*). This was written by occupational and physical therapists who specialized in working with people with arthritis. Although originally intended for the person with arthritis, it has been widely used by health professionals to help their patients with other conditions to explore the possibilities of maintaining independence with the use of assistive devices.

Agencies

There are unique agencies that specialize in prescribing and designing (when necessary) assistive devices to suit individual needs. An example of this is *Project Threshold*. This agency is located in a medical center, although it operates independently. Patients can be referred here who have functional problems at home, school, or work. Most often, the referrals are made by state department rehabilitation counselors, although referrals from multiple other sources are accepted. Another agency that designs assistive devices is the *Harrington Arthritis Research Center*. This agency provides research and development in the design of assistive devices and evaluates existing devices. Other agencies that might assist with provision of assistive devices are *Centers for Independent Living*. These are centers that exist to help people with disabilities in the community with various problems. They may be able to help with resources for obtaining assistive devices. *Occupational therapy departments* typically can make simple assistive devices, as needed, if there are no other available resources. Creative therapists design or adapt a commercially available device to solve individual problems. Occupational therapy departments may engage volunteers to help with building assistive devices, if it is difficult to obtain these through third-party payers or other means.

SUMMARY AND CONCLUSION

The array of assistive devices available for people with disabilities has grown in the last four decades. Through ingenious designs, people have been able to experience independence through the use of this equipment.

There is a continuing need for research on product use to prevent purchase of equipment that goes unused. Cost of products needs to decrease. It is hoped that third-party payers for medical insurance or other agencies will increasingly see that the use of assistive devices is cost-effective in returning individuals to productive living.

SELECTED RESOURCE LIST

ABLEDATA
Macro International
Silver Springs, MD
Information Specialists: (800)346-2742
(Produces HYPERABLE software)

Guide to Independent Living for People with Arthritis
Arthritis Foundation
1313 Spring St., NW
Atlanta, GA 30309
(Photos and descriptions of devices for people with joint problems)

Fred Sammons Inc.
PO Box 32
Brookfield, IL 60513-0032
(Catalog of assistive devices)

AliMed
297 High Street
Dedham, MA 02026-9135
(Catalog of assistive devices)

Smith and Nephew Rolyan Inc.
N93W14475 Whittaker Way
Menomonee Falls, WI 53051
(Catalog of assistive devices)

North Coast Medical, Inc.
187 Stauffer Boulevard
San Jose, CA 95125-1042
(Catalog of assistive devices)

Project Threshold
Rancho Los Amigos Medical Center
7601 E. Imperial Highway
500 Hut
Downey, CA 90242
(Evaluates/recommends/custom-designs for assistive device needs of individuals)

Harrington Arthritis Center Assistive Devices Program
1800 East Van Buren
Phoenix, AZ 85006
(Primarily research, development, and evaluation of assistive devices)

Team Rehab
6133 Bristol Parkway
P.O. Box 3640
Culver City, CA 90231-3640
(Business magazine devoted to the assistive technology market)

BIBLIOGRAPHY

1. Axtell LA, Yasuda YL: Assistive devices and home modifications in geriatric rehabilitation, Geriatr Rehabil 9:803–821, 1993.
2. Batavia AL, Hammer GS: Toward the development of consumer based criteria for the evaluation of assistive devices, J Rehabil Res Dev 27:425, 1990.
3. Caudrey DJ, Seeger BR: Rehabilitation engineering service evaluation: A follow-up survey of device effectiveness and patient acceptance, 44:80–85, 1983.
4. Cooper BA, Hasselkus: Independent living and the physical environment: Aspects that matter to residents, Can J Occup Ther 59:6–15, 1992.
5. Geiger CM: The utilization of assistive devices by patients discharged from an acute rehabilitation setting, Phys Occup Ther Geriatr 9:3–53, 1990.
6. George J, et al: Aids and adaptations for the elderly at home: Underprovided, underused, and undermaintained, BMJ 296: 1365–1366, 1988.
7. Hadley E, Radebaugh TS, Suzman R: Falls and gait disorder among the elderly, Clin Geriatr Med 1:497–500, 1985.
8. Karpman RR: Problems and pitfalls with assistive devices, Top Geriatr Rehabil 8:1–5, 1992.
9. Mitchell SCM: Dressing aids, BMJ 302:167–169, 1991.
10. Pensiero M, Adams M: Dress and self-esteem, J Gerontol Nurs 13:11–17, 1987.
11. Phillips B, Zhao H: Predictors of assistive technology abandonment, Assist Technol 5:36–45, 1993.
12. PSI International, Inc: Assistive technology, Rehab Brief 14:1–4, 1993.
13. Redford JB: Assistive devices. In Leek JC, editor: Principles of physical medicine and rehabilitation in the musculoskeletal diseases, New York, 1986, Grune & Stratton.
14. Rogers JC, Home MB: Assistive technology device use in patients with rheumatoid disease: A literature review, Am J Occup Ther 46:120, 1992.
15. Watzke JR, Kemp B: Safety for older adults: The role of technology and the home environment, Top Geriatr Rehabil 7:9, 1992.
16. Wilson DJ, McKenzie MW, Barber LM: Spinal cord injury: A treatment guide for occupational therapists, Thorofare, NJ, 1974, Charles B. Slack.
17. Yasuda YL: Arthritis: A challenge for rehabilitation, Geriatr Rehabil Prev 4:1–6, 1992.
18. Yasuda YL, Bowman KB, Hsu JD: Mobile arm supports: Criteria for successful use in muscle disease patients, Arch Phys Med Rehabil 67:253–256, 1986.

Electronic Aids and Robotics

Tariq Rahman
William S. Harwin
Richard Foulds

One of the primary objectives of rehabilitation robotics is to provide a person who has a manipulative disability with an interactive aid to carry out personal and vocational tasks, thus increasing his or her level of independence.[11] The robotic manipulator differs from the more familiar prosthesis or orthosis in that the device is not physically attached to the user. The device is controlled *remotely* via some input device, such as a switch, joystick, speech, or one of a range of possible devices.[17]

Rehabilitation robotics, as a field, is still in its infancy. Critical issues such as safety, the human/machine interface, sensors, and reliability of robots have yet to be adequately resolved. These issues are ongoing areas of research at various establishments around the world and are addressed in the following sections. The few devices that have reached the market are also described in detail later in this chapter.

DESIGN CHALLENGES

Robotics technology has traditionally been applied almost exclusively to industrial environments. Efforts have been made to extend the technology into other applications, one of which is rehabilitation. The use of robotics in rehabilitation, however, presupposes a unique set of design criteria:[9]

Safety

The most important human factors issue is the presence of a person within the working envelope of the manipulator. If a robot is to be used as an assistive device, especially in activities of daily living (ADL), it follows that the person using the arm is not only within the working envelope of the system but may well be the object of the manipulator's activities (i.e., combing hair, feeding, brushing teeth). For this reason, it is essential that the design of the robotic aid provides for the greatest possible margin of safety for the user.

Human/machine interaction

The human is a creature of spontaneous desire, shifting needs, and unpredictable responses. This need for a user to interact thoughtfully and spontaneously with the environment, combined with the role of the robotic aid as an assistive device, requires that the robot be flexible and responsive to human input. That interaction is complicated by the fact that the user, by definition, has a disability that affects his or her ability to communicate with the host processor through standard input channels (i.e., keyboard, joystick, voice command).

Task complexity/volume

Although differences exist in terms of the types of tasks carried out, each routine of the day requires its own series of motions and thoughtful interaction with the tools of that task. These tasks tend to be highly complex in structure and organization. In addition, few human activities are considered to be high volume. Eating, combing hair, and brushing teeth are activities that occur with a limited frequency in a given day.

Environment

Human beings exist and function in a generally unstructured environment. It is within this setting that the rehabilitation robot must operate. Any system that is intended to serve as an assistive tool, in order to be readily accepted by the user, must be capable of responding and functioning within a volatile environment. To modify the environment to meet the limitations of the system, rather than to adapt the system to the needs of the individual, is to make the person an object being acted on, rather than the actor in control of his or her own world.

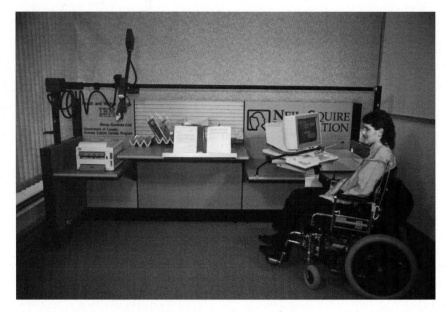

Fig. 44.1.   Neil Squire Foundation Robotic Workstation. *(Courtesy of Neil Squire Foundation.)*

Other less critical, yet important factors are also common to rehabilitation environments. Robotic systems are designed on a human scale and should be aesthetically pleasing in appearance and operation. Cost limitations require efficient and well-engineered planning, design, and construction. Finally, robot systems are often required to exist in the context of a larger, processor-controlled environment system. These are the criteria that challenge the rehabilitation robotics designer and are some of the issues with which a user must contend.

TYPES OF REHABILITATION ROBOTS

Rehabilitation robots fall into three broad classifications. The *workstation*-based system consists of a manipulator that is fixed to a single location or mounted on a linear track. The workstation consists of the robot and typically an environment that includes vocation-related items, such as a computer, telephone, printer, and bins in which to place books and papers. Because the environment in a workstation is usually structured, the robot can be programmed to perform tasks, using object locations stored in memory. A structured environment does offer an ease of control because complex movements can be stored in the computer and called repeatedly by the touch of a button or the utterance of a sound. Superior control, however, is gained at the expense of flexibility. Because the user may not have direct control over robot movements, any change in the environment would have to be "taught" to the robot. There are also

workstation-based systems that offer a combination of programmed and interactive modes of control with varying levels of autonomy.

The main alternative to a fixed-location robot is the *wheelchair-mounted* manipulator, which is usually mounted to the side of a powered wheelchair. The wheelchair-mounted arm has a greater degree of flexibility in that it can easily be transported from place to place. This benefit, however, is accompanied by an increased complexity in controlling the robot because of the changing nature of its environment.

The third type of rehabilitation robot is the *mobile robot*, which consists of a remotely controlled mobile platform that may have a robotic manipulator arm mounted on it. This type of system is still mainly in the research and development stage owing to the complexity of the human interface. The mobile robot, however, has vast potential to affect the lives of people with disabilities and the elderly.

APPLICATIONS

The successful use of robotic devices as functional aids for individuals with disabilities has been demonstrated for a number of different application areas. Because independence in all environments is the major objective in rehabilitation robotics, there is a natural interest in developing systems for ADL applications. Assistive tools in vocational settings is another application where the potential exists for making previously unemployable persons self-supporting or at least allowing them to contribute to their own financial support. A number of workstations have been developed for this area, and some are already commercially available.[2,5,20] Other less prevalent applications for robots to aid people with disabilities include recreational,[15] educational,[14] and therapeutic[7] applications.

REHABILITATION ROBOTS

This section describes seven rehabilitation robots that are currently on the market. All are a result of many years of research and development and range from human-powered mechanical systems to computer-controlled workstations operated by voice commands.

Neil Squire Foundation arm

The Neil Squire Foundation arm is a workstation-based, six-joint robot that uses interchangeable modules for its joints (Fig. 44.1). The arm was initiated 9 years ago by the Foundation's research and development group[2] and was based on work done on telemanipulators in the nuclear industry. It has evolved into a commercial product currently marketed by the Regenisis Corporation, Vancouver, Canada.

The Neil Squire arm can be operated by a standard IBM-compatible PC through the serial port. It can be controlled through voice, expanded keyboard, or Morse code. Currently, there are eight manipulators being used at various universities, hospitals, and rehabilitation centers in North America, mainly for field trials.

The manipulator may be verbally commanded to perform vocational tasks, such as "get paper from printer." The task is then executed automatically and the paper presented to the user. The user may also use a keyboard to direct the robot's motions more interactively.

Papworth arm

The Papworth arm is a wheelchair-mounted robotic arm that uses pneumatics for actuation. The arm has been under development at Inventaid in Bedford, England, since 1987. It is being built and marketed by the Papworth Group of Papworth, England.[13]

The manipulator is powered by compressed air and uses the Flexator air muscles to move its five joints plus a gripping action. Some of the advantages offered by the system include ease of repair; high durability and reliability because of the lack of electronic components; relative low cost; and inherent compliance because of its having pneumatic actuators, which is an important feature considering it operates close to the human.

The controls are provided through an array of switches on a control box. Each joint movement corre-

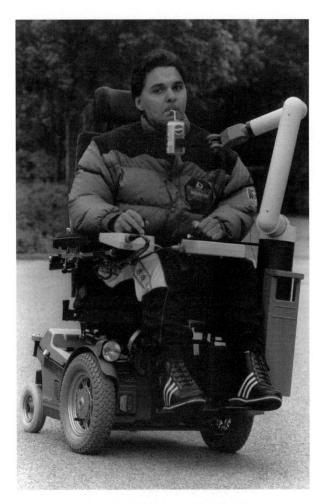

Fig. 44.2. Manus wheelchair-mounted manipulator. *(Courtesy of TNO-TPD.)*

sponds to two switches (one for forward and one for backward movements). Six of these units have been built and are in use by various individuals and spinal cord injury centers.

Manus

The Manus manipulator is a wheelchair-mounted robotic arm designed specifically for people with severe physical disabilities (Fig. 44.2). The Manus is a Dutch project that started in 1984.[16]

The Manus is a computer-controlled, motorized, eight-joint arm that is capable of picking objects off the floor or reaching up and flicking a light switch. The electronics and computer hardware are housed in a control box permanently attached to the wheelchair. The software is designed to allow a professional the ability to modify the interface to the robot. Some of the input devices that have been used include joysticks, a trackball, Unicorn keyboard, and a Nintendo sip-and-puff controller, in addition to a standard 4 × 4 matrix keypad.

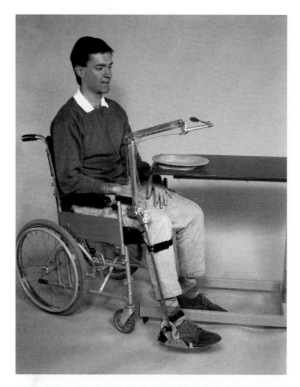

Fig. 44.3. Cable-controlled Magpie robot. *(Courtesy of Mervyn Evans, Oxford Orthopaedic Engineering Centre.)*

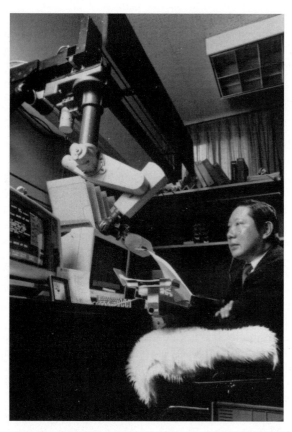

Fig. 44.4. DeVAR (Desktop Vocational Assistant Robot for Independent People with Special Needs). *(Courtesy of Independence Works, Inc.)*

The manipulator is commercially available through Exact Dynamics, Zevenaar, The Netherlands. It continues to be improved in terms of functionality, human/machine interface, and safety. A third-generation device will shortly be introduced.

Magpie

The Magpie is a mechanical linkage that attaches to the wheelchair and is controlled by coordinated movements of the foot. Its primary use is as a feeding device.[8] Magpie was initiated in 1983 at the Mary Marlborough Lodge at the Nuffield Orthopaedic Center in England (Fig. 44.3). It was designed to fill a void between "high-tech" robotic equipment and the more basic devices such as rotating feeding plates.

About 10 of the 500 patients admitted each year to Mary Marlborough Lodge at the Nuffield Orthopaedic Centre, Oxford, England, have no use in either arm or hand, yet maintain control of a leg and foot, suffering from motor neurone disease, syringomyelia, poliomyelitis, cerebral palsy, congenital reduction deformities of the limbs, or bilateral brachial plexus injuries. It was decided to maximize the remaining physical ability of these people by designing a system that would be operated by leg and foot movements, giving the patient direct control and feedback.

Magpie underwent extensive trials with a number of subjects. One of the users has had a Magpie since 1984 and still uses it daily to feed himself. He also has an adaptation for shaving with a battery-powered electric shaver.

DeVAR

Five years ago, Stanford University and the Palo Alto VA medical center began a collaborative effort to commercialize a voice-controlled robotic assistant (Fig. 44.4) for individuals with physical disabilities. This effort culminated in the Desktop Vocational Robot.[20,21]

DeVAR uses a small, anthropomorphic manipulator, the PUMA-260, which runs upside-down on a 4-inch motorized overhead transverse track. The PUMA uses an Otto Bock Greifer, a prosthetic hand, retrofitted with a finger position sensor for servo control. The track and arm are mounted in a 4×8 foot landscape furniture office and provide manipulation of small objects (paper, diskettes, cups, medication, throat lozenges) to and from the side shelves, desktop, and the user's face, as appropriate. The user interface is by voice recognition and digitized speech output, augmented by a monitor for visual status and cues.

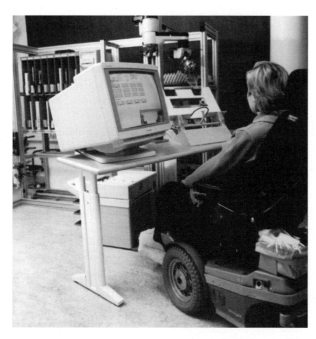

Fig. 44.5. RAID robotic workstation. *(Courtesy of Oxford Intelligent Machines.)*

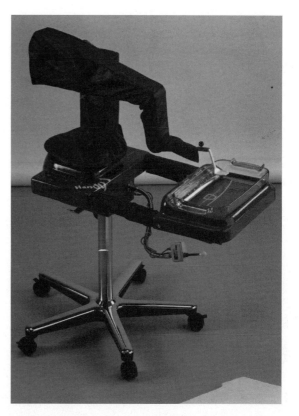

Fig. 44.6. Handy 1 robotic eating assistant. *(Courtesy of Department of Biomedical Engineering and Medical Physics/ Department of Design, Keele University.)*

Over several years since 1988, DeVAR has been tested at the VA and then was the subject of a 2-year field study in the San Francisco office of a programmer. Currently, it is part of the VA-sponsored vocational training facility in Palo Alto and is undergoing clinical trials under the auspices of the Baltimore-based VA Technology Transfer Section (TTS). At this time, six units are operational: three in office settings at the VA, two built by Independence Works for the TTS, and one as a research prototype for interface and control development by Stanford University and the Palo Alto VA.

Independence Works, Inc., a small Palo Alto company, has been assigned the rights to the DeVAR software by the VA. The technology transfer process, which started two years ago as part of a Cooperative R&D Agreement (CRDA) with the Rehabilitation R&D Center of the Palo Alto VA, has been 90% completed. The ongoing effort to complete the detailed documentation will give Independence Works complete control of further developments of the technology. A new CRDA covers further development, including a second-generation controller and user interface.

RAID

Robot for Assisting the Integration of the Disabled (RAID) is a European Economic Community collaborative project (Fig. 44.5), funded through the TIDE (Technology Integration of the Disabled and Elderly) initiative.[19] RAID is a vocational robotic workstation for use by people with disabilities in an office environment, currently focusing on CAD/CAM job tasks.

The target group of users has been defined by the collaborators as being wheelchair users who have insufficient motor functions to be able to operate a computer workstation unaided but who have at least two degrees of movement available—enough to operate a joystick, roller ball, or chin switch.

The workstation is designed around a commercial RT200 robot and includes bins and shelves offering extensive book and paper handling facilities. The system is modular, capable of accessing up to 60 separate books or folders and 24 different reams of paper or magazines, which are presented to the user as a computer interface. The computer running the entire system is an IBM-compatible 486 PC with all the control and application software running in the well-supported Windows environment.

The system has undergone extensive user trials at various rehabilitation centers in Europe. OXIM, Oxford, England, plans to take the current prototype into production and, following extensive trials in the three countries involved (France, Sweden, and England), will produce the specification for the workstation to be used in the final phase of the project.

Handy 1

The Handy 1 (Fig. 44.6) was initially developed in 1988 as a feeding tool specifically to assist a 12-year-old boy with cerebral palsy.[12] The system was designed in the Department of Biomedical Engineering, at Keele University, England, which also markets the system. It consists of a Cyber 310 robotic arm that has five degrees of freedom plus a gripper. A BBC microcomputer was used to program movements for the system, and a concept keyboard was used as the human/machine interface.

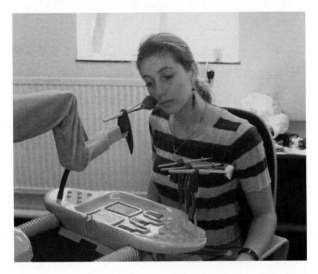

Fig. 44.7. Handy 1 shown with makeup application module. *(Courtesy of Department of Biomedical Engineering and Medical Physics/Department of Design, Keele University.)*

Over a period of four years, 60 prototype versions were produced and placed on a full-time basis with several different disability groups with a wide age range. The disability groups currently using the equipment are cerebral palsy, motor neurone disease, stroke, muscular dystrophy, and multiple sclerosis. The ages range from 3 to 84 years.

Handy 1 in its standard form comes with a wobble switch fitted to its casing via a length of flexible gooseneck tubing. In this form, the robot can be used by any individual using the hands, arm, or lower body movement. The gooseneck may also be repositioned on a wheelchair allowing for control through upper body or head movements.

A scanning LED indicator strip on the tray provides the user with a choice of food to pick up. Handy 1 allows a maximum of seven different types of food from which to choose. The pace at which the meal is taken is also under direct control of the user. Many users have commented on how patient the system is with them, allowing them to enjoy their meal more readily.

The food is placed on the glass dish and warmed if necessary. At this point, the LED indicator strip behind the dish begins to scan from left to right along the length of the dish. The user then simply waits for the light to be lit behind the section of food he or she wants to eat. The user then activates the single switch, and the robot proceeds onto the dish, scoops up a section of that food and brings it back to a preset comfortable mouth position. The user then takes the food from the spoon and the process starts over again. The system logs

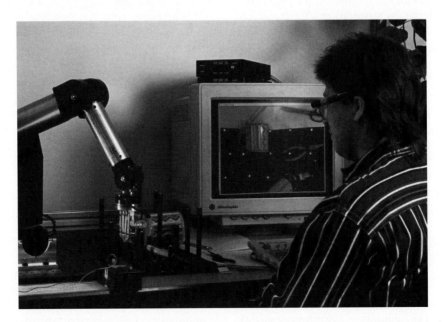

Fig. 44.8. Multi-modal project at the A.I. duPont Institute. The robotic arm is being guided by a head-mounted laser pointer. A vision system surveys the scene, and commands are issued to the robot to move to a desired location or to perform a desired task. *(Courtesy of A.I. duPont Institute and the University of Delaware.)*

where the robot has been and does not allow it to return to an area from which food has been removed. The Handy 1 has recently seen the introduction of a module to apply makeup (Fig. 44.7).

RESEARCH ISSUES

Although there are a number of commercially available rehabilitation robotic systems, as described previously, the field has yet to see widespread acceptance of a robotic aid in the home or workplace. Some reasons are high cost; poor human/machine interface, which results in a directly controlled robot being too slow or a programmed robot being inflexible to a changing environment; and, to a lesser degree, aesthetics and reliability.

A number of research institutions are addressing these problems. The University of Delaware and the A.I. duPont Institute jointly administer the Rehabilitation Robotics program, which includes the National Rehabilitation Engineering Research Center in rehabilitation robotics. Projects the center is researching include interface issues such as providing enhanced sensory feedback to persons with spinal cord injury and cerebral palsy[18] and control of a powered orthosis for people with muscular dystrophy. A major emphasis of the center is to investigate devices that are simpler to use and control for various applications, such as vocational, educational, and ADL (Fig. 44.8). Consumers are included in the appropriate stages of research and, in fact, initiate some of the projects.

A number of other North American,[6,21,22] European,[3,4,5,10] and Japanese universities and institutes are performing basic and applied research in an attempt to advance the field of rehabilitation robotics.

REFERENCES

1. Alexander MA, et al: Rehabilitation technology for disabled children, Phys Med Rehab 5:365–387, 1991.
2. Birch G: Rehabilitation robotics at the Neil Squire Foundation, Rehab Robotics Newsletter, A.I. duPont Institute 3(3), 1991.
3. Casals A: TOU: A friendly assistant arm, Rehab Robotics Newsletter, A.I. duPont Institute 5(2), 1993.
4. Dario P: URMAD: A mobile robotic unit for the assistance to the disabled, Rehab Robotics Newsletter, A.I. duPont Institute 5(3), 1993.
5. Detriche JM, Lesigne B: MASTER: The robotized system to assist handicapped people, Rehab Robotics Newsletter, A.I. duPont Institute 4(3), 1992.
6. Echard, et al: Pattern recognition techniques for cortical control of a robotic arm, Proceedings of the Southern Biomedical Engineering Conference, Washington, DC, 1994.
7. Erlandson RF, et al: A robotic system as a remedial tool in rehabilitation, Proc of the Second International Conference on Rehab Robotics, Atlanta, 1991.
8. Evans E: MAGPIE, Rehab Robotics Newsletter, A.I. duPont Institute 5(4), 1993.
9. Gilbert M, et al: Development of a programming environment for rehabilitation robotics, Proceedings of the Twelfth Annual RESNA Conference, Washington, DC, 1989, RESNA.
10. Gosine RG, et al: Interactive robotics to aid physically disabled people in manufacturing tasks, Proc Instn Mech Engrs 205:241–245, 1991.
11. Heckathorne CW: Augmentative manipulation. In Foulds R, editor: Interactive robotic aids—one option for independent living: An international perspective, Monogr 37, New York, 1986, World Rehabilitation Fund.
12. Hegarty JR, Topping MJ: HANDY 1: A low-cost robotic aid to eating, Proceedings of the Second International Conference on Rehabilitation Robotics, Atlanta, 1991.
13. Hennequin J, Platts R, Hennequin Y: INVENTAID: Putting technology to work for the disadvantaged, Rehab Robotics Newsletter, A.I. duPont Institute 4(3), 1992.
14. Howell R, et al: Design issues in the use of robotics as cognitive enhancement aids for disabled individuals: Transitions in mental retardation, Monograph of the American Association for Mental Deficiency, Norwood, NJ, 1988, Ablex Publishing.
15. Kassler M: Robotics for health care: A review of the literature, Robotica 11:495–516, 1993.
16. Kwee HH, Stanger C: The MANUS manipulator, Rehab Robotics Newsletter, A.I. duPont Institute 5(2), 1993.
17. Leifer L: Rehabilitative robots, Robotics Age, May/June:4–1, 1981.
18. Rahman T, Harwin WS: Bilateral control in teleoperation of a rehabilitation robot, Proceedings of SPIE—Telemanipulator Technology, Boston, 1992.
19. Upton C: The RAID workstation, Rehab Robotics Newsletter, A.I. duPont Institute 6(1), 1994.
20. Van der Loos M: DeVAR, Rehab Robotics Newsletter, A.I. duPont Institute 6(1), 1994.
21. Van der Loos M, Hammel JM: Designing rehabilitation robots as household and office equipment, Proceedings of the International Conference on Rehabilitation Robotics, Wilmington, DE, 1990.
22. Verburg, et al: An evaluation of the Manus wheelchair-mounted manipulator, Proceedings of the Fifteenth Annual RESNA Conference, Toronto, 1989.

EPILOGUE

THE FUTURE
Bertram Goldberg
John D. Hsu

In a society that is becoming more mobile every day, we, as health care practitioners and providers, must face the challenge of seeing that individuals with disabilities are given the means to function not only as patients in their own environment but as wage earners in the workplace. This demands the development of orthotic systems that will be increasingly lighter in weight, more cosmetically acceptable, and, in this era of cost containment, more affordable to the patient and society as a whole.

Pain, deformity, and decreased functional abilities prevent the physically challenged individual from achieving a better quality of life. Creative use of new materials and designs helps the orthotist meet the challenge of overcoming these obstacles.

Today's Certified Orthotist has the education and skills to offer high-technology answers to patient's problems. The ability to create specific designs for individual needs allows an improved quality of life for those who rely on orthotic solutions to meet their functional needs.

The American Board for Certification in Orthotics and Prosthetics (ABC), in existence since 1948, has continued to raise the educational standards by which practitioners are credentialed. There are a variety of programs available to train orthotic practitioners. Programs accredited by the National Commission for Orthotic-Prosthetic Education (NCOPE) offer entry-level education leading to a postgraduate residency, the combination of which prepare an individual to sit for the ABC certification examinations. In recent years, mandatory continuing education has become a requirement to maintain certified status.

As the last chapter demonstrates, the age of robotics is upon us. We must look to the future with imagination and provide those who have the ability to make their ideas a reality the means to develop orthoses for all who want and need them. In the long run, money spent today for research and development will reap significant benefits and money saved in the future.

INDEX